Oral and maxillofacial surgery in dogs and cats

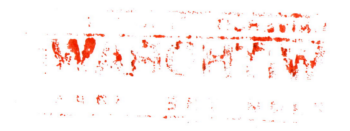

Commissioning Editor: *Robert Edwards*
Development Editors: *Catherine Jackson, Sally Davies*
Project Manager: *Sukanthi Sukumar*
Designer: *Charles Gray*
Illustration Manager: *Merlyn Harvey*
Illustrators: *Samantha J Elmhurst, Jennifer Rose*

Oral and maxillofacial surgery in dogs and cats

Edited by

Frank J M Verstraete DrMedVet BVSc(Hons) MMedVet Diplomate AVDC ECVS and EVDC

Professor of Dentistry and Oral Surgery, Department of Surgical and Radiological Sciences, School of Veterinary Medicine, University of California, Davis, California, USA; Adjunct Professor, Department of Orofacial Sciences, Division of Oral Medicine, Oral Pathology and Oral Radiology, School of Dentistry, University of California, San Francisco, California, USA

Milinda J Lommer DVM Diplomate AVDC

Aggie Animal Dental Service, San Francisco, California, USA; Clinical Assistant Professor Volunteer, Department of Surgical and Radiological Sciences, School of Veterinary Medicine, University of California, Davis, California, USA

Consulting Editor (Surgical Anatomy): Abraham J Bezuidenhout BVSc DVSc

Senior Lecturer, Department of Biomedical Sciences, College of Veterinary Medicine, Cornell University, Ithaca, New York, USA

Foreword by

M Anthony Pogrel DDS MD FRCS FACS Diplomate ABOMS

William Ware Endowed Professor and Chairman, Department of Oral and Maxillofacial Surgery; Associate Dean for Hospital Affairs, School of Dentistry, University of California, San Francisco, California, USA

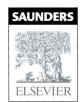

SAUNDERS

ELSEVIER

Edinburgh   London   New York   Oxford   Philadelphia   St Louis   Sydney   Toronto   2012

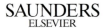

10067975779
ISBN 978-0-7020-4618-6
Reprinted 2012 (twice)

British Library Cataloguing in Publication Data
A catalogue record for this book is available from the British Library

Library of Congress Cataloging in Publication Data
A catalog record for this book is available from the Library of Congress

Notices

Knowledge and best practice in this field are constantly changing. As new research and experience broaden our understanding, changes in research methods, professional practices, or medical treatment may become necessary.

Practitioners and researchers must always rely on their own experience and knowledge in evaluating and using any information, methods, compounds, or experiments described herein. In using such information or methods they should be mindful of their own safety and the safety of others, including parties for whom they have a professional responsibility.

With respect to any drug or pharmaceutical products identified, readers are advised to check the most current information provided (i) on procedures featured or (ii) by the manufacturer of each product to be administered, to verify the recommended dose or formula, the method and duration of administration, and contraindications. It is the responsibility of practitioners, relying on their own experience and knowledge of their patients, to make diagnoses, to determine dosages and the best treatment for each individual patient, and to take all appropriate safety precautions.

To the fullest extent of the law, neither the Publisher nor the authors, contributors, or editors, assume any liability for any injury and/or damage to persons or property as a matter of products liability, negligence or otherwise, or from any use or operation of any methods, products, instructions, or ideas contained in the material herein.

ELSEVIER your source for books, journals and multimedia in the health sciences

www.elsevierhealth.com

Working together to grow libraries in developing countries

www.elsevier.com | www.bookaid.org | www.sabre.org

ELSEVIER   BOOK AID International   Sabre Foundation

The publisher's policy is to use paper manufactured from sustainable forests

Printed in China

Contents

Contents

Foreword

It gives me a great pleasure to write this foreword for Dr. Verstraete and Dr. Lommer's important new textbook. Human surgeons and veterinary surgeons live in a symbiotic relationship with each other. In many cases, surgical techniques utilized on humans are first evaluated in an animal model before being transferred to humans. In other cases, surgical techniques evolve in humans before the basic biology of the technique is later evaluated in animal models. On the reverse side of the coin, techniques that have been perfected in humans are often then transferred back to the animal world to become options for animal surgery. This has been particularly applicable in the field of oral and maxillofacial surgery, and in particular with domestic cats and dogs. In particular, techniques for fracture fixation, mandibular and maxillary resection and reconstruction, particularly with the use of plates, screws and bone grafts, are now commonplace in animal surgery, and have evolved from human technique and utilize the same instrumentation. Restoration of form and function have become more important in domestic animal oral and maxillofacial surgery over the years due to improved prognosis in the management of disease and increased expectations on behalf of both the surgeon and the animal guardian.

Differences, however, still remain with regard to expectations following similar animal and human surgical procedures. In particular, long-term goals are often different in that in humans we are often looking at 20, 30 and 40-year follow-up results, whereas in cats and dogs, a success over a 2 to 3-year period is often all that is desired or required.

This is an important textbook and addition to the literature, and although it is mainly of value to veterinary surgeons, it will also be of value to human surgeons as we continue our close relationship. As the father of a veterinarian trained by Dr. Verstraete, I wish this textbook the best of success.

M. Anthony Pogrel DDS MD FRCS FACS Diplomate ABOMS
William Ware Endowed Professor and Chairman
Department of Oral and Maxillofacial Surgery;
Associate Dean for Hospital Affairs
School of Dentistry
University of California
San Francisco

Preface

Oral and maxillofacial surgery is an exciting and rewarding field, offering practitioners numerous opportunities to improve their patients' quality of life. Because oral diseases and maxillofacial lesions are often painful and debilitating, treating these conditions can have a huge impact on an animal's well-being. Unfortunately, although oral diseases are prevalent among companion animals, and veterinarians are expected to diagnose and treat them, the anatomy, physiology, and pathology of the oral cavity are discussed only cursorily in veterinary school. This textbook aims to provide students, general practitioners, residents and specialists with a comprehensive survey of oral and maxillofacial surgery. Each chapter includes the 'why' as well as the 'how', and the procedures described range from non-surgical, single-rooted tooth extraction to major resection of maxillary and mandibular tumors. It is important to note that the text is not intended to be a 'step-by-step' guide to performing these procedures, and that practitioners interested in learning a particular procedure described in the text should pursue additional training with a board-certified specialist before attempting an unfamiliar surgical procedure on a patient.

We also wish to point out that procedures which we feel are ethically questionable (performed for the purpose of pleasing the client or demonstrating the technical prowess of the operator rather than to improve the patient's quality of life) are not included in this book. We specifically refer to orthognathic surgery and dental implants. Orthognathic surgery is complicated, puts the animal at risk of serious complications, and is rarely justifiable. While we aim to restore a comfortable and functional occlusion to our patients, the goal of correcting a malocclusion through orthognathic surgery is misguided, particularly since malocclusions causing discomfort can typically be treated by orthodontic means or by selective extractions. Regarding the replacement of missing teeth, although dogs have been used extensively in dental implant research, it is very difficult to provide ethical justification for implant surgery in client-owned animals given how well dogs and cats function with missing teeth.

This textbook was compiled with the contribution of experts in human oral pathology and maxillofacial surgery as well as board-certified veterinary surgeons and dentists. The information contained is based on reviews of relevant literature and the clinical expertise of the authors. We have attempted to make the text comprehensive, authoritative, and easy to read. Every effort has been made to ensure that the nomenclature used in this textbook is correct and in agreement with *Nomina Anatomica Veterinaria*. Intentional repetition of some material is present throughout several chapters to allow for complete presentation of the material in the individual chapters, and to reinforce basic surgical principles relative to the specific procedures described.

We believe that oral and maxillofacial surgery should be taken seriously by the veterinarian, and should not be delegated to staff members. A well-planned and skillfully performed procedure will result in minimal postoperative discomfort, reduced healing time, and rapid return to function for the patient. As veterinarians, our primary goal is to improve our patients' well-being; this can best be achieved by continuing to educate ourselves, to improve our skills, and to share our knowledge with others.

Acknowledgments

We are grateful to the contributing authors for sharing their knowledge, for their generous commitment of time to this project, and for their patience. We also wish to acknowledge the contributions of John Doval, Senior Artist with the Department of Surgical and Radiological Sciences at the University of California – Davis School of Veterinary Medicine, for many of the illustrations throughout the text. We would also like to thank the patient and highly professional team of Elsevier who enabled us to bring this book to completion.

Dedications

I dedicate this book to the individuals from whom I have learned, and thank the two universities that I have been affiliated with in my career, the University of Pretoria in South Africa and the University of California at Davis, which have given me the opportunity to develop my skills and practice veterinary dentistry and oral surgery.

A mind grows by what it feeds upon - associates, books, teachers, and an atmosphere encouraging to scholarly pursuits – Owen H. Wangensteen*

Frank J. M. Verstraete

To those individuals who have guided me throughout my education and my life: I continue to strive to be an excellent clinician and an exceptional person. Thank you for your patience and support.

For my husband, Edward, and our daughters, Margaret and Ella: your love and laughter are the light of my life.

Milinda J. Lommer

---

*Wangensteen OH. Credo of a surgeon following the academic line. *J Am Med Assoc* 1961;177:558–563.

Contributors

Jamie G. Anderson RDH DVM MS Diplomate AVDC and AVCIM
San Francisco, California, USA
Co-author for chapter(s):
20 – Osteoconductive and osteoinductive agents in periodontal surgery

Boaz Arzi DVM Diplomate AVDC
Postdoctoral Fellow, Department of Biomedical Engineering, and Staff
Clinician, Department of Surgical and Radiological Sciences, University of
California, Davis, California, USA
First author for chapter(s):
38 – Clinical staging and biopsy of maxillofacial tumors
Co-author for chapter(s):
27 – Surgical approaches for mandibular and maxillofacial trauma repair

Janusz Bardach (deceased) MD
Formerly Professor Emeritus of Plastic Surgery, Division of Plastic and
Reconstructive Surgery, Department of Surgery, University of Iowa, Iowa
City, Iowa, USA
Co-author for chapter(s):
35 – Biologic basis of cleft palate and palatal surgery

Abraham J. Bezuidenhout BVSc DVSc
Senior Lecturer, Department of Biomedical Sciences, College of Veterinary
Medicine, Cornell University, Ithaca, New York, USA
Co-author for chapter(s):
27 – Surgical approaches for mandibular and maxillofacial trauma repair

Dea Bonello MedVet SRV PhD Diplomate EVDC
Torino, Italy
First author for chapter(s):
42 – Non-neoplastic proliferative oral lesions

Randy J. Boudrieau DVM Diplomate ACVS and ECVS
Professor of Surgery, Section Head – Small Animal Surgery, Department
of Clinical Sciences, Cummings School of Veterinary Medicine, Tufts
University, North Grafton, Massachusetts, USA
First author for chapter(s):
25 – Principles of maxillofacial trauma repair
30 – Maxillofacial fracture repair using intraosseous wires
31 – Maxillofacial fracture repair using miniplates and screws
Co-author for chapter(s):
2 – Maxillofacial bone healing

Thomas P. Chamberlain MS DVM Diplomate AVDC
Animal Dentistry and Oral Surgery, Inc, The Life Center, Leesburg,
Virginia, USA
First author for chapter(s):
41 – Clinical behavior of odontogenic tumors
47 – Clinical behavior and management of odontogenic cysts

Edward R. Eisner DVM Diplomate AVDC
Chief of Dental Services, Animal Hospital Specialty Center, Highlands
Ranch, Colorado, USA
First author for chapter(s):
23 – Principles of endodontic surgery
24 – Apicoectomy techniques

Patricia Frost Fitch DVM Diplomate AVDC
Veterinary Dental Consulting, Battle Ground, Washington, USA
Co-author for chapter(s):
19 – Periodontal flaps and mucogingival surgery

Cecilia E. Gorrel BSc MA VetMB DDS Diplomate EVDC
Veterinary Dentistry and Oral Surgery Referrals, Pilley Nr. Lymington,
Hants, UK
First author for chapter(s):
17 – Principles of periodontal surgery
18 – Gingivectomy and gingivoplasty

Margherita Gracis MedVet Diplomate AVDC and EVDC
Clinica Veterinaria Gran Sasso, Milan; Clinica Veterinaria Città di
Codogno, Codogno (Lodi), Italy
First author for chapter(s):
22 – Management of periodontal trauma

Clare R. Gregory DVM Diplomate ACVS
Emeritus Professor, Department of Surgical and Radiological Sciences,
School of Veterinary Medicine, University of California, Davis, California,
USA; Staff Surgeon, PetCare Veterinary Hospital, Santa Rosa, California,
USA
Co-author for chapter(s):
9 – Microvascular techniques in maxillofacial surgery

Fraser A. Hale DVM Diplomate AVDC
Hale Veterinary Clinic, Guelph, Ontario, Canada
First author for chapter(s):
21 – Crown-lengthening
Co-author for chapter(s):
17 – Principles of periodontal surgery
18 – Gingivectomy and Gingivoplasty

Franz Härle MD DMD
Professor Emeritus, Klinik für Mund-, Kiefer- und Gesichtschirurgie,
Universitätsklinikum Kiel, Kiel, Germany
First author for chapter(s):
2 – Maxillofacial bone healing

Contributors

Steven E. Holmstrom DVM Diplomate AVDC
Chief of Staff, Animal Dental Clinic, San Carlos, California, USA
First author for chapter(s):
52 – Inferior labial frenoplasty and tight-lip syndrome

Kevin M. Kelly PhD
Associate Research Scientist and Adjunct Associate Professor, Department of Occupational and Environmental Health, College of Public Health, University of Iowa, Iowa City, Iowa, USA
First author for chapter(s):
35 – Biologic basis of cleft palate and palatal surgery

Roberto Köstlin DrMedVet DrMedVet habil Diplomate ECVS
Associate Professor of Surgery and Ophthalmology, Center of Clinical Veterinary Medicine, Ludwig-Maximilians-University, Munich, Germany
Co-author for chapter(s):
28 – Symphyseal separation and fractures involving the incisive region

J. Geoffrey Lane BVetMed DESTS FRCVS
Cedars Surgical Services, The Cedars, Cross, Axbridge, Somerset, UK
First author for chapter(s):
50 – Surgical treatment of sialoceles

Gary C. Lantz DVM Diplomate ACVS and AVDC
Professor of Surgery and Dentistry, Department of Veterinary Clinical Sciences, School of Veterinary Medicine, Purdue University, West Lafayette, Indiana, USA
First author for chapter(s):
33 – Fractures and luxations involving the temporomandibular joint
45 – Maxillectomy techniques
46 – Mandibulectomy techniques
55 – Temporomandibular joint dysplasia
57 – Pharyngotomy and pharyngostomy

Anh D. Le DDS PhD Diplomate ABOMS
Associate Professor, Oral and Maxillofacial Surgery, Herman Ostrow School of Dentistry, Los Angeles County and USC Medical Center, California Hospital Medical Center, Los Angeles, California, USA
Co-author for chapter(s):
1 – Oral soft tissue wound healing

Loïc F.J. Legendre DVM Diplomate AVDC and EVDC
Northwest Veterinary Dental Services Ltd, North Vancouver, British Columbia, Canada
First author for chapter(s):
54 – Management of unerupted teeth
Co-author for chapter(s):
29 – Maxillofacial fracture repair using noninvasive techniques

Milinda J. Lommer DVM Diplomate AVDC
Aggie Animal Dental Service, San Francisco; Clinical Assistant Professor Volunteer, Department of Surgical and Radiological Sciences, School of Veterinary Medicine, University of California, Davis, California, USA
First author for chapter(s):
11 – Principles of exodontics
12 – Simple extraction of single-rooted teeth
14 – Extraction of multirooted teeth in dogs
15 – Special considerations in feline exodontics
16 – Complications of extractions
20 – Osteoconductive and osteoinductive agents in periodontal surgery
43 – Principles of oral oncologic surgery
Co-author for chapter(s):
13 – Extraction of canine teeth in dogs
41 – Clinical behavior of odontogenic tumors
53 – Management of maxillofacial osteonecrosis

Sandra Manfra Marretta DVM Diplomate ACVS and AVDC
Professor of Small Animal Surgery and Dentistry, Department of Veterinary Clinical Medicine, University of Illinois, Urbana, Illinois, USA
First author for chapter(s):
34 – Maxillofacial fracture complications
36 – Cleft palate repair techniques
37 – Repair of acquired palatal defects
53 – Management of maxillofacial osteonecrosis

Stanley L. Marks BVSc PhD Diplomate ACVIM and ACVN
Professor of Small Animal Medicine, Department of Medicine and Epidemiology, School of Veterinary Medicine, University of California, Davis, California, USA
First author for chapter(s):
5 – Enteral nutritional support

Kyle G. Mathews DVM MS Diplomate ACVS
Professor of Small Animal Soft Tissue and Oncologic Surgery, Department of Clinical Sciences, College of Veterinary Medicine, North Carolina State University, Raleigh, North Carolina, USA
First author for chapter(s):
56 – Correction of overlong soft palate
58 – Oral approaches to the nasal cavity and nasopharynx
59 – Tonsillectomy

Ulrike Matis DrMedVet DrMedVet habil Diplomate ECVS
Professor of Surgery, Faculty of Veterinary Medicine, Ludwig-Maximilians-University, Munich, Germany
First author for chapter(s):
28 – Symphyseal separation and fractures involving the incisive region

Margaret C. McEntee DVM Diplomate ACVIM ACVR(RO)
Professor of Oncology and Chair, Department of Clinical Sciences, College of Veterinary Medicine, Cornell University, Ithaca, New York, USA
First author for chapter(s):
40 – Clinical behavior of nonodontogenic tumors

Peter J. Pascoe BVSc DVA Diplomate ACVA and ECVAA
Professor of Veterinary Anesthesiology, Department of Surgical and Radiological Sciences, School of Veterinary Medicine, University of California, Davis, California, USA
First author for chapter(s):
4 – Anesthesia and pain management

George M. Peavy DVM Diplomate ABVP
Director of Comparative Medicine Programs, Beckman Laser Institute and Medical Clinic, College of Medicine, University of California, Irvine, California, USA
First author for chapter(s):
8 – Laser surgery

Marijke E. Peeters DVM PhD Diplomate ECVS
Senior Lecturer in Surgery, Department of Clinical Sciences of Companion Animals, Faculty of Veterinary Medicine, Utrecht University, Utrecht, The Netherlands
First author for chapter(s):
49 – Principles of salivary gland surgery

M. Anthony Pogrel DDS MD FRCS FACS Diplomate ABOMS
William Ware Endowed Professor and Chairman, Department of Oral and Maxillofacial Surgery; Associate Dean for Hospital Affairs, School of Dentistry, University of California, San Francisco, California, USA
First author for chapter(s):
10 – Use of the dog and cat in experimental maxillofacial surgery

Joseph A. Regezi DDS MS Diplomate ABOP
Professor Emeritus, School of Dentistry, University of California, San Francisco, California, USA
First author for chapter(s):
39 – Clinical–pathologic correlations

Celeste G. Roy DVM Diplomate AVDC
Veterinary Specialty Center of Tucson, Tucson, Arizona, USA
Co-author for chapter(s):
42 – Non-neoplastic proliferative oral lesions

Eva M. Sarkiala-Kessel DVM PhD Diplomate AVDC and EVDC
Docent, Department of Clinical Veterinary Sciences, Faculty of Veterinary Medicine, University of Helsinki, Helsinki, Finland
First author for chapter(s):
3 – Use of antibiotics and antiseptics

Bernard Séguin DVM MS Diplomate ACVS
Associate Professor, Department of Clinical Sciences, College of Veterinary Medicine, Oregon State University, Corvallis, Oregon, USA
First author for chapter(s):
44 – Surgical treatment of tongue, lip, and cheek tumors

Vivek Shetty DDS DrMedDent
Professor, Section of Oral and Maxillofacial Surgery, UCLA School of Dentistry, Los Angeles, California, USA
First author for chapter(s):
1 – Oral soft tissue wound healing

Daniel D. Smeak DVM Diplomate ACVS
Professor of Small Animal Surgery, James Voss Veterinary Teaching Hospital, College of Veterinary Medicine and Biomedical Sciences, Colorado State University, Fort Collins, Colorado, USA
First author for chapter(s):
51 – Cheiloplasty

Mark M. Smith VMD Diplomate ACVS and AVDC
Center for Veterinary Dentistry and Oral Surgery, Gaithersburg, Maryland, USA
First author for chapter(s):
29 – Maxillofacial fracture repair using noninvasive techniques
48 – Advanced maxillofacial reconstruction techniques

Barry B. Staley DDS Diplomate ABP
Aptos, California, USA
First author for chapter(s):
19 – Periodontal flaps and mucogingival surgery

Steven F. Swaim DVM MS
Professor Emeritus, Department of Clinical Sciences and Scott-Ritchey Research Center, College of Veterinary Medicine, Auburn University, Auburn, Alabama, USA
First author for chapter(s):
26 – Facial soft tissue injuries

Cheryl H. Terpak BSDH RDH MS
Oral Health Consultant, Maternal, Child and Adolescent Health, California Department of Public Health, Sacramento, California, USA
First author for chapter(s):
6 – Instrumentation, patient positioning and aseptic technique

Anson J. Tsugawa VMD Diplomate AVDC
Chief of Staff, Dog and Cat Dentist, Inc., Culver City, California, USA
First author for chapter(s):
7 – Suture materials and biomaterials
13 – Extraction of canine teeth in dogs
32 – Maxillofacial fracture repair using external skeletal fixation
Co-author for chapter(s):
14 – Extraction of multirooted teeth in dogs

Frank J.M. Verstraete DrMedVet BVSc(Hons) MMedVet Diplomate AVDC ECVS and EVDC
Professor of Dentistry and Oral Surgery, Department of Surgical and Radiological Sciences, School of Veterinary Medicine, University of California, Davis; Adjunct Professor, Department of Orofacial Sciences, Division of Oral Medicine, Oral Pathology and Oral Radiology, School of Dentistry, University of California, San Francisco, California, USA
First author for chapter(s):
27 – Surgical approaches for mandibular and maxillofacial trauma repair
Co-author for chapter(s):
6 – Instrumentation, patient positioning and aseptic technique
7 – Suture materials and biomaterials
12 – Simple extraction of single-rooted teeth
13 – Extraction of canine teeth in dogs
14 – Extraction of multirooted teeth in dogs
25 – Principles of maxillofacial trauma repair
32 – Maxillofacial fracture repair using external skeletal fixation
33 – Fractures and luxations involving the temporomandibular joint
38 – Clinical staging and biopsy of maxillofacial tumors
39 – Clinical–pathologic correlations
42 – Non-neoplastic proliferative oral lesions
43 – Principles of oral oncologic surgery
47 – Clinical behavior and management of odontogenic cysts

Peter J. Walsh DVM MVSc Diplomate ACVS
Northern California Veterinary Specialty Group, West Sacramento, California, USA
First author for chapter(s):
9 – Microvascular techniques in maxillofacial surgery

Xudong Wang DDS MD
Associate Professor, Department of Oral and Maxillofacial Surgery, Ninth People's Hospital, Shanghai, P.R. China
Co-author for chapter(s):
10 – Use of the dog and cat in experimental maxillofacial surgery

Robert W. Wiggs (deceased) DVM Diplomate AVDC
Formerly at Coit Road Animal Hospital, Dallas, Texas, USA
Co-author for chapter(s):
20 – Osteoconductive and osteoinductive agents in periodontal surgery

Petra E. Wilder-Smith BDS(Hons) LDS RCS PhD Diplomate RCSGB and BBDS
Associate Professor and Director of Dentistry, Beckman Laser Institute, University of California, Irvine, California, USA
Co-author for chapter(s):
8 – Laser surgery

Chapter | **1** |

Oral soft tissue wound healing

Vivek Shetty & Anh D. Le

DEFINITIONS

A *wound*, regardless of the cause of injury, is a disruption of normal tissue continuity. *Healing* is simply the process of restoring the integrity of the wounded tissue. If the result is tissue that is structurally and functionally the same as the original tissue, then *regeneration* has taken place. However, if tissue integrity is reestablished primarily through the formation of a fibrous, connective-tissue scar, then *repair* has occurred. The nature of the native tissue involved determines whether regeneration or repair will ensue and the surgeon's expectations should be correspondingly realistic. Whereas a fibrous scar may be normal for dermal healing, it is suboptimal in the case of bone healing.

GENERAL CONSIDERATIONS

Every injury initiates an orderly, but complex sequence of orchestrated events that reestablish the integrity of the damaged tissue. Despite the body's innate ability to heal, surgical intervention is often used to optimize the healing process and favorably modulate the outcome. Interventions may include adequate debridement of devitalized tissue, removal of diseased tissue or foreign materials, securing adequate hemostasis, and apposing severed tissues with mechanical means until such time the wound is capable of withstanding functional stresses.

From a surgical viewpoint, the nature of wound healing depends upon the site, type of tissue involved, and the surgeon's ability to approximate the wound margins. Healing by *first intention* usually occurs when early primary closure can be achieved by accurately reapproximating the wound margins. Such a wound heals quickly with no separation of the wound edges, and with minimal scar formation. Absent favorable conditions, wound healing is prolonged and occurs through a filling of the tissue defect with granulation and connective tissue. This process is called healing by *second intention* and is frequently encountered following avulsive injury, wound infection, or poor apposition of the wound margins. In instances of infected or contaminated traumatic wounds with severe tissue loss, the surgeon may attempt healing by *third intention*. This is a staged procedure wherein the wound is allowed to granulate and heal by second intention before a delayed primary closure is carried out by bringing together the two surfaces of granulation tissue.

WOUND HEALING PHASES

The healing of soft tissue wounds occurs in a cascade of overlapping phases. Beginning with the inflammatory phase precipitated by the injury, the wound eventually restores itself through sequentially occurring proliferative and remodeling phases. While the rates and patterns of healing depend on a host of local, systemic and surgical factors, the phases of oral soft tissue healing are typical for all other tissues as well. In general, wounds in the oral cavity seem to heal faster than wounds to the skin. Oral wounds, despite being exposed to a bacteria-laden, moist, seemingly hostile environment, heal perfectly well and reepithelialize rapidly with minimal or no scar formation.

Inflammatory phase

The wounded area attempts to restore its normal state (homeostasis) immediately following injury. Disrupted blood vessels constrict and thrombose, and the thromboplastin released by the injured cells initiates the coagulation process. The accumulating platelets help form a fibrin clot to control bleeding. Additionally, the injured tissue and platelets begin to release key mediators of wound healing, particularly platelet-derived growth factors (PDGFs) and transforming growth factor β (TGF-β). These chemoattractants recruit inflammatory cells that begin to remove damaged tissue and bacteria from the injured area. Clinical signs include localized edema, pain, redness, and increased warmth at the wound site. Neutrophils are the predominant inflammatory cells during the initial 2 to 3 days following injury, but are rapidly outnumbered by macrophages derived from mobilized monocytes. As the primary source of modulating cytokines such as PDGF and vascular endothelial growth factor (VEGF), the macrophages regulate the formation of the granulation tissue that is distinctive of the proliferation phase.[1]

DOI: 10.1016/B978-0-7020-4618-6.00001-4

Proliferation phase

The proliferation phase is a period of intense replication of cells and is characterized by the migration and proliferation of fibroblasts and smooth muscle cells into the wound milieu. The fibroblast is the major cell responsible for the production of collagen and proteoglycans. Fibroblasts interact with their surrounding matrix via receptors known as integrins that regulate the level of collagen gene expression and collagenase induction. Collagen restores the strength and integrity of the repaired tissue, whereas the proteoglycans function as moisture storage. Concurrent with these events is the process of neoangiogenesis, whereby new blood vessels are formed and lymphatics are recanalized in the healing tissues. This essential process reestablishes transport of the nutrients and oxygen to the local injured site. In a synergistic way, the new capillaries supply nourishment to the developing collagen, while the collagen fibers structurally support the new capillary beds. Epithelial cells originating from hair follicles, sebaceous glands and margins of the wound edges proliferate and resurface the wound above the basement membrane. In contrast to skin, the process of reepithelialization progresses more rapidly in the oral mucosal wound. The oral epithelial cells migrate directly onto the moist, exposed surface of the fibrin clot instead of under the dry exudate (scab) of the dermis as in dry skin.[2] The rapid reepithelialization limits further insults from the oral cavity environment such as food debris, foreign particles and microorganisms.

Maturation/remodeling phase

The remodeling phase is the final stage of tissue repair and is distinguished by a continual turnover of collagen molecules as precursor collagen is broken down and new collagen synthesized. The tensile strength of the wound gradually restores as the collagen fibers are realigned and increasingly cross-linked to each other. The maximal tensile strength of a healed wound is reached in 6 to 12 months post injury but never reaches the strength of unwounded tissue. Eventually, active collagen synthesis achieves equilibrium with collagenolysis. However, disruptive processes such as poor oxygen perfusion, lack of nutrients, and wound infection can shift the balance to favor collagen breakdown and wound dehiscence.

HEALING OF EXTRACTION WOUNDS

The healing of a dental extraction wound is a specialized example of healing by second intention (Fig. 1.1).[3] Immediately after the removal

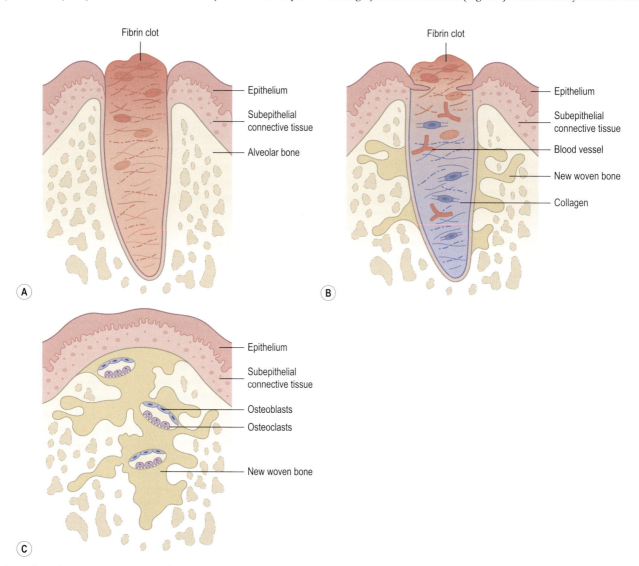

Fig. 1.1 Healing of an extraction wound after: (**A**) 24–48 hours; (**B**) 1 week; (**C**) 2–4 weeks.

of the tooth from the alveolus, blood fills the extraction site. Both intrinsic and extrinsic pathways of the clotting cascade are activated. The resultant fibrin meshwork containing entrapped red blood cells seals off the torn blood vessels and reduces the size of the extraction wound. Organization of the clot begins within the first 24 to 48 hours with engorgement and dilation of blood vessels within the periodontal ligament remnants, leukocytic migration and formation of a fibrin layer. In the first week, the clot forms a temporary scaffold upon which inflammatory cells migrate. Epithelium at the wound periphery grows over the surface of the organizing clot. Osteoclasts accumulate along the alveolar bone crest (in humans) or margin (in animals) setting the stage for active crestal or marginal resorption. Angiogenesis begins in the remnants of the periodontal ligaments. In the second week, the clot continues to get organized through fibroplasia and neoangiogenesis that begin to penetrate towards the center of the clot. Trabeculae of osteoid slowly extend into the clot from the alveolus and osteoclastic resorption of the cortical margin of the alveolus is more distinct. By the third week, the extraction socket is filled with granulation tissue and poorly calcified bone forms around the periphery of the wound. The surface of the wound is completely reepithelialized with minimal or no scar formation. Active bone remodeling by deposition and resorption continues for several more weeks. Radiographic evidence of bone formation does not become apparent until 6 to 8 weeks following tooth extraction. As bone remodeling proceeds, the extraction site becomes less distinct and is inconspicuous after 6–8 months.

Occasionally, the blood clot fails to form or may disintegrate, causing a localized alveolar osteitis. In such instances, healing is delayed considerably and the socket fills gradually. Because of the absence of a healthy granulation tissue matrix, the apposition of regenerate bone to remaining alveolar bone takes place at a much slower rate. Compared to a normal alveolus, the infected alveolus remains open or partially covered with hyperplastic epithelium for extended periods.

FACTORS AFFECTING HEALING

Infection

Wound infection is the most common cause of impaired wound healing. Though oral wounds are always colonized by bacteria, infection occurs only when the virulence or the number of the bacteria exceeds the ability of local tissue and host defenses to control them. The likelihood of wound infection increases substantially when the bacteria proliferate to levels beyond 10^5 organisms per gram of tissue.[4] Bacteria provoke various degrees of inflammation at the wounded tissue by releasing endotoxins, metalloproteinases, and breakdown products that inhibit the activities of regenerating cells and the scavenger macrophages. In addition to systemic diseases, local factors such as inadequate tissue perfusion and the presence of necrotic tissue or foreign bodies facilitate deterioration of a contaminated wound into an infected wound. The most important factor in minimizing the risk of infection is meticulous surgical technique, including thorough debridement, adequate hemostasis and elimination of dead space. Proper postoperative care, including stringent wound hygiene and absence of reinjury, further reduces the risk of infection.

Tissue perfusion and oxygenation

Adequate tissue perfusion is critical to the healing process. To a certain degree, hypoxia stimulates the cells to produce angiogenic growth factors. However, severe tissue hypoxia combines together with lactic acid produced by bacteria to lower tissue pH and contributes to tissue breakdown or necrosis.[5-7] Wounds in hypoxic tissues are more easily infected and heal poorly as leukocytic, fibroblastic and epithelial proliferation is depressed by low oxygen concentration. Poor oxygenation also interferes with the synthesis of collagen since oxygen is required for the hydroxylation of lysine and proline.[8] Furthermore, studies have shown that collagen deposition and wound tensile strength are limited by tissue perfusion and oxygen tension.[9]

The impaired healing associated with conditions such as diabetes mellitus, radiation damage, vasculitis, venous stasis, arteriosclerosis, and chronic infection can be largely ascribed to a faulty oxygen delivery system. Ischemic tissues produced by improper surgical techniques are poorly perfused and are excessively prone to infection. Tissue edema, remnants of necrotic tissues or a systemic perfusion defect such as hypovolemia, all impair wound healing. It follows that the natural resistance of the wound can also be enhanced by the maintenance of an adequate body fluid volume and satisfactory arterial oxygen tension. The use of hyperbaric oxygen to maintain the wound in a state of hyperoxia is based on this rationale.

Age

In general, oral wound healing is faster in the young animal than in the elderly. The influence of age on wound healing probably results from the general reduction of tissue metabolism that may be manifested by multiple physiologic problems as the animal ages. The major processes that drive soft tissue healing are diminished or damaged with progressive age. As a result, free oxidative radicals continue to accumulate and are deleterious to the dermal enzymes responsible for the integrity of the dermal or mucosal composition. In addition, the regional vascular support may be subjected to extrinsic deterioration and systemic disease decompensation, resulting in poor perfusion capability.[10]

Diabetes mellitus

Most of the complications related to diabetes, particularly poor wound healing, can be attributed to the development of diabetic microangiopathy. Local ischemia, secondary to poor oxygen delivery at the tissue level, and small vessel occlusion play an essential role in the pathogenesis and delayed healing of diabetes. Glycosylated hemoglobin has a higher binding affinity to oxygen molecules, which further impairs oxygen delivery to ischemic tissues. In addition, granulocyte function in uncontrolled diabetes is impaired, rendering these animals more susceptible to wound infection. Poor healing has also been related to the metabolic problems related to hyperglycemia, insulin deficiency and/or insulin resistance. The wound in the diabetic animal often demonstrates a decreased inflammatory response, fibroblast proliferation and collagen deposition, resulting in a healing product with reduced tensile strength. A stringent regulation of blood sugar is therefore essential in the diabetic patient undergoing surgery to optimize the wound healing potential.

Malnutrition

Nutritional deficiencies that produce hypoproteinemia hinder wound healing and impair the immune defense by limiting the availability of the amino acids critical for the synthesis of collagen and other proteins. Methionine, in particular, is a key amino acid in wound healing. It is metabolized to cysteine, and plays a vital role in the inflammatory, proliferative and remodeling phases of wound healing. As long as a state of protein catabolism exists, the wound heals very slowly. Several vitamins and trace minerals play a significant role in wound healing. Vitamin C and iron are essential cofactors for the hydroxylation of lysine and proline during collagen synthesis. Absent adequate compensatory collagen synthesis, scars may dissolve if collagenolytic activity continues unabated. Vitamin A is essential for normal immune function, epithelialization, and proteoglycan synthesis and healing is impaired when vitamin A is deficient. The B-complex vitamins and cobalt are essential cofactors in the antibody formation, white blood cell function and bacterial resistance. Vitamin D, thiamin and riboflavin deficiencies also result in poor repair.

Copper is needed for lysyl amine oxidase, whereas calcium is required for the normal function of granulocyte collagenase and other collagenases at the wound site. Zinc deficiency retards both fibroplasia and reepithelialization.[11] Zinc is required for DNA replication and serves as a coenzyme for DNA-polymerase and reverse-transcriptase. However, pharmacologic overdosing of zinc levels can exert a distinctly detrimental effect on healing by inhibiting macrophage migration and interference with collagen cross-linking.

CURRENT TRENDS IN WOUND CARE

An increased understanding of the wound healing processes has generated heightened interest in manipulating the wound microenvironment to facilitate healing. The traditional passive ways of treating wounds are rapidly giving way to approaches that actively modulate wound healing. These approaches include treatments that selectively jump-start the wound into the healing cascade, increase oxygenation and perfusion of the local tissues, or mechanically protect the wound.

Growth factors

A variety of topical exogenous recombinant growth factors have been investigated as agents to accelerate the wound healing process. These include platelet-derived growth factor (PDGF), angiogenesis factor, epidermal growth factor (EGF), transforming growth factor (TGF), fibroblast growth factor (bFGF), tumor necrosis factor (TNF), and interleukin-1 (IL-1). However, the potential of these extrinsic agents has not been realized clinically and may relate to figuring out which growth factors to put into the wound – and when and at what dose. To date, only a single recombinant growth factor – recombinant human platelet derived growth factor-BB form (PDGF-BB: Becaplermin, Ortho-McNeil Pharmaceutical, Raritan, NJ) – has been approved by the United States Food and Drug Administration for the treatment of cutaneous ulcers, specifically diabetic foot ulcers. Results from several controlled clinical human trials show that platelet derived growth factor-BB form gel was effective in healing lower extremity diabetic ulcers and significantly decreased their healing time when compared to the placebo group.[12,13]

More recently, recombinant human keratinocyte growth factor 2 (KGF-2: Repifermin, Human Genome Sciences, Inc., Rockville, MD)

has been shown to accelerate wound healing in experimental animal models. It enhances both the formation of granulation tissue in both young and old rabbits and wound closure of the human meshed skin graft explanted on athymic nude rats.[14,15] The safety assessment of the drug showed that keratinocyte growth factor 2 was well tolerated in human with no differences in adverse events.[16]

Topical chitosan, a derivative of chitin, is increasingly used in veterinary clinical medicine as a wound-healing accelerator for large open wounds. Chitosan appears to stimulate a rapid infiltration of inflammatory cells and granulation tissue formation along with an increased production of biological mediators and cytokines and fibroblastic proliferation.[17] Typical complications associated with the application of large doses of chitosan (above 50 mg/kg) in dogs include leukocytosis, elevated serum LDH2, LDH3 isoenzymes and severe hemorrhagic pneumonia.

Hyperbaric oxygen therapy

Hyperbaric oxygen therapy (HBOT) is occasionally used in veterinary medicine to raise tissue oxygen tension to a level that facilitates healing. In HBOT, 100% oxygen is delivered to the patient at pressures between 1.5 and 2.4 atmospheres. This stimulates the growth of fibroblasts and endothelial cells, increases the killing ability of leukocytes and is lethal for anaerobic bacteria. Multiple studies in HBOT in the treatment of human diabetic patients suggest that HBOT can be an effective adjunct in the management of diabetic wounds.[18] Animal studies suggest that HBOT could be beneficial in the treatment of osteomyelitis and soft tissue infections.[19,20] Adverse effects of HBOT are barotrauma of the ear, seizure and pulmonary oxygen toxicity.

Skin substitutes

Immediate wound coverage is critical for the acceleration of wound healing. When the surface area is large, wounds can be covered by synthetic and natural dressings. The human skin substitutes available are grouped into three major types and serve as excellent alternatives to autografts. The first type consists of grafts of cultured epidermal cells with no dermal components (Epicel: Epicel, Genzyme Tissue Repair Corp., Cambridge, MA). The second type has only dermal components (AlloDerm Regenerative Tissue Matrix: AlloDerm, Life-Cell Corp., Woodlands, TX; Dermagraft: Dermagraft, Advanced Bio-Healing, Inc., La Jolla, CA). The third type consists of a bilayer of both dermal and epidermal elements (Apligraf: Apligraf, Organogenesis Inc., Canton, MA, Integra: Integra, Johnson & Johnson Medical Integra Life Sciences Corp., Plainsboro, NJ). The chief effect of most skin substitutes is to promote wound healing by stimulating the recipient host to produce a variety of wound-healing cytokines. The use of cultured skin to cover wounds is particularly attractive inasmuch as the living cells already know how to produce growth factors at the right time and in the right amounts.

REFERENCES

1. Singer A, Clark R. Cutaneous wound healing. N Engl J Med 1999;341: 738–46.
2. Gustafson GT. Ecology of wound healing in the oral cavity. Scand J Haematol Suppl 1984;40:393–409.
3. Huebsch RF, Hansen LS. A histopathologic study of extraction wounds in dogs. Oral Surg Oral Med Oral Pathol 1969;28: 187–96.
4. Robson MC, Krizek TK, Heggers JP. Biology of surgical infection. In: Ravitch MM, editor. Current problems in surgery. Chicago, IL: Yearbook Medical Publishers; 1973. p. 1–62.
5. Hunt TK, Conolly WB, Aronson SB, et al. Anaerobic metabolism and wound healing: a hypothesis for the initiation and cessation of collagen synthesis in wounds. Am J Surg 1978;135:328–32.
6. Knighton DR, Silver LA, Hunt TK. Regulation of wound-healing angiogenesis effect of oxygen gradients and inspired oxygen concentration. Surgery 1981;90:262–70.
7. LaVan FB, Hunt TK. Oxygen and wound healing. Clin Plast Surg 1990;17:463–72.
8. Chvapil M, Hurych J, Ehrlichova E. The influence of varying oxygen tensions upon

proline hydroxylation and the metabolism of collagenous and non-collagenous proteins in skin slices. Hoppe Seylers Z Physiol Chem 1968;349:211–17.

9. Jonsson K, Jensen JA, Goodson WH, et al. Tissue oxygenation, anemia, and perfusion in relation to wound healing in surgical patients. Ann Surg 1991;214:605–13.

10. Fenske NA, Lober CW. Structural and functional changes of normal aging skin. J Am Acad Dermatol 1986;15:571–85.

11. Tengrup I, Ahonen J, Zederfeldt B. Granulation tissue formation in zinc-treated rats. Acta Chir Scand 1980; 146:1–4.

12. Steed DL. Clinical evaluation of recombinant human platelet-derived growth factor for the treatment of lower extremity diabetic ulcers. Diabetic Ulcer Study Group. J Vasc Surg 1995;21:71–81.

13. Wieman TJ, Smiell JM, Su Y. Efficacy and safety of a topical gel formulation of recombinant human platelet-derived growth factor-BB (Becaplermin) in patients with non healing diabetic ulcers: a phase III, randomized, placebo-controlled, double-blind study. Diabetes Care 1998;21:822–7.

14. Xia YP, Shao Y, Marcus J, et al. Effects of keratinocyte growth factor-2 (KGF-2) on wound healing in an ischemia-impaired rabbit ear model and on scar formation. J Pathol 1999;1888:431–8.

15. Soler PM, Wright TE, Smith PD, et al. In vivo characterization of keratinocyte growth factor-2 as a potential wound healing agent. Wound Rep Reg 1999;7: 172–8.

16. Robson M, Phillips T, Falanga V, et al. Randomized trial of topically applied repifermin (recombinant human keratinocyte growth factor-2) to accelerate wound healing in venous ulcers. Wound Rep Reg 2001;9:347–52.

17. Ueno H, Murakami M, Okumura M, et al. Chitosan accelerates the production of osteopontin from polymorphonuclear leukocytes. Biomaterials 2001;22: 1667–73.

18. Faglia E, Favales F, Aldeghi A, et al. Adjunctive systemic hyperbaric oxygen therapy in the treatment of severe prevalently ischemic diabetic foot ulcers. A randomized study. Diabetes Care 1996; 19:1338–43.

19. Mader JT, Guckian JC, Glass DL, et al. Therapy with hyperbaric oxygen for experimental osteomyelitis due to *Staphylococcus aureus* in rabbits. J Infect Dis 1978;138:312–18.

20. Bakker DJ. Selected aerobic and anaerobic soft tissue infections. In: Kindwall EP, Whelan HT, editors. Hyperbaric Medicine Practice. 2nd ed. Flagstaff, AZ: Best Publishing Company; 1999. p. 575–601.

Chapter | 2 |

Maxillofacial bone healing

Franz Härle & Randy J. Boudrieau

STRUCTURE OF FACIAL BONE

The structure of facial bone is determined by its material properties and by its mechanical role. The bone marrow cavity, the cortex and the spongiosa of the mandible and the midface are similar with respect to their material composition. The major difference is the geometric distribution of the bone. The canine mandible differs from the long bones in that it does not have a medullary canal. Instead, the cortex surrounds the cancellous bone and the mandibular canal, which contains the inferior alveolar neurovascular structures but no hematopoietic cells typical for a medullary canal.[1,2] The structure of the feline mandible closely resembles the canine mandible. The midfacial skeleton differs from the mandible in that it consists of a single, thin lamina of bone. The basic composition of bone is that of a dynamic tissue constantly undergoing resorption and remodeling.[3–5] Bone cell types consist of osteoblasts, osteocytes and osteoclasts.

Osteoblast

Osteoblasts are derived from pluripotential precursor cells. They produce osteoid, the organic matrix of bone, which is transformed into calcified bone. A layer of 1 μm of osteoid may be produced per day, followed by a maturation phase of 10 days before calcification.

The microscopic structure of the osteoid is differentiated between woven and lamellar bone. In woven bone, the collagen fibrils are randomly orientated and have a felted texture. In lamellar bone, the collagen fibrils are arranged in parallel bundles. Woven bone mineralizes immediately after osteoid deposition. In fracture healing, woven bone is formed first to clinically unite the bone, and then is transformed into lamellar bone.

Osteocyte

Osteocytes are derived from osteoblasts. Osteocytes essentially are entombed osteoblasts within the mineralized matrix of bone. They transform into osteocytes after they become surrounded within the osteoid. The newly trapped osteocytes are connected with other deeper osteocyte cell layers by long branching processes, which extend into radiating canaliculi for some distance in the mineralized matrix, to the lacunae of neighboring cells. The osteocytes lie between the concentric lamellae.

Osteoclast

Osteoclasts are multinucleated giant cells derived from mononuclear macrophages. Osteoclasts have a specialized role of bone breakdown. These cells are found on the surface of bone in concavities called Howship's lacunae. Howship's lacunae are small subcellular chambers with a low pH. The pH is maintained by hydrochloric acid, which dissolves the mineral. The organic matrix is degraded by proteases and collagenases, which are thought to be secreted by the osteoclasts. Osteoclasts are capable of resorbing 50–100 μm of bone per day.

Osteon (Haversian canal)

Osteons are cylindrical vascular tunnels formed by an osteoclast-rich tissue. They contain pluripotential precursor cells and endosteum known as the cutting cone. The bone removed by the cutting cone is replaced by osteoblast-rich tissue. This is known as the closing cone, which forms concentric layers of lamellar bone that surround the vascular Haversian canal. Volkmann canals also contain nutritional vessels arising from the periosteal and endosteal bone surface, which connect with the Haversian vessels within the osteons.[6] The size of the osteonal transport system is 100 μm, which limits the width of an osteon to approximately 200 μm. The mean width of a lamella is 3–7 μm (Fig. 2.1).

The three most important conditions necessary for bone formation and bone mineralization are: pluripotential precursor cells, ample blood supply and mechanical stability.[7]

FRACTURE HEALING

Fracture healing undergoes the same general processes as with soft tissue healing: inflammation, removal of organic debris, cellular proliferation and granulation tissue formation. Fracture healing differs in

DOI: 10.1016/B978-0-7020-4618-6.00002-6

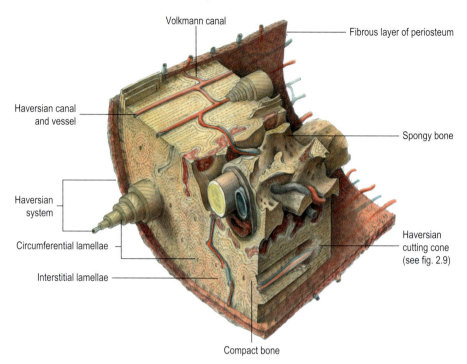

Fig. 2.1 Normal bone structure. *(From: Härle F. Bone repair and fracture healing. In: Härle F, Champy M, Terry BC, eds. Atlas of craniomaxillofacial osteosynthesis: miniplates, microplates, and screws. Stuttgart: Thieme; 1999: 8–14. Reprinted by permission.)*

that there is necrotic bone present, which is difficult to remove, with subsequent proliferation of osteogenic precursor cells, and the transformation of the granulation tissue into callus and finally into reconstituted bone. Bone thus is fully reconstituted without the formation of a scar.[3–5]

There are two types of fracture healing, namely indirect and direct bone healing.[3–6] Indirect bone healing occurs via the pluripotential cells located within the cortical and cancellous bone, periosteum, endosteum, and associated soft tissues. Indirect bone healing results from mechanical instability of the fracture, caused by resorption of fracture ends and callus formation. In the case of direct bone healing, the close apposition of the fracture segments provides mechanical stability. Consequently, the osteons of the fracture ends are in direct contact, allowing transverse bridging of the Haversian system with no intervening callus formation (Fig. 2.2). Two different forms of direct bone healing are described: contact healing and gap healing.[6,8] Direct bone healing also comprises a synergism between contact and gap healing.

The preferred objective in maxillofacial bone healing is for direct bone healing. Direct bone healing will occur only with anatomic reduction and absolutely rigid fixation. This form of bone healing results in quicker function, and without the adverse consequences associated with a large callus (that occurs with indirect bone healing).

Indirect bone healing

Bone fracture leads to initiation of the inflammatory phase of fracture repair. The fracture causes rupture of blood vessels, torn periosteum and disruption of the cortex and marrow; contraction and thrombosis of the blood vessels usually limits blood loss. Subsequently, ischemic necrosis of the bone ends occurs within the Haversian and Volkmann's canals a few millimeters from the fragment's ends (Fig. 2.3). As a result of this trauma, a protein-rich exudate forms within the fracture site. There is activation of the osteogenic cells of the periosteum and endosteal lining of the Haversian canals and marrow cavity. In

addition, a proliferative vascular response ensues (initially a transient extraosseous circulation from the adjacent soft tissues), which also furnishes inflammatory cells and osteogenic progenitor cells to the site. Fibroblastic proliferation occurs within the clot, with accumulation of a cellular infiltrate composed of neutrophils and macrophages. These cells participate in the removal of the debris at the fracture. The osteoprogenitor cells differentiate into fibroblasts and chondroblasts (formation of fibrocartilaginous callus), osteoblasts (formation of new bone), and osteoclasts (resorption of dead bone). These proliferating cells lay down callus, a fibrous matrix of collagen, which thereby forms a bridge across the fracture. A number of contiguous, and overlapping, stages of callus formation can be distinguished. Initially, the formation of periosteal callus leads to a decrease of interfragmentary strain, which is followed by interfragmentary and endosteal callus formation. Granulation tissue invasion replaces the initial hematoma and is transformed into interfragmentary connective tissue (Fig. 2.4) while the ends of the bone fragments are resorbed by osteoclasts (Figs 2.4 and 2.5).

The reparative phase of fracture repair consists of consolidation, proliferation and maturation of this callus. Depending upon the local microenvironment, oxygen tension, pH, tensile or compressive stresses, the cells within the gap differentiate accordingly. In well-vascularized areas, usually nearest the bone surface, the osteogenic cells transform directly into osteoblasts and lay down a cartilaginous matrix that calcifies directly into bone. In less well-vascularized areas, the osteogenic cells transform into chondroblasts and form cartilage. The more interfragmentary connective tissue is remodeled into fibrocartilage (Fig. 2.6). Since fibrocartilage is more rigid than fibrous tissue, the interfragmentary tissue becomes stiffer and increases the resistance against motion of the fragments. Subsequently, the fibrocartilage undergoes mineralization. Vascular invasion of fibrocartilage is combined with resorption of mineralized matrix. Calcified fibrocartilage must undergo resorption before osteoblasts can start to produce osteoid as a base for new bone deposition (Fig. 2.7). Initially, the calcified fibrocartilage is replaced by woven bone. After the fracture is

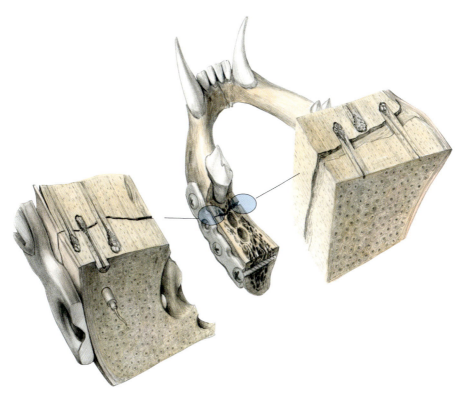

Fig. 2.2 A feline mandibular body fracture with miniplate osteosynthesis on the ventral side of the bone (the bone adjacent to the teeth has been cut away in this diagrammatic representation). Direct bone healing (contact healing) is observed in the buccal cortex of the mandible directly adjacent to (under) the implants (see Fig. 2.9). Direct bone healing (gap healing) is observed in the lingual cortex of the mandible opposite the implants (see Figs 2.11 & 2.12). Areas with large gaps (>800 μm), or without this degree of rigid fixation, will heal by indirect bone healing.

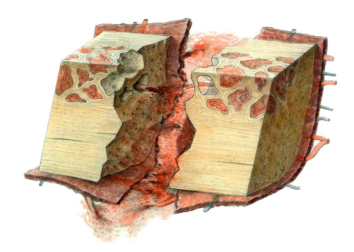

Fig. 2.3 Indirect bone healing: fracture of the bone with rupture of the blood vessels and a hematoma in the surrounding soft tissues. *(From: Härle F. Bone repair and fracture healing. In: Härle F, Champy M, Terry BC, eds. Atlas of craniomaxillofacial osteosynthesis: miniplates, microplates, and screws. Stuttgart: Thieme; 1999: 8–14. Reprinted by permission.)*

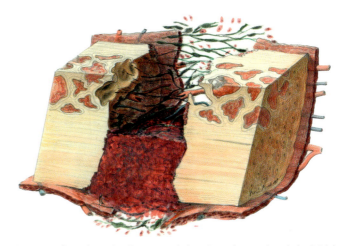

Fig. 2.4 Indirect bone healing: granulation tissue has replaced the initial hematoma within the fracture site; the necrotic ends of the bone fragments subsequently will be resorbed by osteoclasts. Remaining hematoma is shown only in the ventral part of the fracture site. *(From: Härle F. Bone repair and fracture healing. In: Härle F, Champy M, Terry BC, eds. Atlas of craniomaxillofacial osteosynthesis: miniplates, microplates, and screws. Stuttgart: Thieme; 1999: 8–14. Reprinted by permission.)*

bridged by woven bone, stability is obtained and function is possible.[9] This process whereby the cartilage is removed and then replaced with bone is termed endochondral ossification. The increase in this tissue strength, as it is replaced with bone, results in the clinically healed fracture.

The healed fracture undergoes a further increase in strength as the remodeling process restores the bone into its original shape over a prolonged period of time. Redundant bone trabeculae are removed at the same time new structural trabeculae of lamellar bone are formed. This bony deposition in a more advantageous orientation and location is influenced by the stresses within the bone (Wolff's law) to eventually restore the normal pre-fracture bony architecture.[10] This process is termed Haversian remodeling of bone, replacing the woven bone with lamellar bone (Fig. 2.8). It is the identical process whereby

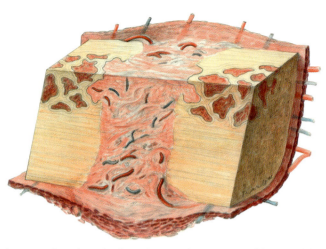

Fig. 2.5 Indirect bone healing: the granulation tissue will be remodeled into interfragmentary connective tissue. *(From: Härle F. Bone repair and fracture healing. In: Härle F, Champy M, Terry BC, eds. Atlas of craniomaxillofacial osteosynthesis: miniplates, microplates, and screws. Stuttgart: Thieme; 1999: 8–14. Reprinted by permission.)*

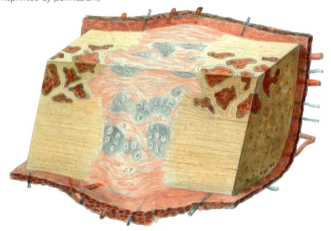

Fig. 2.6 Indirect bone healing: the interfragmentary connective tissue will be remodeled into fibrocartilage. *(From: Härle F. Bone repair and fracture healing. In: Härle F, Champy M, Terry BC, eds. Atlas of craniomaxillofacial osteosynthesis: miniplates, microplates, and screws. Stuttgart: Thieme; 1999: 8–14. Reprinted by permission.)*

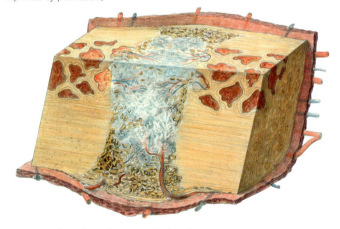

Fig. 2.7 Indirect bone healing: calcified fibrocartilage must partially be resorbed before osteoblasts can start to produce osteoid. *(From: Härle F. Bone repair and fracture healing. In: Härle F, Champy M, Terry BC, eds. Atlas of craniomaxillofacial osteosynthesis: miniplates, microplates, and screws. Stuttgart: Thieme; 1999: 8-14. Reprinted by permission.)*

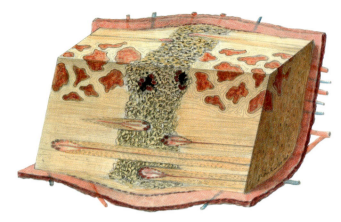

Fig. 2.8 Indirect bone healing: Haversian remodeling begins to reconstruct the lamellar orientation of the bone. *(From: Härle F. Bone repair and fracture healing. In: Härle F, Champy M, Terry BC, eds. Atlas of craniomaxillofacial osteosynthesis: miniplates, microplates, and screws. Stuttgart: Thieme; 1999: 8–14. Reprinted by permission.)*

bone constantly is remodeled over the animal's lifetime. Haversian remodeling of cortical bone begins with osteoclastic resorption. Several osteoclasts bore a longitudinally oriented cavity (the 'cutting cone'). These osteoclasts are followed closely by a vascular loop and osteoprogenitor cells that differentiate into osteoblasts. These cells produce osteoid on the inside wall of the resorption cavity. This osteoid then mineralizes and these successive layers of mineralized osteoid become layers of lamellar bone – leaving a narrow central vascular channel, the Haversian canal.

Direct bone healing

Direct bone healing is the process of bone union in which bone is the only type of connective tissue to form between the fracture fragments.[6] Direct bone healing was first described radiographically after perfect anatomic repositioning and stable fixation. Healing of fractures was observed with a lack of callus formation and simultaneous disappearance of the fracture lines. This was originally described as 'soudure autogène' (autogenous welding).[11] Callus-free direct bone healing requires what is often called 'absolute stability by interfragmentary compression.'[12] The biological signal responsible for recruitment of osteogenic progenitor cells, which contributes to callus formation in indirect bone healing, apparently is eliminated with precise reduction and fixation; therefore, direct bone healing occurs with unimpeded cellular function and vascularization via Haversian remodeling.[13] Bone is the only type of connective tissue to form between fracture fragments with direct bone healing; however, the deposition of bone varies depending upon whether contact or a small gap is present.

If no gap is present, and direct cortical contact is present, contact healing occurs whereby bone union and Haversian remodeling occur simultaneously. If a small gap is present, <800 μm, gap healing occurs whereby bony union and Haversian remodeling are separate sequential processes (with gaps >800 μm indirect bone healing occurs as previously described).

Contact healing

Contact healing of the bone means that healing of the fracture line occurs after stable anatomic repositioning with perfect interfragmentary contact, without the possibility for any cellular or vascular ingrowth.[6,8] Haversian cutting cones are able to cross this interface

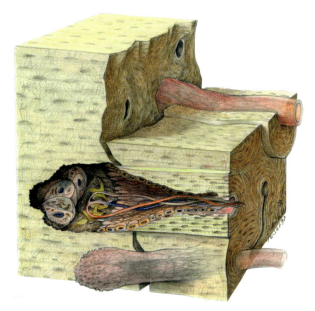

Fig. 2.9 Direct bone healing (contact healing): cutting cones cross the interface from one bone fragment to the other by remodeling the Haversian canal (compare with Fig. 2.2, directly adjacent to the implants). *(After: Härle F. Bone repair and fracture healing. In: Härle F, Champy M, Terry BC, eds. Atlas of craniomaxillofacial osteosynthesis: miniplates, microplates, and screws. Stuttgart: Thieme; 1999: 8–14. Reprinted by permission.)*

from one bone fragment to the other by immediate remodeling of the Haversian canal. As previously noted, Haversian canal remodeling is the main mechanism to restore the internal architecture of compact bone (Fig. 2.9). Contact healing takes place over the entire fracture line after perfect anatomical reduction, osteosynthesis and absolute mechanical stability (Fig. 2.10). Contact healing generally is observed only directly beneath the fixation, where such direct contact, and interfragmentary compression, can be obtained.

Gap healing

Gap healing takes place in stable or 'quiet' gaps with a width of >200 μm osteonal diameter, but <800 μm.[6,8] Ingrowth of vessels and mesenchymal cells starts after surgical stabilization. Osteoblasts deposit osteoid on the fragment ends without osteoclastic resorption. The gaps are filled exclusively with primarily formed, transversely orientated lamellar bone. Replacement is usually completed within 4 to 6 weeks (Fig. 2.11). In the second stage the transversely-oriented bone lamellae are replaced by axially-oriented osteons, i.e., Haversian remodeling (Fig. 2.12). After approximately 10 weeks, the fracture is replaced by newly reconstructed cortical bone. Gap healing plays an important role in direct bone healing, as small gaps are far more extensive than contact areas. Contact areas, on the other hand, are essential for stabilization by interfragmentary friction, as these contact areas protect the gaps against deformation. Gap healing usually can be observed far from the fixation, e.g., the opposite bone cortex, or areas where interfragmentary compression is not obtained.

Craniomaxillofacial bone healing

Bone repair and fracture healing to restore original integrity (*restitutio ad integrum*) can be achieved with the use of wire, standard plates (DCP or reconstruction) and miniplates, the latter of which provide the optimum environment for direct bone healing. In the mandible, the plates must be placed at the most biomechanically favorable sites

to neutralize the tension forces and torsional movements which cause fracture distraction (see Chs 25, 30 & 31). Bone plate fixation provides both contact and gap bone healing. Contact bone healing generally is observed between compressed bone fragments, either adjacent to the plate or where interfragmentary compression can be applied, e.g. miniplate (see Fig. 2.2 on the bone window in the fracture line on the lateral cortex of the mandible). Gap bone healing generally is observed remotely from the plates, e.g. transcortex to the plate, e.g. miniplate (see Fig. 2.2 on the bone window in the fracture line on the inner cortex of the mandible).

Mandibular fracture healing in the dog and cat essentially is identical to healing of long bones.[1,2] The obvious primary difference is the presence of the teeth and the mandibular canal. In the dog and cat the tooth roots occupy a considerable volume of the mandible, >40% of the dorsoventral mandibular volume. Because of the presence of the teeth, it is difficult to provide the conditions of rigid stabilization along the alveolar margin, i.e., the tension-band side of the bone, which is the biomechanically preferred location to place implants (see Ch. 25). In humans, implants are placed below the tooth roots and also below the level of the mandibular canal, but remain on the tension-band side of the bone because of the overall large dorsoventral mandibular height.[14,15] Despite the biomechanical advantage of implant (mini- or microplate) location at this level, a second implant (miniplate) is placed parallel to, and a few millimeters apart from, the tension-band device for added stability. In the dog and cat, the dorsoventral mandibular height is much more limited, and simultaneously has a much larger tooth root volume compared to humans. Despite these anatomic constraints, implants still may be placed along the alveolar margin, in this preferential location, between the tooth roots using similar small implants (wire or miniplates – see Chs. 30 & 31).

One principle of application of these implants along the alveolar margin is to avoid penetration of the tooth roots; the implication is that such penetration will lead to tooth death.[16] Despite these recommendations, it is likely that both major (>50% of screw diameter penetrating the tooth root) and minor (<50% of screw diameter penetrating the tooth root) contacts with a tooth occur. It is unknown whether significant clinical problems manifest in the dog and cat should this occur; however, studies in humans have shown minimal morbidity in a large series of clinical patients.[17,18]

Because of the large size of the tooth roots in the dog and cat, and the bony area that they occupy, the teeth play an important role in maintaining fracture stability, which directly affects subsequent bone healing. Removal of teeth may increase complications that adversely affect bone healing. Further dissection to excise apical fragments may lead to additional disruption of the blood supply, cause iatrogenic trauma to the adjacent tissues (e.g., further fragment displacement), eliminate available structures for possible fracture fixation, eliminate occlusal landmarks used to realign bone segments to provide for functional occlusion, and create large bony defects that prevent adequate fracture stabilization. In order to enhance the environment for bone healing (and maximize the stability of the fracture repair), teeth that are present within a fracture line generally are not removed unless they cannot be stabilized.[16]

Additionally, implant placement to avoid the mandibular canal is recommended. This is very difficult in the dog and cat because of the short dorsoventral mandibular height and the large size of the tooth roots. Again, it is very likely that this area is penetrated with implant placement, but with minimal patient morbidity despite the few specific studies to investigate this potential problem.[19] Experimental studies have demonstrated that despite disruption of the nutrient vessel within the mandibular canal (inferior alveolar artery) the teeth remain unaffected, i.e., without evidence of pulpal necrosis or diseased teeth.[19] This is likely due to the rapid reconstitution of the

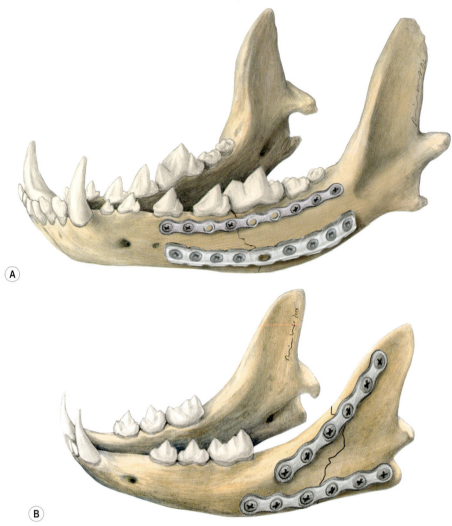

(A)

(B)

Fig. 2.10 Perfect anatomical reconstruction of: (**A**) mandibular body fracture in a dog, miniplate and reconstruction plate osteosynthesis along the alveolar margin (tension-band) and ventral mandibular margin, respectively; (**B**) mandibular ramus fracture in a cat using miniplate osteosynthesis along the coronoid crest (tension-band) and ventral mandibular margin. Areas of direct (contact) healing occur adjacent to the implants (compare with Figs 2.2 & 2.9).

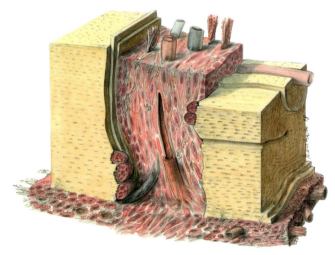

Fig. 2.11 Direct bone healing (gap healing): osteoblasts deposit osteoid and the gaps are filled with primary formation of transversely-oriented lamellar bone (compare with Fig. 2.2, the lingual cortex of the mandible opposite the implants). *(From: Härle F. Bone repair and fracture healing. In: Härle F, Champy M, Terry BC, eds. Atlas of craniomaxillofacial osteosynthesis: miniplates, microplates, and screws. Stuttgart: Thieme; 1999: 8–14. Reprinted by permission.)*

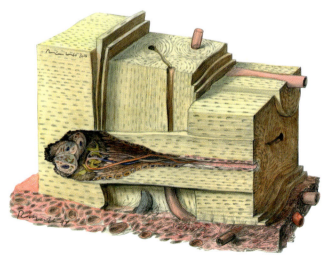

Fig. 2.12 Direct bone healing (gap healing): transversely-oriented bone lamellae are replaced by axially-oriented osteons (Haversian remodeling). *(After: Härle F. Bone repair and fracture healing. In: Härle F, Champy M, Terry BC, eds. Atlas of craniomaxillofacial osteosynthesis: miniplates, microplates, and screws. Stuttgart: Thieme; 1999: 8–14. Reprinted by permission.)*

vascular supply from the transient extraosseous circulation (from the surrounding soft tissues) that becomes established shortly after fracture.[1,2]

The midfacial skeleton differs from the mandible in that it consists of a thin lamina of bone, which provides an increased surface area to bone:volume ratio as compared with the mandible; consequently, the closer proximity of nutritional vessels provides a superior blood supply to the bone. The result is an increased healing rate of these midfacial bones. A combination of direct and indirect bone healing also occurs in the maxilla, following the principles of miniplate osteosynthesis when applied to this region. However, in the craniomaxillofacial skeleton, interfragmentary compression for direct bone healing is not necessarily required in order to obtain direct bone healing, as demonstrated experimentally and clinically.[20-24] Identical principles of repair applied to human maxillofacial fixation using miniplate osteosynthesis can be applied to the dog and cat (see Ch. 31). All of the same issues with regard to the teeth exist in the maxilla as with the mandible in the dog and cat.

REFERENCES

1. Roush JK, Howard PE, Wilson JW. Normal blood supply to the canine mandible and mandibular teeth. Am J Vet Res 1989;50:904–7.

2. Wilson JW. Blood supply to developing, mature, and healing bone. In: Sumner-Smith G, editor. Bone in clinical orthopaedics. 2nd ed. New York: Thieme; 2002. p. 23–116.

3. Schenk RK. Biology of fracture repair. In: Browner BD, Jupiter JB, Levine AM, et al, editors. Skeletal trauma. Philadelphia, PA: Saunders; 1992. p. 31–75.

4. Brand RA, Rubin CT. Fracture healing. In: Albright JA, Brand RA, editors. The scientific basis of orthopaedics. 2nd ed. Norwalk, CT: Appleton and Lange; 1987. p. 325–45.

5. Ham AW, Cormack DH. Bone and bones. In: Ham AW, Cormack DH, editors. Histology. 8th ed. Philadelphia, PA: Lippincott, 1979. p. 377–462.

6. Schenk R, Willenegger H. Zur Histologie der primären Knochenheilung. Arch Klin Chir 1964;308:440–52.

7. Pauwels F. Grundriss einer Biomechanik der Frakturheilung. Verh Dtsch Orthop Ges 1940;34:62–108.

8. Schenk R, Willenegger H. Zum histologischen Bild der sogenannten Primärheilung der Knochenkompakta nach experimentellen Osteotomien am Hund. Experimentia 1963;19:593–614.

9. Philipps JH, Rahn BA. Bone healing. In: Yaremchuk MJ, Gruss JS, Manson PN, editors. Rigid fixation in the craniomaxillofacial skeleton. Boston, MA: Butterworth-Heinemann; 1992. p. 3–6.

10. Perren SM. Primary bone healing. In: Bojrab MJ, editor. Disease mechanisms in small animal surgery. 2nd ed. Philadelphia, PA: Lea and Febiger; 1993. p. 663–70.

11. Danis R. Théorie et pratique de l'ostéosynthèse. Paris: Masson; 1949.

12. Steinemann SG. Implants for stable fixation of fractures. In: Rubin LR, editor. Biomaterials in reconstructive surgery. St. Louis, MO: Mosby; 1983. p. 283–311.

13. O'Sullivan ME, Chao EYS, Kelly J. The effect of fixation on fracture healing. J Bone Joint Surg 1989;71A:306–10.

14. Champy M, Blez P. Anatomical aspects and biomechanical considerations. In: Härle F, Champy M, Terry BC, editors. Atlas of craniomaxillofacial osteosynthesis: miniplates, microplates and screws. Thieme: Stuttgart; 1999. p. 3–7.

15. Pape H-D, Gerlach KL, Champy M. Mandibular fractures including atrophied mandible. In: Härle F, Champy M, Terry BC, editors. Atlas of craniomaxillofacial osteosynthesis: miniplates, microplates and screws. Thieme: Stuttgart; 1999. p. 31–9.

16. Henney LHS, Galburt RB, Boudrieau RJ. Treatment of dental injuries following craniofacial trauma. Semin Vet Med Surg (Small Anim) 1992;7:21–35

17. Fabbroni G, Aabed S, Mizen K, et al. Transalveolar screws and the incidence of dental damage: a prospective study. Int J Maxillofac Surg 2004;33:442–6.

18. Borah GL, Ashmead D. The fate of teeth transfixed by osteosynthesis screws. Plast Reconstr Surg 1996;97:726–9.

19. Kern DA, Smith MM, Stevenson S, et al. Evaluation of three fixation techniques for repair of mandibular fractures in dogs. J Am Vet Med Assoc 1995;206:1883–90.

20. Ikemura K, Kouno J, Shibata H, et al. Biomechanical study on monocortical osteosynthesis for the fracture of the mandible. Int J Oral Surg 1984;13:307–12.

21. Ewers R, Härle F. Osteotomieheilung im Unterkiefer nach Kontakt- und Spaltheilung sowie nach kortiko-kortikaler Heilung. Dtsch Zahnärztl Z 1983;38:361–2.

22. Ewers R, Härle F. Biomechanics of the midface and mandibular fractures: Is a stable fixation necessary? In: Hjørting-Hansen E, editor. Oral and maxillofacial surgery. Chicago, IL: Quintessence; 1985. p. 207–11.

23. Champy M, Lodde JP. Etude des contraintes dans la mandibule fracturée chez l'homme. Mesures théoriques et vérification par jauges extensométriques in situ. Rev Stomatol 1977;78:545–56.

24. Kahn JL, Khouri M. Champy's system. In: Yaremchuk MJ, Gruss JS, Manson PN, editors. Rigid fixation of the craniomaxillofacial skeleton. Boston, MA: Butterworth-Heinemann; 1992. p. 116–23.

In dogs, streptococci, the most common cause of IE, most often infect the mitral valve and are likely to be associated with polyarthritis and fever. By contrast, dogs with IE secondary to *Bartonella* spp. infection are often afebrile, are more likely to develop congestive heart failure, rarely have mitral valve involvement, and have shorter survival time.[14] Although periodontal disease has been associated with histologic abnormalities in a variety of organs in dogs, including the myocardium and left atrioventricular valves,[15,16] the influence of oral disease or dental procedures on the development of endocarditis in dogs remains controversial. Periodontal pathogens are obligate anaerobic bacteria and are not likely to survive in the highly oxygenated blood of the heart and arterial system. They also lack the surface adhesion factors that are a major factor in the propensity of streptococci and staphylococci to attach to damaged cardiac valves.[3] Current veterinary literature does not support the association between bacterial endocarditis and either dental/oral surgical procedures or oral infection in dogs.[17,18] One recent study suggested an association between the severity of periodontal disease and the risk of 'cardiovascular-related events,' and found that dogs with stage 3 periodontal disease (defined as up to 50% attachment loss, presence of periodontal pockets and/or gingival recession and root exposure) were nearly six times as likely to have endocarditis as dogs with no periodontal disease or stage 1 periodontal disease (defined as gingival inflammation with no attachment loss).[19] In this study, diagnosis of a 'cardiovascular-related event' included non-specific clinical findings, such as a history of coughing or tiring easily and elevated white blood cell count, as well as specific cardiac diagnoses such as cardiomyopathy, endocarditis, and mitral valve insufficiency. The incidence of endocarditis was reported to be 0.01% in the nonperiodontal cohort and 0.15% in the stage 3 periodontal disease patients, but it was not specified how the diagnosis of endocarditis was reached. The mean age of dogs reported to have stage 3 periodontal disease in the study was 9.4 years, while the mean age of dogs in the nonperiodontal cohort was 7.5 years. Dental radiographs were not required to determine the presence or stage of periodontal disease in this study. These factors may have influenced the results, and further research is required to determine whether the conclusions of this study are valid.

The AHA currently recommends IE prophylaxis for dental procedures only for human patients with underlying cardiac conditions associated with the highest risk of adverse outcome from IE: those with prosthetic cardiac valve(s), previous infective endocarditis, congenital heart disease (CHD) and recipients of cardiac transplant with a history of cardiac valvulopathy. For these patients, prophylaxis is recommended for all dental procedures that involve manipulation of gingival tissue or the periapical region of teeth, or perforation of the oral mucosa, with the following exceptions: local anesthetic injection through noninfected tissue, obtaining dental radiographs, placement of a removable prosthodontic or orthodontic appliance, adjustment of an orthodontic appliance, exfoliation of deciduous teeth, and bleeding from trauma to lips or oral mucosa.[20]

The standard regimen in human antibiotic prophylaxis is a high dose of amoxicillin orally 1 hour, or ampicillin intravenously 30 minutes, preoperatively. For patients with penicillin allergy, clindamycin, cephalexin, cefadroxil or azithromycin can be used orally, or clindamycin or cefazolin IV.[3]

Prophylactic antibiotic treatment for patients with orthopedic implants

In 2009, the American Academy of Orthopedic Surgeons (AAOS) published a recommendation that antibiotic prophylaxis be considered for joint replacement patients prior to any invasive procedure that may cause bacteremia.[21] Antibiotic prophylaxis is not indicated for dental patients with pins, plates or screws not within a synovial

joint. This is a change from previous recommendations which stated that antibiotic prophylaxis should be considered for joint replacement patients within 2 years of placement and when high-risk conditions such as immunosuppression, type 1 diabetes, history of joint infection, severe hemophilia or malnourishment are present; routine use of prophylactic antibiotics was not recommended for most dental patients with total joint replacements.[22] Antibiotic prophylaxis is not indicated for healthy dental patients with pins, plates or screws not within a synovial joint.[21]

Prophylactic antibiotic treatment for patients with other conditions

Other conditions in humans where antibiotic prophylaxis has been used in association with dental procedures, but with no national medical organization guidelines or recommendations, are organ transplant recipients, immunocompromised patients (those with HIV/AIDS, agranulocytosis, cancer, leukopenia, leukemia) when neutrophil count < 1000 mm^3 and/or CD4 count < 200 mm^3, and patients on long-term corticosteroid therapy. Antibiotic prophylaxis may also be indicated in poorly controlled type 1 diabetics who require extractions, oral surgery, or periodontal procedures and during the first 6 months following surgery in patients who have undergone splenectomy.[13]

ANTIBIOTICS IN ORAL SURGERY

The aim of antibiotic prophylaxis in oral and maxillofacial surgery is to prevent infection at the surgical wound. Characteristics of the surgery, degree of contamination of the surgical field, or the general state of the patient will determine if antibiotics are indicated. Prophylactic antibiotics may be used in clean-contaminated and contaminated surgeries, and antibiotic treatment is recommended in dirty surgeries.[23]

In the USA, 17.7% of human oral and maxillofacial surgeons reportedly never use antibiotics to prevent infection, while 59.9% responded that they prescribed antibiotics to prevent infection 'half of the time,' 'often' or 'almost always.' The most frequently used antibiotics are penicillin V, amoxicillin and clindamycin.[24]

Extractions

Several studies have compared the rate of postoperative complications after third molar surgery in humans with and without the use of pre- and/or postoperative antibiotics.[25–28] Use of intravenous antibiotics administered prophylactically decreased the frequency of surgical site infections and alveolar osteitis after third molar extraction[25] or third molar surgery.[28] The longer it took to extract the third molar, the higher the rate of infection was (13.8% for long versus 1.6% for short procedures). Also, the difficulty of the procedure increased the rate of infection (with ostectomy, 12.7% versus without ostectomy, 3.5%).[26] The risk of infection in patients who required ostectomy was 24%, 9% and 4% with placebo, presurgical dose of amoxicillin-clavulanate and pre-emptive 5-day postsurgical treatment with amoxicillin-clavulanate, respectively.[26]

The authors of a study involving surgical removal of 528 impacted lower third molars reported that, compared to no antibiotic treatment, postoperative oral antibiotic treatment with amoxicillin-clavulanic acid or clindamycin did not contribute to better wound healing, reduced pain, or increased mouth opening, nor did it prevent inflammatory problems after surgery. They concluded that postoperative oral antibiotic treatment should not be routinely recommended.[27] In a separate study, a single preoperative dose, with or without postoperative multidose clindamycin therapy, failed to demonstrate efficacy in preventing infectious and inflammatory complications in third molar surgery.[29]

Scientific veterinary medical studies reporting the indication for antibiotic therapy in association with extractions are not available. Based on the data from human studies, it can be concluded that antibiotics are not needed for most veterinary patients undergoing extractions. Veterinarians may consider a perioperative dose of antibiotics for patients who require multiple surgical extractions with ostectomy, those with severe, generalized periodontitis, and/or patients with medical conditions which might impair their ability to clear the anticipated bacteremia. (See recommendations for patients with other health problems in Antibiotic Prophylaxis.)

Maxillary and mandibular fractures

Recommendations regarding the use of antibiotics in surgical treatment of mandibular and maxillary fractures vary. Some authors recommend prophylactic perioperative antibiotic administration initiated prior to surgery but not exceeding 24 hours.[30,31] Several studies conclude that postoperative use of antibiotics is often unnecessary in humans and dogs.[30,32–37] Two human studies confirmed that postoperative oral administration of antibiotics (for 5 to 10 days) offered no additional benefit beyond perioperative intravenous antibiotic administration in patients with mandibular fractures.[36,37] Other studies failed to demonstrate any statistically significant benefit with the administration of postoperative antibiotics in patients undergoing open reduction and internal fixation of mandibular fractures.[33,35] Antibiotic therapy had no impact on the development of postoperative complications after repair of mandibular fractures using open reduction internal fixation (ORIF) alone, maxillomandibular fixation (MMF), or with a combination of MMF and ORIF.[34]

In the case of mandibular fractures with communication to the oral cavity, five randomized studies in humans indicate that antibiotics significantly reduce the risk of fracture line infection.[32] Antibiotic prophylaxis is also justified in compound or open fractures and those communicating with paranasal sinuses in humans.[23]

Maxillectomy and mandibulectomy

Proper surgical technique reduces the likelihood of development of postsurgical infection.[38] Oral soft tissues should not be traumatized, electrocoagulation should be used judiciously, and irrigation must be used to prevent thermal necrosis of bone during osteotomy, ostectomy and osteoplasty. Routine periodontal treatment should be performed for dogs and cats prior to major oral tumor surgery if there is a large amount of plaque and calculus present. This results in a cleaner surgical field and less inflamed gingival tissue at the time of the surgery.[38]

A review of 547 patients who had major contaminated oncologic head and neck surgery concluded that perioperative antibiotic administration should be performed, but no evidence exists to support prolonged administration of antibiotics beyond the first 24 hours following surgery.[31] A 1-day antibiotic regimen was as effective as a 3-day regimen in preventing wound or systemic infection in clean-contaminated head and neck cancer surgery without flap reconstruction.[39] Healthy patients undergoing surgery of the salivary glands do not need antibiotic prophylaxis.[23]

Luxated or avulsed teeth

The proper conditioning for a tooth that remains out of the mouth in a dry condition for less than 60 minutes, or is stored in one of the recommended media within the advised time frame, is to coat the root surface with tetracycline and reimplant the tooth. In the event

that 60 minutes have passed in dry conditions, or the tooth remained in a recommended medium longer than the advised time period, then the tooth should be soaked in a fluoride solution before reimplantation.[40] When extracted monkey teeth were treated with topical doxycycline (1 mg/10 mL for 5 min) before reimplantation, infection-related root resorption was reduced or prevented.[32] Postoperatively, patients with laterally luxated or avulsed teeth are prescribed amoxicillin (or clindamycin if allergic to penicillin) for 7 days after tooth reimplantation.[40]

Antibiotic use in periodontal surgery

Ideally, scaling and polishing should be a pretreatment procedure in dogs with severe periodontitis and a postscaling examination should be performed a couple of weeks later. As a result, periodontal tissue would have time to heal, and a determination of surgical treatment would not be done on unhealthy tissue. However, in veterinary dentistry, scaling, polishing and other periodontal treatment is often performed during one anesthetic episode. In some patients with severe periodontitis, antibiotic treatment for several days before a dental procedure may be indicated to reduce the inflammation of periodontal tissues.[41]

Studies in human patients have indicated that the incidence of infection after periodontal surgery is very low in patients treated with or without antibiotics. Therefore, unless there is a medical indication, there is no justification for using prophylactic antibiotic therapy to prevent infection following periodontal surgery.[42,43]

Antimicrobial resistance of subgingival bacterial flora in dogs appears to be increasing, as evidenced by the results of two veterinary studies that were published 11 years apart.[44,45] Subgingival microflora in dogs with severe gingivitis or periodontitis was highly susceptible to commonly used antibiotics in the 1995 study.[44] In that study, amoxicillin-clavulanic acid had the highest in-vitro susceptibility (96%) against all canine isolates tested. In a similar study evaluating bacterial isolates from cats with gingivitis, amoxicillin-clavulanic acid had the highest in-vitro susceptibility against all subgingival isolates, and both amoxicillin-clavulanic acid and clindamycin were effective against all anaerobes.[46]

In a more recent study, antimicrobial resistance of subgingival aerobic and anaerobic flora to commonly used antibiotics in dogs with periodontal disease was high.[45] Anaerobic bacteria appeared to be the most susceptible to amoxicillin-clavulanic acid, doxycycline, and erythromycin; aerobic bacteria appeared to be most susceptible to amoxicillin-clavulanic acid, erythromycin, gentamicin, and sulfatrimethoprim. Although antimicrobial resistance to amoxicillin-clavulanic acid was the lowest of the commonly used antibiotics in dentistry, it was still significant (e.g., *Prevotella intermedia* 33.3%, *P. gingivalis* and *Peptostreptococcus* spp. 25%). *Bacteroides fragilis* was resistant to all antibiotics tested.[45] Susceptibility to clindamycin was not tested in this study, but resistance to metronidazole and doxycycline was high.

Although amoxicillin may still be advocated as a suitable first-line agent in periodontal therapy in humans, reduced susceptibility of *Prevotella* strains remains a matter of concern with penicillins.[47] Recent studies conclude that amoxicillin-clavulanic acid, clindamycin, doxycycline and metronidazole are useful alternatives in combating the anaerobic bacteria involved in dentoalveolar infection and aggressive periodontitis in humans.[47,48]

Locally delivered antibiotics

Subgingival treatment of periodontal pockets with controlled-release tetra- or minocycline is an option for dogs and cats with periodontitis, and in several studies has resulted in substantial improvement of periodontal health in dogs.[49–51] Some studies have failed to show statistically significant clinical or microbiological results between use of subgingival doxycycline in addition to scaling and root planing (SRP) and SRP alone.[52–54] One study reported a 3-month positive effect on clinical parameters with the adjunctive use of locally delivered doxycycline, but repeated applications annually had no clinical or microbiological effect.[52] Subgingivally delivered, sustained-release doxycycline polymer is registered and marketed for veterinary patients (Doxirobe™, Pfizer Animal Health) for treatment of periodontal pockets with probing depths 4 mm or deeper after periodontal debridement.[41]

Even at subantimicrobial doses, doxycycline down-regulates the activity of matrix metalloproteinases (MMPs), key destructive enzymes in periodontal disease.[55] Therefore, subantimicrobial dose doxycycline (SDD), usually 20 mg BID for 9 months, is sometimes used in the treatment of chronic adult periodontitis. Several studies report that SDD as an adjunct to scaling and root planing (SRP) resulted in significantly greater clinical benefits than SRP alone, and appears to be safe and effective in the long-term management of chronic periodontitis.[55–58] In addition, several studies report no evidence of microbiologically significant changes, or development of antibiotic resistance in patients treated with SDD.[55,56,59] However, one author states that the clinical relevance of improvements obtained with SDD beyond those obtained with conventional therapy alone is debatable.[60] SDD might be an option to manage some dogs with chronic periodontitis when professional periodontal treatment and dental home care are not effective enough to control the disease.

Side effects of antimicrobial treatment

Risks associated with antibiotics include hypersensitivity reactions (such as anaphylaxis), development of antibiotic-resistant bacteria, superinfections, antibiotic-associated colitis and/or diarrhea, pseudomembranous colitis (PMC), cross-reactions with other drugs, and death. The costs involved with the use of antibiotics can be significant as well.[3,13]

Allergic reactions to antibiotics are reported less frequently in veterinary medicine than in human patients.[61–63] Acute anaphylaxis is characterized by one or more of the following signs: hypotension, bronchospasm, angioedema, urticaria, erythema, pruritus, pharyngeal and/or laryngeal edema, vomiting and colic. Penicillins, cephalosporins and sulfonamides most frequently cause hypersensitivity reactions in animals.[61] In humans, the most common antibiotic capable of inducing diarrhea, colitis, or PMC is amoxicillin, followed by cephalosporins and clindamycin.[64] Reported allergies alter antibiotic therapy in 30% of human patients.[65]

Bacterial resistance to antimicrobials

The occurrence of bacterial resistance corresponds to an increase in an antibiotic's minimum inhibitory concentration (MIC, the lowest concentration of the antibiotic capable of inhibiting bacterial growth) for a particular bacterial strain.[66] Bacterial resistance to antimicrobials has been an ongoing challenge for clinicians ever since the discovery of antimicrobial agents. Bacteria have succeeded in developing resistance to all antibacterial agents shortly after they have been marketed.[66,67] Bacteria have developed several mechanisms to neutralize the action of antimicrobial drugs; these include enzymatic drug inactivation, modification or replacement of the drug target, active drug efflux, and reduced drug uptake.[1] Improper use of antibiotics, in terms of either dosage (duration of treatment too long or dose too weak) or indication, are major factors in the emergence of antibiotic

resistance.[66,68] Growing concerns regarding antibiotic resistance caused by overprescribing should be balanced with the potential benefits of prophylactic antibiotic administration.

Bacteria in dental plaque are in a biofilm.[41] Concentrations of antibiotics necessary to inhibit subgingival plaque bacteria in steady-state biofilms have been reported to be 250–1000 times greater than the concentrations needed to inhibit the same strains grown planktonically.[69,70] Bacteria also become progressively more resistant as the biofilm matures.[69] Several mechanisms confer greater bacterial resistance in a biofilm: low bacterial metabolic activity within the biofilm limits the assimilation of antibiotics; extracellular matrix of the biofilm limits the diffusion of antimicrobial agents; in addition, extracellular bacterial enzymes involved in deactivating antibiotics are trapped and concentrated in the biofilm.[66] As a result, antibiotic sensitivity tests may be of limited use, given that the behavior of bacteria inside the biofilm is completely different from that observed for the same bacteria in planktonic form.[66] Removal of plaque by mechanical debridement (scaling and polishing) is therefore essential prior to considering antimicrobial therapy in the treatment of periodontal disease.[43]

Antimicrobial resistance in animals also poses a risk to humans. Horses, dogs, cats and exotic animal pets can be reservoirs of resistant bacteria. Companion animals may transfer *S. typhimurium, C. jejuni*, meticillin-resistant *Staphylococcus aureus* (MRSA) or *Staphylococcus intermedius* to people.[71] There is now increasing evidence that MRSA can be transmitted in both directions, from human to animal and from animal to human. Once exposed to MRSA, animals can become colonized, and may serve as reservoirs to transmit the infection to other animals and humans.[72–76] A recent study in a university veterinary hospital reported that certain MRSA genotypes are capable of infecting a wide spectrum of small and exotic animals.[77] MRSA isolates from dogs and cats are indistinguishable from human healthcare isolates.[76]

The emergence and dissemination of multidrug-resistant bacteria is a serious problem in veterinary medicine. Veterinarians should carefully evaluate when antibiotics are indicated in veterinary dentistry and oral surgery.

ORAL ANTISEPTICS

Antiseptics are substances that prevent or arrest the growth or action of microorganisms on living tissue, either by inhibiting their activity or by destroying them.[78]

Chlorhexidine

Chlorhexidine is a cationic bisguanide, available as a solution and a scrubbing agent.[78] Chlorhexidine exhibits a broad spectrum of antibacterial activity; it is highly effective against Gram-positive organisms, less so against Gram-negative ones.[78,79] Oral chlorhexidine gel has been shown to inhibit the formation of plaque and reduce the severity of gingivitis in dogs.[80] The cationic nature of chlorhexidine allows it to bind to negatively charged surfaces in the mouth, such as tooth and mucosa.[78–80] It is then released over time and provides a continuing bacteriostatic effect.[79] Chlorhexidine does not absorb through the oral tissues.[80]

Chlorhexidine is commercially available as a 0.12% oral rinse or gel for animals. Before dental treatment and oral surgical procedures, the mouth should be irrigated with an antiseptic solution, such as chlorhexidine.[38,81] Rinsing the mouth preoperatively with chlorhexidine produced significant reductions in bacterial aerosols during ultrasonic scaling in humans[82] and the number of bacteria entering into the bloodstream in dogs.[83] In the previously mentioned study concluding that postoperative antibiotics do not prevent inflammatory problems after third molar surgery, the mouths of all patients were rinsed with 0.2% chlorhexidine before their extractions, which may have decreased the oral bacterial flora, and possibly prevented infection and dry socket.[27]

In veterinary dentistry, chlorhexidine oral rinse may be used before dental and oral surgical procedures, and postoperatively in some patients with severe oral inflammation or after extractions or other oral surgery. Chlorhexidine may also be used to reduce plaque accumulation on tooth surfaces, since many owners may not be willing or able to brush their pet's teeth. Oral rinses containing chlorhexidine may also be beneficial in the management of chronic feline gingivostomatitis.[84]

Side effects of chlorhexidine in humans include reversible staining of teeth, increased calculus formation, and alteration in taste perception. The incidence of side effects is significantly reduced with 0.12% chlorhexidine compared to 0.2%.[79]

Zinc ascorbate

Zinc ascorbate is available as an oral gel for animals. Cats seem to tolerate the taste of it better than chlorhexidine. One study reported that it decreases bacterial growth, plaque formation, and gingivitis in cats when applied following a professional teeth cleaning procedure.[85]

Povidone-iodine

Elemental iodine and its derivatives (polyvinylpyrrolidone-iodine complex, PVP-iodine) are among the most broad-spectrum and potent antiseptics available. Povidone-iodine is used as an oral antiseptic in humans. In the treatment of periodontal disease, subgingival 10% povidone-iodine application in addition to mechanical debridement reduces pocket depth and total counts of periodontal pathogens and helps to control periodontal disease in man. Povidone-iodine has a broad spectrum of antimicrobial action, and is less likely to induce development of resistant bacteria and adverse host reactions compared to antibiotics.[86,87]

REFERENCES

1. Guardabassi L, Kruse H. Principles of prudent and rational use of antimicrobials in animals. In: Guardabassi L, Jensen L, Kruse H, editors. Guide to antimicrobial use in animals. Oxford, UK: Blackwell Publishing Ltd.; 2008. p. 1–12.
2. Wilcke JR. Use of antimicrobial drugs to prevent infections in veterinary patients. Probl Vet Med 1990;2:298–311.
3. Pallasch TJ. Antibiotic prophylaxis. In: Yagiela JA, Dowd FJ, Neidle E, editors. Pharmacology and therapeutics for dentistry. 5th ed. St. Louis, MO: Elsevier Mosby; 2004. p. 782–95.
4. Beilin B, Shavit Y, Hart J, et al. Effects of anesthesia based on large versus small doses of fentanyl on natural killer cell cytotoxicity in the perioperative period. Anesth Analg 1996;82:492–7.
5. Kitamura T, Ohno N, Bougaki M, et al. [Comparison of the effects of sevoflurane and propofol on changes in leukocyte-count induced by surgical stress]. Masui 2008;57:968–72.
6. Felsburg PJ, Keyes LL, Krawiec DR, et al. The effect of general anesthesia on canine lymphocyte function. Vet Immunol Immunopathol 1986;13:63–70.
7. Anonymous. American Veterinary Dental College Position Statement on the Use of Antibiotics in Veterinary Dentistry. http://avdcorg/position-statementshtml#AB. Accessed 9-30-2009.
8. Lam DK, Jan A, Sandor GK, et al. Prevention of infective endocarditis: revised guidelines from the American Heart Association and the implications for dentists. J Can Dent Assoc 2008;74:449–53.
9. Sakamoto H, Karakida K, Otsuru M, et al. Antibiotic prevention of infective endocarditis due to oral procedures: myth, magic, or science? J Infect Chemother 2007;13:189–95.
10. Oliver R, Roberts GJ, Hooper L, et al. Antibiotics for the prophylaxis of bacterial endocarditis in dentistry. Cochrane Database Syst Rev 2008;CD003813.
11. Maestre Vera JR, Gomez-Lus Centelles ML. Antimicrobial prophylaxis in oral surgery and dental procedures. Med Oral Patol Oral Cir Bucal 2007;12:E44–E52.
12. Tomas I, Pereira F, Llucian R, et al. Prevalence of bacteraemia following third molar surgery. Oral Dis 2008;14: 89–94.
13. Little JW, Falace DA, Miller CS, et al. Antibiotic prophylaxis in dentistry: an update. Gen Dent 2008;56:20–8.
14. Sykes JE, Kittleson MD, Pesavento PA, et al. Evaluation of the relationship between causative organisms and clinical characteristics of infective endocarditis in dogs: 71 cases (1992–2005). J Am Vet Med Assoc 2006;228:1723–34.
15. DeBowes LJ, Mosier D, Logan E, et al. Association of periodontal disease and histologic lesions in multiple organs from 45 dogs. J Vet Dent 1996;13:57–60.
16. Pavlica Z, Petelin M, Juntes P, et al. Periodontal disease burden and pathological changes in organs of dogs. J Vet Dent 2008;25:97–105.
17. Harari J, Besser TE, Gustafson SB, et al. Bacterial isolates from blood cultures of dogs undergoing dentistry. Vet Surg 1993;22:27–30.
18. Peddle GD, Drobatz KJ, Harvey CE, et al. Association of periodontal disease, oral procedures, and other clinical findings with bacterial endocarditis in dogs. J Am Vet Med Assoc 2009;234:100–7.
19. Glickman LT, Glickman NW, Moore GE, et al. Evaluation of the risk of endocarditis and other cardiovascular events on the basis of the severity of periodontal disease in dogs. J Am Vet Med Assoc 2009;234:486–94.
20. Wilson W, Taubert KA, Gewitz M, et al. Prevention of infective endocarditis: guidelines from the American Heart Association: a guideline from the American Heart Association Rheumatic Fever, Endocarditis and Kawasaki Disease Committee, Council on Cardiovascular Disease in the Young, and the Council on Clinical Cardiology, Council on Cardiovascular Surgery and Anesthesia, and the Quality of Care and Outcomes Research Interdisciplinary Working Group. J Am Dent Assoc 2008;139(Suppl): 3S–24S.
21. Anonymous. American Academy of Orthopedic Surgeons Information statement: antibiotic prophylaxis for bacteremia in patients with joint replacements. http://wwwaaosorg/about/papers/advistmt/1033asp. Accessed 11-30-2009.
22. Anonymous. NZDA code of practice: Antibiotic prophylaxis for dental treatment of patients with prosthetic joint replacements (adopted March 2003). N Z Dent J 2003;99:63–4.
23. Salmeron-Escobar JI, del Amo-Fernandez de Velasco A. Antibiotic prophylaxis in oral and maxillofacial surgery. Med Oral Patol Oral Cir Bucal 2006;11:E292–E296.
24. Moore PA, Nahouraii HS, Zovko JG, et al. Dental therapeutic practice patterns in the U.S. II. Analgesics, corticosteroids, and antibiotics. Gen Dent 2006;54:201–7.
25. Halpern LR, Dodson TB. Does prophylactic administration of systemic antibiotics prevent postoperative inflammatory complications after third molar surgery? J Oral Maxillofac Surg 2007;65:177–85.
26. Lacasa JM, Jimenez JA, Ferras V, et al. Prophylaxis versus pre-emptive treatment for infective and inflammatory complications of surgical third molar

removal: a randomized, double-blind, placebo-controlled, clinical trial with sustained release amoxicillin/clavulanic acid (1000/62.5 mg). Int J Oral Maxillofac Surg 2007;36:321–7.

27. Poeschl PW, Eckel D, Poeschl E. Postoperative prophylactic antibiotic treatment in third molar surgery–a necessity? J Oral Maxillofac Surg 2004;62:3–8.

28. Ren YF, Malmstrom HS. Effectiveness of antibiotic prophylaxis in third molar surgery: a meta-analysis of randomized controlled clinical trials. J Oral Maxillofac Surg 2007;65:1909–21.

29. Kaczmarzyk T, Wichlinski J, Stypulkowska J, et al. Single-dose and multi-dose clindamycin therapy fails to demonstrate efficacy in preventing infectious and inflammatory complications in third molar surgery. Int J Oral Maxillofac Surg 2007;36:417–22.

30. Davidson JR, Bauer MS. Fractures of the mandible and maxilla. Vet Clin North Am Small Anim Pract 1992;22:109–19.

31. Johnson JT, Yu VL. Antibiotic use during major head and neck surgery. Ann Surg 1988;207:108–11.

32. Andreasen JO, Jensen SS, Schwartz O, et al. A systematic review of prophylactic antibiotics in the surgical treatment of maxillofacial fractures. J Oral Maxillofac Surg 2006;64:1664–8.

33. Miles BA, Potter JK, Ellis E, III. The efficacy of postoperative antibiotic regimens in the open treatment of mandibular fractures: a prospective randomized trial. J Oral Maxillofac Surg 2006;64:576–82.

34. Furr AM, Schweinfurth JM, May WL. Factors associated with long-term complications after repair of mandibular fractures. Laryngoscope 2006;116: 427–30.

35. Prasad KC, Prasad SC, Mouli N, et al. Osteomyelitis in the head and neck. Acta Otolaryngol 2007;127:194–205.

36. Lovato C, Wagner JD. Infection rates following perioperative prophylactic antibiotics versus postoperative extended regimen prophylactic antibiotics in surgical management of mandibular fractures. J Oral Maxillofac Surg 2009;67:827–32.

37. Abubaker AO, Rollert MK. Postoperative antibiotic prophylaxis in mandibular fractures: A preliminary randomized, double-blind, and placebo-controlled clinical study. J Oral Maxillofac Surg 2001;59:1415–19.

38. Verstraete FJ. Mandibulectomy and maxillectomy. Vet Clin North Am Small Anim Pract 2005;35:1009–39.

39. Righi M, Manfredi R, Farneti G, et al. Clindamycin/cefonicid in head and neck oncologic surgery: one-day prophylaxis is as effective as a three-day schedule. J Chemother 1995;7:216–20.

40. Lin S, Zuckerman O, Fuss Z, et al. New emphasis in the treatment of dental trauma: avulsion and luxation. Dent Traumatol 2007;23:297–303.

41. Harvey CE. Management of periodontal disease: understanding the options. Vet Clin North Am Small Anim Pract 2005; 35:819–36, vi.

42. Pack PD, Haber J. The incidence of clinical infection after periodontal surgery. A retrospective study. J Periodontol 1983; 54:441–3.

43. Herrera D, Alonso B, Leon R, et al. Antimicrobial therapy in periodontitis: the use of systemic antimicrobials against the subgingival biofilm. J Clin Periodontol 2008;35:45–66.

44. Harvey CE, Thornsberry C, Miller BR, et al. Antimicrobial susceptibility of subgingival bacterial flora in dogs with gingivitis. J Vet Dent 1995;12:151–5.

45. Radice M, Martino PA, Reiter AM. Evaluation of subgingival bacteria in the dog and susceptibility to commonly used antibiotics. J Vet Dent 2006;23:219–24.

46. Harvey CE, Thornsberry C, Miller BR, et al. Antimicrobial susceptibility of subgingival bacterial flora in cats with gingivitis. J Vet Dent 1995;12:157–60.

47. Kuriyama T, Williams DW, Yanagisawa M, et al. Antimicrobial susceptibility of 800 anaerobic isolates from patients with dentoalveolar infection to 13 oral antibiotics. Oral Microbiol Immunol 2007;22:285–8.

48. Lakhssassi N, Elhajoui N, Lodter JP, et al. Antimicrobial susceptibility variation of 50 anaerobic periopathogens in aggressive periodontitis: an interindividual variability study. Oral Microbiol Immunol 2005;20:244–52.

49. Hellstrom MK, McClain PK, Schallhorn RG, et al. Local minocycline as an adjunct to surgical therapy in moderate to severe, chronic periodontitis. J Clin Periodontol 2008;35:525–31.

50. Hayashi K, Takada K, Hirasawa M. Clinical and microbiological effects of controlled-release local delivery of minocycline on periodontitis in dogs. Am J Vet Res 1998; 59:464–7.

51. Polson AM, Southard GL, Dunn RL, et al. Periodontal pocket treatment in beagle dogs using subgingival doxycycline from a biodegradable system. I. Initial clinical responses. J Periodontol 1996;67:1176–84.

52. Bogren A, Teles RP, Torresyap G, et al. Locally delivered doxycycline during supportive periodontal therapy: a 3-year study. J Periodontol 2008;79:827–35.

53. Eickholz P, Kim TS, Schacher B, et al. Subgingival topical doxycycline versus mechanical debridement for supportive periodontal therapy: a single blind randomized controlled two-center study. Am J Dent 2005;18:341–6.

54. Jorgensen MG, Safarian A, Daneshmand N, et al. Initial antimicrobial effect of controlled-release doxycycline in subgingival sites. J Periodontal Res 2004;39:315–19.

55. Preshaw PM, Hefti AF, Jepsen S, et al. Subantimicrobial dose doxycycline as adjunctive treatment for periodontitis. A review. J Clin Periodontol 2004;31:697–707.

56. Preshaw PM, Novak MJ, Mellonig J, et al. Modified-release subantimicrobial dose doxycycline enhances scaling and root planing in subjects with periodontal disease. J Periodontol 2008;79:440–52.

57. Lee JY, Lee YM, Shin SY, et al. Effect of subantimicrobial dose doxycycline as an effective adjunct to scaling and root planing. J Periodontol 2004;75: 1500–8.

58. Caton JG, Ciancio SG, Blieden TM, et al. Treatment with subantimicrobial dose doxycycline improves the efficacy of scaling and root planing in patients with adult periodontitis. J Periodontol 2000; 71:521–32.

59. Thomas J, Walker C, Bradshaw M. Long-term use of subantimicrobial dose doxycycline does not lead to changes in antimicrobial susceptibility. J Periodontol 2000;71:1472–83.

60. Greenstein G. Efficacy of subantimicrobial-dose doxycycline in the treatment of periodontal diseases: a critical evaluation. Int J Periodontics Restorative Dent 2004;24:528–43.

61. Maddison JE, Watson AD. Antibacterial drugs. In: Maddison JE, Page SW, Church D, editors. Small animal clinical pharmacology. London: W.B. Saunders; 2002. p. 115–48.

62. Chiou CS, Lin SM, Lin SP, et al. Clindamycin-induced anaphylactic shock during general anesthesia. J Chin Med Assoc 2006;69:549–51.

63. Meropol SB, Chan KA, Chen Z, et al. Adverse events associated with prolonged antibiotic use. Pharmacoepidemiol Drug Saf 2008;17:523–32.

64. Pallasch TJ. Principles of antibiotic therapy. In: Yagiela JA, Dowd FJ, Neidle E, editors. Pharmacology and therapeutics for dentistry. 5th ed. St. Louis, MO: Mosby; 2004. p. 613

65. Lutomski DM, Lafollette JA, Biaglow MA, et al. Antibiotic allergies in the medical record: effect on drug selection and assessment of validity. Pharmacotherapy 2008;28:1348–53.

66. Bidault P, Chandad F, Grenier D. Risk of bacterial resistance associated with systemic antibiotic therapy in periodontology. J Can Dent Assoc 2007;73:721–5.

67. Weber JT, Courvalin P. An emptying quiver: antimicrobial drugs and resistance. Emerg Infect Dis 2005;11:791–3.

68. Al-Haroni M, Skaug N. Incidence of antibiotic prescribing in dental practice in Norway and its contribution to national consumption. J Antimicrob Chemother 2007;59:1161–6.

69. Sedlacek MJ, Walker C. Antibiotic resistance in an in vitro subgingival

biofilm model. Oral Microbiol Immunol 2007;22:333–9.

70. Donlan RM. Role of biofilms in antimicrobial resistance. ASAIO J 2000;46:S47-52.

71. Jensen LB, Angulo FJ, Molbak K. Human health risks associated with antimicrobial use in animals. In: Guardabassi L, Jensen L, Kruse H, editors. Guide to antimicrobial use in animals. Oxford, UK: Blackwell Publishing Ltd.; 2008. p. 13–26.

72. Baptiste KE, Williams K, Willams NJ, et al. Methicillin-resistant staphylococci in companion animals. Emerg Infect Dis 2005;11:1942–4.

73. Hanselman BA, Kruth SA, Rousseau J, et al. Methicillin-resistant *Staphylococcus aureus* colonization in veterinary personnel. Emerg Infect Dis 2006;12:1933–8.

74. Manian FA. Asymptomatic nasal carriage of mupirocin-resistant, methicillin-resistant *Staphylococcus aureus* (MRSA) in a pet dog associated with MRSA infection in household contacts. Clin Infect Dis 2003; 36:e26–e28.

75. Weese JS. Methicillin-resistant *Staphylococcus aureus*: an emerging pathogen in small animals. J Am Anim Hosp Assoc 2005;41:150–7.

76. Leonard FC, Markey BK. Meticillin-resistant *Staphylococcus aureus* in animals: a review. Vet J 2008;175:27–36.

77. Walther B, Wieler LH, Friedrich AW, et al. Methicillin-resistant *Staphylococcus aureus* (MRSA) isolated from small and exotic animals at a university hospital during routine microbiological examinations. Vet Microbiol 2008; 127:171–8.

78. Boothe HW. Antiseptics and disinfectants. Vet Clin North Am Small Anim Pract 1998;28:233–48.

79. Gleason MJ, Molinari JA. Antiseptics and disinfectants. In: Yagiela JA, Dowd FJ, Neidle E, editors. Pharmacology and therapeutics for dentistry. 5th ed. St. Louis, MO: Elsevier Mosby; 2004. p. 756–61.

80. Davies RM, Hull PS. Plaque inhibition and distribution of chlorhexidine in beagle dogs. J Periodontal Res Suppl 1973;12:22–7.

81. Seymour RA, Hogg SD. Antibiotics and chemoprophylaxis. Periodontol 2000 2008;46:80–108.

82. Klyn SL, Cummings DE, Richardson BW, et al. Reduction of bacteria-containing spray produced during ultrasonic scaling. Gen Dent 2001;49:648–52.

83. Bowersock TL, Wu CC, Inskeep GA, et al. Prevention of bacteremia in dogs undergoing dental scaling by prior administration of oral clindamycin or chlorhexidine oral rinse. J Vet Dent 2000;17:11–16.

84. Lyon KF. Gingivostomatitis. Vet Clin North Am Small Anim Pract 2005;35:891–911, vii.

85. Clarke DE. Clinical and microbiological effects of oral zinc ascorbate gel in cats. J Vet Dent 2001;18:177–83.

86. Hoang T, Jorgensen MG, Keim RG, et al. Povidone–iodine as a periodontal pocket disinfectant. J Periodont Res 2003;38: 311–17.

87. Sahrmann P, Puhan MA, Attin T, et al. Systematic review on the effect of rinsing with povidone-iodine during nonsurgical periodontal therapy. J Periodontal Res. 2010;45:153–64.

Chapter | 4 |

Anesthesia and pain management

Peter J. Pascoe

DEFINITIONS

Pain has been defined by the International Association for the Study of Pain as 'an unpleasant sensory and emotional experience associated with actual or potential tissue damage or described in terms of such damage.' One of the notes appended to this states, 'The inability to communicate in no way negates the possibility that an individual is experiencing pain and is in need of appropriate pain relieving treatment.' For veterinarians this is an important qualification since our patients cannot 'describe' their pain. A specific definition of animal pain has been given as 'an aversive sensory emotional experience representing an awareness by the animal of damage or threat to the integrity of its tissues (note, there may not be any damage): it changes the animal's physiology and behavior to reduce or avoid the damage, to reduce the likelihood of recurrence and to promote recovery; non-functional pain occurs when the intensity or duration of the experience is not appropriate for the damage sustained (especially if none exists) and when physiological and behavioral responses are unsuccessful in alleviating it.'[1] This definition addresses both the survival function of pain and chronic pain where the animal has exhausted its ability to deal with the problem and is condemned to suffer. As veterinarians we are dedicated to the comfort of our patients and so the provision of analgesia is a primary goal in the management of any animal.[2,3]

Hyperalgesia is present when there is an exaggerated response to a stimulus that would normally be noxious. This can either be *primary*, where it is related to changes in sensitivity of the peripheral neurons, or *secondary*, where it is due to changes in central processing of the neuronal input. When a noxious stimulus is applied to tissue, there is a release of various mediators such as histamine, bradykinin, prostaglandins and various cytokines that reduce the threshold for further stimulation of the nociceptors in the injured area (primary hyperalgesia). Secondary hyperalgesia occurs because the nociceptive input into the spinal cord interacts with adjacent neurons and sensitizes them to further stimuli. This is manifested clinically as a change in nociceptive threshold outside the area of injury.[4] *Allodynia* is defined as 'pain due to a stimulus which does not normally provoke pain' and this would apply to the pain associated with hot or cold liquids on

exposed dentin as opposed to the lack of pain to such a stimulus on normal enamel.

PRINCIPLES OF PAIN MANAGEMENT

Assessment of pain

Since pain can only be felt by the individual who has been injured, and our patients cannot communicate verbally, our assessment of pain depends on observation of the behavior of the animal and our clinical acumen. It must be assumed that animals that are brought into a strange environment (a veterinary hospital) are anxious and stressed and therefore less likely to tolerate pain. The second part of being able to assess pain is to know the behavior of the animal. In general terms, cats and dogs tend to respond in different ways: a cat in pain is more likely to crawl to the back of the cage and curl up into a ball whereas a dog is much more likely to vocalize and draw attention to its discomfort. There are breed differences as well as differences related to each individual patient. Animals may show gross signs of being in pain (howling, guarding some particular site, restlessness) or the signs may be more subtle (e.g., adoption of a particular posture, retreating to the back of the cage, a change in temperament – usually becoming more aggressive, failure to interact normally with the caregiver).[5,6] These signs must be assessed in light of the analgesics the animal has already received and the level of consciousness of the patient. There have been no studies in dogs and cats looking at behavior following dental extractions.

Efforts to develop a satisfactory scale for the objective assessment of pain in animals are ongoing. The Glasgow University Composite Measure Pain Score[7] may be useful for postoperative pain assessment, but was found to be less accurate than a visual analog scale for assessing pain in dogs undergoing radiation therapy[8] due to the initial influence of anxiety in these patients early in the course of treatment.

Regardless of the scale employed, it is best for all hospital employees to use a standardized method for assessing pain, since it is likely that individuals using a particular approach will develop their skills and will be motivated to assess pain routinely.[4,9–11] Such an approach has been embodied in veterinary medicine by the adoption of pain

DOI: 10.1016/B978-0-7020-4618-6.00004-X

management standards by the American Animal Hospital Association in 2007.[12]

Management of pain

Pain is the result of a complex series of interactions in the nervous system. Since there are systems that facilitate and inhibit the passage of nociception to the cerebral cortex, it is possible for a noxious stimulus to be perceived with equanimity or as the most horrible experience. This complexity allows us to intervene to reduce the input, reduce the result of that input, minimize facilitation within the central nervous system (CNS) or to block perception.[13]

Reducing the input

Continuous stimulation of C-fiber input tends to produce central sensitization or facilitation to further stimulation, which is largely responsible for secondary hyperalgesia. The simplest way to block the input is to use a local anesthetic such that none of the stimulated neurons deliver their impulses to the CNS. Drugs blocking prostaglandin production (nonsteroidal antiinflammatory drugs – NSAIDs), stimulating opioid receptors and blocking alpha-1 adrenergic receptors can also affect the input.

Reducing the result of the input

The powerful descending inhibitory systems use opioid, alpha-2 receptors and serotonin as well as other neurotransmitters and these decrease what reaches the cerebral cortex. Part of the secondary hyperalgesia is mediated by N-methyl D-aspartate (NMDA) glutamate receptors in the spinal cord. Ketamine is an NMDA antagonist and so may prevent this facilitation.

Minimizing facilitation

The central processing of nociception can be enhanced by pathways descending from the brain to the spinal cord. These are triggered by anxiety, stress and sleeplessness and thus any actions to minimize these for the patient may decrease their experience of pain. This could be very simple things such as handling the animal gently or could involve the use of drugs to minimize the anxiety and stress (e.g., phenothiazines, benzodiazepines).

Blocking perception

Any anesthetic will make it impossible to feel pain since any feeling requires consciousness. It should be noted that many anesthetics do not alter the input into the CNS from a surgical site and therefore, while the animal may not perceive the pain at the time, facilitation may occur, making the animal more susceptible to pain postoperatively.

The complexity of the system also allows us to try to attack it at several different points at the same time. This is the principle of *balanced analgesia* – using several different drugs to block the perception of pain at various points throughout the system. For example, a balanced analgesia approach might include premedication with a phenothiazine and an opioid, induction with a dissociative drug (NMDA antagonist), administration of a local anesthetic prior to the first incision to block input to the CNS, and postoperative administration of an opioid and an NSAID.

PREOPERATIVE CONCERNS

The success of an anesthetic depends on adequate preparation. Dental disease may be a manifestation of systemic disease and may be the cause of some systemic changes.[14] In addition, many patients presented for oral surgical procedures are geriatric, owing to the association between age and the progression of dental disease[15] and the fact that maxillofacial neoplasia is common in older pets. These factors therefore make it imperative to examine the patient carefully and to carry out any ancillary tests to confirm the diagnosis before undertaking the procedure. It is also important to ensure that, if the procedure is elective, the animal should be in the best health possible. For example, if hypothyroidism is diagnosed based on preoperative blood test results, the procedure should be postponed and the patient should be treated with thyroid hormone for sufficient time to counter this metabolic derangement. Hypothyroid animals do not handle stress well, and the outcome can be fatal if they are anesthetized and stressed by a surgical procedure. Old age is not by itself a contraindication to anesthesia but many older patients have concomitant disease, are on other medications and have poor reserves to combat the effects of the anesthetic drugs, hypothermia and the stress of the procedure.[16,17] The clinician should be cognizant of the possible interactions between the medications being received and the planned anesthetic drugs. These include direct pharmacological interactions such as the effect of aminoglycosides or organophosphates on the activity of neuromuscular blocking drugs, pharmacokinetic interactions, such as the effects of two highly protein-bound drugs competing for the same binding sites, or pharmacodynamic alterations where one drug increases or decreases the effect of another drug.[18] In today's practice it is also important to ask the client if the animal is on any herbal therapies or nutritional supplements. Garlic and gingko biloba have been associated with bleeding problems in people and there may be interactions between these herbal supplements and other drugs, such as NSAIDs, that can affect coagulation.[19] Some of the herbal preparations that have central nervous system effects (e.g., St. John's wort, valerian) may alter the duration of action of anesthetics. In human medicine it is common for patients not to disclose their use of herbal supplements; it is likely that pet owners do not disclose such use for fear of disapproval by the veterinarian, or because they do not think a 'natural remedy' could have any significant impact on the anesthetic.[19] The clinician must therefore ask specific questions and explain why it is important to know of all the substances the animal is receiving. The American Society of Anesthesiologists suggests a two-week withdrawal period for herbal supplements prior to anesthesia in humans.[20]

Before deciding on a course of action with regard to analgesia, it is necessary to consider what the expected level of pain is likely to be for the planned procedure. A young dog that requires dental scaling and polishing is unlikely to need postoperative analgesics. However, if extractions or other oral surgical procedures are planned, administration of analgesics is indicated.

Since one of the approaches to treating pain is to reduce the nociceptive input, techniques which reduce this input before it occurs are often employed. This idea has been termed preemptive analgesia. From a biological perspective it makes sense, and the idea has been proven many times in a laboratory setting.[21,22] When it comes to clinical proof, the evidence is less convincing, and a recent meta-analysis of the data available in people concluded that a preemptive approach has minimal benefit for most treatments used.[23] Drugs commonly used for premedication may provide some preemptive benefit. Phenothiazine tranquillizers, such as acepromazine, reduce the patient's anxiety and, while acepromazine is not an analgesic in its own right, this reduced anxiety may decrease the descending facilitation of pain that can occur when the patient is stressed by the hospital environment. Opioids are analgesics that can reduce the nociceptive input by their effects at both primary and secondary nociceptive neurons.[24] The presence of opioid receptors in peripheral tissues, particularly inflamed tissue, means that opioids may also act to reduce nociceptive input at the tissue level. The cyclohexanones (e.g., ketamine) affect both the descending inhibition of pain as well as having a direct effect at the N-methyl D-aspartate receptor (NMDA) to prevent wind-up or facilitation. Alpha-2 agonists have analgesic effects in the brain, the spinal cord and, to some extent, in the periphery (by reducing the release of norepinephrine), and these drugs may also be used preemptively. Nonsteroidal antiinflammatory drugs are used to reduce the release of prostaglandins in peripheral tissues, thus reducing peripheral sensitization of nociceptors, but there is increasing evidence that they also have activity in the CNS as analgesics. In the past, there have been major concerns about the use of NSAIDs in the perioperative period because of concerns about gastric ulceration, renal insufficiency and platelet dysfunction, but the advent of newer drugs with greater specificity for cyclooxygenase-2 (COX-2) has revolutionized the potential for their use in this context (see below). Finally, local anesthetic techniques applied before the incision will tend to reduce the overall nociceptive input into the CNS and therefore reduce facilitation. *Whether a preemptive approach is chosen or not, the clinician should provide treatment of pain on an ongoing basis after the procedure.*

INDUCTION AND MAINTENANCE OF ANESTHESIA

General anesthetics

The induction technique used should be appropriate for the individual patient. Many practitioners use a single technique (e.g., diazepam/ketamine) and become very proficient with this method. However, despite the safety of some such methods in most patients, there are some where a particular technique may be inappropriate or contraindicated (e.g., the use of ketamine as part of an induction technique was associated with a high mortality rate in cats with hyperthyroidism).[25] If an appropriate technique is not available, or the clinician is unfamiliar with alternative induction agents, consideration should be given to referring the patient to a clinic with the required expertise.

Venous access and intubation

In most cases, venous access with a catheter should be established prior to induction in order to provide fluids and pharmacological support if needed (e.g., antibiotics, positive inotropes or vasopressors). Patients that are very difficult to handle prior to induction and cannot be catheterized should have a catheter placed as soon as possible after they are anesthetized. The animal should be intubated with a cuffed endotracheal tube and the cuff carefully inflated. Reports of tracheal rupture in cats have been largely associated with dental procedures.[26,27] There has been no specific explanation for this association but the size of the cuff in relation to the tube may play a role (many of the ruptures in one study were associated with low-pressure/high-volume endotracheal tubes) and the method of inflation may also be a factor. The preferred technique is to connect the tube to the breathing circuit and fill the rebreathing bag with oxygen. A breath is then given manually (to a maximum pressure of 25 cm H_2O) and the anesthetist should listen at the mouth for escaping gas. If there is some gas escaping, a small amount of air is added to the cuff and the procedure repeated until no gas escapes. Once this has been achieved, the vaporizer can be turned on (It is better to turn the vaporizer on after the cuff is sealed to prevent the escape of inhalant into the room.).

In carrying out dental procedures, there is often water and debris in the mouth which could enter the airway. While an endotracheal tube cuff may prevent gross debris from getting beyond it, it will not prevent all liquid from running down into the distal airway.[28] Hence

it is important to position the patient in such a way that fluid does not run into the larynx, to use pharyngeal packing to soak up any liquid, or to use suction in such a way that fluid does not reach this area (see Ch. 6).

If it is known or suspected that fluid has gone down between the endotracheal tube and the larynx then extubation at the end of the procedure should be performed without deflating the cuff. This should squeeze most of the fluid out of the airway and minimize the risk of aspiration.

If it is necessary to check the patient's occlusion during a procedure and the presence of the endotracheal tube in the mouth will impair this assessment, there are three options:

1. Removal of the tube each time the occlusion needs to be assessed. This is the least desirable because it leaves the airway unprotected during this time, increases the risk of introducing debris into the trachea and increases the risk of laryngeal trauma if the tube has to be removed and replaced several times.

2. Creation of a pharyngotomy incision and replacement of the endotracheal tube into the larynx via this pharyngeal incision. It is best to carry out this procedure with a wire-reinforced endotracheal tube, which will not kink when curved or bent, in order to minimize the possibility of airway occlusion (see Ch. 57).

3. Placement of a short endotracheal tube with an adapter that fits on the end to lengthen the tube. The endotracheal tube is then positioned such that the proximal end of the tube is in the caudal part of the mouth. The adapter is attached such that the end of this part is just rostral to the incisors. When it is necessary to check the occlusion the adapter is removed and the mouth can be closed with the short endotracheal tube remaining in the back of the mouth (Fig. 4.1). The animal should be watched carefully when this technique is used because it is possible for the airway to be occluded by the tongue pushing into the end of the tube when the adapter is removed. The adapter can also become disconnected when the mouth is being manipulated, so it must be handled carefully.

Maintenance of anesthesia

Maintenance of anesthesia with inhalants is the most common method for oral surgical procedures. Currently available inhalants include isoflurane, sevoflurane and desflurane. The clinical differences between isoflurane, sevoflurane and desflurane are relatively subtle, with a tendency toward more rapid mask inductions with sevoflurane compared with isoflurane. Desflurane has not reached the veterinary market because it currently requires a vaporizer which is 4–5 times the cost of the standard units used with the other agents. Nitrous oxide (N_2O) has been applied widely to reduce the concentration of inhalant used. A concentration of 50–67% is typically used; it is imperative to monitor the concentration of oxygen being delivered to ensure that a hypoxic mixture is not being delivered; inclusion of pulse oximetry in the monitoring of these patients is also advantageous. The addition of N_2O (compared to an equivalent dose of inhalant alone) has been shown to improve cardiac output in dogs[29] but not in cats.[30] Injectable adjuncts (e.g., opioids) to inhalant anesthetic agents may decrease the nociceptive input during the procedure, and may allow the use of less inhalant. In order to achieve a particular plasma concentration of the drug, it is usually necessary to give a loading dose before the constant rate infusion (CRI). It is generally estimated that it takes five elimination half-lives to reach a steady state, so the need for a loading dose is dependent on this variable. As an example, one report gives the elimination half-life of fentanyl as 46 minutes[31] so it would take 230 minutes to reach a steady state at any particular infusion rate. Opioids

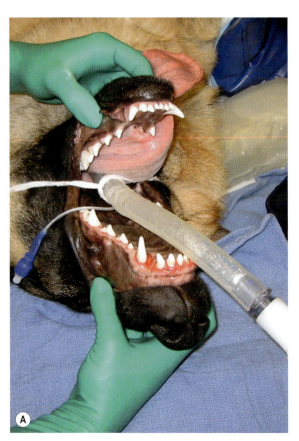
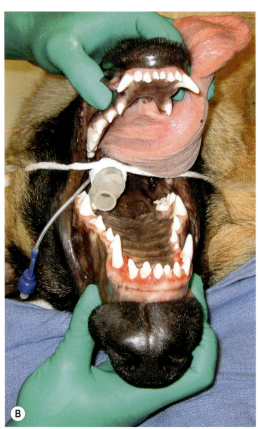

Fig. 4.1 Endotracheal tube adapter technique allowing the occlusion to be evaluated during the dental procedure: (**A**) Endotracheal tube and adapter connected to the anesthetic machine during the procedure; (**B**) Endotracheal tube disconnected and adapter removed to check the occlusion.

are often used, as they provide good analgesia with minimal effect on the cardiovascular system; these include morphine, oxymorphone, hydromorphone, methadone, fentanyl, alfentanil, sufentanil and remifentanil. These can be given as intermittent boluses (e.g., oxymorphone 0.02–0.05 mg/kg, fentanyl 1–2 μg/kg, sufentanil 0.1–0.2 μg/kg q 15–20 minutes) or as a continuous infusion (fentanyl 10 μg/kg loading dose with 0.1–1 μg/kg/min constant rate infusion (CRI), sufentanil 1 μg/kg loading dose with 0.01–0.1 μg/kg/min CRI, alfentanil 40 μg/kg loading dose with 1–3 μg/kg/min CRI – halve these doses for cats, remifentanil, no loading dose required, 0.1–1.0 μg/kg/min CRI) with the major disadvantage being the degree of respiratory depression associated with these drugs. If this technique is used, controlled intermittent positive-pressure ventilation should be instituted. These doses of opioids will also cause bradycardia in dogs, which typically responds to administration of atropine (0.02 mg/kg IM) or glycopyrrolate (0.01 mg/kg IM). Lidocaine has also been used as an infusion, and has been reported to result in a 20–30% reduction in the amount of inhalant needed.[32] This is less likely to produce respiratory depression than the opioids. In the dog, a loading dose of lidocaine at 1–2 mg/kg can be followed by an infusion of 100–120 μg/kg/min. This technique is not useful in the cat, where lidocaine linearly reduces the amount of inhalant needed but also linearly decreases cardiac output.[33,34] Ketamine has also been reported to reduce the amount of inhalant used by 45–75% in cats and 11–95% in dogs.[35,36] However, the doses used in these laboratory studies exceed those that would be practical in a clinical setting, and currently a dose of 10–20 μg/kg/min is recommended with a loading dose of 2 mg/kg. A combination of an opioid (morphine), lidocaine and ketamine has become popular, providing a decrease in nociceptive input from multiple mechanisms. Intraoperatively, the lidocaine and ketamine don't

seem to add any benefit, in terms of reducing the inhalant dose beyond that provided by the morphine,[37] but continuing this infusion into the postoperative period may provide some advantage. The doses used in the intraoperative study were morphine (3.3 μg/kg/min), lidocaine (50 μg/kg/min) and ketamine (10 μg/kg/min).

Monitoring the patient

Monitoring cardiovascular function

Although the inhalants are not supposed to cause excessive cardiopulmonary depression at regular clinical doses, they may produce profound hypotension in some patients and at higher concentrations.[38–40] Given this disturbing effect on the cardiovascular system, it is important to monitor blood pressure and to be able to treat hypotension if necessary. Several techniques are available to monitor blood pressure; these include Doppler ultrasound and sphygmomanometry, indirect blood pressure measurement via oscillometric or photoacoustic technique, and direct blood pressure measurement using an arterial catheter. A Doppler technique is the least expensive and most robust of these methods, but requires someone to read the pressures at regular intervals throughout the procedure. Machines that read pressures automatically using an oscillometric or photoacoustic technique are more expensive, but can be programmed to read at set time intervals, freeing the clinician to do other things. These devices have not functioned well in small patients but technological developments are improving their sensitivity and one unit has been validated for the measurement of blood pressure in cats.[41] The placement of an arterial catheter with the use of direct pressure measurement is generally more accurate than the use of indirect techniques. The placement of such catheters requires practice and is not advocated for the routine measurement of blood pressure in all patients. However, in some patients it is a valuable method because it allows for moment-to-moment analysis of the blood pressure and provides access to the arterial blood for blood gas analysis in the assessment of ventilatory and metabolic acid–base status.

Hypotension is defined as a systolic pressure <90 mmHg or a mean pressure of <70 mmHg. Consideration should be given to treating pressures below these values, and the first step is to assess the depth of anesthesia and turn down the vaporizer as much as possible, given the necessity of providing adequate anesthesia for the procedure. The second step is to increase the rate of fluid administration, usually to the maximum allowed by gravity and the limitations of the fluid administration set and catheter. An initial bolus of 20 mL/kg of a balanced electrolyte solution is a good starting point to increase the blood volume, with further volumes given as needed. Crystalloid solutions redistribute rapidly and less than 50% of the volume administered will remain in the vascular space.[42] Colloid solutions remain in the vascular space and increase the circulating volume for a longer period than crystalloids and can also be used in the hypotensive patient. A bolus of hetastarch or a polygelatin solution at 5–10 mL/kg would rapidly expand vascular volume and may be more effective than a crystalloid, but is also much more expensive.[38] If these measures fail to increase the blood pressure into the normal range, then a positive inotrope should be used to try to increase cardiac output and thereby increase perfusion pressure. The most commonly used inotropes in dogs and cats are dopamine, dobutamine and ephedrine. The first two need to be given as infusions while the ephedrine is normally given as a bolus. Table 4.1 gives details of how to prepare these solutions and administer them.

The infusion rates of dopamine and dobutamine should be altered in response to the change in blood pressure. Dopamine, in particular, is known to have highly variable individual pharmacokinetics, so if the initial dose is not working within 5 minutes it is appropriate to increase it to a higher rate.[43] Arrhythmias or tachycardia probably indicate a relative overdose, in which case the infusions should be decreased or stopped. Repeated doses of ephedrine may be associated with some tachyphylaxis. Another approach to the management of hypotension during inhalant anesthesia is to replace the inhalant with a drug that produces less cardiovascular depression. Nitrous oxide (N_2O) is one example and can be given in concentrations of 50–67% which should allow a 25–33% reduction in the amount of inhalant required to maintain an appropriate anesthetic plane. Nitrous oxide will often cause a slight increase in blood pressure and may increase respiratory rate in some patients. The concentration of oxygen in the breathing circuit should be monitored to ensure that a hypoxic mixture is not delivered; it is also prudent to monitor arterial hemoglobin saturation with oxygen (SpO_2) using a pulse oximeter.

Central venous pressure

Central venous pressure (CVP) is underutilized as a monitor in veterinary patients despite being simple to measure and providing valuable information about the state of the patient's circulation. A catheter is placed in the jugular vein such that the tip of the catheter is at the entrance to the right atrium. This can then be attached to a water manometer or to a pressure transducer zeroed to the level of the right atrium. Central venous pressure is a reflection of vascular volume, intrathoracic pressure and the ability of the right heart to pump blood forward. In a dog with real or potential congestive heart failure, the CVP will increase if the rate of fluid administration exceeds the ability of the heart to pump the fluids forward. This allows the clinician to adjust the fluid administration to the clinical condition of the animal. Many animals with heart failure receiving diuretics may be relatively dehydrated, but it is very difficult to assess this clinically; central venous pressure measurement allows a more accurate assessment of the patient's ability to tolerate a given fluid volume.

Monitoring respiratory function

Monitoring of respiratory function can be carried out using several methods such as direct observation of the frequency and quality of respiration, breath detection/apnea alerting, respirometry, capnometry, and blood gas analysis. The latter is the gold standard for determining the efficiency of ventilation, while capnometry provides a noninvasive method for the assessment of carbon dioxide elimination. The advantages of capnometry are that it can be applied routinely to all patients and it provides immediate and continuous information. However, there can be significant discrepancies between the end-tidal CO_2 measured by the capnometer and the actual $PaCO_2$, making capnometry a less accurate method than blood gas analysis. Hypoventilation is present when the $PaCO_2$ is above the normal reference interval (≈ 43 mmHg for the dog and 35 mmHg for cats) but it is not common to treat hypoventilation until the animal becomes acidemic and the $PaCO_2 > 65$ mmHg. Although positive-pressure ventilation may be performed by hand, a ventilator will provide much more reliable results. A respirometer gives quantitative information on the amount of gas the animal is breathing but does not measure gas exchange, thus making it a less reliable technique than capnometry or blood gas analysis. Breath rate monitors ('apnea alert' monitors) simply indicate whether the animal is breathing and give no quantitative information on the effectiveness of ventilation.

Pulse oximetry is often difficult to use in dental patients because the most reliable site in dogs and cats is the tongue, and the pulse oximeter probe is not a welcome addition to the confined oral space during these procedures. In addition, some pulse oximeters are affected by movement of the site, and will not read if the tongue is being manipulated. Technological improvements in signal processing can account for motion, and newer generations of pulse oximeters may be able to function despite movement of the tongue. If the tongue is not accessible, the probe can be placed on an ear, paw or tail, but failure rates are much higher in these sites, especially if there is dense pigment of the skin. The measurement of arterial oxygen saturation is also of limited value in patients who are breathing 95–100% oxygen and have no pulmonary pathosis, because the saturation will not

Table 4.1 Concentrations and dilutions used for infusions of positive inotropes in dogs and cats

Drug	Concentration	Dilution	Dose	Infusion rate
Dopamine	40 mg/mL	75 mg (1.825 mL)/250 mL	5–10 µg/kg/min	1–2 mL/kg/h
Dobutamine	12.5 mg/mL	75 mg (6 mL)/250 mL	2.5–5 µg/kg/min	0.5–1 mL/kg/h
Ephedrine	50 mg/mL	5 mg (0.1 mL)/1 mL	50 –100 µg/kg boluses	0.01–0.02 mL/kg per 15–20 minutes

change significantly until the PaO$_2$ decreases to values below 80 mmHg. Since this is a rare event and the technology is prone to artifact, it is likely that the practitioner will be alerted to many false events before a real desaturation occurs. This leads people to believe that the machine is at fault and needs 'fixing' when it gives a low reading and not that there is a real problem. The result is that there is a tendency to fiddle with the pulse oximeter, by moving the probe to a different site for example, rather than looking at the patient to see if the number could be real.

Accurate assessment of the anesthetic status of dental patients may also be challenging because the intense work around the head limits access to the eyes (palpebral response), jaws (muscle tone) and tongue (lingual pulse, blood gas sampling from the lingual vessels). If there is any doubt about the status of the patient, the dental procedure should be discontinued until the animal can be assessed. It is also important to monitor the size of the tongue because it may become swollen due to decreased venous/lymphatic drainage (pharyngeal packs) or due to prolonged manipulation. A swollen tongue may be more prone to injury, and may interfere with ventilation during recovery. Treatment for lingual swelling is symptomatic, using osmotic techniques (sugar applied externally, mannitol IV), diuretics (furosemide IV) and/or corticosteroid injections. These treatments have not been examined for efficacy in dogs and cats.

Temperature and renal function

Although dental patients do not have a major body cavity exposed, flushing the oral cavity and wetting the head with fluids throughout the procedure increases the likelihood of hypothermia,[44,45] and it is advisable to make sure they are on a heating pad and wrapped up in a blanket or warm air heating blanket. Body temperature should be monitored regularly to ensure that it remains within normal limits.

Many dental patients are old and have some degree of renal insufficiency. It is important that the anesthetic should not cause any further damage to the kidneys. For these patients it is therefore even more crucial to monitor blood pressure and the addition of CVP for those patients with concurrent cardiac insufficiency is advisable. The use of drugs to enhance renal perfusion during the procedure is controversial, there being no scientific evidence to suggest either negative or positive effects. This author routinely uses mannitol (0.25 g/kg over 20 minutes followed by 0.1 g/kg/h). Animals treated in this way should be carefully monitored postoperatively and kept on fluids for 24 hours after the procedure. If this is not feasible, subcutaneous fluids can be given to prevent dehydration.

Local anesthetics

Local anesthetics can be used as part of the anesthetic regimen for dental patients. Whenever an invasive procedure is being carried out, the use of a nerve block will decrease the nociceptive input into the CNS, which may have a preemptive analgesic effect. A bigger advantage is that by removing the noxious stimulation, less of the general (inhalant) anesthetic is needed to maintain an adequate anesthetic plane, thus decreasing all the negative effects of these central depressants. Appropriate administration of a long-acting local anesthetic will also delay the need for other analgesic administration;[46] when combined with the need for less general anesthetic, this should allow a more rapid recovery.

Pharmacology

Local anesthetics have a lipophilic and a hydrophilic moiety joined by either an amide or ester linkage. The ester local anesthetics (procaine, tetracaine, benzocaine and cocaine) are metabolized by cholinesterases in the blood but are rarely used in clinical practice. The amide local anesthetics (which include articaine, bupivacaine, etidocaine, lidocaine, mepivacaine, prilocaine and ropivacaine) are generally metabolized in the liver and generally have longer half-lives than the esters. Only the most commonly used amide local anesthetic agents will be discussed here; information on the others is summarized in Table 4.2. The particular choice of drug is dependent on desired onset of effect and duration of action. However, the duration of action is dependent on the site of injection – a more vascular site will have a shorter duration of action due to rapid removal of the drug. To counter this, it is common to add a vasoconstrictor to the local anesthetic agent to reduce the rate of absorption and thus prolong the block. Epinephrine is the most commonly used vasoconstrictor; there is no advantage to using concentrations greater than 5 µg/mL (1 : 200 000), as higher concentrations do not slow the reabsorption of the drug and thus do not prolong the block. This concentration is also less likely to lead to significant absorption and subsequent systemic effects. Even with a consistent site of injection the duration of action can be highly variable. In 4 of 6 dogs a block with chloroprocaine lasted less than 90 minutes, but in one dog one tooth was desensitized for more than 24 hours.[47] The activity of local anesthetics is dependent on the diffusion of the unionized form through the cell membrane, and the amount of the unionized form is pH-dependent. Tissues with a low pH will promote the presence of the ionized molecule, thus decreasing the action of the drug; therefore local anesthetics injected into infected tissue may be ineffective due to the local acidosis.

Table 4.2 Local anesthetics that might be used for dental anesthesia

Drug	Trade names	Concentrations	Onset (minutes)	Duration (hours)
Lidocaine	Xylocaine® Anestacaine™	0.5–4%	2–5	0.5–3
Bupivacaine	Marcaine® Sensorcaine®	0.25–0.75%	5–10	2–10
Mepivacaine	Carbocaine®, Isocaine®, Polocaine®, Scandonest™	2–3% ± levonordefrin	2–4	0.5–3
Prilocaine	Citanest®	4%	2–4	1–2
Etidocaine	Duranest®	1.5% + epinephrine	2–5	2–4
Ropivacaine	Naropin®	0.2–1%	10–15	2–4
Articaine	Septocaine™	4% + epinephrine	2–5	2–4

Lidocaine is the most commonly used local anesthetic and it has a rapid onset of action (2–5 minutes) with a duration of 30–120 minutes. It is normally used as a 2% solution in veterinary medicine with or without epinephrine. Dental cartridges may contain lidocaine 2% with various concentrations of epinephrine. The maximum dose of lidocaine recommended for dogs and cats is 4 mg/kg, although toxicity is rarely seen at doses < 10 mg/kg. Because lidocaine is metabolized in the liver, care should be taken in obese patients or those with hepatic insufficiency. An obese patient will have a smaller hepatic capacity than its weight would suggest. Lidocaine is used as an antiarrhythmic drug, so accidental intravenous administration is not a problem unless a massive dose is given.

Bupivacaine is a longer-acting local anesthetic, often providing a duration of anesthesia 2–3 times as long as lidocaine. It takes about twice as long as lidocaine to reach peak effect. It is supplied in concentrations ranging from 0.25% to 0.75%, but is most commonly used at 0.25–0.5% for dental anesthesia. Dental cartridges may also contain epinephrine (1 : 200 000). Bupivacaine is more cardiotoxic than lidocaine, and should not be given at doses exceeding 2 mg/kg. Levobupivacaine (the S-isomer of bupivacaine) has recently been marketed and is supposed to be less cardiotoxic than the racemic mixture with similar efficacy and duration.[48] Its use has not been evaluated in veterinary dentistry. The information above is a compilation of general facts about these drugs but when applied to dental techniques these 'facts' may not apply. In a series of experiments (unpublished) looking at the infraorbital, middle mental and inferior alveolar blocks in dogs using electrophysiological techniques similar to the ones described by Gross et al.[47] the author has found that:

1. The onset of effect with both lidocaine and bupivacaine is usually within 5 minutes so there would seem to be little advantage to mixing lidocaine with bupivacaine.
2. The duration of effect with lidocaine in the infraorbital canal is 2–3 hours and with bupivacaine it is at least 8 hours and may be > 12 hours.

3. The duration of effect is much shorter with the middle mental block than with the infraorbital block (e.g., 1–2 hours with lidocaine and 2–3 hours with bupivacaine).
4. The lateral gingival tissue over the molar teeth for both the infraorbital and middle mental blocks is largely unaffected and remains sensitive.

Mepivacaine has a slightly slower onset of action than lidocaine, and a slightly longer duration of action (2–3 hours). It is marginally less toxic than lidocaine. It is supplied as a 2% or 3% solution and is sold with a vasoconstrictor (levonordefrin 1 : 20 000) in dental cartridges.

Technique

The greatest concerns when using local anesthetics are damage to a nerve, hematoma and intravascular injection. The likelihood of damage to a nerve can be minimized by the use of a gentle technique where the needle is not moved very much from side to side once it is in tissue. In conscious human dental patients, penetration of the nerve is accompanied by paresthesia, so the patient can usually warn the clinician that this has occurred. This is not the case if the injection is carried out in the anesthetized patient, so the clinician must be particularly careful about the technique used. The use of atraumatic needles may also assist in preventing nerve damage. Various pencil point needles are available (Gertie-Marx, Whitacre and Sprotte spinal needles: International Medical Development, Park City, UT) but have not been used widely in veterinary medicine. Ideally, a fine needle with a short bevel should be used in order to minimize the likelihood of trauma to the nerve. The bevel should be oriented in the same direction as the nerve fibers in order to reduce the chance of cutting through the nerve fibers (Fig. 4.2).[49] Penetration of a blood vessel is a frequent, minor complication due to the presence of large vessels associated with many of the involved nerves. Again, the use of a fine needle will minimize the risk of hematoma, but the clinician should

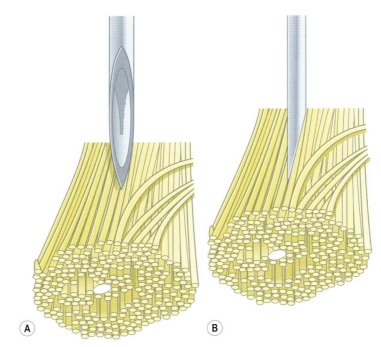

Fig. 4.2 Diagram showing the needle (**A**) parallel to, and (**B**) perpendicular to the nerve fibers.

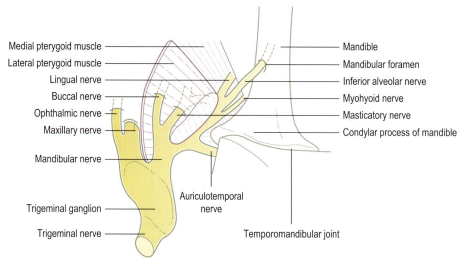

Fig. 4.3 Topographical anatomy of the lingual nerve, mandibular nerve and the mandibular foramen.

always be aware of this possibility and apply pressure to the injection site to limit the extent of bleeding, should it occur. Most hematomas resolve without causing any serious sequelae. Of greater concern is the intravascular injection of local anesthetics, because this has been associated with serious, even fatal, outcomes in people from doses that would not normally be considered dangerous. This may be because inadvertent injection into a facial artery could be associated with retrograde flow into the internal carotid artery, with immediate access to the cerebral circulation. Such reactions have not been described in dogs or cats, but it is wise to be aware of such a possibility. Aspiration, using negative pressure on the syringe, is a simple and effective method for diagnosing vessel penetration and should be carried out before *every* injection of a local anesthetic. Ideally, the needle should be turned and a second aspiration carried out, as it is possible to be in a vessel and have a negative aspiration because the bevel of the needle is positioned against the vessel wall. Other minor considerations with the injection of local anesthetics are the possibility of introducing infection into the tissue. This appears to be a rare complication despite the lack of applying disinfectants to the injection site. Allergies have been described to amide local anesthetics in humans, but not in dogs or cats.

The use of regular disposable plastic syringes versus dental syringes is a matter of personal preference. Dental syringes, with their cartridges, were developed to provide a simple, rapid method for loading and delivering the local anesthetic with one hand. The glass cartridges are prefilled with 1.8 mL of local anesthetic solution. They are more expensive than the usual disposable syringes used by most veterinarians, and carry few advantages when the patient is under general anesthesia. The size and length of the needle is also a matter of choice. As indicated above, a fine needle is less likely to cause significant trauma but very fine needles can break off if any stress is placed on them during the injection, so this author usually uses 25–27-gauge needles.

Neuroanatomy

Two branches of the trigeminal nerve provide sensory innervation of the teeth and associated soft tissues: the infraorbital nerve, which is a direct continuation of the maxillary nerve, and the inferior alveolar nerve, which is a branch of the mandibular nerve.

Medial to the condylar process of the mandible, one of the main branches of the mandibular nerve, gives off the auriculotemporal

nerve and subsequently divides into three nerves: the lingual nerve (medially), the inferior alveolar nerve and the mylohyoid nerve (caudally) (Fig. 4.3). The lingual nerve is sensory to the rostral two-thirds of the tongue. In cats it has been shown that the lingual nerve may carry pulpal fibers to the canine tooth.[50] The mylohyoid nerve runs medial to the ramus and body of the mandible and gives off motor branches to the rostral belly of the digastric muscle and the mylohyoid muscle, and two sensory branches to the caudal two-thirds of the intermandibular region. The inferior alveolar nerve enters the mandibular canal through the mandibular foramen, where alveolar sensory branches are given off to the teeth. The local anesthetic agent should be deposited right at the mandibular foramen, in order to affect only the inferior alveolar nerve. If injected further caudally, all three branches may be affected, which may result in numbness of the tongue. Three cutaneous branches exit from the three mental foramina (caudal, middle and rostral), which are sensory to the lower lip and rostral third of the intermandibular region. It is important to note that the inferior alveolar nerve at the level of the middle mental foramen has already given off its branches supplying the teeth. From there on, the nerve is sensory for the lower lip. Therefore, injecting local anesthetic at the level of the middle mental foramen (sometimes referred to as a 'mental block') will not provide anesthesia to the canine or incisor teeth; to achieve anesthesia of these teeth, the needle must be introduced into the middle mental foramen and advanced caudally. This technique is discussed below.

The infraorbital nerve passes over the medial pterygoid muscle before entering the maxillary foramen (Fig. 4.4). Prior to entering the infraorbital canal through the maxillary foramen, the infraorbital nerve gives off a number of caudal superior alveolar branches, which enter the maxillary bone through small alveolar foramina to supply the maxillary molar teeth and possibly the distal root of the fourth premolar tooth. Once within the infraorbital canal, the middle superior alveolar branches are given off on the ventral aspect, mainly to supply the maxillary fourth premolar tooth. Just before the infraorbital nerve exits the infraorbital foramen, the well-defined rostral superior alveolar branch is given off, which enters the alveolar canal to supply the rostral premolar, canine and incisor teeth. The infraorbital nerve as it exits the infraorbital foramen has already given off its branches supplying the teeth. From there the nerve is sensory for the upper lip and nose. In order for an infraorbital block to be successful for dental extractions, the needle must be inserted *into* the foramen and penetrate deeply, as discussed below.

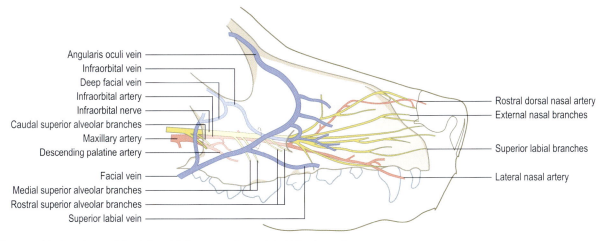

Fig. 4.4 Topographical anatomy of the infraorbital nerve and associated blood vessels.

- Angularis oculi vein
- Infraorbital vein
- Deep facial vein
- Infraorbital artery
- Infraorbital nerve
- Caudal superior alveolar branches
- Maxillary artery
- Descending palatine artery
- Facial vein
- Medial superior alveolar branches
- Rostral superior alveolar branches
- Superior labial vein

- Rostral dorsal nasal artery
- External nasal branches
- Superior labial branches
- Lateral nasal artery

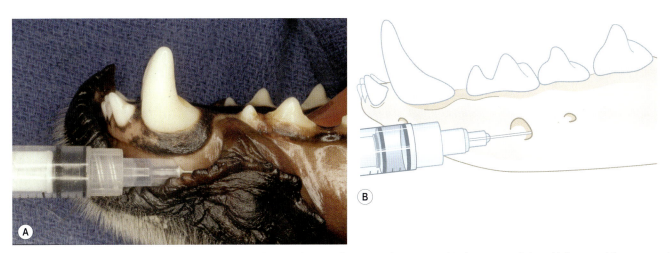

Fig. 4.5 Mental nerve block: (**A**) Clinical photograph, and (**B**) line drawing illustrating the topographical anatomy of the middle mental foramen and its relationships with teeth, lower lip frenulum and mandible.

Technique for performing regional intraoral nerve blocks

The volumes of drug mentioned below should be modified by accounting for the maximum dose of the drug that should be used. For example, if a four-quadrant block is planned (using both infraorbital and inferior alveolar nerve blocks) in a 5-kg dog, the total volume used would be 2.12 mL. With bupivacaine (0.5%) this would amount to 10.6 mg, which is slightly over the recommended maximum dose of 2 mg/kg. The volume used for each quadrant could be reduced slightly or the drug diluted up to the recommended volume. In larger animals, the volumes used are unlikely to exceed the maximum recommended dose.

Middle mental nerve

The middle mental nerve is anesthetized for procedures involving the rostral part of the mandible. In one study, anesthesia was established at least as far caudally as the first molar tooth within 10 minutes of injecting 1 mL of 2% chloroprocaine into the middle mental foramen in five out of six dogs.[47] The middle mental foramen is located ventral to the mesial root of the second premolar tooth, medial to the lower lip frenulum (Fig. 4.5). The foramen can be palpated through the frenulum (or the latter can be moved rostrally or caudally) in the

ventral third of the vertical distance from the gingival margin to the ventral border of the mandible.[51] Once the landmark has been located, the needle is introduced into the foramen in a rostral to caudal direction. The canal in which the nerve lies is slightly curved, so the needle may need to be manipulated a little for it to advance far into the canal. The author has found it possible to advance a 1.5-inch, 27-gauge needle fully into this canal in 20-kg dogs. Injecting this deep into the canal will anesthetize the canine and premolar teeth but does not routinely remove sensitivity from the lateral gingival area over the molar teeth. With the needle in place, the syringe is aspirated before injecting the local anesthetic into the site. Injection should be relatively easy, and there should be no swelling over the site. If it starts to swell as the injection is made, digital pressure should be applied over the area to prevent the drug from escaping into the tissue surrounding the foramen. There are no studies which have defined how much should be injected into this canal. In the study quoted above[47] a volume of 1 mL was used in dogs weighing an average of 20.5 kg, suggesting a dose of about 0.05 mL/kg. It is likely that the volume of the canal is not linearly related to body weight, so this author suggests using a scaled dose of $0.13 \text{ mL/kg}^{2/3}$, although even this will not account for the differences in the length of the canal between animals of similar weight but different skull types. For example, it is expected that a lower dose would be used in a 30-kg English bulldog compared with a 30-kg collie. This dose translates to approximately 0.4 mL for a 5-kg dog, 0.8 mL for a 15-kg dog and 1.75 mL for a 50-kg dog. In cats and small dogs it can be difficult to gain access to the canal so a block of the mental nerve as it egresses from the canal can be achieved by injecting a small volume (0.1–0.2 mL) of anesthetic over the middle mental foramen under the lower lip frenulum if the goal is to anesthetize the soft tissues rostral to this site.

Inferior alveolar nerve

Anesthetizing this nerve will remove sensation over the hard and soft tissues of the body of the mandible. There are two approaches to this block: intraoral and extraoral. In both cases the mandible is palpated on the lingual aspect, caudal and ventral to the last molar in an attempt to locate the mandibular foramen. It is often hard to appreciate the foramen itself, but it is usually possible to feel the neurovascular bundle as a thin string-like structure as it enters the foramen. With the intraoral technique, the nerve is palpated with one hand while the syringe and needle are held in the other hand (Fig. 4.6). The needle penetrates the mucosa overlying the mandible rostral to the nerve, and is advanced caudally until it is next to the nerve. The syringe is aspirated before injecting. In using this technique the tongue tends to be pushed medially so that there is less likelihood of blocking the lingual nerve at the same time. With the extraoral approach the landmarks are slightly different in the dog and the cat (Fig. 4.7). In the dog the deepest part of the depression on the caudal ventral border of the mandible is usually directly over the mandibular foramen with the dog in dorsal recumbency. In the cat, palpation of the nerve/

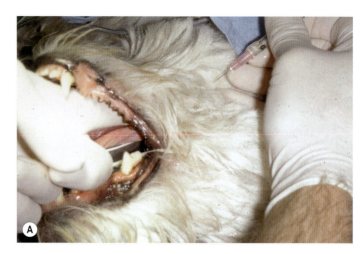

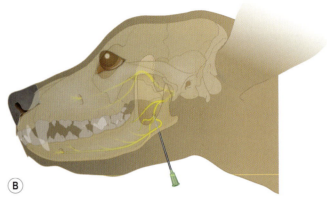

Fig. 4.7 Extraoral technique for administering the inferior alveolar block: (**A**) Clinical photograph, and (**B**) line drawing illustrating the positioning of the needle at the mandibular foramen.

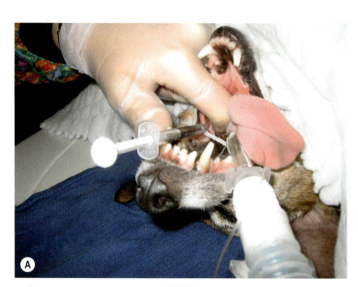

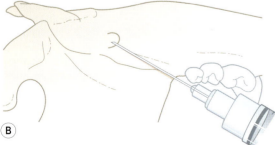

Fig. 4.6 Intraoral technique for administering the inferior alveolar block: (**A**) Clinical photograph, and (**B**) line drawing illustrating the positioning of the needle at the mandibular foramen.

foramen from inside the mouth becomes the best landmark, since the ventral border of the mandible is relatively flat. Alternatively, the foramen is located approximately halfway on an imaginary line drawn from the last molar tooth to the angle of the mandible in both cats and dogs.[52] The needle should first be advanced perpendicularly on to the most ventral surface of the mandible, then walked medially, advancing towards the foramen as close to the bone as possible. Once in place, the syringe is aspirated before injecting. Volumes of local anesthetic required for this block will be higher than those used for the mental or infraorbital blocks, because the injection is not made into a bony canal. A suggested dose is 0.18 mL/kg$^{2/3}$. In the feline study by Gross et al[53] a volume of 0.25 mL, 2% chloroprocaine, was used with the extraoral approach and there was a failure rate of 50% for blockade of the mandibular first molar tooth but the reasons for these failures were not elucidated. In the author's experiments (unpublished) the extraoral approach with this block failed to provide adequate anesthesia in most subjects.

There are anecdotal reports of tongue and lip chewing secondary to an inferior alveolar nerve regional block. This has been observed rarely in our practice, but may be explained by depositing the local anesthetic too far caudally, thereby blocking the lingual and mylohyoid nerves in addition to the inferior alveolar nerve. In our worst case, a dog with a mandibular fracture that had been stabilized using an intraoral composite splint over the incisor, canine and first premolar teeth, the tongue lacerations were sufficiently damaging that part of the tongue had to be resected. Although the inferior alveolar block may have contributed to this problem, it is not certain that this was the only factor in this injury.

Infraorbital nerve

This branch of the trigeminal nerve supplies the teeth and gingiva of the upper jaw. The nerve exits from the infraorbital foramen which is located dorsal to the distal root of the maxillary third premolar tooth. The foramen can easily be palpated from the mucosal surface as a distinct, vertically oriented, elliptical indentation in the maxillary bone. A needle is introduced into the foramen by advancing it caudally, with the axis of the needle parallel to the bone of the maxilla (Fig. 4.8). The length of needle introduced into the canal should be tailored to the length of the infraorbital canal. This can be estimated by palpating the junction of the zygomatic bone with the maxilla, which is immediately dorsal to the caudal end of the infraorbital canal. In cats and brachycephalic dogs the canal may only be a few millimeters in length and if a long needle is use it may end up penetrating the globe of the eye. In dolichocephalic dogs the canal may be 20–30 mm in length and a longer needle is required to achieve the desired effect. It is thought that solution injected into the infraorbital canal will spread caudally along the nerve; in the study by Gross et al[47] the first molar tooth was blocked using this approach,

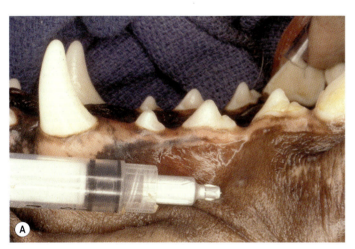

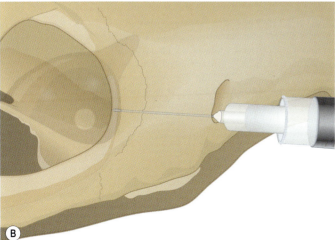

Fig. 4.8 Technique for administering the infraorbital block with the patient in dorsal recumbency: (**A**) Clinical photograph, and (**B**) line drawing illustrating the positioning of the needle in the infraorbital canal.

suggesting that the drug will diffuse back to the caudal superior alveolar nerve. Although a catheter was placed into the infraorbital canal in that study, diffusion of a liquid injected into the canal with a needle appears to provide a similar distribution (personal observations). Even with the needle passed to the end of the canal the second molar tooth may not be adequately blocked using this technique. Once the needle is in place, the syringe is aspirated and, if no blood is aspirated, the solution injected over 20–30 seconds. Resistance to injection should be absent or minimal. If considerable resistance is detected, the needle may be in the periosteum and should be repositioned before continuing. The volume of the solution used for this block should be the same as for the mental nerve block – $0.11 \text{ mL/kg}^{2/3}$. Some authors advocate using very small doses of the desired anesthetic agent (0.1–0.3 mL) deposited more specifically over the preferred site for the teeth involved by advancing a long needle to that location.[54] This approach may provide a shorter duration of action. The large infraorbital vein and artery also travel through the infraorbital canal, and it is more common to contact one of these vessels when performing this block compared with the others described here. Despite the size of these vessels, and their location proximate to the nerves, it appears to be an uncommon problem clinically.

Maxillary nerve

This nerve is anesthetized when it is difficult to achieve an infraorbital block (e.g., a tumor or abscess over the site) or certainty about anesthetizing the last molar tooth is required. The block can be performed extra- or intraorally. One landmark for the extraoral block is the notch between the caudal border of the cranial ventral aspect of the zygomatic arch and the maxilla. The needle should be advanced from this point, parallel to the plane of the hard palate and slightly rostrally, until it touches the perpendicular lamina of the palatine bone (Fig. 4.9). It should then be retracted 2–3 mm before aspirating and injecting, as the nerve is located dorsal to the medial pterygoid muscle. The palatine bone may be very thin at this point, so care must be taken not to put too much pressure on the bone. The volume for this block should also be at the higher value used for the extraoral inferior alveolar block ($0.18 \text{ mL/kg}^{2/3}$). A second approach is to use a dorsal approach, passing the needle either through the conjunctiva or through the skin close to the lateral canthus of the eye. The needle is advanced a short distance ventrally at right angles to the axis of the hard palate so that it sits directly over the entrance to the infraorbital canal. For the intraoral approach the needle is inserted behind the last molar tooth slightly towards the palatine side of the tooth[55] or at the point where the zygomatic arch meets the bone around the last molar.[51] The needle is advanced at a 40°[55] or a 90°[51] angle with the palate parallel to the teeth and this will intersect with the maxillary nerve before it gives off the caudal superior alveolar branches. Another approach is to use a curved needle to try to place the tip of the needle closer to the entrance to the infraorbital canal. The starting point is the same but the needle head is rotated as it is being advanced to bring the tip up caudal to the foramen.

Major palatine foramen approach to the maxillary nerve

This approach is sometimes used to anesthetize the maxillary nerve. Because of the thickness of the palatine soft tissue it is difficult to palpate this foramen. It lies at the midpoint between the mesial border of the maxillary first molar tooth and midline. A needle is passed through the major palatine foramen and the injection made into the rostral part of the orbit where the maxillary nerve is located.[52,53] Trauma to the major palatine artery may occur with this approach, in which case severe hemorrhage may result; therefore this technique is not recommended. Some authors have recommended blocking the palatine nerve as it exits from the canal by depositing 0.1–0.2 mL of

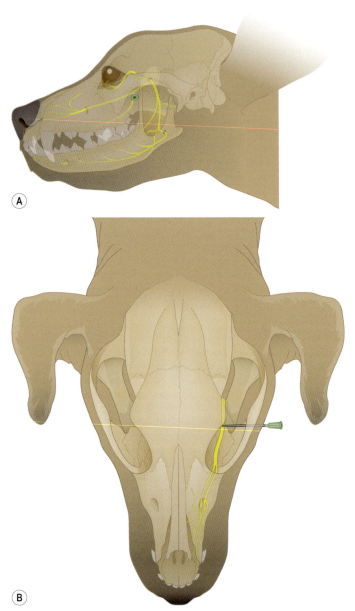

Fig. 4.9 (**A**, **B**) Diagrams showing the needle placement for the lateral extraoral approach to the maxillary nerve block.

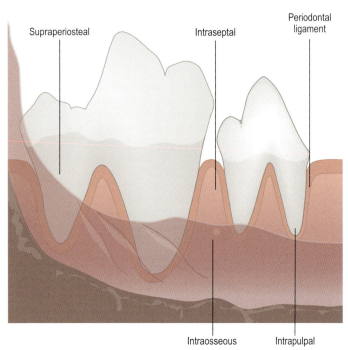

Fig. 4.10 Supraperiosteal, periodontal ligament, intraseptal, intraosseus (note hole drilled into bone) and intrapulpal injection techniques.

0.5% bupivacaine to provide maximal analgesia of the palate during invasive procedures in this region.[56]

Local infiltration

In humans, five local infiltration techniques are described:[57] supraperiosteal, periodontal ligament, intraseptal, intraosseus and intrapulpal injection (Fig. 4.10). Supraperiosteal injection involves the injection of the local anesthetic over the periosteum adjacent to the tooth root. This is most effective in young people with less dense bony tissue because it relies on diffusion of the drug through the periosteum and bone to reach the tooth root. It is thought that this will not work for canine and feline mandibles because the bone is too dense.[58] In humans, a volume of 0.6 mL is suggested. Injection into the periodontal ligament is carried out by inserting the needle down the periodontal ligament towards the root of the tooth. It is

suggested that the bevel of the needle face the tooth and that an injection of 0.1–0.2 mL of local anesthetic be used. Since this is dense tissue, it can require considerable force to inject the agent into this region (pressures exceeding 17 000 mmHg have been recorded).[59] The high pressures used for such injections may increase osteoclastic activity and cause temporary bone resorption.[60] An injection should be made over each tooth root affected by the procedure. An experiment carried out in young dogs (3–9 months) demonstrated that local anesthetic agent diffused down the paths of least resistance to the vascular channels and intertrabecular spaces, but did not appear to penetrate into the permanent tooth buds.[61] Injection of local anesthetic containing epinephrine can be absorbed rapidly by this route, which may result in a decrease in blood pressure.[62] Intraseptal injection requires the placement of the needle in the cortical plate of bone adjacent to the tooth root. The needle is advanced into this plate from the gingiva and 0.3–0.5 mL of local anesthetic deposited. Again, there is a high resistance to injection, and injection of lidocaine with epinephrine can cause up to a 90% reduction in pulpal blood flow using this technique.[63] Intraosseus anesthesia requires the penetration of the bone using a drill and then advancing the needle through this hole into the subcortical bone. This is performed over the tooth of interest using a lateral approach and 0.45–0.6 mL of drug is injected. Intrapulpal injection is only performed when the pulp has been exposed (for example, during an acute complicated crown fracture). A small volume of solution (0.2–0.3 mL) is injected under pressure, directly into the exposed pulp.

POSTOPERATIVE CARE

If an opioid analgesic agent was not employed as a premedicant, it is appropriate to administer an opioid towards the end of any oral surgical procedure. Also, if the procedure has been prolonged it may be appropriate to give a second dose of opioid analgesic to a patient who

Table 4.3 Opioid/NSAID doses for perioperative pain

Drug	Dose	Species	Route	Duration of action
Morphine	0.5–1.0 mg/kg	Dog	IM SC	3–4 hours
	0.5 mg/kg loading dose, followed by 0.1–1.0 mg/kg/h	Dog	IM, slow IV IV	Duration of CRI*
	0.05–0.1 mg/kg	Cat	IM SC	3–4 hours
Meperidine	3–5 mg/kg	Dog/Cat	IM SC	1–2 hours
Methadone	0.1–0.5 mg/kg	Dog/Cat	IM SC	2–4 hours
Oxymorphone	0.05–0.1 mg/kg	Dog	IM IV SC	3–4 hours
	0.03–0.05 mg/kg	Cat	IM SC	3–4 hours
Hydromorphone	0.05–0.15 mg/kg	Dog Cat	IM IV SC IM SC	2–4 hours
Fentanyl	5 µg/kg +3–6 µg/kg/h 2–3 µg/kg +2–3 µg/kg/h	Dog Cat	IV IV	Duration of CRI*
Tramadol	1–6 mg/kg	Dog	Oral	6–12 hours
	1–2 mg/kg	Cat	Oral	12 hours
Butorphanol	0.1–0.2 mg/kg	Dog/Cat	IM IV SC	3–4 hours
	0.1–1.0 mg/kg	Dog/Cat	Oral	3–4 hours
Pentazocine	1–3 mg/kg	Dog/Cat	IM IV SC	2–4 hours
Nalbuphine	0.03–0.1 mg/kg	Dog/Cat	IM IV SC	2–4 hours
Buprenorphine	5–30 µg/kg	Dog/Cat	IM IV SC	8–12 hours
	5–30 µg/kg	Cat	Oral transmucosal	8–12 hours
Ketamine	1–2 mg/kg loading dose, followed by 1–2 mg/kg/h	Dog/Cat	IV	Duration of CRI*
Carprofen	2–4 mg/kg	Dog/Cat	Oral, IV or SC	6–12 hours
Ketorolac	0.25–0.3 mg/kg	Dog	IM IV	8–12 hours
Ketoprofen	2 mg/kg	Dog/Cat	IM IV SC	12–24 hours
Meloxicam	0.2 mg/kg	Dog/Cat	IV SC	24 hours

*Constant rate infusion

has received an opioid preoperatively. The intensity of the pain is likely to be at its greatest in the early part of recovery, so an opioid is usually recommended at this stage to cover this period (Table 4.3). Mu agonists, such as morphine, hydromorphone or oxymorphone, provide more intense analgesia than agonist/antagonists, such as butorphanol, or partial agonists such as buprenorphine; choice of opioid agent should be tailored to the degree of pain expected. The drug should be administered at such a time that it will reach peak effect by the time the animal is recovering. For most opioids, this means 10–15 minutes before the end of the procedure. The exception is buprenorphine, which should be given about 30 minutes before the end of the procedure, because it takes longer to reach its maximal effect. Further treatment beyond this initial period will depend on reassessing the animal periodically and administering further analgesics as needed. As indicated below, NSAIDs can be very useful as an adjunct to opioids. Ideally, a technique is chosen which will provide continuous analgesia. This might be a continuous infusion of an opioid, a transdermal administration system or, as indicated above, an opioid combined with an NSAID. Since there is a great deal of

variation from patient to patient in terms of response to opioids, it is important to reassess the patient frequently to ensure that the amounts and dose intervals used are appropriate. If local anesthetics have been used, the animal should also be monitored for signs of ongoing paralysis or self-mutilation.

With the new information about NMDA receptors and their role in central facilitation, there have been studies of existing NMDA antagonists such as ketamine and tiletamine for use in postoperative analgesia. Several studies in humans have examined ketamine as an analgesic. At low doses it can provide preemptive analgesia, and provides postoperative analgesia in some cases. There are still concerns over the hallucinogenic effects of the drug, and this has limited its use in humans. It may have a place for providing analgesia in combination with other drugs when they are individually ineffective. Intravenous infusions of ketamine have been used to provide analgesia for dogs and cats[64] (see Table 4.3), usually in combination with opioids.[65] The addition of ketamine to an opioid regimen has provided superior pain relief under some circumstances (e.g., burn patients).[66] Amantadine is a drug that was originally developed as an antiviral compound but it appears to have NMDA antagonist properties as well.[67] One clinical study in dogs with osteoarthritis showed efficacy with this drug at 3–5 mg/kg once daily.[68]

Gabapentin is another drug that is increasingly being used to manage perioperative and postoperative pain, especially chronic and/ or neuropathic pain.[69–71] Gabapentin is an analog of GABA, but it does not appear to act like GABA in the central nervous system. It is an antiepileptic drug that can also be used to manage pain in dogs and cats. The mechanism of action is thought to be inhibition of the alpha-2-delta subunits of voltage-gated calcium channels, which are related to signal transduction. Gabapentin is highly bioavailable, minimally protein-bound, and in dogs about 35% of the dose is metabolized in the liver to n-methylgabapentin and the rest is excreted unchanged by the kidneys.[72] The plasma half-life is 3–4 hours in dogs and 2.0–2.5 hours in cats.[73] Although it has been used with success in the perioperative period in humans[69] the only veterinary trial with gabapentin did not show any analgesic benefit.[74] Recommended oral doses start at 4–5 mg/kg BID (8–10 mg/kg BID or TID for severely painful patients). Doses in some animals may need to be escalated further (e.g., 60 mg/kg/day) to maintain comfort if the lower doses worked but pain has become more severe. The most common side effect is sedation, and this will usually abate within a few days; the dose can be reduced and then increased again as the animal begins to tolerate the drug. It is important to note that there may be some rebound pain if gabapentin is stopped abruptly, so patients receiving gabapentin should be weaned off the drug with gradually decreasing doses over 2–3 weeks.

Other antiepileptic drugs and antidepressants have also been found to be useful for the management of animal pain. Feline oral pain syndrome (FOPS), observed primarily in Burmese cats, has not responded well to traditional analgesics. The most successful pharmacological treatment of this syndrome has been the use of phenobarbital or diazepam.[75] The tricyclic antidepressants such as imipramine and amitryptyline have been useful adjuncts for neuropathic pain but very little is documented about their use in dogs and cats.[71]

Alpha-2 agonists are very effective analgesics. However, the marked sedation caused by alpha-2 agonists may limit their utility for the management of ongoing pain in small animals.[76] In some cases the degree of sedation provided by these drugs may be desirable. In cats recovering from extensive surgery it may be difficult to give enough opioid to provide analgesia without promoting further excitation. Dexmedetomidine at 0.5–2.5 µg/kg will often calm these cats enough for an uneventful recovery. Similarly, dexmedetomidine at low doses (0.5–1.5 µg/kg IV) may provide enough analgesia and sedation to improve the recovery of dogs displaying postoperative excitation or dysphoria.

Use of opioids for the maintenance of analgesia

Oral administration

Opioids are metabolized in the liver, which results in a significant loss of any orally administered opioid agent before it reaches the brain. Hydromorphone has a bioavailability of about 60% when given orally and can be a useful analgesic (0.2–0.6 mg/kg PO q6–8 h). Oxycodone is twice as potent as morphine with a 3–6-hour duration in humans. It appears to be effective in dogs at 0.3 mg/kg (increase if required) PO q 6–8 h and may be administered with a nonsteroidal antiinflammatory analgesic (personal communication, K. Mathews). Codeine appears to be a poor choice since it has an oral:parenteral ratio of 6.5% in dogs – about one tenth of that in humans.[77] In humans, about 10% of codeine is metabolized to morphine, and it is thought that most of the analgesic action of codeine comes from this conversion.

In the dog and cat less than 1.5% is converted to morphine and the intrinsic analgesic action of codeine is thought to be low.[78] However, in a tooth pulp assay in dogs, 4 mg/kg codeine SC was equivalent to about 0.15 mg/kg morphine.[79]

An oral sustained-release morphine has been studied in dogs and found to be absorbed over about 6 hours, with a 20% bioavailability. The terminal elimination half-life for this preparation was 8–10 hours, suggesting that it could be given twice a day at a dose of 2–5 mg/kg. It should be noted, however, that oral administration of the morphine was associated with vomiting in several dogs.[80,81] Methadone has a very low oral bioavailability in dogs with none detected in plasma after a 1.9 mg/kg oral dose.[82]

The author has also used oral butorphanol in dogs, assuming that the bioavailability is of the order of 20–30% (0.5–2 mg/kg). This has been given every 6–8 hours.

Recently, the transmucosal administration of buprenorphine has been described in cats and dogs.[83,84] At 20 µg/kg and a standard 0.3 mg/mL formulation, the resulting per-dose volume is very small, and the tasteless solution is well accepted by most patients. The drug is absorbed into the bloodstream through the mucosa and the reported bioavailability was >100% in cats and 38% in dogs.[83,84] An increase in thermal threshold was present from 30 to 360 minutes after administration in cats.[85]

Tramadol is being used with increasing frequency in canine and feline patients. This drug and its major metabolite (O-desmethyl-tramadol) have mu opioid activity, but also interact with serotonin and alpha-2 adrenergic receptors to produce analgesia. To date, it is not regarded as a drug of abuse and so is not a scheduled substance. The pharmacokinetics of the drug have been examined in the dog[86] and cat.[87,88] It is supplied as a 50-mg tablet and doses range from 1–6 mg/kg BID to QID for the dog and 1–2 mg/kg BID for the cat. Using thermal and mechanical threshold testing, one study was unable to show significant analgesic effects with tramadol (1 mg/kg) in cats[89] while a more comprehensive study of thermal thresholds showed a dose-related increase in threshold and duration.[90] With oral administration of 0.5–4 mg/kg the peak plasma concentration of tramadol occurred between 1 and 3 hours and the peak concentration of O-desmethyl-tramadol occurred between 1 and 4 hours. With doses above 2 mg/kg the increase in thermal threshold lasted for at least 6 hours.[90] In a clinical trial in cats undergoing ovariohysterectomy, tramadol was not much better than placebo but when combined with vedaprofen (an NSAID) it improved pain control.[91] A study in dogs undergoing maxillectomy or mandibulectomy compared tramadol, codeine and ketoprofen and combinations of the opioids with ketoprofen. According to the pain scoring system, the tramadol gave adequate analgesia but there were no significant differences between the treatment groups.[92]

Transdermal administration

Highly lipid-soluble drugs such as fentanyl can be absorbed through the skin, resulting in the development of transdermal delivery systems. The original transdermal patches consisted of a drug reservoir containing fentanyl, alcohol gelled together with hydroxyethyl cellulose and an ethylene-vinyl acetate copolymer membrane which controlled the rate of delivery of fentanyl to the skin. The newer patches have the fentanyl in the glue matrix so there is no reservoir. The original patches (Duragesic, Janssen Pharmaceutica Products, Titusville, NJ) are available in four sizes releasing fentanyl at the rate of 25, 50, 75 and 100 µg/h with surface areas of 10, 20, 30 and 40 cm², containing 2.5, 5, 7.5 and 10 mg of fentanyl, respectively. The matrix patches (Mylan Pharmaceuticals Inc., Morgantown, WV) are smaller (3.13, 6.25, 12.5, 18.75 and 25 cm² for the 12.5, 25, 50, 75 and 100 µg/kg/h patches, respectively).

Fentanyl is a schedule II drug and as such is subject to DEA regulation. Initially licensed for human cancer patients, fentanyl patches are labeled with an explicit warning that they are not for perioperative use. Since there are significant dangers to humans exposed to this drug, it is very important that veterinarians prescribing these patches for outpatients have an understanding of the environment in which the dog or cat is living. A young child could tear a patch off a pet and, by licking the patch or sticking it on himself/herself, be exposed to a fatal dose of fentanyl.[93] Additionally, deaths have been reported following attempts to inject fentanyl extracted from a patch.[94] It is therefore recommended that clients sign an 'informed consent' document stating that they understand the risks involved in bringing home a pet with a transdermal fentanyl delivery system in place.

Initial absorption of fentanyl is relatively slow and it takes approximately 6 to 24 hours to reach peak plasma concentrations in cats and dogs, respectively.[95-99] Once the peak value is obtained, the plasma concentrations remain fairly constant until removal of the patch (or until the reservoir runs out). In canine studies the patches have been removed at 72 hours, whereas in one feline study the patches were left on until 104 hours, with documented maintenance of plasma concentrations.[100] After removal of the patch, plasma concentrations decay more slowly than after intravenous administration because there is thought to be a reservoir of drug in the dermis which continues to be absorbed. In dogs it takes 2–12 hours for concentrations to decay below a therapeutic value.[95,97,101] Bioavailability of fentanyl delivered transdermally is high (>90%) and there appears to be little degradation of the drug by the skin or its microflora.[102] Several studies have demonstrated the effectiveness of the system as a contribution to postoperative analgesia in humans, but it is not being advocated as a sole approach to pain management.[101,103-105] In humans there have been a number of fatalities caused by heating the patch; this has occurred when a patient had been lying on a heating pad, which increases the rate of absorption of fentanyl from the patch. One study in dogs (22±7 kg) found comparable levels of analgesia after ovariohysterectomy between a fentanyl patch (50 μg/h) and oxymorphone (about 0.05 mg/kg IM as a preanesthetic and at 6,12 and 18 hours).[106] In two feline studies comparing fentanyl patches versus butorphanol following onychectomy there appeared to be some benefit in one study[96] but minimal difference in the second one.[107] In cats undergoing ovariohysterectomy the fentanyl patch treatment decreased the cortisol response but did not alter pain scores.[108]

Dose recommendations are:

Cats
    25–50 μg/h
Dogs
    3–10 kg = 25 μg/h
    10–20 kg = 50 μg/h
    20–30 kg = 75 μg/h
    >30 kg = 100 μg/h

When using the original patches it is extremely important not to cut them. The diffusion of fentanyl into the animal is limited by the membrane on the patch and direct exposure to the gel may cause rapid uptake. If it is necessary to use a smaller area, then the covering on the adhesive surface of the patch could be peeled back and cut so that part of it remains covering the adhesive, and only a half or a quarter of the patch is adhered to the skin.[109] With the matrix patches it is acceptable to cut them into smaller pieces, as the dose will be proportional to the size of patch applied. A variety of sites have been used for these patches but all of the above studies were carried out with the patches applied to the lateral thorax or the back of the neck. It is not clear how the uptake of the drug might be affected by sites on the back or the leg although it is likely that these other sites will work well. Before applying these patches, the skin should be gently cleaned with water

and allowed to dry. Soap or detergent should not be used as any residue may prevent the patch from sticking and will increase the likelihood of a skin reaction. If a detergent or alcohol is used these will remove oils from the skin and this may alter the uptake of this lipid-soluble drug. Once the area has been prepared, the patch is applied firmly and held for about 2 minutes. It is preferable to apply a bandage over the patch to decrease the likelihood of the patch being removed by a person or the animal. The bandage should be labeled with the size/dose of the patch and the time and date of application.

An Elizabethan collar (or equivalent) should be considered, as the animal may try to remove the patch, and ingestion of part or all of the patch could lead to a relative overdose.[110]

Local administration

Recently, it has been demonstrated that, in addition to central nervous system opioid receptors, there are opioid receptors on nociceptive nerve terminals which are activated by trauma or inflammation.[111] This knowledge has been put to use for treatment of human dental patients with the demonstration that morphine administered into inflamed tissue surrounding a dental lesion provided better analgesia than when it was not administered or when the same dose of morphine (1 mg) was administered subcutaneously.[112,113] The combination of local anesthetics and opioids has also provided prolonged postoperative analgesia in some instances. In one human study the addition of buprenorphine (7.5 μg/mL) to bupivacaine for intraoral nerve blocks increased the duration of postoperative analgesia from 8 to 28 hours without apparently prolonging the local anesthetic effect.[114] Other studies using local anesthetics and opioids given submucosally for dental procedures have not shown a difference with the addition of the opioid, but this may be related to dose or site of administration.[115,116]

Nonsteroidal antiinflammatory drugs (NSAIDs)

These drugs may be useful for perioperative analgesia for more minor procedures but they should be given preoperatively for maximal benefit. The peripheral action has been alluded to earlier and further evidence suggests that there is also a central action.[117,118] The cyclooxygenase enzymes involved in prostaglandin production have now been divided into two isoforms: cyclooxygenase 1 and 2 (COX-1, COX-2). COX-1 is constitutively expressed in many sites including the stomach, kidney and platelets, accounting for the most common side effects of COX-1 inhibitors – gastric ulceration,[119] renal pathosis and increased bleeding. COX-2 expression is increased during inflammation in many sites in the body but is also constitutively expressed in the kidneys and spinal cord, the latter supporting a role for COX-2 inhibition in acute pain. These discoveries suggest that drugs that have less activity on COX-1, the constitutive form, and more specificity for the induced COX-2 form, would be less likely to cause the side effects described above. An increased tendency to bleed during and after oral surgery is particularly important due to the vascularity of many oral structures. This is particularly relevant with aspirin since it binds irreversibly with platelets.[120] Other COX-1 inhibitors bind reversibly and their effect on platelets decreases as the plasma concentration of the drug decreases, so surgery can be carried out within 24 hours of discontinuing the drug in most cases.

Given this lack of life-threatening side effects, the use of COX-2 inhibitors in perioperative care is becoming more routine. However, the role of COX-2 in renal function suggests that animals that suffer from hypotension during anesthesia may be more at risk of renal pathosis if the drug has been given before the procedure. For this reason, together with the small benefit evident with

dobutamine, epinephrine, and phenylephrine in healthy anesthetized cats. Am J Vet Res 2006;67:1491–9.

44. Cabell LW, Perkowski SZ, Gregor T, et al. The effects of active peripheral skin warming on perioperative hypothermia in dogs. Vet Surg 1997;26:79–85.

45. Hale FA, Anthony JM. Prevention of hypothermia in cats during routine oral hygiene procedures. Can Vet J 1997;38: 297–9.

46. Chapman PJ, Ganendran A. Prolonged analgesia following preoperative bupivacaine neural blockade for oral surgery performed under general anesthesia. J Oral Maxillofac Surg 1987;45:233–5.

47. Gross ME, Pope ER, O'Brien D, et al. Regional anesthesia of the infraorbital and inferior alveolar nerves during noninvasive tooth pulp stimulation in halothane-anesthetized dogs. J Am Vet Med Assoc 1997;211:1403–5.

48. McLeod GA, Burke D. Levobupivacaine. Anaesthesia 2001;56:331–41.

49. Hirasawa Y, Katsumi Y, Kusswetter W, et al. Experimentelle Untersuchungen zur peripheren Nervenverletzung durch Injektionsnadeln. Reg Anesth 1990;13: 11–15.

50. Holland GR, Robinson PP. Evidence for the persistence of axons at the apex of the cat's lower canine tooth after section of the inferior alveolar nerve. Anat Rec 1984;208:175–83.

51. Beckman B, Legendre L. Regional nerve blocks for oral surgery in companion animals. Compend Contin Ed Pract Vet 2002;24:439–44.

52. Lantz GC. Regional anesthesia for dentistry and oral surgery. J Vet Dent 2003;20:181–6.

53. Gross ME, Pope ER, Jarboe JM, et al. Regional anesthesia of the infraorbital and inferior alveolar nerves during noninvasive tooth pulp stimulation in halothane-anesthetized cats. Am J Vet Res 2000;61:1245–7.

54. Gengler B. Pain Management for Dentistry. American College of Veterinary Internal Medicine Forum 2005.

55. Goldstein GS. Dental nerve blocks. Ontario Veterinary Medical Association 2010 Conference 2010;51–7.

56. Carmichael D. Using intraoral regional anesthetic nerve blocks. Vet Med 2004: 766–70.

57. Malamed SF. Management of Pain and Anxiety In: Cohen S,Burns RC, editor. Pathways of the Pulp. 8 ed. St Louis, MO: Mosby; 2002. p. 727–48.

58. Rochette J. Regional anesthesia and analgesia for oral and dental procedures. Vet Clin North Am Small Anim Pract 2005;35:1041–58, viii–ix.

59. Pashley EL, Nelson R, Pashley DH. Pressures created by dental injections. J Dent Res 1981;60:1742–8.

60. Pertot WJ, Dejou J. Bone and root resorption. Effects of the force developed during periodontal ligament injections in dogs. Oral Surg Oral Med Oral Pathol 1992;74:357–65.

61. Tagger E, Tagger M, Sarnat H, et al. Periodontal ligament injection in the dog primary dentition: Spread of local anaesthetic solution. Int J Paed Dent 1994;4:159–66.

62. Smith GN, Pashley DH. Periodontal ligament injection: evaluation of systemic effects. Oral Surg Oral Med Oral Pathol 1983;56:571–4.

63. Kim S, Edwall L, Trowbridge H, et al. Effects of local anesthetics on pulpal blood flow in dogs. J Dent Res 1984;63: 650–2.

64. Cairns BE, McErlane SA, Fragoso MC, et al. Tooth pulp- and facial hair mechanoreceptor-evoked responses of trigeminal sensory neurons are attenuated during ketamine anesthesia. Anesthesiology 1999;91:1025–35.

65. Wagner AE, Walton JA, Hellyer PW, et al. Use of low doses of ketamine administered by constant rate infusion as an adjunct for postoperative analgesia in dogs. J Am Vet Med Assoc 2002;221: 72–5.

66. Joubert K. Ketamine hydrochloride – an adjunct for analgesia in dogs with burn wounds. J South Afr Vet Med Assoc 1998; 69:95–7.

67. Blanpied TA, Clarke RJ, Johnson JW. Amantadine inhibits NMDA receptors by accelerating channel closure during channel block. J Neurosci 2005;25: 3312–22.

68. Lascelles BD, Gaynor JS, Smith ES, et al. Amantadine in a multimodal analgesic regimen for alleviation of refractory osteoarthritis pain in dogs. J Vet Intern Med 2008;22:53–9.

69. Ho KY, Gan TJ, Habib AS. Gabapentin and postoperative pain – a systematic review of randomized controlled trials. Pain 2006;126:91–101.

70. Wiffen PJ, McQuay HJ, Edwards JE, et al. Gabapentin for acute and chronic pain. Cochrane Database Syst Rev 2005: CD005452.

71. Cashmore RG, Harcourt-Brown TR, Freeman PM, et al. Clinical diagnosis and treatment of suspected neuropathic pain in three dogs. Aust Vet J 2009;87: 45–50.

72. Radulovic LL, Turck D, von Hodenberg A, et al. Disposition of gabapentin (neurontin) in mice, rats, dogs, and monkeys. Drug Metab Dispos 1995; 23:441–8.

73. Siao KT, Pypendop BH, Ilkiw JE. Pharmacokinetics of gabapentin in cats. Am J Vet Res 2010;71:817–21.

74. Wagner AE, Mich PM, Uhrig SR, et al. Clinical evaluation of perioperative administration of gabapentin as an adjunct for postoperative analgesia in dogs undergoing amputation of a forelimb. J Am Vet Med Assoc 2010;236: 751–6.

75. Rusbridge C, Heath S, Gunn-Moore DA, et al. Feline orofacial pain syndrome (FOPS): a retrospective study of 113 cases. J Feline Med Surg 2010;12: 498–508.

76. Ansah OB, Vainio O, Hellsten C, et al. Postoperative pain control in cats: Clinical trials with medetomidine and butorphanol. Vet Surg 2002;31:99–103.

77. Findlay JW, Jones EC, Welch RM. Radioimmunoassay determination of the absolute oral bioavailabilities and O-demethylation of codeine and hydrocodone in the dog. Drug Metab Dispos 1979;7:310–4.

78. Yeh SY, Woods LA. Excretion of codeine and its metabolites by dogs, rabbits and cats. Arch Int Pharmacodyn Ther 1971; 191:231–42.

79. Skingle M, Hayes AG, Tyers MB. Effects of opiates on urine output in the water-loaded rat and reversal by beta-funaltrexamine. Neuropeptides 1985;5: 433–6.

80. Dohoo S, Tasker R. Pharmacokinetics of oral morphine sulfate in dogs: a comparison of sustained release and conventional formulations. Can J Vet Res 1997;61X:251–255X.

81. Dohoo S, Tasker R, Donald A. Pharmacokinetics of parenteral and oral sustained-release morphine sulphate in dogs. J Vet Pharmacol Ther 1994;17X: 426–433X.

82. Kukanich B, Lascelles BD, Aman AM, et al. The effects of inhibiting cytochrome P450 3A, p-glycoprotein, and gastric acid secretion on the oral bioavailability of methadone in dogs. J Vet Pharmacol Ther 2005;28:461–6.

83. Abbo LA, Ko JC, Maxwell LK, et al. Pharmacokinetics of buprenorphine following intravenous and oral transmucosal administration in dogs. Vet Ther 2008;9:83–93.

84. Robertson SA, Lascelles BD, Taylor PM, et al. PK-PD modeling of buprenorphine in cats: intravenous and oral transmucosal administration. J Vet Pharmacol Ther 2005;28:453–60.

85. Lascelles BDX, Roberston SA, Taylor PM. Comparison of the pharmacokinetics and thermal antinociceptive pharmacodynamics of 20 µg kg^{-1} buprenorphine administered sublingually or intravenously in cats. Vet Anaesth Analg 2003;30:100–20.

86. KuKanich B, Papich MG. Pharmacokinetics of tramadol and the metabolite O-desmethyltramadol in dogs. J Vet Pharmacol Ther 2004;27: 239–46.

87. Cagnardi P, Villa R, Zonca A, et al. Pharmacokinetics, intraoperative effect

and postoperative analgesia of tramadol in cats. Res Vet Sci 2010.

88. Pypendop BH, Ilkiw JE. Pharmacokinetics of tramadol, and its metabolite O-desmethyl-tramadol, in cats. J Vet Pharmacol Ther 2008;31: 52–9.

89. Steagall PV, Taylor PM, Brondani JT, et al. Antinociceptive effects of tramadol and acepromazine in cats. J Feline Med Surg 2008;10:24–31.

90. Pypendop BH, Siao KT, Ilkiw JE. Effects of tramadol hydrochloride on the thermal threshold in cats. Am J Vet Res 2009;70:1465–70.

91. Brondani JT, Luna SP, Marcello GC, et al. Perioperative administration of vedaprofen, tramadol or their combination does not interfere with platelet aggregation, bleeding time and biochemical variables in cats. J Feline Med Surg 2009;11:503–9.

92. Martins TL, Kahvegian MA, Noel-Morgan J, et al. Comparison of the effects of tramadol, codeine, and ketoprofen alone or in combination on postoperative pain and on concentrations of blood glucose, serum cortisol, and serum interleukin-6 in dogs undergoing maxillectomy or mandibulectomy. Am J Vet Res 2010;71: 1019–26.

93. Hardwick W, King W, Palmisano P. Respiratory depression in a child unintentionally exposed to transdermal fentanyl patch. South Med J 1997; 90:962–4.

94. Marquardt K, Tharratt R. Inhalation abuse of fentanyl patch. J Toxicol Clin Toxicol 1994;32:75–8.

95. Egger CM, Duke T, Archer J, et al. Comparison of plasma fentanyl concentrations by using three transdermal fentanyl patch sizes in dogs. Vet Surg 1998;27:159–66.

96. Franks JN, Boothe HW, Taylor L, et al. Evaluation of transdermal fentanyl patches for analgesia in cats undergoing onychectomy. J Am Vet Med Assoc 2000; 217:1013–20.

97. Kyles AE, Papich M, Hardie EM. Disposition of transdermally administered fentanyl in dogs. Am J Vet Res 1996;57:715–19.

98. Scherk-Nixon M. A study of the use of a transdermal fentanyl patch in cats. J Am Anim Hosp Assoc 1996;32:19–24.

99. Schultheiss PJ, Morse BC, Baker WH. Evaluation of a transdermal fentanyl system in the dog. Contemporary Topics 1995;34:75–81.

100. Yackey M, Ilkiw JE, Pascoe PJ, et al. Effect of transdermally administered fentanyl on the minimum alveolar concentration of isoflurane in cats. Vet Anaesth Analg 2004;31:183–9.

101. Gourlay GK, Kowalski SR, Plummer JL, et al. The efficacy of transdermal fentanyl in the treatment of postoperative pain:

a double-blind comparison of fentanyl and placebo systems. Pain 1990;40: 21–8.

102. Varvel JR, Shafer SL, Hwang SS, et al. Absorption characteristics of transdermally administered fentanyl. Anesthesiology 1989;70:928–34.

103. Caplan RA, Ready LB, Oden RV, et al. Transdermal fentanyl for postoperative pain management. A double-blind placebo study. JAMA 1989;261:1036–9.

104. Gourlay GK, Kowalski SR, Plummer JL, et al. The transdermal administration of fentanyl in the treatment of postoperative pain: pharmacokinetics and pharmacodynamic effects. Pain 1989;37:193–202.

105. Latasch L, Luders S. Transdermal fentanyl against postoperative pain. Acta Anaesthesiol Belg 1989;40:113–19.

106. Kyles AE, Hardie EM, Hansen BD, et al. Comparison of transdermal fentanyl and intramuscular oxymorphone on post-operative behaviour after ovariohysterectomy in dogs. Res Vet Sci 1998;65:245–51.

107. Gellasch KL, Kruse-Elliott KT, Osmond CS, et al. Comparison of transdermal administration of fentanyl versus intramuscular administration of butorphanol for analgesia after onychectomy in cats. J Am Vet Med Assoc 2002;220:1020–4.

108. Glerum LE, Egger CM, Allen SW, et al. Analgesic effect of the transdermal fentanyl patch during and after feline ovariohysterectomy. Vet Surg 2001;30: 351–8.

109. Davidson CD, Pettifer GR, Henry JD, Jr. Plasma fentanyl concentrations and analgesic effects during full or partial exposure to transdermal fentanyl patches in cats. J Am Vet Med Assoc 2004;224: 700–5.

110. Schmiedt CW, Bjorling DE. Accidental prehension and suspected transmucosal or oral absorption of fentanyl from a transdermal patch in a dog. Vet Anaesth Analg 2007;34:70–3.

111. Stein C. Peripheral mechanisms of opioid analgesia. Anesth Analg 1993; 76:182–91.

112. Dionne RA, Lepinski AM, Gordon SM, et al. Analgesic effects of peripherally administered opioids in clinical models of acute and chronic inflammation. Clin Pharmacol Ther 2001;70:66–73.

113. Likar R, Koppert W, Blatnig H, et al. Efficacy of peripheral morphine analgesia in inflamed, non-inflamed and perineural tissue of dental surgery patients. J Pain Symptom Manage 2001;21:330–7.

114. Modi M, Rastogi S, Kumar A. Buprenorphine with bupivacaine for intraoral nerve blocks to provide postoperative analgesia in outpatients after minor oral surgery. J Oral Maxillofac Surg 2009;67:2571–6.

115. Bhananker SM, Azavedo LF, Splinter WM. Addition of morphine to local anesthetic infiltration does not improve analgesia after pediatric dental extractions. Paediatr Anaesth 2008;18:140–4.

116. Rattan V, Arora S, Grover VK. Assessment of the effectiveness of peripheral administration of fentanyl with lidocaine in inflamed dentoalveolar tissues. Int J Oral Maxillofac Surg 2007;36:128–31.

117. Shyu KW, Lin MT. Hypothalamic monoaminergic mechanisms of aspirin-induced analgesia in monkeys. J Neural Transm 1985;62:285–93.

118. Willer JC, De Broucker T, Bussel B, et al. Central analgesic effect of ketoprofen in humans: electrophysiological evidence for a supraspinal mechanism in a double-blind and cross-over study. Pain 1989;38:1–7.

119. Wallace MS, Zawie DA, Garvey MS. Gastric ulceration in the dog secondary to the use of nonsteroidal antiinflammatory drugs. J Am Anim Hosp Assoc 1990;26:467–71.

120. Rackear DG. Drugs that alter the hemostatic mechanism. Vet Clin North Am Small Anim Pract 1988;18:67–77.

121. Holtsinger RH, Parker RB, Beale BS, et al. The therapeutic efficacy of carprofen (Rimadyl-V™) in 209 clinical cases of canine degenerative joint disease. Vet Comp Orth Traum 1992;5:140–4.

122. Lascelles BD, Cripps PJ, Jones A, et al. Efficacy and kinetics of carprofen, administered preoperatively or postoperatively, for the prevention of pain in dogs undergoing ovariohysterectomy. Vet Surg 1998;27:568–82.

123. Nolan A, Reid J. Comparison of the postoperative analgesic and sedative effects of carprofen and papaveretum in the dog. Vet Rec 1993;133:240–2.

124. Balmer TV, Irvine D, Jones RS, et al. Comparison of carprofen and pethidine as postoperative analgesics in the cat. J Small Anim Pract 1998;39:158–64.

125. Mathews KA, Paley DM, Foster RA, et al. A comparison of ketorolac with flunixin, butorphanol, and oxymorphone in controlling postoperative pain in dogs. Can Vet J 1996;37:557–67.

126. Mathews KA. Nonsteroidal anti-inflammatory analgesics in pain management in dogs and cats. Can Vet J 1996;37:539–45.

127. Pibarot P, Dupuis J, Grisneaux E, et al. Comparison of ketoprofen, oxymorphone hydrochloride, and butorphanol in the treatment of postoperative pain in dogs. J Am Vet Med Assoc 1997;211:438–44.

128. Budsberg SC, Johnston SA, Schwarz PD, et al. Efficacy of etodolac for the treatment of osteoarthritis of the hip joints in dogs. J Am Vet Med Assoc 1999;214:206–10.

129. Panciera DL, Johnston SA. Results of thyroid function tests and concentrations of plasma proteins in dogs administered etodolac. Am J Vet Res 2002;63:1492–5.

130. Inoue T, Ko JCH, Mandsager RE, et al. Analgesic effect of pre-operative etodolac and butorphanol administration in dogs undergoing overiohysterectomy. Vet Anaesth Analg 2003;30:110–11.

131. Nell T, Bergman J, Hoeijmakers M, et al. Comparison of vedaprofen and meloxicam in dogs with musculoskeletal pain and inflammation. J Small Anim Pract 2002;43:208–12.

132. Lascelles BD, Henderson AJ, Hackett IJ. Evaluation of the clinical efficacy of meloxicam in cats with painful locomotor disorders. J Small Anim Pract 2001;42:587–93.

133. Doig PA, Purbrick KA, Hare JE, et al. Clinical efficacy and tolerance of meloxicam in dogs with chronic osteoarthritis. Can Vet J 2000;41: 296–300.

134. Budsberg SC, Cross AR, Quandt JE, et al. Evaluation of intravenous administration of meloxicam for perioperative pain management following stifle joint surgery in dogs. Am J Vet Res 2002;63:1557–63.

135. Mathews KA, Pettifer G, Foster R, et al. Safety and efficacy of preoperative administration of meloxicam, compared with that of ketoprofen and butorphanol in dogs undergoing abdominal surgery. Am J Vet Res 2001;62:882–8.

136. Lafuente MP, Franch J, Durall I, et al. Comparison between meloxicam and transdermally administered fentanyl for treatment of postoperative pain in dogs undergoing osteotomy of the tibia and fibula and placement of a uniplanar external distraction device. J Am Vet Med Assoc 2005;227:1768–74.

137. Gunew MN, Menrath VH, Marshall RD. Long-term safety, efficacy and palatability of oral meloxicam at 0.01–0.03 mg/kg for treatment of osteoarthritic pain in cats. J Feline Med Surg 2008;10:235–41.

138. Busch U, Schmid J, Heinzel G, et al. Pharmacokinetics of meloxicam in animals and the relevance to humans. Drug Metab Dispos 1998;26:576–84.

139. Murison PJ, Tacke S, Wondratschek C, et al. Postoperative analgesic efficacy of meloxicam compared to tolfenamic acid in cats undergoing orthopaedic surgery. J Small Anim Pract 2010.

140. Smith SA. Deracoxib. Compend Contin Ed Pract Vet 2003;25:452–5.

141. Lascelles BD, Blikslager AT, Fox SM, et al. Gastrointestinal tract perforation in dogs treated with a selective cyclooxygenase-2 inhibitor: 29 cases (2002–3). J Am Vet Med Assoc 2005;227:1112–17.

142. Case JB, Fick JL, Rooney MB. Proximal duodenal perforation in three dogs following deracoxib administration. J Am Anim Hosp Assoc 2010;46: 255–8.

143. Hanson PD, Brooks KC, Case J, et al. Efficacy and safety of firocoxib in the management of canine osteoarthritis under field conditions. Vet Ther 2006; 7:127–40.

144. Ryan WG, Moldave K, Carithers D. Clinical effectiveness and safety of a new NSAID, firocoxib: a 1,000 dog study. Vet Ther 2006;7:119–26.

145. Bosmans T, Gasthuys F, Duchateau L, et al. A comparison of tepoxalin-buprenorphine combination and buprenorphine for postoperative analgesia in dogs: a clinical study. J Vet Med A Physiol Pathol Clin Med 2007; 54:364–9.

146. Clark TP. The clinical pharmacology of cyclooxygenase-2-selective and dual inhibitors. Vet Clin North Am Small Anim Pract 2006;36:1061–85, vii.

147. Curry SL, Cogar SM, Cook JL. Nonsteroidal antiinflammatory drugs: a review. J Am Anim Hosp Assoc 2005;41:298–309.

148. Lascelles BD, McFarland JM, Swann H. Guidelines for safe and effective use of NSAIDs in dogs. Vet Ther 2005;6: 237–51.

149. Lascelles BD, Court MH, Hardie EM, et al. Nonsteroidal anti-inflammatory drugs in cats: a review. Vet Anaesth Analg 2007;34:228–50.

150. Nagatsuka C, Ichinohe T, Kaneko Y. Preemptive effects of a combination of preoperative diclofenac, butorphanol, and lidocaine on postoperative pain management following orthognathic surgery. Anesthesia Progress 2000;47:119–24.

151. Chang DJ, Fricke JR, Bird SR, et al. Rofecoxib versus codeine/acetaminophen in postoperative dental pain: a double-blind, randomized, placebo- and active comparator-controlled clinical trial. Clin Ther 2001;23:1446–55.

Chapter 5

Enteral nutritional support

Stanley L. Marks

THERAPEUTIC DECISION-MAKING

Rationale for enteral nutritional support

Enteral feeding is indicated in patients who cannot ingest adequate amounts of calories, but have sufficient gastrointestinal function to allow digestion and absorption of feeding solutions delivered into the gastrointestinal tract via an enteral feeding device. The rationale for prescribing enteral nutrition rather than parenteral nutrition (TPN) is based on the superior maintenance of intestinal structure and function, safety of administration, and reduced cost of enteral alimentation. The average daily cost of TPN for maintaining the caloric requirements of a 20-kg dog at the University of California, Davis, Veterinary Medical Teaching Hospital, is US$50.00 (excluding catheter costs) compared with US$5.00 for a commercial liquid enteral formula (Hill's Prescription diet® a/d, Hill's Pet Nutrition, Topeka, KS), and US$3.00 for a commercial canned diet (Hill's Prescription diet® canine p/d, Hill's Pet Nutrition, Topeka, KS). The most important stimulus for mucosal cell proliferation is the direct presence of nutrients in the intestinal lumen. Bowel rest due to starvation or administration of TPN leads to villous atrophy, increased intestinal permeability, and a reduction in intestinal disaccharidase activities.[1,2] Prolonged fasting in the stressed, critically ill patient can lead to intestinal barrier failure and increased permeability to bacteria and endotoxins.

Patient selection for nutritional support

Efforts to assess nutritional status, and attempts to decide whether nutritional support is required on the basis of a single biochemical measurement or body weight determination are simplistic and of limited value. Objective methods of assessing nutritional status such as body composition measurement (anthropometry, impedance measurements, dual energy X-ray absorptiometry) are still in their infancy in veterinary medicine, with the result that a subjective global assessment of the patient's nutritional status needs to be performed. This technique is based on easily collected historical information (changes in oral intake, degree of weight loss, presence of vomiting or diarrhea) and changes found on physical examination (muscle wasting, body condition, and presence of edema or ascites). Although body weight is routinely determined in sick animals, it is important to appreciate its limitations. One cannot equate the appearance of the animal with its state of nourishment because body weight does not differentiate between fat, lean tissue, and extracellular water. Determination of the animal's serum albumin concentration and total lymphocyte count are insensitive determinants of nutritional status because of the large number of disease processes that influence these parameters unrelated to the effects of malnutrition. Nutritional support should be considered for animals demonstrating recent weight loss exceeding 10% of optimal body weight or for those whose oral intake has been or will be interrupted for more than 5 days. Animals with increased nutrient losses from chronic diarrhea or vomiting, wounds, renal disease, or burns should also be considered for nutritional support. Specific maxillofacial indications include long-term mouth closure, less-than-optimal fracture fixation, multiple fractures and major oral tumor resections. Postoperative inappetence is especially common in cats with maxillofacial trauma or surgical procedures involving the nasal cavity, and these patients greatly benefit from enteral nutritional support.

ENTERAL FEEDING ACCESS DEVICES

Most feeding tubes today are made of polyurethane or silicone. These materials have tended to replace the older polyvinylchloride feeding tubes that tend to stiffen when exposed to digestive juices and are more irritating to patients, necessitating frequent tube replacement. Silicone is softer and more flexible than other tube materials with a greater tendency to stretch and collapse. Polyurethane is stronger than silicone, allowing for a tube of this material to have thinner walls and thus a larger internal diameter, despite the same French size.[3] The flexibility and decreased internal diameter of silicone tubes may lead to clogging or kinking of the tube.[4] Both polyurethane and silicone do not rapidly disintegrate or embrittle in situ, providing a longer 'wear'. The French (F) unit measures the outer lumen diameter of a tube (one French unit is equal to 0.33 mm). Tubes that are too flexible may be chilled before placement to increase stiffness.

© 2012 Elsevier Ltd
DOI: 10.1016/B978-0-7020-4618-6.00005-1

Nasoesophageal tubes

Nasoesophageal tubes are a simple and efficient choice for the short-term (less than 10 days) nutritional support of most anorectic hospitalized animals that have a normal nasal cavity, pharynx, esophagus, and stomach.[5,6] Nasoesophageal tube feeding is contraindicated in animals that are vomiting, comatose, or lack a gag reflex; it is also contraindicated with maxillary fractures. Polyvinylchloride (Infant Feeding Tube, Argyle Division of Sherwood Medical, St. Louis, MO) or red rubber tubes (Sovereign Feeding Tube, Monoject Division of Sherwood Medical, St. Louis, MO) are the least expensive tubes for dogs and cats, although the polyvinylchloride tubes may harden within 2 weeks of insertion and cause irritation or ulceration of the pharynx or esophagus. Tubes made of polyurethane (MILA International, Inc., Florence, KY) or silicone (Global Veterinary Products, Inc., New Buffalo, MI) are more expensive; however, they are less irritating and more resistant to gastric acid, allowing prolonged usage. An 8–10 F by 109 cm (43 inch) tube (preferably with a guide wire) is suitable for dogs weighing more than 15 kg. A 5–8 F by 56–109 cm (22–43 inch) tube is recommended for dogs weighing less than 15 kg and for cats.

The length of tube to be inserted into the distal esophagus is determined by measuring the distance from the tip of the nose to the eighth or ninth rib. This will help verify the correct placement of the tube in the distal esophagus rather than the stomach, and decrease the likelihood of reflux esophagitis.[7] Desensitization of the nasal cavity with four or five drops of 0.5% proparacaine hydrochloride is recommended. The tube tip should be lubricated with a water-soluble lubricant or 5% lidocaine ointment to facilitate passage. The tube is passed by maintaining the animal's head in the normal angle of articulation and gently directing the tip of the tube in a ventromedial direction. The tube should move with minimal resistance through the ventral meatus and nasopharynx and into the esophagus. In dogs, the presence of a small ventral ridge at the proximal end of the nasal passage necessitates directing the tip of the tube dorsally initially to allow passage over the ventral ridge and into the nasal vestibule (Fig. 5.1).[5] Nasoesophageal intubation is more difficult to perform in dogs because of their long, narrow nasal passages and extensive turbinate structures. In the dog, the tube is directed in a ventromedial direction while pushing the external nares dorsally.[8] This maneuver opens the ventral meatus and guides the tube into the oropharynx.

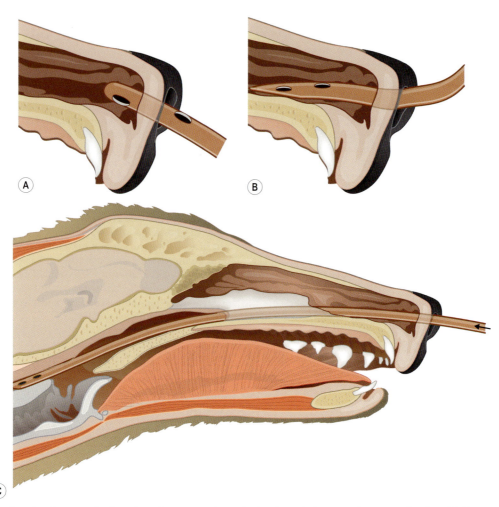

Fig. 5.1 Parasagittal section showing stepwise insertion of a nasoesophageal tube through the ventral meatus of a dog: (**A**) The presence of a small ventral ridge at the rostral end of the nasal passage necessitates directing the tip of the tube dorsally to clear the protuberance; (**B**) Once past the protuberance, the tube is aimed medially and ventrally and advanced into the ventral meatus; (**C**) Tube through ventral meatus and nasal pharynx (NP). Structures identified: nasal vestibule (NV), cartilaginous septum (CS), maxilla (M), dorsal meatus (DM), middle meatus (MM), ethmoidal conchae (EC), ventral nasal conchae (VNC), dorsal nasal conchae (DNC), and alar fold (AF). *(After Crowe DT. Clinical use of an indwelling nasogastric tube for enteral nutrition and fluid therapy in the dog sand cat. J Am Anim Hosp Assoc 1986;22: 675–682.)*

If the tube is unable to be passed with minimal resistance into the oropharynx, it should be withdrawn and redirected because it could be positioned in the middle meatus with its tip encountering the ethmoid turbinate. Once the tube has been passed to the level of the attached 'butterfly' tape, it should be secured as close to the nostril as possible, with either suture material or glue (Superglue, Loctite Corp., Cleveland, OH). A second tape tab should be secured to the skin on the dorsal midline between the eyes (Fig. 5.2). An Elizabethan collar is usually required for dogs to prevent inadvertent tube removal; however, most cats do not require such a device. Removal of the tube is facilitated by clipping the hair that is attached to the glue.

After placement, the tube position is checked by injecting 5–10 mL of air while auscultating the cranial abdomen for borborygmi, or by infusing 3–5 mL of sterile saline or water through the tube and

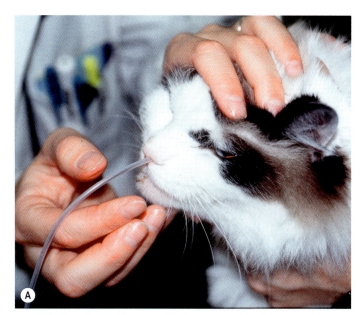

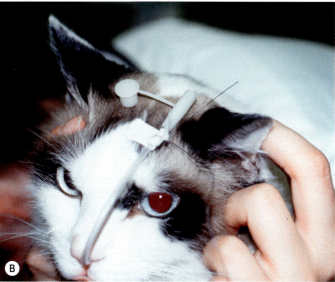

Fig. 5.2 (**A**) The tip of the nasoesophageal tube has been lubricated and passed into the ventral meatus by positioning the animal's head in a normal angle of articulation; (**B**) The nasoesophageal tube can be secured to the skin on the dorsal midline between the eyes with tape 'butterflies.' A second tape tab should be secured as close to the nostril as possible, with either suture material or glue.

observing for a cough response.[5] Confirmation of correct tube placement can also be obtained by obtaining a lateral survey thoracic radiograph and observing the position of the radiopaque tube in the esophagus. The most common complications associated with the use of nasoesophageal tubes include epistaxis, dacrocystitis, rhinitis, tracheal intubation and secondary pneumonia, and vomiting.[5]

A major disadvantage of nasoesophageal feeding tubes is their small diameter, necessitating the use of liquid enteral formulas. Commercially available canned pet foods that are diluted with water will invariably clog the feeding tube. The caloric density of most human and veterinary liquid enteral formulas varies from 1.0 to 1.5 kcal/mL. Diets are fed full strength on continuous (pump infusion) or bolus feeding schedules.

Pharyngostomy tubes

The increasing availability of endoscopic equipment and the advantages of esophagostomy and percutaneous gastrostomy tube placement have resulted in pharyngostomy tubes becoming virtually obsolete. Nevertheless, the introduction of placement modifications has resulted in a dramatic reduction in complications associated with the interference of epiglottic movement and partial laryngeal obstruction.[9,10] The indications for pharyngostomy tube placement are similar to those for nasoesophageal tube placement; however, the procedure requires general anesthesia (see Ch. 57).

Esophagostomy tubes

Esophagostomy feeding tubes are easily inserted, and insertion only requires light general anesthesia with isoflurane or heavy sedation, and intubation with a cuffed endotracheal tube. The technique is minimally invasive and no specialized endoscopic equipment is needed. The patient should be placed in right lateral recumbency, and the left lateral cervical region clipped and aseptically prepared for tube placement.[11-13] A 14–20-F red rubber catheter (Sovereign Feeding Tube, Monoject Division of Sherwood Medical, St. Louis, MO), silicone catheter (Global Veterinary Products, Inc., New Buffalo, MI), or polyurethane catheter (MILA International, Inc., Florence, KY) should be premeasured from the mid-cervical esophagus to the eighth rib, and marked with a permanent marker to ensure the distal end of the catheter terminates in the distal esophagus.[7] Three basic techniques for placement of a midcervical esophagostomy tube have been described.[11-13]

Technique using curved Rochester–Carmalt, Mixter, or Schnidt forceps

Advance the right-angle forceps into the mid-cervical esophagus from the oral cavity. Use the angle of the jaw and the point of the shoulder for landmarks to help ensure that the tip of the forceps can be palpated externally in the mid-cervical region. Push the curved tips of the Rochester–Carmalt forceps laterally at the mid-cervical esophagus, so they can be palpated below the skin. Use a number 11 scalpel blade to make a stab incision through the skin only, exposing the subcutaneous tissue and muscle layers of the esophagus. Be careful to avoid the jugular and maxillofacial veins when selecting the stoma site. Exteriorize the tip of the forceps from the esophageal lumen through the skin incision. Guide the advancing forceps through the esophageal muscle layers and carefully dissect the esophageal mucosa off the tip of the forceps with a scalpel blade. Use the tip of the forceps to grasp the distal end of the feeding tube, and draw the tube out of the oral cavity. Secure the distal end of the feeding tube using the forceps to ensure that the tube remains exteriorized while the proximal end of the tube is pulled out of the animal's mouth. Retroflex the proximal tip of the feeding tube and advance it in an aboral direction across the pharynx and down the esophagus, while slowly retracting on the external end of the tube 20–40 mm. A wire guide can be used to facilitate pushing the proximal tip of the feeding tube into the esophagus. The exteriorized portion of the tube will be observed to rotate in a cranial direction as the tube moves down the esophagus, indicating correct placement of the tube in the esophagus. Retention sutures (Chinese finger-trap suture) using 3–0 polypropylene are used to secure the distal end of the tube to the skin. An additional method of securing the tube involves passing a heavy suture on a tapered needle through the skin next to the tube and into the periosteum of the wing of the atlas. Antibiotic ointment and gauze dressing is placed at the incision site, and the tube and entrance site is loosely bandaged with conforming gauze wrap. The correct placement of the tube in the mid-to-distal esophagus should be confirmed radiographically. It is important to ensure that the tube does not traverse the lower esophageal sphincter, as the tube can cause irritation, and predispose the patient to vomiting and gastroesophageal reflux. Feeding can be instituted immediately following full recovery of the patient from anesthesia. The tube esophagostomy–skin interface should be examined at least daily during the first week for evidence of infection or leakage of food or saliva. The stoma site can be kept clean with a topical antiseptic solution (1 : 100 povidone-iodine solution in 0.9% saline). The tube can easily be removed once nutritional support is no longer needed by cutting the Chinese finger-trap anchoring suture and pulling the tube. The wound should be allowed to heal by second intention.

Percutaneous feeding tube applicator technique

An alternative tube esophagostomy technique utilizing an ELD percutaneous feeding tube applicator (Jorgensen Laboratories, Loveland, CO) or similar device can be used.[13] The applicator is inserted into the mid-cervical esophagus via the oral cavity. The distal tip is palpated, and an incision is made through the skin and subcutaneous tissue over the tip of the ELD. The trocar is advanced through the esophageal wall and directed through the incision. The distal end of the feeding tube is secured to the eyelet of the trocar with suture material. The ELD device and attached feeding tube are retracted into the esophagus and exteriorized out of the oral cavity. The feeding tube is redirected into the mid-cervical esophagus after inserting a wire stylet into the distal tip of the feeding tube. The tube is secured to the skin as mentioned above.

Percutaneous needle catheter technique

This method incorporates the use of an esophagostomy introduction tube (Van Noort oesophagostomy tube set, Global Veterinary Products, Inc., New Buffalo, MI) that is introduced into the mid-cervical esophageal area (Fig. 5.3). The slot in the distal portion of the tube is palpated, and a Peel-away® sheath needle (Global Veterinary Products, Inc., New Buffalo, MI) is introduced into the distal portion of the tube. The needle is removed from the sheath, and a 10-F catheter is introduced through the sheath to the distal third of the esophagus. The sheath is peeled away and the esophagostomy tube is carefully removed. The feeding tube is secured as described above. This technique has limitations as the small diameter of the feeding tube (10 F) only allows for the administration of fluids and liquid enteral formulas.

Complications

Despite the potential for esophageal scarring and stricture formation, esophageal stricture or a persistent esophagocutaneous fistula has not developed. The most common minor complication is peristomal

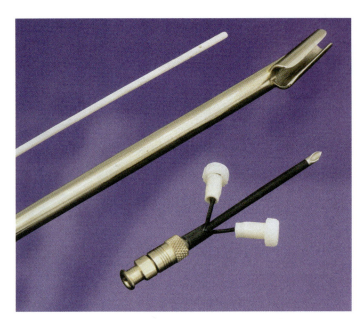

Fig. 5.3 An esophagostomy tube set, illustrating the esophagostomy introduction tube, 10-gauge, 50-mm-long needle with Peel-away® sheath needle, and a 10-French silicone catheter.

inflammation, with peristomal abscessation occurring infrequently.[11–14] Most of the inflammatory reactions are mild and respond to thorough cleansing with topical antibiotics. Other less common complications include regurgitation of the tube into the oral cavity and tube obstruction.[11–14]

Gastrostomy tubes

Gastrostomy tube feeding is indicated for long-term (weeks to months) nutritional support of anorectic or dysphagic animals. Gastrostomy feeding tubes are of comparatively large diameter (20–24 F), allowing the economic use of blended pet foods and the direct administration of medications. Gastrostomy tube feeding is contraindicated in animals with persistent vomiting, decreased consciousness, or gastrointestinal obstruction. Caution should be exercised in conditions under which the stomach cannot be apposed to the body wall (severe ascites, adhesions, space-occupying lesions).

Gastrostomy tubes can be placed percutaneously or during laparotomy. Placement is usually accompanied via a percutaneous endoscopic gastrostomy (PEG) technique, or a blind percutaneous gastrostomy (BPG) technique.[15–18] There are a variety of feeding tubes that can be utilized for gastrostomy feeding including latex (Bard Urological Division, Murray Hill, NJ), polyurethane (MILA International, Inc., Florence, KY), and silicon (Global Veterinary Products, Inc., New Buffalo, MI; US Endoscopy, Mentor, OH) tubes with French–Pezzer mushroom, balloon, bumper, or silicone dome tips (Fig. 5.4). One can modify the catheters by cutting off and discarding the flared open end of the catheter and cutting off two 20-mm pieces of tubing (to be used as internal and external flanges) from the same end of the catheter. The end of the catheter opposite the mushroom tip is trimmed to facilitate its introduction into the larger opening of a disposable plastic micropipette. Make a small stab incision through the center of each flange and fit one flange over the cut end of the catheter, sliding it down until it rests against the mushroom tip. The other 20-mm piece of tubing will be used as an external flange that lies against the abdominal wall. It is not recommended to cut the small nipple on the mushroom tip to enhance the flow of food

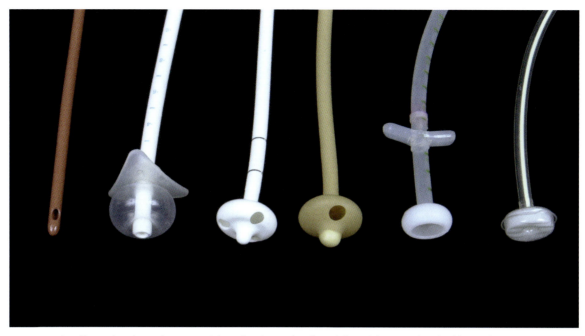

Fig. 5.4 Gastrostomy tubes illustrating the various materials and catheter tips; from left to right: French red rubber catheter, silicone balloon catheter, silicone mushroom catheter, latex mushroom catheter, silicone catheter with dome, polyurethane catheter with bumper.

through the tube. Removing the tip of the mushroom compromises the integrity of the mushroom and hinders percutaneous removal of the tube.

Percutaneous endoscopic gastrostomy (PEG) technique

Endoscopic and blind placement of gastrostomy tubes necessitates brief anesthesia. The animal should be placed in right lateral recumbency so that the stomach tube can be placed through the greater curvature of the stomach and the left body wall. Patient preparation for both percutaneous procedures is identical and involves a surgical preparation of the skin caudal to the left costal arch. The endoscope is introduced into the stomach and the stomach is carefully inflated until the abdomen is distended but not drum tight. The left body wall is transilluminated with the endoscope to ensure that the spleen is not positioned between the stomach and body wall. An appropriate site for insertion of the tube is determined by endoscopically monitoring digital palpation of the gastric wall. A small incision is made in the skin with a scalpel blade, and an intravenous catheter (16–18G, 38–51 mm) is stabbed through the body wall into the lumen of the stomach (Fig. 5.5A). The stylet is removed and nylon or polyester suture is threaded through the catheter into the lumen of the stomach. The suture material is grasped with the endoscopic biopsy forceps (Fig. 5.5B), and the endoscope and forceps are carefully withdrawn through the esophagus and out of the mouth. The suture material is secured to the feeding tube and gentle traction is applied to the suture material at its point of exit from the abdominal wall (Fig. 5.5C). The feeding tube is pulled out through the body wall, allowing the mushroom end to draw the stomach wall against the body wall (Fig. 5.5D). The feeding tube is anchored in this position by the external flange placed over the catheter at the skin surface (Fig. 5.5E). The endoscope is then reinserted into the stomach to verify the correct placement of the mushroom against the gastric mucosa. If blanching of the mucosa is observed, less tension should be applied to the tube, otherwise necrosis of the gastric wall may ensue as a result of ischemia. A plastic clamp is placed over the tube and the tube is capped with a Y-port

connector. A jacket made from stockinette (San Jose Surgical Supply, Inc., San Jose, CA) is fitted to protect the tube (Fig. 5.5F).

Complications related to PEG tubes include those associated with placement of the tube (splenic laceration, gastric hemorrhage, and pneumoperitoneum), and delayed complications such as vomiting, aspiration pneumonia, tube extraction, tube migration, and stoma infection.[15,16,19] Splenic laceration can be minimized by insufflating and transilluminating the stomach prior to placement of the needle or catheter into the abdominal wall. The author has recognized a discordant number of large-breed dogs that have had major complications secondary to the stomach falling off the silicone dome at the end of the gastrostomy tube. The stoma appeared normal in all dogs, with the unfortunate consequence that food was introduced intraperitoneally in several dogs. This complication occurred despite the placement of an internal flange between the dome and the gastric mucosa. For this reason, the author recommends that all dogs heavier than 30 kg do not have a PEG procedure, and instead have a gastrostomy tube placed surgically. Minor complications include pressure necrosis at the stoma site and cellulitis.[15,16,19]

Blind percutaneous gastrostomy (BPG) technique

An alternative technique for non-endoscopic and non-surgical gastrostomy tube placement has been described.[17,18] The gastrostomy tube placement device can be prepared with a length of vinyl or stainless steel tubing (diameter 12–25 mm) purchased from a hardware store, or an ELD gastrostomy tube applicator (Jorgensen Laboratories, Loveland, CO) or Cook gastrostomy tube introduction set (Global Veterinary Products, Inc., New Buffalo, MI) can be used. The ELD gastrostomy tube applicator is the only device that utilizes an internal trocar, whereas the Cook gastrostomy tube introduction set contains a wire that is threaded through an introduction needle. The distal tip of a stainless steel tube can be flared and deflected 45 degrees to the long axis of the tube to help displace the lateral body wall. The lubricated tube is passed through the mouth and into the stomach. The tube is advanced until the end of the tube displaces the stomach and lateral abdominal wall. Positioning the animal with its head over the edge of the table and lowering the proximal end of the tube will facilitate

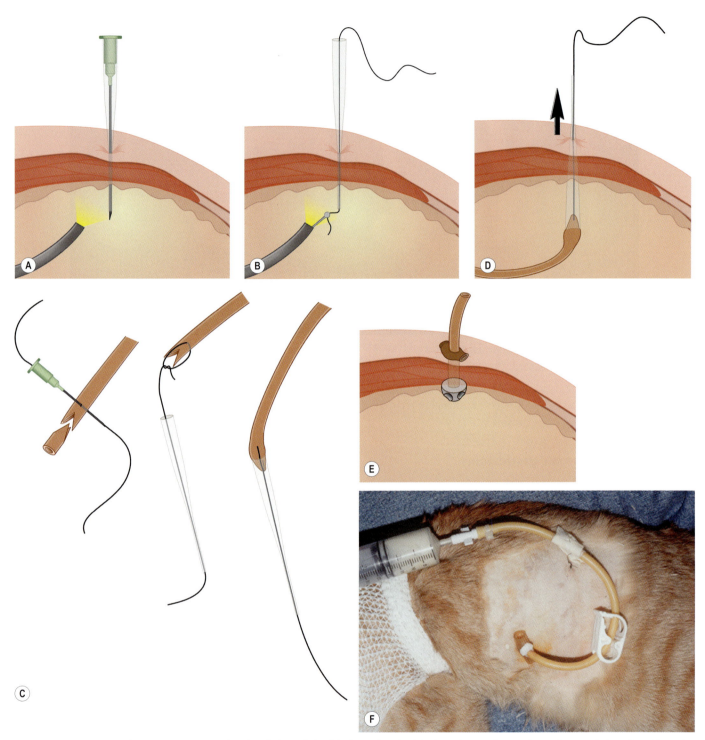

Fig. 5.5 Percutaneous endoscopic gastrostomy (PEG) technique: (**A**) With the patient in right lateral recumbency, the endoscope is introduced into the stomach, and the stomach is insufflated with air. The left body wall is transilluminated with the endoscope to ensure that the spleen is not between the stomach and the body wall. A 16–18G sheathed catheter is pierced transabdominally into the insufflated stomach lumen; (**B**) The catheter stylet is removed, and nylon suture is advanced through the catheter until it can be grasped with endoscopic retrieval forceps. The nylon suture is pulled out through the mouth as the endoscope is withdrawn; (**C**) The suture material is secured to the feeding tube and water-soluble jelly is applied liberally to the catheter sheath and the mushroom-tip catheter; (**D**) The lubricated catheter is drawn down the esophagus and into the stomach as the assistant applies traction on the suture exiting the abdominal wall; (**E**) The catheter is advanced until the mushroom tip rests gently against the gastric mucosa. Endoscopy should be repeated to confirm the correct position of the mushroom tip. An external flange is fitted down the tube against the skin to prevent the tube from slipping into the stomach; (**F**) Gastrostomy feeding tube in place, with the clamp in the open position. The stockinette jacket is pulled over the gastrostomy tube once feeding is completed.

identifying the tube tip through the body wall. For the Cook gastrostomy introduction set or similarly prepared device, a percutaneous needle is introduced into the lumen of the introduction tube while the assistant firmly holds the distal tip of the tube between two fingers. A skin nick is made over the end of the tube and a 14-G over-the-needle catheter advanced into the lumen of the tube. Proper positioning of the catheter is confirmed by moving the hub from side to side and feeling the catheter tip strike the inside of the tube. A guide wire prepared from a banjo string is attached to suture material that is 60 cm longer than the stomach tube. The guide wire is threaded through the catheter, into the tube, and out the mouth of the patient. The attached suture is pulled through the tube and cut from the wire at the mouth. The tube and catheter are removed and the suture is attached to a gastrostomy tube which is secured in an identical fashion to the PEG tube procedure.

The reported complication rate for BPG is similar to that of PEG; however, the risk of penetrating the spleen, stomach, or omentum is greater when the stomach is not insufflated with air prior to positioning the tube against the lateral abdominal wall.[20,21] Contraindications to using the blind technique include severe obesity precluding accurate palpation of the tube against the abdominal wall and esophageal disease. Surgical placement of gastrostomy tubes should be reserved for these patients.

Surgical tube gastrostomy technique

Surgical placement of gastrostomy tubes has been superseded by the percutaneous techniques because of the ease and speed of placement, lower cost, and decreased patient morbidity associated with the nonsurgical techniques. A surgical approach is indicated in obese patients, patients with esophageal obstruction, or in situations where the patient requires a laparotomy for reasons other than tube placement.[21] Surgical tube gastrostomy can be performed either via a routine celiotomy, or by a left paracostal flank approach 10–20 mm caudal to the last rib.[22,23] The use of a mushroom-tipped catheter is recommended because the self-retaining tip is more resistant to acid damage than the balloon-tipped urethral catheters (Foley Catheter, Bard Urological Division of C.R. Bard, Covington, GA).

Patient anesthesia and preparation of the left paracostal region is the same as the PEG tube procedure. A 30–50-mm skin incision is made just caudal and parallel to the last rib, beginning 20–40 mm below the ventral edge of the epaxial muscles. Blunt dissection is used to separate the external and internal oblique muscles in the direction of their fibers, and the transverse abdominal muscle and peritoneum are incised. The greater curvature of the stomach is located digitally and retracted toward the incision with Allis or Babcock tissue forceps. Location of the stomach can be facilitated by having an assistant insufflate the stomach with air using an orogastric tube.

The stomach is examined to identify the left lateral aspect of the gastric body or the caudal aspect of the fundus for the ostomy site. The stomach is packed off with moistened gauze sponges and temporary stay sutures are placed in the seromuscular layers at the 12 o'clock and 6 o'clock positions. Two full-thickness purse-string sutures are placed around the selected ostomy site. A stab incision is made in the middle of the purse string and the feeding tube is introduced into the stomach. The purse-string sutures are tightened and tied, starting with the inner suture. A layer of omentum is placed around the ostomy site between the stomach and the body wall to help prevent leakage of gastric contents. The stomach is then sutured to the body wall using simple interrupted or continuous 2-0 nylon or polypropylene sutures placed around the ostomy site. The tube may exit through the initial grid incision or via a separate stab incision. Securing of the tube outside the stomach is the same as for the PEG tube procedure.

Enterostomy tubes

Enterostomy tubes are indicated in patients unable to tolerate intragastric or intraduodenal feeding, despite having normal distal small intestine and colon function.[24,25] Specific indications for feeding via jejunostomy tube include gastric outlet obstruction, gastroparesis, recurrent/potential aspiration, proximal small bowel obstruction, and partial gastrectomy.[24] Jejunal tube feeding minimizes the stimulation of pancreatic secretion and is a viable route for patients with severe pancreatitis.[25] Jejunostomy tube feeding is rarely if ever indicated in oral surgery patients, and detailed descriptions of the technique are readily available for the reader if indications for enterostomy tube placement are present.[24,26]

POSTOPERATIVE CARE AND ASSESSMENT

Nutrition

Calculation of nutritional requirements

Nutritional support provides substrates for gluconeogenesis and protein synthesis, and provides the energy needed to meet the additional demands of host defense, wound repair, and cell division and growth. An estimate of an animal's nutrient requirements is needed to determine the minimum amount of food necessary to sustain critical physiologic processes (Table 5.1). The resting energy requirement (RER) is the animal's energy requirement at rest in a thermoneutral environment and in a postabsorptive state. A linear formula can be applied to determine the RER of dogs and cats weighing at least 2 kg. Alternatively, one can utilize an allometric formula that can be applied to dogs and cats of all body weights (BW).

$$\text{Linear formula: RER (kcal/day)} = (30 \text{ H } BW_{kg}) + 70$$
$$\text{Allometric formula: RER (kcal/day)} = 70 (BW_{kg}^{0.75})$$

Accurate, direct measurements of energy expenditure in sick or traumatized dogs and cats are not available. Despite the paucity of data on energy requirements of these animals, it is conceivable that the requirements of critically ill animals are less than normal maintenance amounts (MER), but greater than RER. Hospitalized patients should be fed at their calculated RER initially, realizing that their

---

Table 5.1 Enteral feeding worksheet for dogs and cats

1. Calculate resting energy requirement (RER):
   Body weight 2 to 45 kg: RER (kcal) = 30 Wt_{kg}+70
   Body weight <2 or >45 kg: RER = 70($Wt_{kg}^{0.75}$)
   Body weight = _____ kg   RER = _____ kcal
2. Calculate illness energy requirement (IER)*:
   Illness factor = 1.1 to 1.2 for dogs and cats
   IER = RER* illness factor   IER = _____ kcal
3. Calculate amount of diet to feed:
   Daily volume to feed: IER) energy density (kcal/mL)
   Daily volume = _____ mL
4. Evaluate responses and modify as needed:
   Weight changes often reflect fluid dynamics in the early period following injury. Caloric requirement may need to be increased or decreased depending on animal's metabolic rate and response to nutritional support.

*Animals should be fed their RER initially, and have their body weights, physical examination findings, and ongoing losses carefully evaluated before gradually increasing their caloric intake based on the IER formula.
Modified from Marks SL. The principles and practical application of enteral nutrition. Vet Clin North Am Small Anim Pract 1998;28:677–708.

actual energy requirement is likely to change over the course of the disease process through recovery. Use of 'fudge factors' extrapolated from the human literature to calculate the energy requirements of critically ill animals is discouraged, particularly in the early phase of nutritional support. Close observation of changes in body weight, physical examination findings (decreased subcutaneous fat stores, muscle wasting, and presence of edema or ascites), and ongoing losses (diarrhea, vomiting, exudative wounds) will help determine whether to increase or decrease the patients caloric intake towards the illness energy requirement (IER) or RER, respectively. The term 'illness energy requirement' (IER) is used to determine caloric requirements of critically ill animals and can be determined from these formulas:

$$\text{Canine and feline IER (kcal/day)} = 1.1{-}1.2 \times \text{RER}$$

Diet selection

The type of formula to feed the patient will depend on the selected route of feeding, the functional status of the gastrointestinal tract, and the animal's nutrient requirements. Other factors, such as cost, availability, and ease of use may also be important. Patients fed via nasoesophageal or jejunostomy feeding tubes are limited to receiving liquid enteral formulas that have a caloric density of approximately 1 kcal/mL. When selecting a liquid formula for feeding, one should pay particular attention to the amount of protein in the formula, the type of protein (intact proteins, peptides, and amino acids) and the quality of the protein. Whole egg has the highest biologic value, followed by cow milk, lactalbumin, beef, soy and casein. Most human liquid formulas contain less than 20% protein calories, precluding their use for the long-term (longer than 2 weeks) feeding of cats. The lower-protein formulas should be supplemented with protein modules such as Promod (Ross Laboratories, Columbus OH), Casec (Mead-Johnson, Evansville, IN), or Promagic (Animal Nutrition Laboratories, Burlington, NJ) at 15–30 g casein or whey powder per 240 mL can. Almost all human liquid enteral formulas lack taurine, an essential amino acid in cats, necessitating its supplementation (approximately 250 mg taurine per 240 mL can) in this species. High-protein commercial human liquid formulations contain between 21% and 30% protein calories and include Impact (Sandoz Nutrition, Minneapolis, MN), Immun-Aid (McGaw, Inc., Irvine, CA), Alitraq (Ross Laboratories, Columbus OH), Promote (Ross Laboratories, Columbus OH) and Traumacal (Mead-Johnson, Evansville, IN).

Polymeric solutions contain macronutrients in the form of isolates of intact protein (casein, lactalbumin, whey, egg white), triglycerides and carbohydrate polymers. The carbohydrates are usually glucose polymers in the form of starch and its hydrolysates and the fats are of vegetable origin. The osmolality varies between 300 and 450 mOsm/kg in solutions with a caloric density of 1 kcal/mL; however, the osmolality may reach 650 mOsm/kg in solutions with a greater caloric density. Monomeric solutions contain protein as peptides or amino acids, fat as long-chain triglycerides (LCT) or a mixture of LCT and medium-chain triglycerides (MCT), and carbohydrates as partially hydrolyzed starch maltodextrins and glucose oligosaccharides. These solutions require less digestion and their absorption is more efficient than regular foods or polymeric solutions; however, the partially digested macronutrients contribute to the higher osmolality, which is between 400 and 700 mOsm/kg.

Commercial blended pet food diets are recommended for feeding via pharyngostomy, esophagostomy, or gastrostomy tubes. In select cases, the feeding of a liquid enteral formulation may be indicated (nasoesophageal or jejunostomy tube feeding). There are a number of complete and balanced veterinary enteral formulations (Table 5.2) that contain adequate amounts of protein, taurine, and micronutrients, precluding the need for supplementation in most situations.

Feeding should be delayed for 24 hours after placing a gastrostomy tube, to allow return of gastric motility and allow formation of a fibrin seal. In contrast, feeding can be instituted immediately following pharyngostomy or esophagostomy tube placement once the animal has fully recovered from anesthesia. Diet can be administered as bolus feedings or continuous infusion when feeding via esophagostomy and gastrostomy tube. Improved weight gain and decreased gastroesophageal reflux have been reported in human patients given continuous feedings, although similar studies are lacking in the veterinary literature.[27] If continuous feeding is employed, it should be interrupted every 8 hours to determine the residual volume by applying suction to the feeding tube. If the residual volume is more than twice the volume infused in 1 hour, feeding should be discontinued for 2 hours, and the rate of infusion decreased by 25% to prevent vomiting. Treatment with metoclopramide (1–2 mg/kg/24 hour as a continuous infusion) may be used to enhance gastric emptying and prevent vomiting.[28]

With bolus feeding, the required daily volume of food should be divided into four to six feeds. Patients are usually fed approximately 25% of their caloric requirement on the first day of feeding, with a gradual increase of 25% of the caloric requirement per day. Most patients are able to reach their energy requirement by the fourth or fifth day of feeding. The food should be warmed to room temperature and fed slowly through the tube to prevent vomiting. Flushing of the tube with 15–20 mL of lukewarm water helps prevent clogging. Before each feeding, aspirate the tube with an empty syringe to check for residual food left in the stomach from the previous feeding. If more than half of the last feeding is removed from the stomach, skip the feeding and recheck residual volume at the next feeding.

Removal and replacement

Esophagostomy tube removal

Unlike gastrostomy tubes, an esophagostomy tube can be removed the same day it is placed if necessary without concern for leakage and development of secondary complications. The dressing and sutures are removed while the tube is held in place. The tube is then occluded by kinking and pulled out using gentle traction. The ostomy site should be cleaned, antibiotic ointment applied, and a light dressing placed around the neck. The dressing should be removed in 24 hours, and the ostomy site inspected. The ostomy site should close within 24–36 hours. Skin sutures are not needed for closure of the ostomy site.

Gastrostomy tube removal

For percutaneously placed tubes, it is recommended that the tube be left in place for a minimum of 14 days. Animals receiving immune-suppressive therapy or patients that are severely debilitated may require longer for a peritoneal seal to form. The tube should only be removed when oral food intake is sufficient to meet the patient's caloric requirement. One of two methods of Pezzer tube removal can be applied. The tube can be cut at the body wall and the mushroom tip pushed into the stomach to be passed in the feces. This method is safe in medium to large dogs, because the mushroom and internal flange should be easily passed in the stool. Alternatively, a stylet can be inserted into the tube to flatten the mushroom tip, while exerting firm traction on the tube. This method is recommended for cats and small dogs, because the mushroom can cause intestinal obstruction. Removal of the MILA catheter (MILA International, Inc., Florence, KY) is accomplished by deflating the bumper which occurs once the Y-port adapter is removed. Catheters with a dome (Bard Urological Division, Murray Hill, NJ) are removed by gentle but firm traction on the tube.

Table 5.2 Macronutrient composition of selected veterinary liquid enteral formulations

Product	Protein type	Caloric density (kcal/mL)	Nutrients (% of total kcal)			Formula characteristics
			Protein	Fat	Carbohydrate	
Prescription diet Canine & Feline a/d (Hill's Prescription diet® a/d, Hill's Pet Nutrition, Topeka, KS)	Liver, chicken, corn flour, casein	1.3	34	55	11	Isotonic, lactose free, fiber 1.3 % DM, adequate taurine, fatty acid ratio (n6 : n3 = 2.2 : 1)
Eukanuba Maximum-Calorie Canine & Feline (The Iams Company, Dayton, OH)	Chicken, chicken by-product meal	2.1	29	66	5	Isotonic, lactose free, fiber 1.6 % DM, adequate taurine, fatty acid ratio (n6 : n3 = 8.3 : 11)
CliniCare Canine (Abbott Laboratories, North Chicago, IL)	80% casein 20% whey	1.0	20	55	25	Isotonic (230 mOsm/kg), lactose free, fiber free, fatty acid ratio (n6 : n3 = 6.4 : 1)
Clinicare Feline (Abbott Laboratories, North Chicago, IL)	60% casein 40% whey	1.0	30	45	25	Isotonic (235 mOsm/kg) , lactose free, fiber free, adequate taurine, fatty acid ratio (n6 : n3 = 6.4 : 1)
Clinicare RF Specialized Feline (Abbott Laboratories, North Chicago, IL)	80% casein 20% whey	1.0	22	57	21	Isotonic (165 mOsm/kg), lactose free, fiber free, adequate taurine, fatty acid ratio (n6 : n3 = 6.4 : 1)
Purina CV Feline Formula (Nestle Purina Veterinary Diets, St. Louis, MO)	Liver, beef, ground yellow corn, fish	1.4	31.5	50.5	18	Isotonic, lactose free, 140 mg of taurine/can, 30 mg of magnesium/can, 15 mg of carnitine/can, 600 mg of potassium/can (can size is 165 mL)
Select Care Canine Development Formula (Innovative Veterinary Diets, Pittsburgh, PA)	Beef, chicken liver, chicken, poultry by-products, egg product, cornmeal, salmon	0.9	28	30	42	Isotonic, lactose free, fatty acid ratio (n6 : n3 = 10.3 : 1), 80 mg of magnesium/can, 510 mg of potassium/can (can size is 360–420 mL)

Modified from Marks SL. The principles and practical application of enteral nutrition. Vet Clin North Am Small Anim Pract 1998;28: 677–708.

The gastrocutaneous tract should seal with minimal or no leakage within 24 hours.

Gastrostomy and esophagostomy tube replacement

The PEG tube may malfunction or be prematurely removed by the patient, requiring replacement. If the gastrostomy tube is removed within 14 days of placement (before establishment of the gastrocutaneous tract), a PEG procedure should be performed to evaluate the gastric mucosa and verify correct positioning of the replacement gastrostomy tube. If the tube is inadvertently removed once the gastrocutaneous tract is well healed, one can replace the original catheter with a balloon-type catheter (Flexiflo: Ross Laboratories, Columbus OH) or a low-profile gastrostomy device (LPGD) (Bard Interventional Products Division, Murray Hill, NJ) (Fig. 5.6A).[29] Both catheter types do not require an endoscopic procedure or anesthesia for placement. The gastrostomy 'button' is a small, flexible silicone device that has a mushroom-like dome at one end and two small wings at the other end that lies flush with the outer abdominal wall (Fig. 5.6B). A one-way antireflux valve prevents reflux of gastric contents through the top of the tube. There are two types of LPGDs: obturated and non-obturated. The obturated device has an enlarged mushroom tip that must be stretched for placement in the stomach by using a special introducer (Fig. 5.6C).[30] The non-obturated tube works like a Foley catheter and does not require forceful entry into the gastrostomy stoma.[30] The length of the gastrocutaneous fistula must be precisely determined to guide correct selection of the appropriate 'button' shaft length. This is accomplished with a special stoma measuring device provided with the kit. The main advantages of the LPGD include its durability due to the silicon material, decreased likelihood of inadvertent removal by the patient, and the aesthetically pleasing appearance to the clients.

COMPLICATIONS

Gastric pressure necrosis

Gastric pressure necrosis can occur from either the mushroom of the PEG tube or flange eroding the mucus layer of the stomach due to excessive tension being exerted on the PEG tube during placement. In addition, overzealous traction of the PEG tube followed by placement of the external flange flush against the skin of the patient can also cause pressure necrosis characterized by redness, swelling, and moistness of the skin. To minimize this problem from occurring, ensure that the PEG tube can be rotated following its placement and leave a 5-mm space between the external flange and the skin.

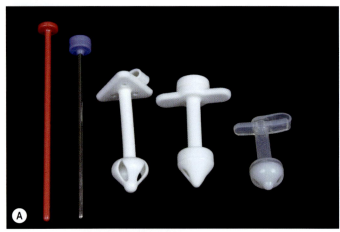

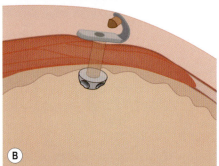

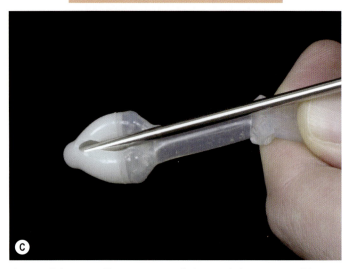

Fig. 5.6 (**A**) Low-profile gastrostomy devices and obturators used for stretching the dome-shaped tip of the device. From left, the Stomate low-profile device (Ross Laboratories, Columbus OH), The Cook low profile device (Global Veterinary Products, Inc., New Buffalo, MI), and the Button® low-profile device (Bard Interventional Products Division, Murray Hill, NJ); (**B**) Low-profile gastrostomy device with small outer wings of the device lying flush against the skin of the abdominal wall. For feedings, the small plastic plug is removed and a feeding adapter is connected to a syringe; (**C**) Correct technique for stretching the dome-shaped tip of the low profile gastrostomy device with an obturator. The dome should not be stretched by passing the obturator through the lumen of the device as it will compromise the integrity of the anti-reflux valve located adjacent to the dome.

Feeding tube displacement

This is a relatively common problem, particularly with nasoesophageal tubes. Displacement of the tube can lead to aspiration, diarrhea or, in the case of gastrostomy tubes, peritonitis. Gastrostomy tubes should be marked with tape or a marking pen at the level of the skin to help verify the position of the tube. Detachment of the stomach from the abdominal wall with consequent intraperitoneal leakage of gastric contents can occur in large-breed dogs, and an internal flange should be placed in these animals to minimize dislodgement of the tube.

Tube obstruction

Obstruction of the feeding tube is one of the most common complications of enteral feeding.[31] Most obstructions are secondary to coagulation of formula, although obstruction by tablet fragments, tube kinking, and precipitation of incompatible medications can also result in tube obstruction. Nasoesophageal tubes are prone to obstruction because of their small diameter, and obstruction also occurs up to three times more frequently in patients fed by continuous versus bolus feedings.[32] Sucralfate and antacids have been reported to precipitate with enteral formulas and cause tube obstruction.[32] Several 'remedies' have been advocated to relieve tube obstruction. Warm water injected with gentle pressure and suction will relieve most obstructions. For more unyielding obstructions, carbonated water is instilled into the tube and allowed to sit for 1 hour before applying gentle pressure and suction. Pancreatic enzyme infusions and meat tenderizer have also been advocated to dissolve tube obstructions.[31] On rare occasions, the passage of an angiographic wire down the lumen is needed to unclog the tube. Tube obstructions can be minimized by flushing the feeding tube with warm water before and after administering medications or enteral feedings. The tube should also be flushed after checking for gastric residuals, because the acid pH will cause the formula to coagulate in the tube. Elixir forms of medication should be used rather than crushed tablet forms whenever possible. Tablets should be crushed and dissolved in water prior to administration through the feeding tube, if no alternative form of medication is available.

Leakage through stoma sites

Mild leakage at the stoma site can occur for the first few days following placement of the feeding tube. Persistent leakage may indicate tube dysfunction, peristomal infection, or a stoma site greater than necessary for the tube. Signs of inflammation with or without discharge or fever may indicate infection of the stoma site. This must be differentiated from fasciitis, as a simple wound infection can usually be treated locally with dilute povidone-iodine solution, topical povidone-iodine antibacterial ointments, and more frequent dressing changes. Systemically administered antibiotics are usually reserved for patients with systemic signs of infection.

Aspiration

Pulmonary aspiration is a common complication of enteral feeding, although the actual incidence of this complication is difficult to determine due to the lack of consistency in how aspiration is defined. Risk factors for aspiration include impaired mental status, neurologic injury, absence of a cough or gag reflex, mechanical ventilation, and previous aspiration pneumonia.[33,34] The source of the aspirated material should be identified because withholding gastrostomy feedings or placing a jejunostomy feeding tube in a patient will have no benefit if the patient aspirated oropharyngeal secretions. Although controversial, most authors agree that postpyloric feeding reduces the risk of aspiration.[35] In addition, the use of continuous versus bolus feedings has been shown to induce less gastroesophageal reflux than bolus feedings.[27]

Diarrhea

Diarrhea is the most commonly sited complication associated with tube feeding in human and animal patients, with an incidence ranging from 2.3% to 63%.[36] The clinical implications of enteral feeding-related diarrhea are significant. Severe diarrhea leads to fluid, electrolyte, and nutrient loss, and can cause considerable distress to the patient. Diarrhea in tube-fed patients occurs due to multiple factors, including hypoalbuminemia, hyperosmolar or high fat diets, infected diets, and concomitant antibiotic therapy.[37] The incidence of diarrhea in enterally fed patients taking antibiotics far exceeds the incidence in normally fed patients taking the same antibiotics.[38] Antibiotic-associated diarrhea may arise from overgrowth of enterobacteria (*Klebsiella*, *Proteus*, *Pseudomonas*) or from proliferation of *Clostridium difficile*. Antibiotic administration is also associated with decreased concentrations of fecal short-chain fatty acids, occurring as a result of decreased colonic carbohydrate fermentation.[39]

REFERENCES

1. Levine GM, Deren JJ, Steiger E, et al. Role of oral intake in maintenance of gut mass and disaccharide activity. Gastroenterology 1974;67:975–83.

2. Raul F, Norieger R, Doffeol M. Modification of brush border enzyme activities during starvation in the jejunum and ileum of adult rats. Enzyme 1982; 28:328–35.

3. Geraghty ME. Tube feeding equipment update. Dietitians in Nutrition Support Newsletter 1989;July/Aug:1.

4. Metheny N, Eisenberg P, McSweeney M. Effect of feeding tube properties and three irrigants on clogging rates. Nurs Res 1988;37:165–9.

5. Crowe DT. Clinical use of an indwelling nasogastric tube for enteral nutrition and fluid therapy in the dog and cat. J Am Anim Hosp Assoc 1986;22:675–82.

6. Ford RB. Nasogastric intubation in the cat. Compend Cont Ed Pract Vet 1980;1: 29–32.

7. Balkany TJ, Baker BB, Bloustein PA, et al. Cervical esophagostomy in dogs. Endoscopic, radiographic and histopathologic evaluation of esophagitis induced by feeding tubes. Ann Otol Rhinol Laryngol 1977;86:588–93.

8. Abood SK, Buffington CA. Improved nasogastric intubation technique for administration of nutritional support in dogs. J Am Vet Med Assoc 1991;199: 577–9.

9. Crowe DT, Downs MO. Pharyngostomy complications in dogs and cats and recommended technical modifications: Experimental and clinical investigations. J Am Anim Hosp Assoc 1986;22: 493–503.

10. Lantz GC. Pharyngostomy tube installation for the administration of nutritional and fluid requirements. Compend Contin Educ Pract Vet 1981;3: 135–42.

11. Crowe DT, Devey JJ. Esophagostomy tubes for feeding and decompression: Clinical experience in 29 small animal patients. J Am Anim Hosp Assoc 1997; 33:393–403.

12. Levine PB, Smallwood LJ, Buback JL. Esophagostomy tubes as a method of nutritional management in cats: A retrospective study. J Am Anim Hosp Assoc 1997;33:405–10.

13. Devitt CM, Seim HB. Clinical evaluation of tube esophagostomy in small animals. J Am Anim Hosp Assoc 1997;33: 55–60.

14. Ireland LM, Hohenhaus AE, Broussard JD, et al. A comparison of owner management and complications in 67 cats with esophagostomy and percutaneous endoscopic gastrostomy feeding tubes. J Am Anim Hosp Assoc 2003;39:241–6.

15. Armstrong PJ, Hardie EM. Percutaneous endoscopic gastrostomy. A retrospective study of 54 clinical cases in dogs and cats. J Vet Int Med 1990;4:202–6.

16. Matthews KA, Binnington AG. Percutaneous incisionless placement of a gastrostomy tube utilizing a gastroscope: Preliminary observations. J Am Anim Hosp Assoc 1986;22:601–10.

17. Fulton RB, Dennis JS. Blind percutaneous placement of a gastrostomy tube for nutritional support in dogs and cats. J Am Vet Med Assoc 1992;201: 697–700.

18. Mauterer JV, Abood SK, Buffington CA, et al. New technique and management guidelines for percutaneous nonendoscopic tube gastrostomy. J Am Vet Med Assoc 1994;205:574–9.

19. Bright RM, Burrows CF. Percutaneous endoscopic tube gastrostomy in dogs. Am J Vet Res 1988;49:629–33.

20. Clary EM, Hardie EM, Fischer WD, et al. Nonendoscopic antegrade percutaneous gastrostomy: The effect of preplacement gastric insufflation on tube position and intra-abdominal anatomy. J Vet Intern Med 1996;10:15–20.

21. Michel KE. Practice guidelines for gastrostomy tubes. Compend Cont Educ Pract Vet 1997;19:306–9.

22. Williams JM, White RAS. Tube gastrostomy in dogs. J Small Anim Pract 1993;34:59–64.

23. Crane SW. Placement and maintenance of a temporary feeding tube gastrostomy in the dog and cat. Compend Contin Educ Pract Vet 1980;2:770–6.

24. Orton EC. Enteral hyperalimentation administered via needle catheter – jejunostoma as an adjunct to cranial abdominal surgery in dogs and cats. J Am Vet Med Assoc 1986;188: 1406–11.

25. Ryan Jr JA, Page CP. Intrajejunal feeding: development and current status. J Parenter Enteral Nutr 1984;8:187–98.

26. Crowe DT. Methods of enteral feeding in the seriously ill or injured patient: Part I and Part II. J Vet Emerg Crit Care 1986;3:1–17.

27. Coben RM, Weintraub A, DiMarino AJ, et al. Gastroesophageal reflux during gastrostomy feedings. Gastroenterology 1994;106:13–8.

28. Graves GM, Becht JL, Rawlings CA. Metoclopramide treatment of the contractile and myoelectric alterations in canine paralytic ileus (abstract). Vet Surg 1986;15:121.

29. Kadakia S, Cassaday M, Shaffer R. Comparison of Foley catheter as a replacement gastrostomy tube with commercial replacement gastrostomy tube: A prospective randomized trial. Gastrointest Endosc 1994;40:188–93.

30. Faller N, Lawrence K. Comparing low-profile gastrostomy tubes. Nursing 1994;12:1–3.

31. Marcuard SP, Stegall KS. Unclogging feeding tubes with pancreatic enzyme. J Parenter Enteral Nutr 1990;14:198–200.

32. Carrougher JG, Barrilleaux CN. Esophageal bezoars: the sucralith. Crit Care Med 1991; 19:837–9.

33. Atherton ST, White DJ. Stomach as source of bacteria colonizing respiratory tract during artificial ventilation. Lancet 1978;2:968–9.

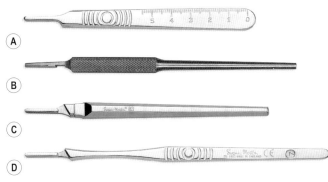

Fig. 6.1 Scalpel handles used in oral surgery: (A) No. 3; (B) No. 5; (C) No. B3; (D) No. 7. *(A, C and D courtesy of Swann-Morton Limited, Owlerton Green, Sheffield, UK; B courtesy of Hu-Friedy Mfg. Inc., Chicago, IL.)*

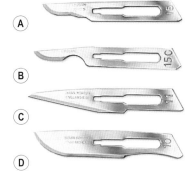

Fig. 6.3 Scalpel blades used in oral surgery: (A) #15; (B) #15c; (C) #11; (D) #10. *(Courtesy of Swann-Morton Limited, Owlerton Green, Sheffield, UK.)*

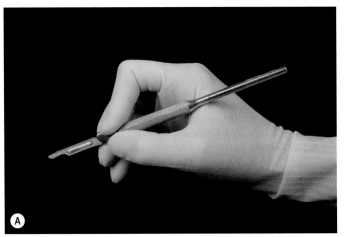

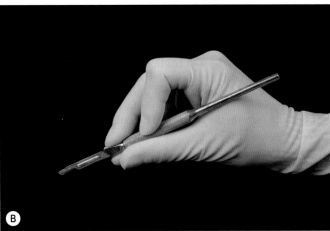

Fig. 6.2 A no. 5 scalpel held in the (A) pen grip and (B) modified pen grip.

this purpose or sturdy general surgical scissors should be utilized when cutting suture material.

Tissue forceps

Tissue forceps are hinged instruments that can either be locking or non-locking. The hinge can either be at the end away from the grasping end, or in the middle, similar to scissors. Tissue forceps that are hinged at the end are also called tissue pliers.

The delicate Adson 1X2 tissue forceps (Fig. 6.5A) is used most commonly in oral surgery for gentle tissue handling, e.g., when stabilizing mucogingival flaps during suturing.[5] The '1X2' refers to the one small sharp point on the one end that fits between the two sharp points on the other end. It causes less tissue trauma compared with the plain Adson forceps and the Adson–Brown forceps, which has multiple teeth. An Adson forceps should be held in a pen grip rather than the finger grip to minimize tissue trauma. An Adson forceps is only 120 mm long. If longer forceps are needed, e.g., to reach the caudal part of the oral cavity, a Gerald 1X2 tissue forceps (Fig. 6.5B), which measures 170–180 mm, can be used.[8]

The Allis tissue forceps (Fig. 6.6) is an example of a locking tissue forceps with a middle hinge. It can only be used on firm tissue that is to be excised, e.g., a large mass of gingival enlargement.[5] It should never be placed on friable tumors, wound edges or mucogingival flaps because it is very traumatic as a result of the crushing action.

Periosteal elevators

Periosteal elevators (also occasionally referred to as 'periosteals') are used to elevate mucoperiosteal flaps.[8] A wide variety of periosteal elevators exist and the choice is often based on personal preference. Many periosteal elevators are double-ended. One end is slightly curved and rounded, while the other end typically is pointed or square. The Molt periosteal elevator #9 (Fig. 6.7A), which is popular both in human and veterinary oral surgery, is a good example. The wax spatula #7 resembles this instrument and is used by some as a periosteal elevator (see Ch. 19). The pointed end of the Molt periosteal elevator is used in a prying motion to elevate the dental papilla between two teeth. However, this instrument end is more applicable to humans than to animals. The rounded end is the most useful one. In humans and in animals with thick gingiva it is gently inserted with the concave side facing the bone in a linear fashion applying small pushing strokes. In animals with thin or friable gingiva, it is safer to insert the instrument under a small increment of tissue, after which it is gently rotated over 45–90 degrees, lifting the tissue up and sideways. This minimizes the risk of slipping and tearing the gingiva, which can easily occur if the push stroke technique is used. The instrument is held in a pen grip or modified pen grip (Fig. 6.8).

The #24G periosteal elevator (Figs 6.7B & 6.8) is a delicate instrument and its rounded end allows mucoperiosteal flaps to be elevated atraumatically, even in very small animals with friable gingiva. The Mead #3 periosteal elevator (Fig. 6.7C) is a sturdy, double-ended periosteal elevator most suitable for thick attached gingiva and hard palatal mucosa. Its round end is used as described above. The square end is knife-like and is occasionally useful for elevating particularly

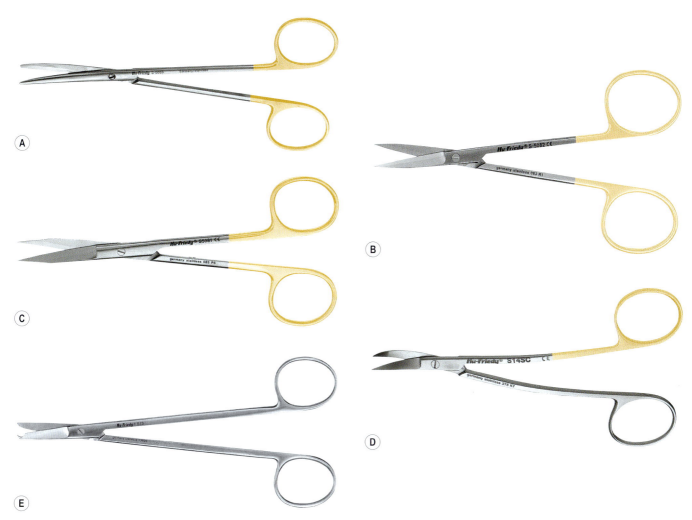

Fig. 6.4 (**A**) Metzenbaum scissors (curved, blunt); (**B**) Iris scissors (straight); (**C**) Goldman–Fox scissors (curved). (**D**) LaGrange scissors. (**E**) Suture scissors. *(Courtesy of Hu-Friedy Mfg. Inc., Chicago, IL.)*

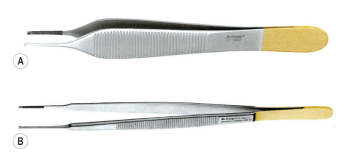

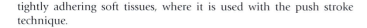

Fig. 6.5 (**A**) Adson 1X2 tissue forceps; (**B**) Gerald 1X2 tissue forceps. *(Courtesy of Hu-Friedy Mfg. Inc., Chicago, IL.)*

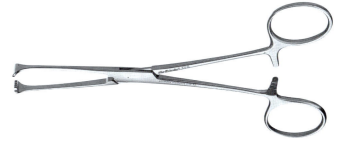

Fig. 6.6 Allis tissue forceps. *(Courtesy of Hu-Friedy Mfg. Inc., Chicago, IL.)*

tightly adhering soft tissues, where it is used with the push stroke technique.

Retractors

Once a mucoperiosteal flap is elevated and bone is exposed, the flap is reflected or retracted using a periosteal elevator, in order to protect it during osseous surgery or sectioning of a tooth. The same periosteal

elevator used for elevating the flap can be used for this purpose, e.g., a Molt #9 or #24G. Periosteal elevators used as retractors are easily scored by burs during this process. If so, these periosteal elevators should no longer be used for lifting flaps but can still be used for retraction. The Seldin retractor (Fig. 6.9A) is an instrument that has evolved from a periosteal elevator to a retractor.[5,8] It is particularly useful for retracting large mucoperiosteal flaps, e.g., in a surgical extraction of a canine tooth.

Some retractors are specifically made for keeping tongue, lips and cheeks away from the surgical site. The Cawood–Minnesota retractor

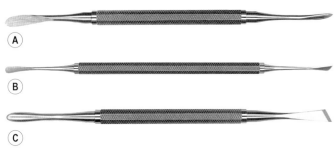

Fig. 6.7 (**A**) Molt #9 periosteal elevator; (**B**) #24G periosteal elevator; (**C**) Mead #3 periosteal elevator. *(Courtesy of Hu-Friedy Mfg. Inc., Chicago, IL.)*

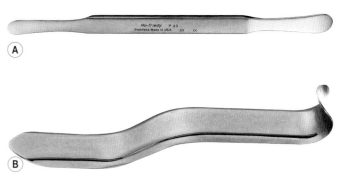

Fig. 6.9 (**A**) Seldin retractor; (**B**) Cawood–Minnesota retractor. *(Courtesy of Hu-Friedy Mfg. Inc., Chicago, IL.)*

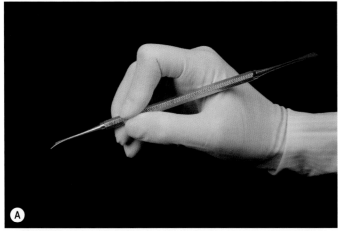

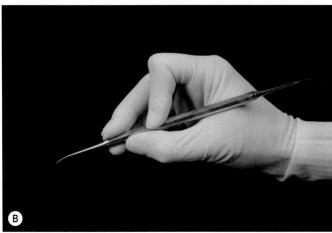

Fig. 6.8 A #24G periosteal elevator held in the (**A**) pen grip and (**B**) modified pen grip.

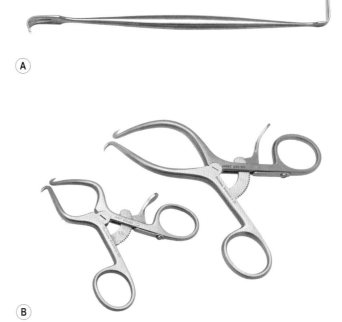

Fig. 6.10 (**A**) Senn retractor; (**B**) A 89-mm (left) and a 140-mm (right) pediatric Gelpi perineal retractor.

(Fig. 6.8B) and the very similar University of Minnesota retractors are typical examples of these. A dental mirror is also occasionally used for this purpose.[5]

During major oral surgery finger-held retractors, such as the Senn retractor (Fig. 6.10A) are very useful instruments to be held by an assistant. The Senn retractor is a double-ended instrument with three relatively sharp or rounded, bent prongs on the one end and a right-angled finger-plate on the other. The sharp-ended version is preferred, as it less likely to slip and therefore less traumatic.[2] Stay sutures and skin hooks are also commonly used in maxillofacial surgery. If no assistant is available, a self-retaining retractor such as a pediatric

Gelpi perineal retractor (Fig. 6.10B) can be used, especially when the surgical site is relatively deep and the access small, such as in a con-dylectomy of the temporomandibular joint.

Needle holders

A needle holder has a short, relatively stout beak, usually with serrated faces, and a locking handle. Fine suture material with small swaged-on needles is generally used in oral surgery (see Ch. 7). The needle holders indicated in oral surgery are therefore delicate to match the size of the needles. The Halsey needle holder (Fig. 6.11A) is a very versatile needle holder well suited for most intraoral procedures. This needle holder is 130 mm in length. Occasionally, a slightly longer instrument is needed, especially for surgery in the caudal oral cavity of large dogs, and a DeBakey needle holder (Fig. 6.11B), which measures 180 mm but still has a relatively slender beak, would be a good

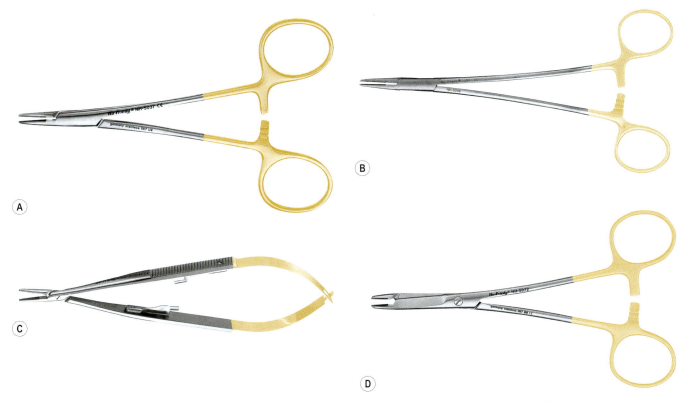

Fig. 6.11 (**A**) Halsey needle holder; (**B**) DeBakey needle holder; (**C**) Castroviejo needle holder; (**D**) Olson-Hegar needle holder. *(Courtesy of Hu-Friedy Mfg. Inc., Chicago, IL.)*

choice. These needle holders are all held with the wide-based tripod grip (Fig. 6.12). The needle should be grasped at two-thirds of its length away from the tip of the needle.[4,5]

In periodontal surgery a Castroviejo needle holder (Fig. 6.11C) is occasionally used.[7] This is a very delicate instrument that can only be used with very small needles. It is held with a pen grip.[4]

Some surgeons working without assistants prefer a needle holder with built-in scissors such as the Olson–Hegar needle holder (Fig. 6.11D).

It should be noted that needle holders cannot be used for wire twisting as this would damage the gripping surface; specifically designed ligature twisters should be used for this purpose.[8] Conversely, hemostats are not strong enough to be used as needle holders, and needles can cause permanent damage to these instruments.

Ancillary instruments

Suction tips

As hemorrhage may be brisk and copious irrigating fluids may be used in oral and maxillofacial surgery, it is imperative to have a well-functioning suctioning device. The Frazier suction tip (typically a # 10) (Fig. 6.13) is the suction tip of choice in oral surgery.[5] It is small and precise and has a decompression opening at the end of the handle. Maximum suction is achieved when the opening is occluded by the index finger of the operator. Suction can be reduced by lifting the finger, which is indicated when working in the vicinity of anatomical structures that could be damaged by the suction. In addition, the Frazier tip comes with a wire stylet that is used for unblocking the tip, should this occur.

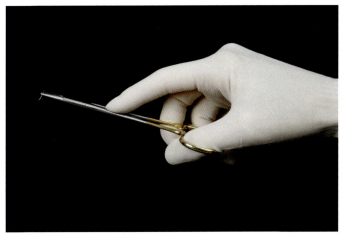

Fig. 6.12 A Halsey needle holder held in the wide-based tripod grip.

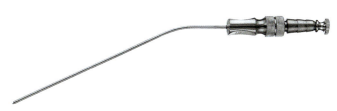

Fig. 6.13 Frazier #10 suction tip. *(Courtesy of Hu-Friedy Mfg. Inc., Chicago, IL.)*

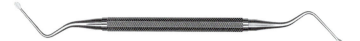

Fig. 6.14 Miller #10 surgical curette. *(Courtesy of Hu-Friedy Mfg. Inc., Chicago, IL.)*

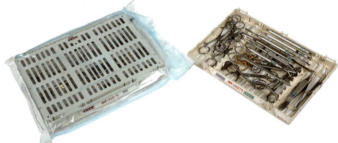

Fig. 6.16 A wrapped and autoclaved instrument cassette (*left*) and an unwrapped cassette with the lid removed (*right*) containing a basic oral surgery instrument set (contents are listed in Table 6.1).

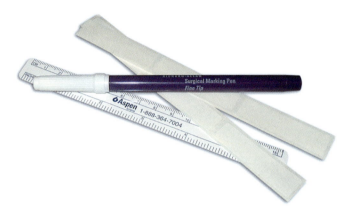

Fig. 6.15 Sterile surgical marker pen with ruler and labels. *(Courtesy of Aspen Surgical Products, Caledonia, MI.)*

Surgical curette

A small surgical curette is used for removing unwanted soft tissue and debris from a bony surface or defect, such as gently debriding an extraction wound if deemed necessary, or removing soft tissue present between two bone fragments in a longstanding fracture. A Miller curette (Fig. 6.14) is an example of a double-ended, spoon-shaped curette that is very versatile.

Surgical marker pen

A sterile surgical marker pen (Fig. 6.15) is a small but important tool in major oral and maxillofacial surgery. It is used for planning skin or oral mucosa flaps for repair of oronasal fistula, and cleft lip and palate. It is also used for outlining the surgical margins in tumor excision. The use of the marker pen helps the surgeon to plan the incisions more carefully and before tissues are distorted once the first incision is made.

Instrument organization

It is practical to have standard sets of instruments for various procedures.[9] Open tray systems are commonly used in veterinary dentistry but are incompatible with aseptic technique desirable in oral surgery. Instrument cassettes greatly facilitate the organization, cleaning, sterilization and storage of instruments (Fig. 6.16). Cassettes are made from plastic or stainless steel and come in various sizes. Instruments are cleaned, autoclaved, and stored in closed cassettes, which are then placed chairside on a sterile field and opened ready for use. Each cassette should contain a selection of instruments that are likely to be used in a given procedure. Certain instruments are used in essentially every oral and maxillofacial surgery procedure, e.g., scalpel handle, needle holder, Metzenbaum scissors, suture scissors, periosteal elevator, Adson tissue forceps, etc. It is practical to group these in a 'basic oral surgery' cassette and have a relatively large number of these available (Table 6.1). In addition, there can then be cassettes for exodontics

Table 6.1 UC Davis basic oral surgery instrument set	
Description	Hu-Friedy (Hu-Friedy Mfg. Inc., Chicago, IL)* item number
IMS resin cassette (18 instruments)	IMS-1118
Adson tissue forceps 1X2	TP5042
Backhaus towel clamps – small (6)	TC3
Cawood-Minnesota retractor	CRM2
Curved baby Allis forceps (2)	TFB
Halsey needle holder	NH-5036
Hartman hemostat straight (2)	HHS
Mead periosteal elevator #3	P3
Metzenbaum scissors – small	S5055
Miller curette #10	CM10
Periosteal elevator 24G	P24G
Scalpel handle #5	10-130-05
Seldin retractor #23	P23
Suture scissors	S13
*Many other companies have some or all of these or similar instruments.	

(see Ch. 11), periodontal surgery, apicoectomy, etc. Infrequently used instruments can be individually packed in standard autoclavable pouches and stored in an organized fashion to be readily available if needed.

Power equipment

Rotary instruments

Rotary instruments are used in oral and maxillofacial surgery for sectioning teeth, removing and smoothing alveolar bone, cutting bone and drilling into bone.

A high-speed handpiece with a tapered diamond bur or a carbide crosscut fissure bur is indicated for sectioning multirooted teeth into single-rooted units (see Ch. 11). An autoclavable straight surgical handpiece, with built-in sterile saline or lactated Ringer's solution irrigation and a round carbide or diamond bur, is the instrument of choice for bone removal (Fig. 6.17A).[5,10] The maximum speed of these

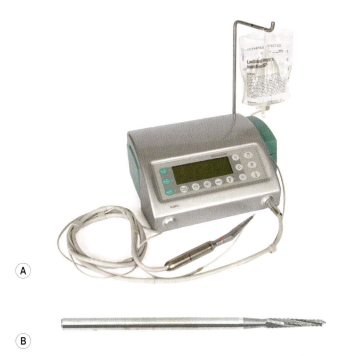

Fig. 6.17 (**A**) INTRAsurge 500 oral surgery unit and handpiece (KaVo Dental Corporation, Lake Zurich, IL); (**B**) Lindemann osteotomy bur (*Hu-Friedy Mfg. Inc., Chicago, IL.*).

oral surgery units is 40 000 rpm and the torque is adjustable. A high-speed handpiece with a round diamond or carbide bur is generally used in veterinary dentistry for removing and smoothing bone.[11] This practice is frowned upon in human oral surgery, as the air exhausted from this type of handpiece may be forced into deeper tissue planes and produce tissue emphysema.[5] Emphysematous complications have been documented in humans but not in animals.[12] In addition, most dental units to which the high-speed handpieces are connected use regular tap water or deionized water as irrigation fluid and the tubing is not sterilizable. It has been shown that tap water is harmful to canine fibroblasts in vitro.[13] The microorganisms that may be present in tap water and the biofilm that may form in the waterline can result in a contaminated irrigation fluid, which is cause for concern.[14,15]

This oral surgery unit with either a straight or contra-angle handpiece combined with an Lindemann osteotomy bur (Hu-Friedy Mfg. Inc., Chicago, IL) (Fig. 6.17B) is the instrument of choice for performing a precision osteotomy and ostectomy, e.g., mandibulectomy and maxillectomy.[16] While an oscillating or reciprocating orthopedic saw can be used for this purpose, turbinate damage and transection of the neurovascular bundle in the mandibular canal are almost impossible to avoid with these instruments.

Electrosurgery and radiosurgery

Electrosurgery and radiosurgery can be used instead of the scalpel to cut soft tissues, with the goal of reducing hemorrhage.[4] However, both methods have been shown to cause lateral thermal damage to skin, compared with the scalpel.[17] Radiosurgery is associated with less damage than electrosurgery.[17] Scalpel incision of oral mucosa results in faster reepithelialization and greater tissue strength than electrosurgery incisions.[18] When electrosurgery is used to incise oral soft tissues in the vicinity of bone, gingival recession, bone necrosis and loss of bone height may occur.[19,20] The same occurs when electrosurgery is used in the vicinity of teeth, in addition to trauma to the cementum.[21]

Electrosurgery is not discussed in a recent leading human oral surgery textbook, which is consistent with its infrequent use.[5] There is some limited application in human periodontal surgery, namely for superficial procedures at a safe distance away from bone and teeth, e.g., the excision of gingival enlargement and frenoplasty.[22]

There are veterinary practices where electrosurgery and radiosurgery are used.[17] The disadvantages of electrosurgery and radiosurgery with regard to delayed wound healing and hard tissue damage would seem to outweigh the advantage of better hemostasis when used in the oral cavity. A possible indication would be gingivectomy/gingivoplasty in an animal with impaired hemostasis (see Ch. 18). The technical details pertaining to the kind and type of waveform, shape and size of electrode, and speed of the electrode through the tissue should be fully understood if these methods are selected for making incisions.[4,23]

Piezosurgery

Piezosurgery is a new surgical technique used in maxillofacial surgery to cut hard tissues without damaging soft tissues.[24] Nerves, blood vessels, and soft tissue are not injured by the microvibrations, which are optimally adjusted to target only mineralized tissue.[25] The piezo-electric handpiece has a built-in sterile irrigation line. The cavitation effect resulting from the ultrasonic vibration and irrigating solution and the lack of soft tissue trauma reduces hemorrhage considerably.[26] It has been used in a variety of human craniomaxillofacial osteotomies with good results, especially when a precise osteotomy of a relatively thin bone was required.[26,27] It has been used experimentally in dogs for periodontal surgery with very good results.[28]

Surgical loupe and headlamp

A surgical loupe is recommended for delicate surgery and small patients.[9] A headlamp is especially useful for procedures in the caudal aspect of the oral cavity, where it may be difficult to obtain good illumination with standard surgical or dental lighting, e.g., with the patient in sternal recumbency.[9]

ASEPTIC TECHNIQUE

Aseptic technique in dentistry

Sanitation and proper sterilization techniques have been an integral part of human dental practice for many years, but since the 1980s a number of disease-causing organisms, such as HBV and HIV, have made these techniques even more important.[29] Dentists performing oral surgery must adhere to the principles of aseptic techniques for two reasons. First, during most oral surgical procedures, the dentist, assistants and equipment become contaminated with the patient's blood and saliva, which may contain pathogenic microorganisms. Second, to perform surgery, the dentist must penetrate an epithelial surface, the most important barrier the patient has against infection.[1] An opportunistic portal has thereby been created through which a pathogen may enter with sufficient strength and numbers to cause infection.[30]

The use of infection-control techniques, such as barrier precautions and sterilization practices, has been recommended by the American Dental Association (ADA) to reduce exposure and eliminate transmission of pathogenic microorganisms.[31,32] The implementation of many of these techniques by dental professionals is now required by law by the US Occupational Safety and Health Administration (OHSA) as the standard for infection control for dental practice.[31,32] These same

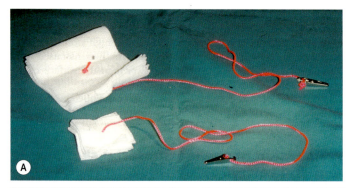

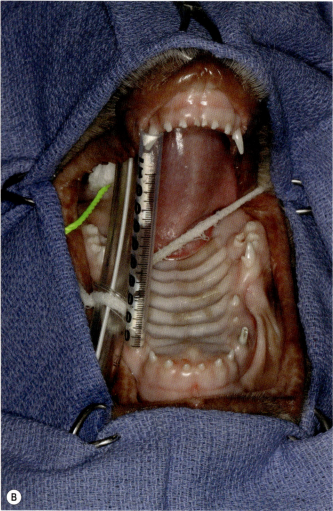

Fig. 6.18 (A) Pharyngeal pack made from exodontia sponges (Exodontia Sponges, Henry Schein, Melville, NY); **(B)** Dog in dorsal recumbency, draped for minor oral surgery using four drapes secured with Backhaus towel clamps. Note the presence of the mouth speculum.

air-sensitive. Therefore it must be kept tightly closed in a light-resistant container until ready for use.

Another oral antimicrobial solution used in dentistry is povidone-iodine. Lower levels of bacteremia among patients treated with povidone-iodine solution have been reported over patients treated with chlorhexidine or sterile water.[56] Iodine exhibits rapid antimicrobial action, even at low concentrations. Available as a 10% povidone-iodine solution (1% free iodine), it may be applied with a syringe or swab to intact oral mucous membranes. A 10-fold dilution (1% povidone-iodine) is used if a laceration is present.[63,64] Some patients may develop a sensitivity or iodine allergy to this solution and must be treated with caution.[61]

Care must be taken not to accidentally spill or spray these antimicrobial solutions into the eyes or ears of the patient.

Maxillofacial skin preparation

The skin and hair of an animal can harbor a significant amount of microbial activity and are known to be a major source of surgical wound infection.[3] Patient preparation techniques, such as hair removal and skin cleansing of the intended surgical site, will kill surface bacteria, but will not completely sterilize the area of all microbes residing in deeper, inaccessible skin structures.[3] The objective of these techniques, however, is to minimize the risk and the potential for surgical site infections in the postoperative period. All initial skin preparation should be performed outside the operating room.

Clipping is the most recommended technique for hair removal for animals.[3] The clip should be thorough yet gentle to prevent trauma or abrasion to the skin. The surgical site should be clipped immediately prior to surgery after the animal has been induced. A wide area of skin should be clipped around the proposed surgical incision. Long hair growing near the periphery of the clipped area should be cut short enough so that it cannot hang over onto the clipped area.[65] Alternatively, the facial hair can be contained by placing a segment of stockinette bandage material around the head caudal to the angle of the mouth. All loose hair and debris should be removed from the skin, and flushed from the oral cavity.

Chlorhexidine and povidone-iodine products have been recommended as the best preoperative skin preparations because they are broad-spectrum bactericidal agents that rapidly kill accessible skin microbes.[3] When these solutions are used in the maxillofacial region, however, possible complications involving the eyes and ears may arise. A review of five antimicrobial skins preparations for the maxillofacial region in humans concluded that povidone-iodine (10%) solution (not the 7.5% surgical scrub with detergent) was the safest and best-suited product.[66]

Before skin preparation of a patient is initiated, the skin should be free of gross debris and dirt. Ophthalmic lubrication should be applied liberally to the patient's eyes. The patient's skin is then prepared by applying an antimicrobial agent in concentric circles, beginning in the area of the proposed incision. The scrubbing action continues outward until the outer margins of the clipped area are reached. This process is repeated using clean sponges each time until dirt and debris are absent.

After the animal is transported to the operating room, and positioning is satisfactory, the surgical site is sprayed with additional antiseptic. If contamination occurred when moving the animal, it will be necessary to re-scrub the area.[3]

Draping of the patient

The placing of sterile drapes to isolate the oral cavity from the rest of the patient is often a neglected part of aseptic technique during oral surgery. A four-drape system may be used by placing each drape along

exhibits broad-spectrum efficacy, substantivity to tooth surfaces and mucosa, low toxicity and dental plaque-inhibiting properties.[61] Chlorhexidine is active against a wide range of Gram-positive and Gram-negative organisms, yeast, fungi, facultative anaerobes and aerobes. Its action is the result of the adsorption of chlorhexidine onto the cell wall of the microorganism, resulting in a leakage of intracellular components.[62] It may be applied to the teeth and oral tissues with the use of a syringe, brush, swab or gauze. Chlorhexidine is both light- and the mucocutaneous junction of the mandible and maxilla (Fig. 6.18B). The drapes are secured to the patient's skin with towel clamps or staples. For major maxillofacial surgery, an additional sterile fenestrated drape should be placed over the surgical site for a greater degree of asepsis.

Drapes act as a barrier, keeping hair and bacteria from hair follicles and skin from contaminating the mouth, instruments, suture material or the surgeon's gloves during a procedure.[1-3,46] They also protect the patient's eyes from oral debris.[1] Sterile drapes are available in either reusable cloth or disposable paper. Cloth is generally less expensive but may absorb bacteria when exposed to blood, tissue fluids and lavage solutions.[3] Cloth drapes are adequate for minor oral surgery. Paper drapes are more expensive, but are water-resistant and are recommended for major oral surgery.

REFERENCES

1. Hupp JR. Infection control in surgical practice. In: Peterson LJ, Ellis E, III, Hupp JR et al, editors. Contemporary oral and maxillofacial surgery. 4th ed. St. Louis, MO: Mosby; 2003. p. 63–74.

2. Piermattei DL, Johnson KA. General considerations. In: Piermattei DL, Johnson KA, editors. An atlas of surgical approaches to the bones and joints of the dog and cat. 4th ed. Philadelphia, PA: Elsevier – Saunders; 2004. p. 1–31.

3. Cockshutt J. Principles of surgical asepsis. In: Slatter DH, editor. Textbook of small animal surgery. 3rd ed. Philadelphia, PA: Elsevier – Saunders; 2003. p. 149–55.

4. Toombs JP, Clarke KM. Basic operative techniques. In: Slatter DH, editor. Textbook of small animal surgery. 3rd ed. Philadelphia, PA: Elsevier – Saunders; 2003. p.199–222.

5. Peterson LJ. Armamentarium for basic oral surgery. In: Peterson LJ, Ellis E, III, Hupp JR et al, editors. Contemporary oral and maxillofacial surgery. 4th ed. St. Louis, MO: Mosby; 2003. p. 76–112.

6. Anonymous. Swann-Morton surgical blades for dentists. http://www.swann-morton.com/dentist.php. Accessed 8-17-2007.

7. Pattison AM, Pattison GL, Takei HH. The periodontal instrumentarium. In: Newman MG, Takei HH, Carranza FA, editors. Carranza's clinical periodontology. 9th ed. Philadelphia, PA: WB Saunders; 2002. p. 567–93.

8. Anonymous. Hu-Friedy product catalog & reference guide. 2nd ed. Chicago, IL: Hu-Friedy Mfg Inc; 2000.

9. Fragiskos FD. Equipment, instruments, and materials. In: Fragiskos FD, editor. Oral surgery. Berlin, Heidelberg & New York: Springer – Verlag; 2007. p. 43–72.

10. Tholen MA. Veterinary oral surgery – 2. Vet Med Small Anim Clin 1982;77: 907–16.

11. Holmstrom SE, Frost P, Eisner ER. Veterinary dental techniques – for the small animal practitioner. 3rd ed. Philadelphia, PA: Elsevier – Saunders; 2004.

12. Heyman SN, Babayof I. Emphysematous complications in dentistry, 1960–1993: an illustrative case and review of the literature. Quintessence Int 1995;26:535–43.

13. Buffa EA, Lubbe AM, Verstraete FJM, et al. The effects of wound lavage solutions on canine fibroblasts: an in vitro study. Vet Surg 1997;26:460–6.

14. Crossley DA. Surgical extraction of the maxillary canine. J Vet Dent 2003;20:136, 138–9.

15. Anonymous. Waterborne disease transmission. Atlanta, GA: Centers for Disease Control, US Department of Health and Human Services; 2000.

16. Verstraete FJ. Mandibulectomy and maxillectomy. Vet Clin North Am Small Anim Pract 2005;35:1009–39.

17. Silverman EB, Read RW, Boyle CR, et al. Histologic comparison of canine skin biopsies collected using monopolar electrosurgery, CO_2 laser, radiowave radiosurgery, skin biopsy punch, and scalpel. Vet Surg 2007;36:50–6.

18. Sinha UK, Gallagher LA. Effects of steel scalpel, ultrasonic scalpel, CO_2 laser, and monopolar and bipolar electrosurgery on wound healing in guinea pig oral mucosa. Laryngoscope 2003;113:228–36.

19. Pope JW, Gargiulo AW, Staffileno H, et al. Effects of electrosurgery on wound healing in dogs. Periodontics 1968;6:30–7.

20. Azzi R, Kenney EB, Tsao TF, et al. The effect of electrosurgery on alveolar bone. J Periodontol 1983;54:96–100.

21. Wilhelmsen NR, Ramfjord SP, Blankenship JR. Effects of electrosurgery on the gingival attachment in rhesus monkeys. J Periodontol 1976;47:160–70.

22. Carranza FA. The gingivectomy technique. In: Newman MG, Takei HH, Carranza FA, editors. Carranza's clinical periodontology. 9th ed. Philadelphia, PA: WB Saunders; 2002. p. 749–53.

23. Williams VD. Electrosurgery and wound healing: a review of the literature. J Am Dent Assoc 1984;108:220–2.

24. Vercellotti T. Technological characteristics and clinical indications of piezoelectric bone surgery. Minerva Stomatol 2004;53: 207–14.

25. Stubinger S, Kuttenberger J, Filippi A, et al. Intraoral piezosurgery: preliminary results of a new technique. J Oral Maxillofac Surg 2005;63:1283–7.

26. Beziat JL, Bera JC, Lavandier B, et al. Ultrasonic osteotomy as a new technique in craniomaxillofacial surgery. Int J Oral Maxillofac Surg 2007;36:493–500.

27. Eggers G, Klein J, Blank J, et al. Piezosurgery: an ultrasound device for cutting bone and its use and limitations in maxillofacial surgery. Br J Oral Maxillofac Surg 2004;42:451–3.

28. Vercellotti T, Nevins ML, Kim DM, et al. Osseous response following resective therapy with piezosurgery. Int J Periodontics Restorative Dent 2005;25: 543–9.

29. Anonymous. Infection control in dentistry – blood disease transmission. Atlanta, GA: National Center for Chronic Disease Prevention and Health Promotion – Oral Health Resources, Centers for Disease Control; 2001.

30. Anonymous. Recommended infection-control practices for dentistry. Atlanta, GA: Centers for Disease Control – Morbidity and Mortality Weekly Report 1993; 42(RR-8):1–10.

31. Anonymous. Infection control recommendations for the dental office and the dental laboratory. ADA Council on Scientific Affairs and ADA Council on Dental Practice. J Am Dent Assoc 1996;127:672–80.

32. Kohn WG, Harte JA, Malvitz DM, et al. Guidelines for infection control in dental health care settings – 2003. J Am Dent Assoc 2004;135:33–47.

33. Mangram AJ, Horan TC, Pearson ML, et al. Guideline for prevention of surgical site infection, 1999. Hospital Infection Control Practices Advisory Committee. Infect Control Hosp Epidemiol 1999; 20:250–78.

34. Emori TG, Gaynes RP. An overview of nosocomial infections, including the role of the microbiology laboratory. Clin Microbiol Rev 1993;6:428–42.

35. Boerlin P, Eugster S, Gaschen F, et al. Transmission of opportunistic pathogens in a veterinary teaching hospital. Vet Microbiol 2001;82:347–59.

36. Brown DC, Conzemius MG, Shofer F, et al. Epidemiologic evaluation of postoperative wound infections in dogs and cats. J Am Vet Med Assoc 1997;210: 1302–6.

37. Fossum TW. Small animal surgery. 3rd ed. St. Louis, MO: Mosby; 2007.

38. Tracy DL. Small animal surgical nursing. 3rd ed. St. Louis, MO: Mosby – Year Book; 2000.

39. Anonymous. Recommendations and reports – guidelines for infection control in dental health-care settings. Atlanta: Centers for Disease Control – Morbidity and Mortality Weekly Report 2003;52 (No. RR-17).

40. Rutala WA. APIC guideline for selection and use of disinfectants. 1994, 1995, and 1996 APIC Guidelines Committee. Association for Professionals in Infection Control and Epidemiology, Inc. Am J Infect Control 1996;24:313–42.

41. Garner JS, Favero MS. Guideline for handwashing and hospital environmental control, 1985. Atlanta, GA: Center for Disease Control; 1987. p. 1–26.

42. AORN Recommended Practices Committee. Proposed recommended practices for sterilization in the practice setting. AORN Journal 1994;60:109–17.

43. Depaola LG, Mangan D, Mills SE, et al. A review of the science regarding dental unit waterlines. J Am Dent Assoc 2002;133: 1199–206.

44. Anonymous. Statement from CDC regarding biofilm and dental unit water quality. Atlanta, GA: Centers for Disease Control, National Center for Chronic Disease Prevention and Health Promotion; 2001.

45. Mills SE. The dental unit waterline controversy: defusing the myths, defining the solutions. J Am Dent Assoc 2000; 131:1427–41.

46. Shmon C. Assessment and preparation of the surgical patient and the operating team. In: Slatter DH, editor. Textbook of small animal surgery. 3rd ed. Philadelphia, PA: Elsevier – Saunders; 2003. p. 162–78.

47. Larson EL. APIC guideline for handwashing and hand antisepsis in health care settings. Am J Infect Control 1995;23:251–69.

48. Anonymous. Guideline for hand hygiene in health-care settings: recommendations of the Healthcare Infection Control Practices Advisory Committee and the HICPAC/SHEA/APIC/IDSA Hand Hygiene Task Force. Atlanta, GA: Centers for Disease Control – Morbidity and Mortality Weekly Report 2002;51 (No. RR-16).

49. Laskin DM. The selection of proper gloves for intraoral surgery [editorial]. J Oral Maxillofac Surg 1999;57:887.

50. Adeyemo WL, Ogunlewe MO, Ladeinde AL, et al. Are sterile gloves necessary in nonsurgical dental extractions? J Oral Maxillofac Surg 2005;63:936–40.

51. Chiu WK, Cheung LK, Chan HC, et al. A comparison of post-operative complications following wisdom tooth surgery performed with sterile or clean gloves. Int J Oral Maxillofac Surg 2006;35:174–9.

52. Rudy RL, Boudrieau RJ. Maxillofacial and mandibular fractures. Semin Vet Med Surg (Small Anim) 1992;7:3–20.

53. Veksler AE, Kayrouz GA, Newman MG. Reduction of salivary bacteria by pre-procedural rinses with chlorhexidine 0.12%. J Periodontol 1991;62:649–51.

54. Walsh TF, Unsal E, Davis LG, et al. The effect of irrigation with chlorhexidine or saline on plaque vitality. J Clin Periodontol 1995;22:262–4.

55. Bowersock TL, Wu CC, Inskeep GA, et al. Prevention of bacteremia in dogs undergoing dental scaling by prior administration of oral clindamycin or chlorhexidine oral rinse. J Vet Dent 2000;17:11–16.

56. Rahn R, Schneider S, Diehl O, et al. Preventing post-treatment bacteremia: comparing topical povidone-iodine and chlorhexidine. J Am Dent Assoc 1995; 126:1145–9.

57. Summers AN, Larson DL, Edmiston CE, et al. Efficacy of preoperative decontamination of the oral cavity. Plast Reconstr Surg 2000;106:895–900.

58. Fine DH, Yip J, Furgang D, et al. Reducing bacteria in dental aerosols: pre-procedural use of an antiseptic mouthrinse. J Am Dent Assoc 1993;124:56–8.

59. Fine DH, Mendieta C, Barnett ML, et al. Efficacy of preprocedural rinsing with an antiseptic in reducing viable bacteria in dental aerosols. J Periodontol 1992;63: 821–4.

60. Robinson JG. Chlorhexidine gluconate – the solution for dental problems. J Vet Dent 1995;12:29–31.

61. Jorgensen MG, Slots J. Practical antimicrobial periodontal therapy. Compend Contin Educ Dent 2000;21: 111–20.

62. Fardal O, Turnbull RS. A review of the literature on use of chlorhexidine in dentistry. J Am Dent Assoc 1986;112: 863–9.

63. Sanchez IR, Nusbaum KE, Swaim SF, et al. Chlorhexidine diacetate and povidone-iodine cytotoxicity to canine embryonic fibroblasts and *Staphylococcus aureus*. Vet Surg 1988;17:182–5.

64. Sanchez IR, Swaim SF, Nusbaum KE, et al. Effects of chlorhexidine diacetate and povidone-iodine on wound healing in dogs. Vet Surg 1988;17:291–5.

65. Davidson JR, Burba DJ. Surgical instruments and aseptic technique. In: McCurnin DM, Bassert JM, editors. Clinical textbook for veterinary technicians. 5th ed. Philadelphia, PA: WB Saunders; 2002. p. 554–89.

66. Morgan III JP, Haug RH, Kosman JW. Antimicrobial skin preparations for the maxillofacial region. J Oral Maxillofac Surg 1996;54:89–94.

Chapter 7

Suture materials and biomaterials

Anson J. Tsugawa & Frank J.M. Verstraete

GENERAL PRINCIPLES

Sutures placed intraorally are exposed to tissues of high vascularity, a constant bathing of saliva, bacteria, fluctuations in temperature and pH and masticatory trauma.[1] The tissue reaction to the placement of sutures in the mouth is different from that seen in other regions of the body.[2] Peak tissue reactions have been reported to occur between the second and seventh days for tissues other than the oral cavity.[3] The physical character of the suture material is the most important consideration in determining intraoral tissue reactivity; in general, monofilament and nonabsorbable sutures are less reactive than multifilament and absorbable suture materials.[2,3] The capillarity of a suture material, the process by which fluid and bacteria are trapped in the interstices of multifilament materials, is also an important consideration for the intraoral placement of sutures, as multifilament sutures are more likely to contribute to the wicking of bacteria and oral fluids deep into the wound.[2,4] Suture materials intended for intraoral use should accumulate little or no bacterial plaque.[1] Furthermore, absorbable suture materials are favored over nonabsorbable materials because they enhance patient comfort and eliminate the need for removal. The additional manipulations required during intraoral suture removal may predispose to bacteremia and endocarditis in the high-risk cardiac patient.[5]

The primary objective of dental suturing is to achieve apposition of wound edges to promote optimal healing.[6] Blood and serum that accumulate beneath the inappropriately apposed flap delay the healing process.[6] Sutures function to appose wound edges until the supported tissues have regained sufficient strength to withstand tensile forces. When their strength is no longer needed, the suture material should absorb completely and predictably to prevent additional delays in healing.[1] The ideal time for suture loss specific to the oral tissues has not been clearly defined.[1] It has been suggested, however, that 4 days is the optimum time for suture removal; by 72 hours, a stratified squamous keratinized epithelial layer has formed in the attached gingiva.[7,8] Connective tissue healing with type III and type I collagen occurs by 96 hours.[9,10]

When selecting a suture material, the surgeon should consider the physical properties of the suture material (capillarity, size, tensile strength, absorbability surface characteristics and tissue reactivity) and the rate of wound healing in the area.[3] All too often, however, the selection of suture material by the surgeon is based on handling properties alone. The minimal requirements for an intraoral suture material are outlined in Table 7.1.

SUTURE CHARACTERISTICS

Suture materials may be absorbable or nonabsorbable, and monofilament or multifilament (see Table 7.1). Absorbable suture materials have been defined by the United States Pharmacopeia (USP) as strands of collagen or synthetic polymers that are capable of absorption in mammalian tissue. In contrast, nonabsorbable sutures are strands of material that are resistant to absorption. Monofilament suture materials are composed of a single strand of material, and multifilament sutures are braided or woven from multiple strands of material.

Physical properties

Handling characteristics

The handling characteristics of a suture material are intimately associated with the intrinsic stiffness of the material. Suture materials that are more pliable and of smaller diameter have favorable handling characteristics to stiff suture materials of large diameter.[11] When cut, the sharp ends of stiff suture materials (e.g., stainless steel or nylon) can result in the mechanical irritation of tissues. As a general rule, multifilament sutures have better handling characteristics than monofilament sutures, as well as uncoated sutures compared to coated ones. Related to stiffness is elasticity. Most suture materials exhibit limited elongation when exposed to increasing loads. Notable exceptions are polypropylene and polybutester, which are relatively elastic. The surface of uncoated braided materials such as polyglycolic acid is rough and causes considerable friction and trauma when going through tissues.

Capillarity

The degree of bacterial transport along suture filaments is determined by the fluid absorption and capillarity of the suture material.[12] Monofilament sutures withstand contamination better than multifilament

DOI: 10.1016/B978-0-7020-4618-6.00007-5

Table 7.1 Minimal physical and biological requirements for intraoral suture materials

1. Fast absorption with minimal tissue reactivity
2. Good short-term tensile/knot strength with sutures of small diameter
3. Minimally plaque retentive
4. Low capillarity and fluid absorption
5. Knots with good security and without injury to the soft tissues
6. Low tissue drag
7. High pliability for favorable handling in confined areas

sutures, and tissue reactivity is minimized with monofilament suture materials.[13] Multifilament sutures have a five- to eightfold higher affinity for bacterial adherence than monofilament nylon sutures.[14]

Tensile strength, knot-pull tensile strength and knot security

The tensile strength of a suture material refers to the strength required to break an untied portion of suture when a force is applied along its length (Table 7.2).[15] Thicker-diameter sutures have greater strength than smaller-diameter sutures, but the thickness also increases the total amount of foreign material in the wound and the severity of associated tissue reaction.[16] The knot is mechanically the weakest link of the suture loop, tension forces are converted into shearing forces at the knot, and the initial tensile strength of a suture is reduced by at least one third.[17,18]

Knot-pull tensile strength is defined as the force in pounds that is required to break a knotted strand of suture material, whereas knot security refers to the knot holding capacity of a suture material expressed as a percentage of the tensile strength. The knot-pull tensile strength is related to the diameter of the suture, the type of suture material and the size of the suture loop.[18,19] Knot security is influenced by the suture diameter, coefficient of friction and the quality of the knot.[18–20]

When induced to failure, secure knots break rather than untie due to slippage of the knot.[21] In general, the use of larger-diameter sutures and the placement of additional throws in the knot will increase the security and reliability of the knot.[16] More specifically, catgut, polyglycolic acid, polyglactin 910 and polypropylene require three throws to ensure knot security; four throws are necessary for polydioxanone and polyamide.[21]

Biologic properties

Suture materials may be derived from natural or synthetic sources. Synthetic sutures account for almost all of the currently used suture materials, and the only naturally derived examples discussed here include catgut and silk (see Table 7.2). Natural and synthetic sutures differ in their mechanism of absorption. Natural sutures are degraded and absorbed by the proteolytic enzymes supplied by macrophages, and synthetic sutures are degraded by hydrolysis in tissue fluid.

Biofilm

Biofilms are complex communities of surface-associated cells enclosed in a polymer matrix containing open water channels that can develop on many different medical devices, including suture materials.[22] Biofilms serve as a reservoir for bacteria. Bacteria growing on the surface of a biofilm have been shown to display a unique phenotype with increased resistance.[23] Within biofilms, bacteria are hidden from the host immune system and are less susceptible to antibiotics.[22] Complete elimination of bacteria from biofilms on suture material may be impossible.[22] The bacteremia created by suture removal and the potential risk of endocarditis has led to the suggestion of antibiotic prophylaxis at the time of suture removal in compromised patients but this is controversial.[24]

Tissue reactivity

All suture materials elicit a foreign body cellular reaction when they are implanted into tissues, but natural sutures exhibit greater tissue reactivity than their synthetic counterparts, and the inflammatory phase of wound healing is prolonged (see Table 7.2). The most inert materials are monofilament synthetics such as nylon and steel. The more material that is implanted in a wound, the greater the tissue reaction, and the knotted portion of the suture loop contains the highest density of foreign material.[25] Suture size contributes more to tissue reaction than extra throws to the knot.[16]

Influence of wound infection

The placement of foreign material in an infected wound can exacerbate or perpetuate infection; therefore, whenever possible, the surgeon should avoid placing sutures in heavily contaminated wounds that require immediate closure.[26] Sutures may potentiate infection by inducing an exudative foreign body response with local tissue autolysis and by physically shielding the bacteria from the host defense.[26] For this reason, multifilament sutures are not recommended for use in contaminated wounds, as the clearance of bacteria from the interstices of multifilament materials is slower than with monofilament materials.[26] Although the physical and chemical structure of a suture material influences the degree of infection, proper surgical technique and wound care also play important roles in minimizing wound infection.[26]

Influence of pH

The pH level in tissues and body fluid varies by location (e.g., gastric juice, 0.9 to 1.5; and pancreatic juice in the duodenum, 7.5 to 8.2), and is influenced by the presence of infection and inflammation. *Proteus*, a urea-splitting bacterium, dissociates urea to ammonia and elevates the pH of urine. The pH of inflamed tissue is generally acidic.[27] The pH of a tissue can affect the retention of tensile strength of suture materials.

The degradation of natural absorbable sutures is accelerated in both acidic and alkaline pH but, in general, only alkaline conditions have a significant effect on synthetic absorbable sutures.[27] Polydioxanone is a notable exception, as it degrades faster in acidic solutions.[28] Silk is the most vulnerable of nonabsorbable sutures to fluctuations in pH, but nylon also exhibits a degradation in tensile strength in acidic environments.[27,28] Polypropylene, a synthetic nonabsorbable suture material, retains its initial tensile strength over a wide range of pH.[28]

SUTURE MATERIALS

Catgut

Plain catgut is a natural suture material derived from the submucosa of sheep intestine or the serosa of cattle intestine. Chromic catgut is a modification of plain catgut that is tanned with chromic salts to improve strength and delay dissolution.[29] Gut is absorbed by phagocytosis, and is associated with a marked tissue inflammation that can

Table 7.2 General characteristics of suture materials used in veterinary oral and maxillofacial surgery

Suture	Trade name	Type	Degradation	Tissue reactivity	Intraoral survival time (days)*	Tensile strength retention (%)	Complete absorption (days)
Catgut (chromic)	Surgical gut[a] / Chromic gut[b]	Absorbable Multifilament	Proteolytic enzymes and phagocytosis	Moderate	3–7[48]; 7–10[35] (variable, shorter in infected wounds)	Unpredictable	45–60
Polyglycolic acid	Dexon S[b] (uncoated) / Dexon II[b] (coated)	Absorbable Multifilament	Hydrolysis	Minimal acute	7–14[48]; 16–20[35]	65% (55% sizes 7–0 or smaller) after 14 d; 35% (20% sizes 7–0 or smaller) after 21 d	60–90
Polyglactin 910	Vicryl[a]	Absorbable Multifilament	Hydrolysis	Minimal acute	28[30]	75% after 14 d	56–70
	Vicryl Rapide[a]		Hydrolysis (phagocytosis)		3[1]	50% after 5 d; 0% at 14 d	42
	Coated Vicryl Plus[a]		Hydrolysis		28[30]	75% after 14 d	56–70
Polydioxanone	PDS II[a] / PDS Plus[a]	Absorbable Monofilament	Hydrolysis	Slight	>28[48]	74% after 14 d; 58% after 28 d; 41% after 42 d	180
Polytrimethylene carbonate	Maxon[b]	Absorbable Monofilament	Hydrolysis	Minimal		81% after 14 d; 59% after 28 d; 30% after 42 d	180
Poliglecaprone 25	Monocryl[a] / Monocryl Plus[a]	Absorbable Monofilament	Hydrolysis	Minimal acute		50–60% after 7 d; 20–30% after 14 d; 0% within 21 d	91–119
Polyamide	Ethilon[a] (monofilament) / Nurolon[a] (multifilament) / Dermalon[b] (monofilament) / Surgilon[b] (multifilament)	Nonabsorbable Monofilament/multifilament	Hydrolysis (slow)	Minimal acute		15–20% loss after 365 d, retains remaining 80% indefinitely	Gradual encapsulation by fibrous tissue
Polybutester	Novafil[b]	Nonabsorbable Monofilament	N/A	Minimal acute		N/A	N/A
Polypropylene	Prolene[a] / Surgipro[b] / Surgipro II[b]	Nonabsorbable Monofilament	N/A	Minimal acute		N/A	N/A
Hexafluoropropylene-VDF	Pronova[a]	Nonabsorbable Monofilament	N/A	Minimal acute		N/A	N/A
Polyester	Mersilene[a] (uncoated) / Ethibond Excel[a] (coated) / Ti-cron[b] / Surgidac[b]	Nonabsorbable Multifilament	N/A	Minimal acute		N/A	Gradual encapsulation by fibrous tissue
Stainless steel	Surgical Stainless Steel[a] (monofilament) / Surgical Stainless Steel[a] (multifilament) / Steel[b] (monofilament) / Flexon[b] (multifilament)	Nonabsorbable Monofilament/multifilament	N/A	Minimal acute		N/A	N/A
Silk	Perma-Hand[a] / Sofsilk[b]	Nonabsorbable Multifilament	Proteolytic enzymes and phagocytosis	Severe		70% after 14 d; 50% after 30 d	Gradual encapsulation by fibrous tissue

*Spontaneous loss
[a]Ethicon, Inc., Somerville, NJ
[b]U.S. Surgical, Norwalk, CT

be detrimental to healing. Conversely, tissue inflammation may lead to a more rapid breakdown of catgut. Plain gut has a median survival time of 4 days in the oral cavity, whereas chromic gut retains its strength for 2 to 3 weeks.[26,30] In moist environments such as the oral cavity, the strength of gut is reduced by 20–30%.[31] Gut is a stiff material that must be moistened in alcohol, and forms knots that can be irritating to the oral tissues.[32,33] Infection rates may increase with the use of gut.[34] The advent of synthetic materials preferable to gut, with less tissue reactivity and more predictable resorption, has almost made catgut obsolete.[25]

Synthetic absorbable suture materials

Polyglycolic acid

Polyglycolic acid is a multifilament suture material derived from a homopolymer of glycolic acid (hydroxyacetic acid), and is available uncoated (Dexon S, U.S. Surgical, Norwalk, CT) or coated (Dexon II, U.S. Surgical, Norwalk, CT) with polycaprolate, a copolymer of glycolide and ε-caprolactone. Polyglycolic acid is absorbed by hydrolysis with less associated tissue inflammation than silk, plain or chromic catgut.[35] The median survival time of polyglycolic acid in the oral mucosa is 15 days (16 to 20).[30,35] The initial tensile strength of polyglycolic acid exceeds that of silk and gut, but is decreased appreciably when placed in oral tissue.[36] The handling characteristics of polyglycolic acid are favorable, similar to silk, but its knot security is poor.[37] Polyglycolic acid also has a tendency to cut through friable tissue, which is not a favorable quality for suturing gingival tissues.[21] Polyglycolic acid has been shown to inhibit bacterial transmission due to the release of monomers.[37]

Polyglactin 910

Polyglactin 910 is a braided suture material that is a copolymer of glycolic and lactic acid. The lactic acid provides water repellence, delaying the loss of tensile strength. Vicryl (Vicryl, Ethicon, Inc., Somerville, NJ) is coated with polyglactin 370 and calcium stearate to decrease tissue drag and bacterial adherence. It is absorbed by hydrolysis, and its intraoral survival rate is approximately 28 days.[30] Complete resorption may take up to 40 to 60 days.[38] Because polyglactin 910 persists much longer than is necessary for intraoral wound healing, it is not an ideal suture material for periodontal procedures.[38] The long absorption time of polyglactin 910 also makes it a potential nidus for infection.

Vicryl Rapide (Vicryl Rapide, Ethicon, Inc., Somerville, NJ) is an irradiated form of polyglactin 910 that is lost from the skin as early as 10 to 14 days. Intraorally, the median time for suture loss of Vicryl Rapide is 3 days.[1] Gamma radiation alters the molecular structure of polyglactin 910 and enhances its in vivo absorption rate.[39] In contrast to nonirradiated polyglactin, Vicryl Rapide may also be absorbed by phagocytosis.[39] Vicryl Rapide remains in the skin longer than 5 days and is not recommended for facial skin closure.[40] Irradiated polyglactin 910, however, satisfies many of the minimal physical and biological requirements for an intraoral suture outlined in Table 7.1; these include fast absorption, ease of handling, good knot security and minimal inflammatory reaction of the surrounding tissues.[41] Although Vicryl Rapide is favorable in terms of its enhanced absorption rate, it has a tendency to be more brittle than nonirradiated polyglactin 910, and break if tugged on suddenly.[41]

Coated Vicryl Plus (Coated Vicryl Plus, Ethicon, Inc., Somerville, NJ) is a recent addition to the Vicryl suture material family that contains the synthetic broad-spectrum antimicrobial agent triclosan (2,2,4′-trichloro-2′-hydroxy-diphenyl ether).[42] Triclosan is an antimicrobial agent found in many personal/oral healthcare products,

and is a potent inhibitor of enoyl acyl carrier protein (ACP) reductase, an essential enzyme in bacterial fatty acid biosynthesis.[43] In general, triclosan is considered more effective against Gram-positive than Gram-negative species.[43] Coated Vicryl Plus exhibits the same physical and functional handling properties as Coated Vicryl and the only difference between the two products is the addition of 100–500 ppm of triclosan to the coating.[44] The addition of triclosan to Coated Vicryl was found to affect neither wound healing nor its absorption pattern.[42] Coated Vicryl Plus exhibits in vitro antimicrobial activity against Staphylococcus aureus and S. epidermidis, the most prevalent organisms associated with surgical wound infection, for up to 7 days in an aqueous environment.[45] Triclosan has shown sustained antimicrobial activity during the period of wound reepithelialization within the early postoperative period.[46] The antimicrobial efficacy of triclosan-coated suture material was unhindered when coated with biologic substrates, 20% bovine serum albumin, that mimics the tissue proteins recruited to the margins of a surgical wound.[46] Besides the obvious bactericidal benefit of antibacterial-coated sutures, coated sutures have also demonstrated an ability to significantly reduce bacterial adherence compared to noncoated suture material.[46] The usefulness of Coated Vicryl Plus in the oral cavity is related to triclosan's ability to control oral plaque, and is supported by studies showing the effectiveness of triclosan in oral rinses and dentrifices.[43] Incorporation of antibacterial agents such as triclosan into suture materials, however, is not without controversy; species such as Pseudomonas aeruginosa have already been found to be resistant to various antiseptic agents, including triclosan.[46]

Polydioxanone

PDS (PDS II, Ethicon, Inc., Somerville, NJ) is a polyester of the monomer paradioxanone. PDS is hydrolyzed much slower than other absorbable suture materials, and retains 74% of its original tensile strength at 2 weeks, 58% at 4 weeks and 41% at 6 weeks.[47] In a comparison study of suture materials in the feline oral cavity, PDS was found to be intact at day 28.[48] When used on the gingiva, the hard ends of the suture material may be abrasive to the buccal mucosa that comes into contact with them. PDS is useful in wounds where a long healing time and extended tensile strength are required.[47,48] Although PDS was developed for use as a resorbable suture material, it has also successfully been used as a resorbable alternative to stainless steel wire in transosseous fixation.[49]

Similar to Vicryl Plus, an antibacterial version of PDS, PDS Plus (PDS Plus, Ethicon, Inc., Somerville, NJ), has recently been introduced. PDS Plus inhibits bacterial colonization of the suture by S. aureus, S. epidermidis, Escherichia coli and Klebsiella pneumoniae.

Polytrimethylene carbonate

Maxon (Maxon, U.S. Surgical, Norwalk, CT) is derived from a copolymer of glycolide and trimethylene carbonate. Maxon is very similar to PDS in terms of tensile strength and long tissue retention but is less rigid.[26] Because of its long retention time, Maxon is less desirable as a suture material for routine intraoral use. Maxon retains 81% of its original tensile strength at 2 weeks, 59% at 28 days and 30% at 42 days.[47] Resorption occurs by hydrolysis between 180 and 210 days.[50]

Poliglecaprone 25

Monocryl (Monocryl, Ethicon, Inc., Somerville, NJ) is an extremely pliable monofilament suture material that is derived from a segmented copolymer of ε-caprolactone and glycolide.[51] The pliability of Monocryl contributes to its excellent handling characteristics.[52] Monocryl loses 20–30% of its original tensile strength after 2 weeks, and is completely absorbed by hydrolysis in 90 days.[51] Similar to other absorbable sutures that resorb via hydrolysis, Monocryl exhibits minimal tissue reaction that is characterized by macrophages, fibroblasts, lymphocytes, plasma cells and giant cells.[51,52] Monocryl has superior tensile strength and is less reactive than polyglactin 910.[52] In a recent study involving human patients undergoing dentoalveolar surgery, microbial adherence to Monocryl was shown to be significantly lower than nonresorbable multifilament and monofilament sutures.[53] A triclosan-coated version of Monocryl, Monocryl Plus (Monocryl Plus, Ethicon, Inc., Somerville, NJ), is also available.

Synthetic monofilament nonabsorbable suture materials

Polyamide

Nylon (Ethilon, Ethicon, Inc., Somerville, NJ) is a synthetic polyamide polymer fiber that is a popular suture for cutaneous closure. Nylon is classified as a nonabsorbable suture, but does exhibit some absorption by hydrolysis and loses 15–20% of its tensile strength per year.[26,29] The hydrolysis of nylon is influenced by the acidity of the milieu, as acids catalyze the hydrolysis of the amide linkages in nylon.[29] The tissue reactivity of nylon is minimal, but its knot security is poor, and multiple throws are required to properly seat a suture. If used as an intraoral suture material, the sharp cut ends of nylon can be irritating to the patient and injurious to the oral soft tissues.[42] Soaking in alcohol may improve pliability.[26]

Polybutester

Novafil (Novafil, U.S. Surgical, Norwalk, CT) is a copolymer composed of polyglycol and polybutylene terephthalate. Compared to nylon, Novafil is less stiff and has a lower memory. Novafil also has greater elasticity then either nylon or polypropylene, and the unique feature of being able to stretch 50% of its length under low loads; as a result, Novafil is able to passively accommodate wound edema, reducing suture marks and cut-throughs.[26,54] Although synthetic nonabsorbable sutures are rarely used intraorally, Novafil can be used safely in the mouth with less patient discomfort than nylon.[55]

Polypropylene

Prolene (Prolene, Ethicon, Inc., Somerville, NJ) is a synthetic nonabsorbable monofilament that is derived from the polymerization of propylene. The absorption of Prolene is virtually nonexistent. Its tissue reactivity is low, and is preferable for treating contaminated sites. In comparison to nylon, Prolene has better knot security, elasticity, and pulls smoothly through tissues. The plasticity of Prolene sutures accommodates tissue swelling and reduces trauma to the sutured tissue.[26]

Hexafluoropropylene-VDF

Pronova (Pronova, Ethicon, Inc., Somerville, NJ) is a new synthetic nonabsorbable monofilament that is uniquely composed of two polymers: polyvinylidine fluoride homopolymer and polyvinylidine fluoride hexafluoropropylene copolymer. Pronova is comparable to polypropylene in terms of biocompatibility, and its advantages are reduced package memory, easier handling, greater tensile and knot strength, and greater resistance to instrument damage. Pronova has been marketed for use in cardiovascular, ophthalmic and neurosurgery, but can also be used for general soft tissue wound closure and ligation.

Synthetic multifilament nonabsorbable suture materials

Polyester

Polyester is a braided suture material that is available uncoated (Mersilene, Ethicon, Inc., Somerville, NJ) or coated (Ethibond Excel, Ethicon, Inc., Somerville, NJ) with polytetrafluoroethane. The coating minimizes capillarity and allows for tissue passage with less friction, but the coating may crack off after knots are tied, resulting in deposition of foreign material in the wound.[3] Because polyester is braided, its handling characteristics are better than monofilament nylon but, as a result, it is predisposed to greater bacterial adherence. Polyester has low tissue reactivity, and is retained within the wound in a fibrous cartilaginous capsule.[56] Due to its high tensile strength and knot security, polyester is an excellent suture for mobile facial areas, tracheal anastomosis and respiratory tract surgery.[26,56]

Stainless steel

Stainless steel sutures are composed of low-carbon, iron-alloy strands, and are available as either a monofilament or a multifilament.[30] Stainless steel has low tissue reactivity, and good tensile strength and knot security. Monofilament stainless steel is difficult to handle, and is used infrequently as a suture material in periodontal surgery, but is occasionally used around the lips to prevent suture removal in dog and cat patients.[39] Its characteristics are very similar to monofilament synthetic nonabsorbable suture materials, and it is used more commonly for the internal fixation of fractures. Multifilament stainless steel is easier to work with, but gives rise to the same problems as multifilament nonabsorbable suture materials, namely wound infection due to capillary action and sinus tract formation when used internally.

Silk

Modern silk sutures are composed of 70% natural silk and 30% extraneous materials (gum, beeswax and silicone).[32] Silk is classified as a nonabsorbable suture material, but it loses 50% of its original strength within 1 month, and is completely absorbed by proteolysis in 2 years.[26] Tensile strength is lost in 1 year.[53] Silk has excellent handling characteristics and knot security, and is still occasionally used in oral surgery, but is known to cause substantial tissue inflammation. Host tissue reactions may lead to encapsulation by granulation tissue.[57] Silk has high capillarity, and should generally be avoided in contaminated sites.

SUTURE SIZE

Currently, the common standard for suture size diameter is that issued by the USP. Size is designated by a numerical code, 11–0 being the smallest size available and 6 the largest. The size of the suture material selected should correlate with the tensile strength of the tissue being sutured, and the smallest diameter suture sufficient to adequately appose the wound margins should be used to minimize the trauma incurred from the passage (friction) of the suture through the tissues and the foreign body reaction created by the material that is retained in the wound.[58] Size 3–0 and 4–0 sutures are the most commonly used sizes for oral and maxillofacial surgical procedures in humans.[58] In most dogs and cats, 5–0 suture material is indicated.

SUTURE NEEDLES

The modern suture needle is constructed of corrosion-resistant surgical-grade stainless steel, and consists of three basic parts: attachment end (swaged or closed eye), body and needle point. Needles for use in oro-maxillofacial surgery are of the swaged-on variety, where the needle has been permanently crimped onto the suture material, as swaged needles facilitate suture handling and reduce tissue trauma during suturing compared to eyed needles.[58] The body shape of the needle may be straight, curved or a combination of both (curved-ended straight) (Fig. 7.1). Needles are further divided into cuticular and plastic varieties; the latter is sharpened 36 times, and is designed for cosmetic closures.[59]

Selection of needle shape is based on accessibility of the area to be sutured and surgeon's preference. For the purposes of oromaxillofacial surgery, the $\frac{3}{8}$-circle needle is the most commonly used, as it requires significantly less wrist pronation and supination in comparison to the other commonly used needle in veterinary medicine ($\frac{1}{2}$-circle). As a general rule, curved needles with a comparatively greater arc ($\frac{1}{2}$- or $\frac{5}{8}$-circle) are more suited for suturing small, deep wounds in confined areas (e.g., vestibule or caudal oropharynx).[59] Cutting, tapered and tapercut are the three basic types of needle points (Fig. 7.1). As their name suggests, cutting needles possess sharp edges (two opposing cutting edges and a third cutting edge along the curvature of the needle) that facilitate penetration through tough keratinized tissues such as the gingiva or skin. Cutting needles may be further subdivided

into conventional- and reverse-cutting needles. Although both are triangular in cross-section, the reverse-cutting needle has a flat surface along its inner curvature; preventing the inadvertent cutting of tissue 'cut-out' as the needle is passed through tissue. The reverse-cutting shape also increases the strength of the needle by 32%.[59] Because of the predisposition for 'cut-out' with conventional-cutting needles, their use is limited within the oral cavity, and the reverse-cutting needle is the most commonly selected needle for general use in dentistry and oromaxillofacial surgery. Tapered point needles are round in cross-section, and result in less tissue damage than cutting point needles, but are poorly suited for use in tough tissues, such as gingiva. Tapercut needles combine the cutting action of the reverse-cutting needle at its tip and the round body of the taper for atraumatic passage through delicate tissues. The tapercut needle is recommended for use in mucogingival surgery.

SUTURE RECOMMENDATIONS FOR SPECIFIC TISSUES

Intraoral tissue

Size 5–0 Monocryl and Vicryl Rapide are currently the most compatible suture materials for intraoral use. For vestibular flap closure following maxillectomy, however, polypropylene is recommended.[60] Both Monocryl and Vicryl Rapide have rapid absorption times that

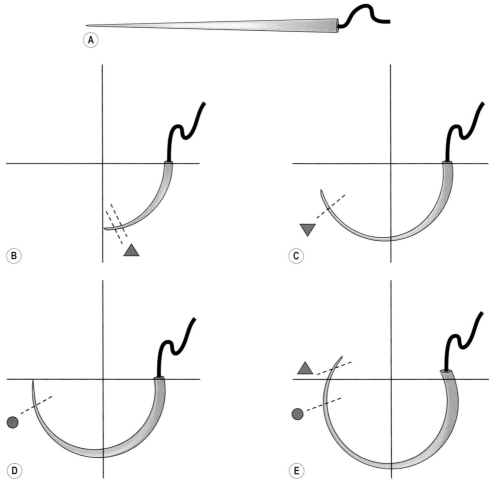

Fig. 7.1 Shapes of surgical needles and types of needle points. (**A**) Straight needle; (**B**) Conventional-cutting $\frac{1}{4}$-circle needle; (**C**) Reverse-cutting $\frac{3}{8}$-circle needle; (**D**) Tapered $\frac{1}{2}$-circle; (**E**) Tapercut $\frac{5}{8}$-circle needle.

approximate the optimum time for removal of nonabsorbable suture materials. The benefits of Monocryl include improved tensile strength, knot security, smoothness and minimal tissue reactivity, previously found only in synthetic monofilament nonabsorbable suture materials. Vicryl Rapide offers the improved handling characteristics of a multifilament, but has a rougher surface and less initial tensile strength, and is more expensive and reactive than Monocryl.[54]

Skin and subcutaneous tissue

The closure of facial skin wounds in the dog or cat is best performed with size 4–0 synthetic monofilament nonabsorbable suture materials such as nylon or polypropylene. A simple interrupted suture pattern is recommended for the most cosmetic closure.[26] Skin sutures placed in areas other than the face are traditionally removed at between 3 and 10 days.[59] Facial skin sutures should be removed in 4 to 6 days to prevent epithelialization of the suture track.[59] The subcutaneous tissues should be approximated with size 4–0 synthetic absorbable suture in a running continuous suture pattern. The use of a continuous suture pattern has the advantage of reducing the quantity of suture buried in the wound.

SURGICAL ADHESIVE TAPE

Cutaneous tapes (Steri-Strips, 3M, St. Paul, MN) are microporous surgical adhesive tapes with a backing of viscous rayon fibers coated with an acrylic copolymer, and are available in ⅛-, ¼- and ½-inch wide strips.[57] The closure of skin wounds with adhesive tape results in excellent wound healing because the skin is not penetrated with a needle, and there is less intrinsic tension on the wound.[26] Approximation of deep tissues cannot be achieved with tape alone, and tape closure is often combined with subcuticular running or interrupted sutures.[26,57] In animals, however, these materials have found little or no application because they are easily removed by the patient. Tincture of benzoin can be applied to the skin surface to enhance adhesion.[26]

SURGICAL STAPLES

Skin clips or staples are useful to expedite closure of scalp or abdominal wounds where cosmesis is less of a concern.[57] Staples maintain wound edges in eversion, but may result in necrosis and edema if used with excessive pressure.[57]

TISSUE ADHESIVES

Cyanoacrylates

Cyanoacrylates (Ethibond Excel, Ethicon, Inc., Somerville, NJ) are liquid adhesives that polymerize in the presence of moisture, and have been used as hemostatic dressings for tongue lacerations, extraction wounds and periodontal surgery.[61–63] Cyanoacrylates are well tolerated by oral tissues, promote healing, and may have bacteriostatic properties.[63] The butyl and isobutyl cyanoacrylates are the most suitable for use in the oral cavity, and the isobutyl form is the least cytotoxic.[39,64] Butyl or isobutyl cyanoacrylates that are applied to mucogingival tissues are exfoliated in 4 to 7 days; however only partial phagocytosis of the adhesive occurs when used in deeper tissues, and may result in granuloma formation.[39]

Fibrin tissue adhesive

Tisseel VH fibrin sealant (Tisseel VH, Baxter Healthcare Corporation, Westlake Village, CA) is a combination of human fibrinogen and bovine thrombin applied with a sterile delivery device.[65] Within 3 to 5 minutes of delivery a solid fibrin clot forms that firmly adheres to soft tissues and promotes hemostasis. It is fully absorbed within 10 to 14 days. It has been used extensively in human surgery, including maxillofacial surgery. Applications include mucogingival flap surgery, cancellous bone grafts, cleft palate repair and oronasal fistula closure.[65,66] It is especially useful for closure of extraction wounds or following cyst enucleation in patients with coagulopathies.[67] Fibrin adhesives do not interfere with wound healing and may, in fact, promote healing.[65,68]

Autologous preparations of fibrin sealants may be prepared by centrifugation of a patient's own whole blood or, if larger quantities are desired, from a cryoprecipitate. As a bioadhesive for the repair of oral mucosal defects, autologous fibrin sealants have been shown to be safe and well-tolerated in cats.[69] Similar to its xenogenous counterpart, autologous fibrin sealants may be used as a hemostatic, but also as an promoter of bone graft healing.[70–72] The substrate provided by the combined interaction of fibronectin, fibrin and factor XIII encourages the migration and growth of mesenchymal cells, accelerates revascularization and slows the multiplication of microorganisms.[70] Healing is accelerated with factor XIII, and fibroblast and osteoblast growth are stimulated by fibrin.[70,73,74] Autologous platelet-rich plasma gel is a modification of autologous fibrin sealants that is formed by mixing platelet-rich plasma from centrifuged autologous whole blood with thrombin and calcium chloride.[75] The primary difference between fibrin sealants and platelet-rich plasma gel is the higher concentration of platelets and a native concentration of fibrinogen in the latter.[75]

BIOMATERIALS FOR HEMOSTASIS

Hemorrhage following flap reflection and exodontia can usually be controlled with aspiration and pressure with moistened gauze, but slow, persistently oozing lesions may require the use of a hemostatic agent. Many hemostatic agents are also used as extraction socket dressings to reduce the volume of the blood clot that is formed and the chance of premature clot dissolution.[76] These agents include bone wax, absorbable gelatin sponge, oxidized cellulose, oxidized regenerated cellulose, microfibrillar collagen and hemostatic sealants.

Bone wax

The present-day formulation for bone wax is a highly purified beeswax that contains isopropyl palmitate as a softening and conditioning agent.[77] The wax functions as a mechanical hemostatic by blocking the vascular openings with plugs of blood and wax.[78] Bone wax is especially useful as a hemostatic during periapical surgery.[77] After hemostasis has been achieved, the bone wax should be removed, as the retained wax will initiate an intense foreign body reaction, characterized by giant cells, plasma cells and fibrous granulation tissue, that will inhibit osteogenesis.[79,80]

Absorbable gelatin sponge

Gelfoam (Gelfoam, Pharmacia & Upjohn, Kalamazoo, MI) is a porous matrix gelatin sponge prepared from partially hydrolyzed pork skin that is intended for use as a hemostatic agent. Gelfoam is provided by the manufacturer in a powder that forms a paste when mixed with a sterile sodium chloride solution. The gelatin sponge is applied directly to the bleeding surface, and is absorbed in 4 to 6 weeks.[81] Due to the potential for embolization, Gelfoam should be used with caution in intravascular compartments. Cube-sized gelatin sponges (Vetspon, Novartis Animal Health US Inc., Greensboro, NC) designed for use in extraction sockets are also available. The use of Gelfoam in extraction sockets is controversial, and has actually been shown to block cancellous bone replacement in dogs.[82] It may also potentiate bacterial growth and serve as a nidus for infection and abscess formation.

Oxidized cellulose

Oxycel (Oxycel, Becton Dickinson and Company, Franklin Lakes, NJ) is a chemically altered form of surgical gauze that functions as an artificial clot.[81] Oxycel should be applied dry and removed from the wound prior to closure. Oxycel inhibits osteogenesis and epithelialization, and should not be used as a surface dressing or placed adjacent to bone.[81] Oxycel will resorb to completion in 1 to 6 weeks.[81]

Oxidized regenerated cellulose

Surgicel (Surgicel, Johnson & Johnson, New Brunswick, NJ) is an absorbable glucose polymer-based sterile knitted fabric that acts as a matrix for clot formation and as a clot stabilizer.[82] Surgicel is prepared by the oxidation of regenerated cellulose, and its function as a hemostatic is dependent upon the bonding of hemoglobin to oxycellulose.[82] Surgicel is resorbed in 7 to 14 days with minimal inflammation, but can swell by up to 135%, resulting in patient discomfort if used as an extraction site packing material.[83] Surgicel has been marketed to control capillary, venous and small arterial hemorrhage, and, because it does not impede epithelialization, can be used as a surface dressing. Surgicel is bactericidal to a wide range of Gram-negative and Gram-positive aerobes and anaerobes, and has been used successfully as a scaffolding material to fill bony defects (e.g., small to moderate-sized clefts of the palate).[84,85]

Microfibrillar collagen

Avitene (Avitene, Davol, Inc., Cranston, RI) is an effective hemostatic agent for use on bleeding surfaces and in extraction sockets that is prepared from edible bovine corium as a water-insoluble, partial acid salt of natural collagen.[86] This microfibrillar collagen product is also useful in the face of certain clotting factor deficiencies and heparinization, and has been reported to shorten the reaction time of the intrinsic clotting pathway by 60%.[87] Avitene, however, does not accelerate new bone formation when implanted in bone defects, and is more prone to bacterial contamination than oxidized cellulose.[86,88]

Thrombin-based hemostatic agents

Bovine-derived thrombin is available in liquid or powder form as a topical hemostat. Thrombin is an enzyme that is active at the end of the coagulation cascade that converts fibrinogen to fibrin. Thrombin products bypass the need for functional platelets, and are useful in thrombocytopenic or thrombocytopathic patients. Since the thrombin is bovine derived, bovine thrombin should be avoided in patients with documented allergic reactions to bovine products.[81] The significance of antibody development to bovine thrombin in veterinary patients is unknown. Synthetic alternatives to bovine thrombin, such as thrombin receptor agonist peptide-6 (TRAP), a synthetic hexapeptide that mimics the effects of thrombin, have been investigated.[90]

FloSeal (FloSeal, Baxter Healthcare Corporation, Westlake Village, CA) is a granular cross-linked collagen-derived matrix that is combined with thrombin to create a flowable gel. In comparison to other topical hemostats (Gelfoam and Surgicel), FloSeal granules swell by only 10–20% upon contact with blood, decreasing patient discomfort when used in extraction sockets. The thrombin that is incorporated with the FloSeal granules converts fibrinogen into a fibrin polymer that forms a clot surrounding the collagen-derived matrix. FloSeal is completely resorbed by the body in 6 to 8 weeks. In a comparison study of FloSeal and Gelfoam plus thrombin for the control of intraoperative hemorrhage, FloSeal provided more rapid and effective hemostasis, 93% of first-site applications, compared to 76% for Gelfoam plus thrombin.[91]

Microporous polysaccharide hemospheres

Microporous polysaccharide hemosphere (MPH) powder (Arista AH, Medafor, Inc., Minneapolis, MN) is a hemostatic wound dressing composed of purified cross-linked starch (potato) particles ranging in size from 10 to 200 micrometers in diameter.[92] When topically applied to a wound bed, the fluid components of blood (low molecular weight) are absorbed into the controlled-size pores of the particles.[92] The high-molecular-weight solids of blood (platelets, red blood cells, albumin, thrombin and fibrinogen) are concentrated between and on the surface of the particles to provide a viscous barrier to blood seepage.[92] Hemostasis with MPH can occur as quickly as 30 seconds. MPH particles are degraded by enzymatic hydrolysis within 24 to 48 hours by endogenous alpha amylase.[92] Potential applications in veterinary oral surgery include placement in areas of diffuse hemorrhage such as oozing extraction sockets and nasal conchae bleeding following maxillectomy.

REFERENCES

1. McCaul LK, Bagg J, Jenkins WM. Rate of loss of irradiated polyglactin 910 (Vicryl Rapide) from the mouth: a prospective study. Br J Oral Maxillofac Surg 2000; 38:328–30.

2. Lilly GE. Reaction of oral tissues to suture materials. Oral Surg Oral Med Oral Pathol 1968;26:128–33.

3. Macht SD, Krizek TJ. Sutures and suturing – current concepts. J Oral Surg 1978;36: 710–12.

4. Lilly GE, Armstrong JH, Salem JE, et al. Reaction of oral tissues to suture materials. II. Oral Surg Oral Med Oral Pathol 1968; 26:592–9.

5. King RC, Crawford JJ, Small EW. Bacteremia following intraoral suture removal. Oral Surg Oral Med Oral Pathol 1988;65:23–8.

6. Silverstein LH, Christensen GJ. Principles of dental suturing: the complete guide to surgical closure. Mahway, NJ: Montage Media Corp; 1999. p. 8–11.

7. Selvig KA, Torabinejad M. Wound healing after mucoperiosteal surgery in the cat. J Endod 1996;22:507–15.

8. Mittleman HR, Toto PD, Sicher H. Healing in human attached gingiva. Periodontics 1964;2:106–14.

9. Harrison JW, Jurosky KA. Wound healing in the tissues of the periodontium following periradicular surgery. I. The incisional wound. J Endod 1991;17: 425–35.

10. Harrison JW. Healing of surgical wounds in oral mucoperiosteal tissues. J Endod 1991;17:401–8.
11. Chu CC, Kizil Z. Quantitative evaluation of stiffness of commercial suture materials. Surg Gynecol Obstet 1989;168:233–8.
12. Blomstedt B, Osterberg B, Bergstrand A. Suture material and bacterial transport. An experimental study. Acta Chir Scand 1977; 143:71–3.
13. Metz SA, Chegini N, Masterson BJ. In vivo and in vitro degradation of monofilament absorbable sutures, PDS and Maxon. Biomaterials 1990;11:41–5.
14. Katz S, Izhar M, Mirelman D. Bacterial adherence to surgical sutures. A possible factor in suture induced infection. Ann Surg 1981;194:35–41.
15. Fossum TW, Hedlund CS, Hulse DA, et al. Small animal surgery. 2nd ed. St. Louis, MO: Mosby; 2002. p. 43–59.
16. van Rijssel EJ, Brand R, Admiraal C, et al. Tissue reaction and surgical knots: the effect of suture size, knot configuration, and knot volume. Obstet Gynecol 1989; 74:64–8.
17. Holmlund DE. Knot properties of surgical suture materials. A model study. Acta Chir Scand 1974;140:355–62.
18. Stashak TS, Yturraspe DJ. Considerations for selection of suture materials. Vet Surg 1978;2:48–55.
19. Thacker JG, Rodeheaver G, Moore JW, et al. Mechanical performance of surgical sutures. Am J Surg 1975;130:374–80.
20. Herrmann JB. Tensile strength and knot security of surgical suture materials. Am Surg 1971;37:209–17.
21. Rosin E, Robinson GM. Knot security of suture materials. Vet Surg 1989;18:269–73.
22. Otten JE, Wiedmann-Al-Ahmed M, Jahnke H, et al. Bacterial colonization on different suture materials – a potential risk for intraoral dentoalveolar surgery. J Biomed Mater Res B Appl Biomater 2005;74:627–35.
23. Marsh PD. Plaque as a biofilm: Pharmacological principles of drug delivery and action in the sub- and supragingival environment. Oral Dis 2003;1:16–22.
24. Giglio JA, Rowland RW, Dalton HP, et al. Suture removal-induced bacteremia: A possible endocarditis risk. J Am Dent Assoc 1992;123:69–70.
25. Hendler BH, Kempers KG. Soft tissue injuries. In: Fonseca RJ, editor. Oral and maxillofacial surgery. Philadelphia, PA: WB Saunders Co; 2000. p. 341–68.
26. Boothe Jr HW. Selecting suture materials for small animal surgery. Compend Contin Educ Pract Vet 1998;20:155–63.
27. Chu CC, Moncrief G. An in vitro evaluation of the stability of mechanical properties of surgical suture materials in various pH conditions. Ann Surg 1983; 198:223–8.
28. Tomihata K, Suzuki M, Ikada Y. The pH dependence of monofilament sutures on hydrolytic degradation. J Biomed Mater Res 2001;58:511–18.
29. Rockwood DP, Miller RI. Characteristics of currently available suture materials. Gen Dent 1988;36:489–93.
30. Shaw RJ, Negus TW, Mellor TK. A prospective clinical evaluation of the longevity of resorbable sutures in oral mucosa. Br J Oral Maxillofac Surg 1996; 34:252–4.
31. Chung H, Weinberg S. Suture materials in oral surgery: a review. Oral Health 1978; 68:31–4.
32. Horton CE, Adamson JE, Mladick RA, et al. Vicryl synthetic absorbable sutures. Am Surg 1974;40:729–31.
33. Laufman H, Rubel T. Synthetic absorbable sutures. Surg Gynecol Obstet 1977;145:597–608.
34. McGeehan D, Hunt D, Chaudhuri A, et al. An experimental study of the relationship between synergistic wound sepsis and suture materials. Br J Surg 1980;67:636–8.
35. Wallace WR, Maxwell GR, Cavalaris CJ. Comparison of polyglycolic acid suture to black silk, chromic and plain catgut in human oral tissues. J Oral Surg 1970;28:739–46.
36. Moser JB, Lautenschlager EP, Horbal BJ. Mechanical properties of polyglycolic acid sutures in oral surgery. J Dent Res 1974;53:804–8.
37. Lilly GE, Osbon DB, Hutchinson RA, et al. Clinical and bacteriologic aspects of polyglycolic acid sutures. J Oral Surg 1973;31:103–5.
38. Levin MP. Periodontal suture materials and surgical dressings. Dent Clin North Am 1980;24:767–81.
39. Duprez K, Bilweis J, Duprez A, et al. Experimental and clinical study of fast absorption cutaneous suture material. Ann Chir Main 1988;7:91–6.
40. Martelli H, Catena D, Rahon H, et al. Skin sutures in pediatric surgery. Use of a fast-resorption synthetic thread. Presse Med 1991;20:2194–8.
41. Aderriotis D, Sandor GK. Outcomes of irradiated polyglactin 910 Vicryl Rapide fast-absorbing suture in oral and scalp wounds. J Can Dent Assoc 1999;65:345–7.
42. Barbolt TA. Chemistry and safety of triclosan, and its use as an antimicrobial coating on Coated VICRYL* Plus Antibacterial Suture (coated polyglactin 910 suture with triclosan). Surg Infect (Larchmt) 2002;3(Suppl 1):S45–53.
43. Gilbert P, McBain AJ. Literature-based evaluation of the potential risks associated with impregnation of medical devices and implants with triclosan. Surg Infect (Larchmt) 2002;3(Suppl 1):S55–63.
44. Storch M, Scalzo H, Van Lue S, et al. Physical and functional comparison of Coated VICRYL* Plus Antibacterial Suture (coated polyglactin 910 suture with triclosan) with Coated VICRYL* Suture (coated polyglactin 910 suture). Surg Infect (Larchmt) 2002;3(Suppl 1):S65–77.
45. Rothenburger S, Spangler D, Bhende S, et al. In vitro antimicrobial evaluation of Coated VICRYL* Plus Antibacterial Suture (coated polyglactin 910 with triclosan) using zone of inhibition assays. Surg Infect (Larchmt) 2002;3(Suppl 1):S79–87.
46. Edmiston CE, Seabrook GR, Goheen MP, et al. Bacterial adherence to surgical sutures: Can antibacterial-coated sutures reduce the risk of microbial contamination. J Am Coll Surg 2006; 203:481–9.
47. Katz AR, Mukherjee DP, Kaganov AL, et al. A new synthetic monofilament absorbable suture made from polytrimethylene carbonate. Surg Gynecol Obstet 1985;161:213–22.
48. DeNardo GA, Brown NO, Trenka-Benthin S, et al. Comparison of seven different suture materials in the feline oral cavity. J Am Anim Hosp Assoc 1996;32:164–72.
49. Quayle AA, El-Badrawy H. Clinical and experimental studies with resorbable transosseous ligature. Br J Oral Maxillofac Surg 1984;22:24–9.
50. Rodeheaver GT, Powell TA, Thacker JG, et al. Mechanical performance of monofilament synthetic absorbable sutures. Am J Surg 1987;154:544–7.
51. Bezwada RS, Jamiolkowski DD, Lee I-Y, et al. Monocryl suture, a new ultra-pliable absorbable monofilament suture. Biomaterials 1995;16:1141–8.
52. LaBagnara Jr J. A review of absorbable suture materials in head & neck surgery and introduction of Monocryl: a new absorbable suture. Ear Nose Throat J 1995;74:409–15.
53. Banche G, Roana J, Mandras N, et al. Microbial adherence on various intraoral suture materials in patients undergoing dental surgery. J Oral Maxillofac Surg 2007;65:1503–7.
54. Rodeheaver GT, Borzelleca DC, Thacker JG, et al. Unique performance characteristics of Novafil. Surg Gynecol Obstet 1987;164:230–6.
55. Pinheiro AL, de Castro JF, Thiers FA, et al. Using Novafil: would it make suturing easier? Braz Dent J 1997;8:21–5.
56. Holt GR, Holt JE. Suture materials and techniques. Ear Nose Throat J 1981;60:12–8.
57. Selvig KA, Biagiotti GR, Leknes KN, et al. Oral tissue reactions to suture materials. Int J Periodont Rest Dent 1998;18:474–87.
58. Hupp JR. Principles of surgery In: Peterson LJ, Ellis III E, Hupp JR et al, editors. Contemporary oral and maxillofacial surgery. 4th ed. St. Louis, MO: Mosby; 2003. p. 42–8.
59. Powers MP, Beck BW, Fonseca RJ. Management of soft tissue injuries In: Fonseca RJ, Walker RV, Betts NJ et al, editors. Oral and maxillofacial trauma.

Philadelphia, PA: WB Saunders Co; 1997, p. 792–854.

60. Salisbury SK, Thacker HL, Pantzer EE, et al. Partial maxillectomy in the dog: comparison of suture materials and closure techniques. Vet Surg 1985; 14:265–76.

61. Ochstein AJ, Hansen NM, Swenson HM. A comparative study of cyanoacrylate and other periodontal dressings on gingival surgical wound healing. J Periodontol 1969;40:515–20.

62. Bhaskar SN, Jacoway JR, Margetis PM, et al. Oral tissue response to chemical adhesives (cyanoacrylates). Oral Surg 1966;22:394–404.

63. Bhaskar SN, Frisch J, Cutright DE, et al. Effect of butyl cyanoacrylate on the healing of extraction wounds. Oral Surg Oral Med Oral Pathol 1967;24:604–16.

64. Forrest JO. The use of cyanoacrylates in periodontal surgery. J Periodontol 1974;45:225–9.

65. Fattahi T, Mohan M, Caldwell GT. Clinical applications of fibrin sealants. J Oral Maxillofac Surg 2004;62:218–24.

66. Davis BR, Sandor GK. Use of fibrin glue in maxillofacial surgery. J Otolaryngol 1998; 27:107–12.

67. Bodner L, Weinstein JM, Baumgarten AK. Efficacy of fibrin sealant in patients on various levels of oral anticoagulant undergoing oral surgery. Oral Surg Oral Med Oral Pathol Oral Radiol Endod 1998;86:421–4.

68. Yucel EA, Oral O, Olgac V, et al. Effects of fibrin glue on wound healing in oral cavity. J Dent 2003;31:569–75.

69. Gaboriau HP, Belafsky PC, Pahlavan N, et al. Closure of mucosal defects over exposed mandibular plates using fibrin glue. Arch Facial Plast Surg 1999;1: 191–4.

70. Tayapongsak P, O'Brien DA, Monteiro CB, et al. Autologous fibrin adhesive in mandibular reconstruction with particulate cancellous bone and marrow. J Oral Maxillofac Surg 1994;52:161–6.

71. Wepner F, Fries R, Platz H. The use of the fibrin adhesion system for local hemostasis in oral surgery. J Oral Maxillofac Surg 1982;40:555–8.

72. Carter G, Goss AN, Lloyd J, et al. Local haemostasis with autologous fibrin glue following surgical enucleation of a large cystic lesion in a therapeutically anticoagulated patient. Br J Oral Maxillofac Surg 2003;41:275–6.

73. Yucel EA, Oral O, Olgac V, et al. Effects of fibrin glue on wound healing in oral cavity. J Dent 2003;31:569–75.

74. Matras H. Fibrin seal: the state of the art. J Oral Maxillofac Surg 1985;43:605–11.

75. Whitman DH, Berry RL, Green DM. Platelet gel: an autologous alternative to fibrin glue with applications in oral and maxillofacial surgery. J Oral Maxillofac Surg 1997;55:1294–9.

76. Olson RA, Roberts DL, Osbon DB. A comparative study of polylactic acid, Gelfoam, and Surgicel in healing extraction sites. Oral Surg Oral Med Oral Pathol 1982;53:441–9.

77. Selden HS. Bone wax as an effective hemostat in periapical surgery. Oral Surg Oral Med Oral Pathol 1970;29:262–4.

78. Geary JR, Frantz VK. New absorbable hemostatic bone wax. Ann Surg 1950; 132:1128–37.

79. Finn MD, Schow SR, Schneiderman ED. Osseous regeneration in the presence of four common hemostatic agents. J Oral Maxillofac Surg 1992;50:608–12.

80. Ibarrola J, Bjorenson J, Austin B, et al. Osseous reactions to three hemostatic agents. J Endod 1985;11:75–83.

81. Klokkevold PR, Carranza FA, Takei HH. General principles of periodontal surgery. In: Newman MG, Takei HH, Carranza FA, editors. Carranza's clinical periodontology. 9th ed. Philadelphia, PA: WB Saunders Co; 2002. p. 725–36.

82. Howard PE, Wilson JW, Ribble GA. Effects of gelatin sponge implantation in cancellous bone defects in dogs. J Am Vet Med Assoc 1988;192:633–7.

83. Halfpenny W, Fraser JS, Adlam DM. Comparison of 2 hemostatic agents for the prevention of postextraction hemorrhage in patients on anticoagulants. Oral Surg Oral Med Oral Pathol Oral Radiol Endod 2001;92:257–9.

84. Petersen JK, Krogsgaard J, Nielsen KM, et al. A comparison between 2 absorbable hemostatic agents: gelatin sponge (Spongostan) and oxidized regenerated cellulose (Surgicel). Int J Oral Surg 1984;13:406–10.

85. Thilander BL, Stenstrom SJ. Bone healing after implantation of some hetero- and alloplastic materials: an experimental study on the guinea pig. Cleft Palate J 1970;7:540–9.

86. Skoog T. The use of periosteum and Surgicel for bone restoration in congenital clefts of the maxilla. A clinical report and experimental investigation. Scand J Plast Reconstr Surg 1967;1: 113–30.

87. Hunt LM, Benoit PW. Evaluation of microcrystalline collagen preparation in extraction wounds. J Oral Surg 1976;34:407–14.

88. Abbott WM, Austen WG. Microcrystalline collagen as a topical hemostatic agent for vascular surgery. Surgery 1974;75: 925–33.

89. Scher KS, Coil JA, Jr. Effects of oxidized cellulose and microfibrillar collagen on infection. Surgery 1982;91:301–4.

90. Landesberg R, Burke A, Pinsky D, et al. Activation of platelet-rich plasma using thrombin receptor agonist peptide. J Oral Maxillofac Surg 2005;63:529–35.

91. Weaver FA, Hood DB, Zatina M, et al. Gelatin-thrombin-based hemostatic sealant for intraoperative bleeding in vascular surgery. Ann Vasc Surg 2002;16: 286–93.

92. Tan SR, Tope WD. Effectiveness of microporous polysaccharide hemospheres for achieving hemostasis in Mohs micrographic surgery. Dermatol Surg 2004;30:908–14.

Chapter | 8 |

Laser surgery

George M. Peavy & Petra E. Wilder-Smith

DEFINITIONS

The word *laser* is an acronym for Light Amplification by the Stimulated Emission of Radiation, which is a description of how a laser beam is generated. *Photons* are the form of electromagnetic energy of which light consists. A photon travels in a straight line, undulating in a waveform that is determined by its energy level. The waveform is characterized by the distance between the crest of two successive wave peaks referred to as the *wavelength* reported in nanometer (nm) or micrometer (μm). Light is further characterized as being *ultraviolet* (UV) (100–400 nm), *visible* (400–750 nm), or *infrared* (IR) (>750 nm).[1-4]

The light emitted from a laser is *monochromatic* (one wavelength), *coherent* (photons traveling parallel and in phase with each other), and *intense* (photons confined within a beam of small diameter). This differs from incandescent light sources where the emitted light is polychromatic (multiple wavelengths), noncoherent (photons travel in many directions away from the source) and not intense (photons distributed over relatively large area).[1-3]

Energy is a measure of work and is reported in *joules* (J). *Power* is a measure of the rate that work is taking place, is measured in J/s and reported in *watts* (W). *Energy density* (also referred to as *fluence*) is a measure of the total amount of energy distributed within a defined area, expressed as J/cm². *Power density* (also referred to as *irradiance*) is a measure of the rate of work within a defined area (W/cm²), and is used to describe the concentration of the power output of the laser as delivered within the area of the beam (Πr²) at a specified beam diameter.[5]

When the beam of photons released from a laser is continuously emitted during the period of activation, the beam is delivered in a *continuous wave mode*. When the beam is emitted in successive bursts of energy of programmed duration, the beam is delivered in a *pulsed mode*. Each individual pulse is emitted for a specified duration of time referred to as the *pulse duration* or *pulse width*. When pulses are released in a successive stream they are emitted in series at a specified time interval referred to as the *pulse interval* that is the time between the onset of two successive pulses (Fig. 8.1), or may be specified as the *pulse repetition rate* (pulses/s) or *pulse frequency* (Hz).

During an individual pulse the energy release starts at zero, increases to a maximum or *peak power*, and then decreases back to zero. During a pulsed laser exposure, energy release occurs during the pulse duration and does not occur between the end of one pulse and the start of the next successive pulse, so the *average power* delivered to tissue over time is the total energy of one pulse divided by the duration of one pulse interval (Fig. 8.1). For a pulse structure where 0.1 J is evenly delivered within a 1 ms pulse with a pulse interval of 4 ms, the peak power of each pulse is 100 W (i.e., $0.1 \text{ J}/1.0 \times 10^{-3}$ s), while the average power delivered to tissue is 25 W (i.e., $0.1 \text{ J}/4.0 \times 10^{-3}$ s).

When beam delivery is made in a succession of very short duration, high frequency, high peak power pulses, the delivery may be referred

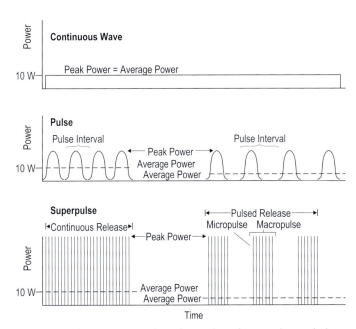

Fig. 8.1 Continuous wave mode, pulse mode and superpulse mode (see text). *(From Peavy GM. Laser and laser-tissue interaction. Vet Clin North Am Small Anim Pract 2002;32:517–534. With permission.)*

DOI: 10.1016/B978-0-7020-4618-6.00008-7

to as a *superpulse mode*. When a succession of very short-duration pulses are delivered for a set time interval, stopped and then repeated for the same time interval, an individual short pulse is referred to as a *micropulse* and the interval of successive micropulse exposures is referred to as a *macropulse* (Fig. 8.1). A typical superpulse mode would be individual 100 W peak power micropulses of 700 μs each, delivered at a frequency of 200 Hz (200 pulses/s). If the micropulses are released in succession for a period of 1 ms at specified intervals, the micropulse duration is 700 μs and the macropulse duration is 1 ms. The peak power during the laser exposure of each micropulse is 100 W, while the average power delivered during the macropulse is 14 W (i.e., 100 J/s × 700 × 10^{-6} s/micropulse × 200 micropulses/s). If a 1 ms macropulse is delivered every 4 ms, the peak power of each micropulse remains the same (100 W); however, the average power delivered to tissue is 3.5 W (i.e., 14 W × 1 ms/4 ms).

SYSTEM SELECTION AND APPLICATION

There are four variables that influence both the mechanism of laser tissue interaction and the resulting effect on tissue. These variables are wavelength, beam intensity, time domain of energy delivery, and tissue handling.[5-13] It is important to understand the principles of these variables not only for the selection of an appropriate laser system, but also to understand how variations in the parameters of beam delivery for the selected system will alter the effects of the application of that laser to tissue.

For any medical laser system, the principal operator is responsible by law for applying the principles of laser safety and for the training of all laser users and support staff in the practice. This includes: (1) standard operating procedures; (2) biological effects of laser radiation on the eye and skin; (3) hazards presented by reflections and inadvertent misdirection of the laser beam; and (4) control measures. This subject is beyond the scope of this text but its understanding is an essential requirement prior to using a laser.[14-17]

Laser–tissue interaction

Mechanisms of action

For most surgical laser systems the mechanism of action for cutting or ablating soft tissue is photothermal (photon energy is absorbed by tissue and transformed into thermal energy that then affects the tissue). Where tissue temperature reaches 60–65°C, proteins are denatured and that area of tissue no longer remains viable. Where tissue temperature reaches or exceeds 100°C, water in the irradiated area expands, creating pressure within the tissue that produces an explosive vaporization event when the internal pressure exceeds the strength of confinement.[11,13,18]

Where photothermal vaporization has been induced, a crater is created by explosive ejection of tissue. This tissue defect may be surrounded by 2–3 zones of altered tissue (Fig. 8.2), the presence and size of which will depend upon the factors that influence both photon and thermal confinement.[9,11] A thin layer of carbonization lining the crater wall may be encountered as the first zone of thermal injury. The carbonization represents an area where the tissue temperature greatly exceeded 100°C, and tissue composition has been broken down into its elemental parts; however, an explosive vaporization event has either not been induced or has been inadequate to carry away all of the debris.

The next area of adjacent thermal influence is a zone of tissue necrosis, where tissue temperature has been elevated above 60–65°C, but has not reached the vaporization threshold. In this zone, protein

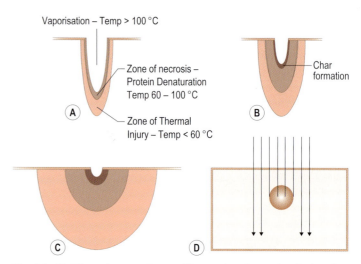

Fig. 8.2 (**A**) When photons of a specific wavelength are absorbed well by a target tissue, they remain confined to a small volume of tissue and rapidly raise the internal tissue temperature to the ablation threshold, minimizing collateral thermal injury caused by photon dispersion; (**B**) and (**C**) When a wavelength is poorly absorbed by the target tissue and photons are dispersed across a large area, or when a well-absorbed wavelength is delivered at a low irradiance that permits diffusion of thermal energy into surrounding tissues before an ablation threshold is reached, shallower areas of vaporization and wider areas of collateral thermal injury are produced; (**D**) Selective photothermolysis uses a wavelength that is transmitted by one tissue to photocoagulate an absorbing tissue located within or under the transmitting tissue. *(From Peavy GM. Laser and laser-tissue interaction. Vet Clin North Am Small Anim Pract 2002;32:517–534. With permission.)*

denaturation has occurred, and while the tissue does retain some structural integrity, it is no longer viable. The third region of collateral thermal injury represents tissue that has been heated, but not high enough or long enough for protein denaturation to occur. This zone of tissue warming will retain viability and will be incorporated in the process of wound healing.

In most cases, one wants to maximize tissue vaporization and minimize collateral thermal injury in order to achieve the highest efficiency of tissue removal while minimizing injury to adjacent tissue. In some cases, an element of collateral thermal influence is desired, particularly where hemostasis is a consideration. Variations in wavelength selection, beam intensity, time domains of energy delivery, and tissue handling will influence both photon and energy confinement, and, thereby, the resulting tissue removal and adjacent tissue injury.

Wavelength selection

There are many different laser sources available, each of which generates a specific wavelength or selection of wavelengths, including excimer (108–353 nm), argon (488 and 514 nm), krypton (647 nm), dye (400–780 nm), semiconductor diode (635–1550 nm), Nd:YAG (1064 nm), Ho:YAG (2120 nm), Er,Cr:YSGG (2780 nm), Er:YAG (2940 nm) and CO_2 (10600 nm).[4,19,20] Wavelength selection is an important consideration, as different wavelengths can have different effects on the same soft tissue. The wavelength-dependent effects on tissue are influenced by the optical properties of the specific tissue, and to what extent those properties reflect, transmit, scatter and/or absorb the incident wavelength.[11,13]

Maximum ablation efficiency occurs when the incident wavelength is highly absorbed by the target tissue, which maximizes energy concentration by confining the photons and their subsequent conversion to thermal energy within a small volume of tissue. When the incident wavelength is poorly absorbed by tissue, photons are more widely disbursed through the tissue before being absorbed. As a result, the subsequent conversion of photon energy into thermal energy is distributed over a larger volume of tissue, making it more difficult to generate temperatures that reach the ablation threshold, resulting in the creation of small ablation craters and large areas of collateral thermal injury.

The components of soft tissue that most commonly serve as photon-absorbing agents are hemoglobin, melanin and water. The distribution of photon absorption in tissue is dependent upon the relative absorption of the incident wavelength by these compounds and both the concentration and distribution of each compound in the tissue.

Hemoglobin and melanin are good absorbers of wavelengths in the ultraviolet to visible blue–green (400–500 nm) region, with decreasing absorption in the near-IR region. Water is a poor absorber in the visible to near-IR regions, but has very good absorption characteristics in the mid- to far-IR regions. While the absorption coefficients for hemoglobin and melanin in the blue–green region are comparable to the absorption coefficients for water in the mid- to far-IR region, the higher concentration of water in soft tissue makes the mid-IR Er:YAG (2940 nm) and the far-IR CO_2 (10 600 nm) lasers more efficient for soft tissue surgery. Near- to mid-IR wavelengths (diode, Nd:YAG and Ho:YAG) are poorly absorbed by water, allowing them to be delivered through optical fibers, but they are similarly poorly absorbed by tissue (Fig. 8.3).

Efficient ablation of dental hard tissues is best achieved by wavelengths that are absorbed well in water and in hydroxyapatite, which are important constituents of enamel, dentine, cementum and bone. Pure thermal ablation mechanisms are enhanced by thermochemical effects caused by high-pressure water vapor on the weakened hard tissues. Lasers producing this dual effect include the Er:YAG and the Er,Cr:YSGG lasers. Generally, thermal damage to collateral tissues during laser ablation is minimized by the use of a carefully timed and calibrated water-cooling spray. This is important because of the extreme thermal sensitivity of some dental structures, such as the dental pulp and periodontal tissues.

Beam intensity

While the power output of the laser is set at a specific level, the surface area of the beam over which the photons are distributed will have a profound effect on the concentration of photons as they reach the tissue, and the resulting effect of the beam on the tissue.[5] Power is the selected energy output of the laser (W) and is divided by the area of the beam (Πr^2) to calculate the power density ($W/\Pi r^2$). Table 8.1 shows the influence on power density of increasing the power output of the laser in comparison to the influence of changing the spot size.

Table 8.1 Power density (W/cm^2) is determined by the power output of the laser and spot size of the beam (see text). When using a CO_2 laser, efficient cutting of tissue resulting in minimal collateral thermal injury requires using a power density of at least 4500 W/cm^2.

Power	Diameter			
	0.2 mm	0.4 mm	0.8 mm	1.0 mm
5 W	16 667	4167	1000	637
10 W	33 333	8333	1992	1274
20 W	66 667	16 667	3984	2547

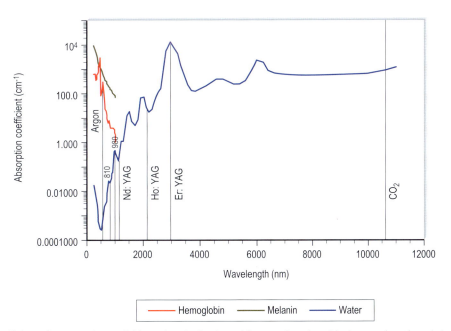

Fig. 8.3 The absorption coefficients for water, hemoglobin and melanin plotted for wavelengths with the wavelength emission of common laser systems noted. The larger the absorption coefficient value the better the wavelength is absorbed by the substance. The coefficient values are plotted in log scale as their values range across eight orders of magnitude. *(From Peavy GM. Laser and laser-tissue interaction. Vet Clin North Am Small Anim Pract 2002;32:517–534. With permission.)*

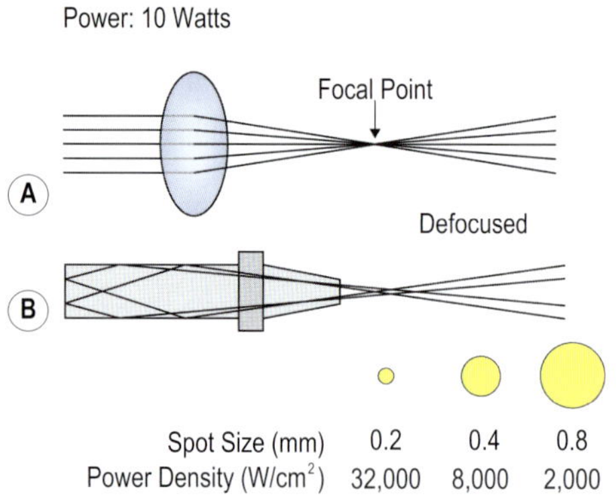

Power: 10 Watts

Fig. 8.4 The area over which photons are distributed influences their concentration and the rate at which energy is deposited into tissue. The beam may be delivered: (**A**) through a lens that focuses the beam into a spot or (**B**) through a fiber or waveguide, where the beam exits through a tip or fiber end. *(From Peavy GM. Laser and laser-tissue interaction. Vet Clin North Am Small Anim Pract 2002;32:517–534. With permission.)*

The power density of a fixed beam diameter changes linearly as the power output of the laser is adjusted, but when the power output is kept constant and the beam diameter is changed by a factor of 2, the power density is inversely changed by a factor of 4.

This is an important concept, which underscores both the necessity to work within the focal point of the beam for maximum efficiency in the cutting of tissue, and the versatility in influencing tissue response through changing power density by working in the focused or defocused portion of the beam (Fig. 8.4). Intuitively, it might seem that a change from a 0.4-mm spot diameter to a 0.8-mm spot diameter would have little effect on the overall influence of the beam on tissue. Practically, the surgeon who feels comfortable in using a 0.4-mm spot at 10 W for the incision of skin and switches to a beam delivery device with a 0.8-mm beam diameter would need to increase the power output of the laser to 40 W in order to maintain the same power density.

The most efficient excision of tissue can be achieved by working at the focal point of the beam. Using the defocused region of the beam by moving the handpiece away from the tissue surface rapidly decreases the power density, permitting superficial tissue ablation, tissue contraction and/or hemostasis without having to adjust the power setting of the laser.

Time domains of energy delivery

Power density will influence the rate of energy deposition within a volume of tissue and subsequently the exposure time required to reach the energy threshold for tissue transformation. Thermal *diffusivity* of a tissue is the speed at which thermal energy will move through that tissue. In a photothermal ablation process, the longer one takes to deposit photon energy into tissue to induce ablation, the more collateral thermal injury will be created as the thermal energy generated at the ablation site has more time to diffuse into adjacent tissue.[8,13]

The time domains of energy delivery to tissue are influenced at two levels, the experience of the surgeon and the mode selection of the laser. In the initial learning phase the laser surgeon tends to select parameters that result in the use of low power densities (large spot size and/or low power output) that will produce slow cutting at an easily controlled rate. As the surgeon increases in proficiency and

confidence there is comfort in proceeding at a more rapid rate, so the surgeon gravitates to higher power densities (small spot size and high power output). With increasing power densities, ablation proceeds at a more rapid rate, reducing the duration of exposure along the incision line and the time available for thermal diffusion to produce collateral thermal injury.

Further enhancing the surgeon's ability to reduce thermal diffusion, lasers may be equipped with pulsing modes that permit the use of higher powers in a succession of pulses. In this manner, ablation thresholds are reached more rapidly because of the high peak powers, but the interval between pulses permits the application to remain controllable. Additionally, pulse modes allow improved precision and control in the removal of small volumes of tissue.

Basic pulse modes can be found in the 1–500-ms range with pulse frequencies of 1–60 Hz. Further reduction in collateral thermal injury can be achieved by using a succession of high peak power pulses that reach the ablation threshold within a time period that is shorter than the time required for thermal energy to diffuse outside of the irradiated volume of tissue. This is referred to as the *thermal relaxation time* (t_r) of tissue, and is both wavelength and thermal diffusivity dependent.[6,9–11,21,22] For the CO_2 laser the t_r values are in the range of 300–700 μs, and for the Er:YAG laser the t_r approximates 2 μs.[6,21]

The superpulse mode of a CO_2 laser generates high peak power pulses (50–500 W) in a time period that approximates the t_r (500–700 μs) in rapid succession (100–1000 Hz) designed to achieve efficient tissue removal while minimizing collateral thermal injury. Using a CO_2 laser with extremely short pulses and high peak powers, collateral thermal damage in oral soft tissues ranged 15–170 μm. Using the same laser system in the continuous mode setting resulted in collateral damage of approximately 600 μm.[23] For the CO_2 laser it is typical to find reported a zone of 300–600 μm for the CW mode, 100–200 μm for pulses of 2–500 ms, and 50 μm or less for pulse durations of 2–600 μs.[21–25]

To minimize collateral thermal injury and maximize ablation efficiency, enough energy to reach the vaporization threshold of water (2500 J/cm^2) must be delivered into the volume of soft tissue irradiated by the CO_2 laser (μ_a=794/cm) within the thermal relaxation time of the tissue (t_r=695 μs). This requires the use of a power density of at least 4500 W/cm^2 (2500 J/cm^3 × 1 cm/794 × 1/695 × 10^{-6} s).[21] While tissue cutting and ablation will occur at lower power densities, it will be accompanied by larger zones of collateral thermal injury because of the longer duration of beam exposure required to achieve tissue vaporization. Table 8.1 outlines power density as a function of power output of the laser and beam diameter at the tissue surface.

Tissue handling

The manipulation of tissue by the surgeon during the application of the laser beam can have a profound influence on the resulting tissue effect. A moderate amount of tension applied across the surgical plane during the laser incision will cause the tissue to separate along the incision line as soon as the tissue is able to part. This moves tissue out of the beam path as it is incised.

Using the separation of the incision line as a visual cue to regulate the speed at which the surgeon moves the beam helps to insure that the tissue surface is completely incised in one pass. If the skin along an incision line is not incised through its full thickness during the initial pass of the beam, repeat passes will be needed to separate the tissue. Each pass of a manually controlled 0.2–0.4 mm focal point along an incision line is not likely to be centered exactly on the original pass, producing otherwise unnecessary heat generation and increased collateral thermal damage.

When the objective is to ablate (vaporize) a volume of tissue rather than make an incision, a power and spot diameter are selected that will allow for the removal of a wide area of tissue. During the ablation process, as tissue is broken down into its elemental components, it is likely that carbon residue (char) will accumulate on the ablation surface. Char formation may be reduced by employing pulsed modes of beam delivery, and/or by passing the beam across the tissue surface at a rapid rate.

The presence of char on the tissue surface will block entry of the beam into tissue. This results in transfer of thermal energy from the heated char into the tissue, inhibiting ablation efficiency and promoting widespread thermal injury.[9] When the wavelength that is being used is poorly absorbed by tissue, such as a near-IR diode, the presence of char may enhance the ablation process of the laser by acting as a primary absorber, confining photons that would otherwise pass through tissue and transferring the thermal energy into the underlying tissue. However, the tissue effect still occurs as a result of thermal transfer, so wide areas of collateral thermal injury should be expected. When using a CO_2 laser to ablate tissue it is important to use a moistened gauze sponge or cotton-tipped applicator to remove char from the ablation site. The surgical technique is to alternate ablating and gently wiping away char.

Beam delivery

Transmission of the beam from the laser to the surgery site requires a delivery system that will facilitate directing the beam to the desired location efficiently (minimal loss of intensity), retain good beam quality (even distribution of photons across the beam) and at a clinically relevant intensity (useful focal point diameter). To accomplish this, the laser will be equipped with one of three delivery mechanisms: optical fiber, articulated arm or waveguide.

Optical fibers

Solid-core, generally silica-based, optical fibers ranging in diameter from 200 to 1000 μm are used with most laser systems that produce wavelengths in the visible to near-IR region. An outer cladding that may be composed of a soft polymer or a hard fluoropolymer covers the silica fiber core. Photons are launched into the fiber at a coupler on the laser and travel through the fiber, exiting through a free cut (cleaved) end, a sculpted tip or a fixed lens.[20]

The beam generally diverges as it moves from the tip, so the narrowest point of the free beam is at the fiber tip and corresponds to the diameter of the fiber core. The beam can be delivered with the fiber either in contact or noncontact with the tissue. A sculpted tip is generally intended for contact, a fixed lens for noncontact, and a cleaved end for either contact or noncontact applications. When used in contact mode the fiber is manually drawn through the tissue during irradiation, adding mechanical force to the photothermal mechanism for the incision of tissue.

Wavelengths that are well absorbed by water (longer than 2.0 μm) are not delivered through silica fibers, as the hydroxyl groups of the silica absorb the beam, resulting in poor transmission efficiency with overheating and breaking of the fibers. While fiber delivery facilitates beam application, especially to difficult-to-access places, their use is limited to wavelengths that are less efficient for soft tissue removal than the wavelengths that are absorbed by water. Fiber applications of visible to near-IR wavelengths are associated with more collateral thermal injury than is experienced with the free beam applications of the Er:YAG or CO_2 lasers except where the laser is able to produce high-intensity, short-pulse beams, or the target tissue has a high concentration of an absorbing chromophore such as melanin or hemoglobin.[9,11,12]

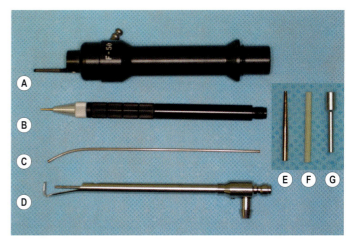

Fig. 8.5 (**A**) The handpiece of an articulated delivery system contains a lens that focuses the beam into a spot of fixed diameter. (**B**) The waveguide delivery handpiece concentrates the beam as the beam exits through a tip. Waveguide delivery tips may be configured to meet specific beam delivery requirements. Extended length tips like (**C**) the 0.8-mm diameter 120-mm long curved tip, and (**D**) the LAUP device with 0.8-mm diameter delivery and backstop, permit focused beam delivery at an extended distance from the handpiece, facilitating surgical procedures in difficult-to-access places. Short insertion tips of (**E**) 0.4-mm diameter, (**F**) 0.8-mm diameter and (**G**) 1.4-mm diameter are most commonly used for general soft tissue surgical applications.

Articulated arm

An articulated arm consists of two hollow tubes connected by an elbow joint that rotates around two parallel mirrors, permitting passage of a collimated beam from the laser through the center of the tubes regardless of their position in respect to each other. The terminal end of the arm assembly will have an articulated handpiece attachment containing a focusing lens of fixed focal length and a specified focal point diameter (Fig. 8.5).

Waveguide

A waveguide is a hollow-core tube with a highly reflective inner surface that attaches to the laser at one end and has either free beam discharge or a handpiece with application tips at the other.[20] Photons traveling through a waveguide exit following their last reflection event from the wall of the waveguide, and are traveling a path of divergence from the tip. They are fairly evenly distributed across the beam as their paths of travel cross while exiting the waveguide, but they are found more on the periphery of the beam at an increasing distance from the point of exit (see Fig. 8.4).

For standardization, the specified diameter of a waveguide tip is the width of the beam measured 1 mm distant from the end of the tip. While there is some ability to move from a focal point (1–3 mm from the end of the tip) to a wider, defocused beam diameter by manually retracting the handpiece away from the tissue surface, retention of an even distribution of photons across the beam at increasingly wider beam diameters requires the changing of tip diameters, usually at intervals where the beam diameter reaches a twofold increase from the tip diameter. An advantage of a waveguide delivery system is the variety of tip configurations and angles that can be incorporated into the system, greatly facilitating delivery of the beam to difficult-to-access places that may be problematic for a lens directed beam with a fixed focal length (Fig. 8.5).

SURGICAL CONSIDERATIONS

Surgical approach

When cutting or ablating tissue with a surgical laser, it is important to consider how the beam will be directed and manipulated to avoid inadvertent tissue exposure. Once the beam penetrates through the targeted tissue it will continue on to the next tissue layer or object in its path. Inadvertent hard tissue exposure at ablative power densities of most clinical lasers will produce charring defects that will remain as permanent etches, and heating of teeth that raises the temperature of dental pulp by $5.5\,°C$, can result in permanent damage to vital pulp.[26]

The placement of a beam diffusing, deflecting or absorbing backstop behind the targeted tissue should be used whenever possible to provide protection to surrounding structures. While backstops are made of a variety of materials, a material that will absorb the selected laser wavelength would be the safest. For the CO_2 laser, water-soaked materials such as gauze sponges, cotton-tipped applicators or tongue depressors make excellent and inexpensive backstops.

Wound healing

The principles of wound healing, management and closure are no different for a laser-induced lesion than for any other wound. Although initial collagen formation and healing of soft tissue may be slightly delayed after CO_2 laser surgery, by 3 weeks post surgery a difference in wound organization and strength is no longer apparent.[27-31] In the long term, CO_2 and Er:YAG laser wound contraction and scar formation are reduced, leading to improved cosmetic results.

The amount of collateral thermal damage created by the laser application is of considerable importance in determining the rate and quality of wound healing. Immediate and final wound contraction tends to increase with greater initial thermal damage and greater depth of ablation. A thick layer of thermal damage at the margins of a wound, especially if char is produced and not removed prior to wound closure, will tend to delay healing and weaken wound cohesive strength.[27,28,30,32]

At the completion of the procedure, the surgery site and especially any wound margins that will be apposed for primary closure should be gently cleaned to remove any debris, particularly any particles of char. When first learning to use a CO_2 laser, one should anticipate that enough collateral thermal injury will occur that primary intention healing will be delayed but, as experience is gained, the healing times will return to those experienced when a scalpel blade is used.

ANESTHETIC CONSIDERATIONS

Laser surgical procedures are not painless, and must be performed in conjunction with an appropriate level of anesthesia and patient immobility. Patient airways should be protected from plume inhalation by use of smoke evacuation and, whenever possible, intubation. When using inhalation anesthesia while working in the oral cavity, endotracheal tubes should be protected from errant beam exposure, and a smoke evacuation system used for the prevention of the accumulation of ignitable oxygen in the surgical field. Where manual or sedated restraint with use of a local anesthetic may be a consideration, the potential complications associated with patient movement during application of the laser are of particular concern, and appropriate safety precautions need to be taken.

ORAL AND MAXILLOFACIAL SURGICAL APPLICATIONS

The following surgical procedures may be performed with standard surgical instrumentation, electro/radiosurgery devices or lasers, and several may be discussed in other sections of this book. These procedures are selected for discussion here because they may illustrate specific techniques of tissue handling associated with laser surgery, or may incorporate modifications of the procedure that are specific to use of a CO_2 laser.

Incision, excision and ablation can be accomplished with the laser. Changes in power density are controlled by adjustments in beam diameter created by movement of the handpiece to adjust the focal distance during the procedure. A tight focal spot (high power density) is used for incision and excision, while a wider, defocused beam (lower power density) is used for ablation and tissue contraction. All procedures are performed under appropriate general anesthesia, patient preparation and in adherence to routine safety precautions.[14-17]

Correction of overlong soft palate

Elongated soft palate is one component of the brachycephalic airway syndrome. The use of a CO_2 laser in the surgical correction of an elongated soft palate was described by Clark and Sinibaldi in 1994.[33] The approach is similar to conventional surgical correction (see Ch. 56). The incised margin of the soft palate is not sutured following the laser excision of tissue, but left to heal by second intention.[33,34] With use of a laser additional attention is given to precautions for protection of the airway, using a smoke evacuator for removal of the vaporization plume, and placement of saline-moistened gauze sponges over the tracheal tube and behind the soft palate to protect the tube and pharyngeal tissues from errant beam exposure during excision.

A CO_2 laser with either an articulated arm or waveguide delivery system may be used for this procedure. However, the approach is facilitated and the visual field less encumbered when an extended-length waveguide tip or a laser-assisted uvuloplasty (LAUP) handpiece is used (see Fig. 8.5). Following intravenous induction of general anesthesia, the oropharynx is inspected and the soft palate marked for resection prior to placement of an endotracheal tube. With the patient in dorsal recumbency and the head supported in a normal position in relation to the neck so that the soft palate and larynx approximate normal alignment with the epiglottis lying under the excess soft palate tissue, the laser beam is directed against the soft palate in a chain of single pulses along the edge of the epiglottis to outline the margins of the segment of soft palate that is to be excised.

Once the excision margin is outlined, a tracheal tube is placed, inhalation anesthesia is administered, and the pharynx is lined by saline-soaked gauze sponges. Tissue forceps, a hook or stay sutures are used on the margins of the soft palate to pull it forward and apply tension across the surgery site during the excision. The laser beam is passed across the soft palate to make a full-thickness incision that is slightly medial to the premarked outline (Fig. 8.6) which allows for some tissue contraction during the procedure and in healing. Considerations for anesthesia recovery and postoperative care are similar to conventional surgical repair.

As some collateral thermal influence on the tissue is desired in order to achieve hemostasis during the excision, a continuous wave mode of delivery is generally preferred over the superpulse mode. The extended waveguide tip and LAUP handpieces usually emit a 0.8-mm diameter beam, which means that the power output of the laser will need to be increased to achieve a cutting efficiency comparable with a 0.2–0.4-mm focal spot.

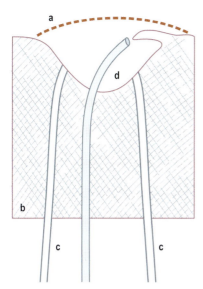

Fig. 8.6 Prior to surgical resection, the soft palate is placed over the epiglottis and individual laser pulses are used to outline the margin of the epiglottis on the soft palate (*a*). The patient is intubated and the end of the soft palate is retracted rostrally over a moistened gauze sponge (*b*) placed to cover the tracheal tube and caudal pharynx. Stay sutures (*c*) and/or Allis forceps are placed on the margin of the soft palate to facilitate the placing of traction across the incision line. The laser beam is used to make a full-thickness incision (*d*) of the soft palate at the marked line.

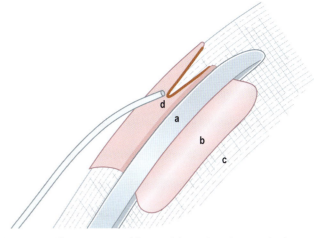

Fig. 8.7 Tonsillectomy: curved forceps (*a*) are placed across the base of the tonsil (*b*) and used to exteriorize the tonsil from the crypt over a moistened gauze sponge (*c*). The laser beam is used to transect the base of the tonsil (*d*). Either an articulated arm or waveguide CO$_2$ laser delivery system may be used for this procedure; however, a narrow extended-length delivery tip (*d*) will facilitate visualization of the surgical field.

Tonsillectomy

Tonsillectomy is occasionally indicated in the dog and cat (see Ch. 59) and hemorrhage is a known complication. Use of a CO$_2$ laser equipped with an extended waveguide tip provides for a quick, easy and generally bloodless approach for the removal of tonsils.

A saline-soaked gauze sponge is placed against the wall of the pharynx just below the crypt to act as a backstop. A curved forceps is passed behind and clamped across the base of the tonsil, and used to extract the tonsil from the crypt, drawing it out and over the gauze sponge. While using the forceps to apply gentle tension to the tonsil, the laser beam is directed across the base of the tonsil, between the forceps and wall of the pharynx, in a caudal to rostral direction. Separation of the tissue is used to gauge the rate of passage of the laser beam so that the tonsil is excised in a single pass of the beam (Fig. 8.7).

Gingivectomy/gingivoplasty

The laser provides a tool for achieving hemostasis while removing gingival tissue, with the added advantage of being able to sculpt gingival tissue during removal (see Ch. 18). Care should be taken to protect the enamel surfaces of teeth from direct exposure to the beam. The removal of hyperplastic gingival tissue by a CO$_2$ laser may be achieved by a combination of excision and ablation techniques. When excising tissue, a margin of the hyperplastic tissue is grasped with thumb forceps while the focused beam is directed in a line parallel to the long axis of the tooth, not perpendicular to the tooth surface (Fig. 8.8A). Vaporization of gingival tissue is achieved by using a defocused beam in a similar manner (Fig. 8.8B). Power density is varied by manually adjusting the focal distance (beam diameter) to control the rate and depth of tissue removal. The beam is moved across the gingival surface in an overlapping, repeating rostral–caudal–rostral pattern, ablating tissue with each pass and removing char as it accumulates on the ablation surface. As the gingival tissue is reduced to the level of the base of the tooth, the handpiece is gradually rotated away from the tooth with each pass in order to sculpt the gingival surface back to a normal conformation (Figs 8.8C and 8.9). Postoperative care is the same as for a routine gingivectomy (see Ch. 18).

Excision of oral mass lesions

Lasers may be used in the treatment of oral mass lesions to remove abnormal tissue by surgical excision, ablation or photothermal coagulation. The laser is used in accordance with the principles of surgical oncology, with reference to the surgical objective (e.g., cure vs. palliation) and surgical margins (see Ch. 43).

In selecting a laser system, consideration should be given to the tissue effect that is desired for the treatment. Where the precise removal of tissue with minimal collateral thermal injury is desired, especially if soft tissue planes are to be preserved or thin layers of tissue vaporized from other structures that are to be preserved without injury, the CO$_2$ or Er:YAG in continuous wave or pulsing modes would be preferred.[35–42] Where coagulation of tissue beyond the margins of surgical excision is desired, or blood vessels 0.5–3.0 mm in diameter are likely to be encountered, a visible or near-IR laser might be selected.[36,39,43–45] Where a large area of tissue coagulation and postsurgical necrosis is intended, similar to cryosurgery or hyperthermia procedures, use of a near-IR wavelength would be the selection of choice.[46–48]

Feline chronic stomatitis

The lack of a full understanding of the pathogenesis of feline chronic stomatitis and the difficulty of achieving control of the disease in many patients lead to both frustration in managing the condition and the susceptibility of practitioners to hold out high expectations for new technologies to conquer this disease. In reality, as the disease appears to have a multifactorial etiology, the treatment is likely to

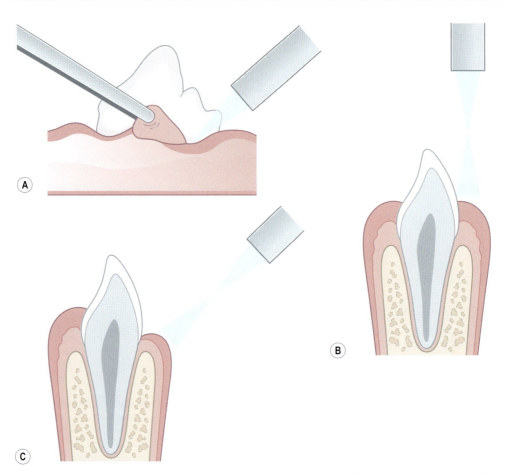

Fig. 8.8 CO_2 laser gingivectomy/gingivoplasty is accomplished by a combination of excision and ablation. (**A**) To excise gingival tissue the margin is grasped with thumb forceps to apply traction while a focused beam is directed in a plane parallel to the long axis of the tooth; (**B**) Vaporization may be used instead of excision to remove hyperplastic gingival tissue by directing a defocused beam parallel to the long axis of the tooth; (**C**) When using either excision or ablation, once the bulk of the hyperplastic tissue has been removed, the remaining gingival tissue can be recontoured using a defocused beam.

remain multifactorial as well. This text will be limited to the potential role that lasers may play in the treatment of feline chronic stomatitis.

Successful treatment is accomplished by selective therapeutic destruction of the diseased tissue, therapeutic control of the pathological process while the body attempts to repair and restore the tissue to normal, or physical removal of the diseased tissue with healing by primary or secondary intention. As with the treatment of infected granulomatous tissue, successful therapy may require a combination of treatment approaches, including both surgical excision and systemic therapy. From this perspective it would seem logical that the surgical removal of the affected tissue would facilitate a shift in the body's focus to healing and restoration; however, if no other therapy is administered concurrently, this presumes that removal of the affected tissue will also arrest the underlying pathological process. In practice, it is likely that the use of a laser to remove stomatitis tissue may be a tool in the armamentarium of things that have a place in the treatment of this condition, but at the present time it would appear that only in limited cases will it be effective as a stand-alone treatment.

Currently, there are no published reports of prospective or retrospective studies regarding the use of a laser for the treatment of chronic stomatitis in cats. The reports of the experiences of using a CO_2 laser for the ablation of stomatitis tissue are anecdotal and mostly verbal. The experiences of these anecdotal reports range between the extremes

of dismal failure with immediate postsurgical pharyngeal swelling and respiratory compromise to uncomplicated and complete resolution in 70–90% of cases.

Where successful management employing laser tissue ablation is reported, there seem to be a few commonalities in the approach that bear consideration if one is going to consider including CO_2 laser ablation as part of a treatment protocol. For these cases, the removal of affected tissue generally is not a stand-alone treatment, but includes at least the systemic use of antimicrobial agents. Complete and aggressive removal of affected tissue is made, and repeated at the earliest signs of recurrence, generally at monthly intervals for at least three successive treatments.

Removal of affected tissue is aggressive, with the objective of removal of all diseased tissue. The alternating ablate and wipe technique is used to remove char accumulation and maintain ablation efficiency during the procedure. Because stomatitis tissue is vascular and friable, the adequacy of tissue removal is judged by the use of a cotton-tipped applicator to physically irritate the ablation surface, and tissue removal is discontinued when hemorrhage is no longer easily induced. Some who advocate this procedure hypothesize that it is not the healing with restoration of normal oral mucosa but its replacement with more fibrous tissue during healing that benefits the resolution, and to achieve this objective they use low power densities and the continuous wave mode so that some collateral thermal injury is produced in the remaining tissue bed.

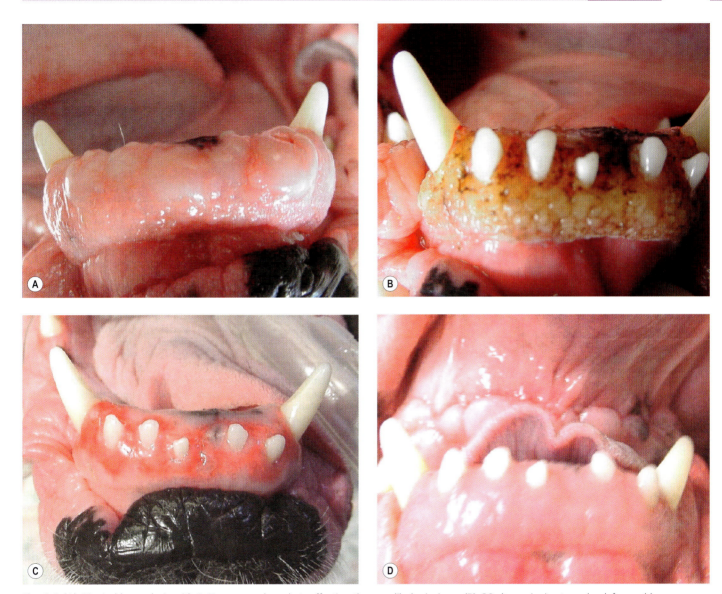

Fig. 8.9 (**A**) Gingival hyperplasia with 3–5-mm pseudopockets affecting the mandibular incisors; (**B**) CO_2 laser gingivectomy by defocused beam ablation; (**C**) Healing 11 days and (**D**) 19 days following treatment. *(Photographs courtesy of Dr. R. Arza)*

REFERENCES

1. Hitz CB. Understanding laser technology. Tulsa, OK: Penn-Well; 1985.

2. Siegman AE. Lasers. Sausalito, CA: University Science Books; 1986.

3. Berns MW, Nelson JS, Wright WH. Laser physics and laser-tissue interactions. In: Achauer BM, Vander Kam VM, Berns MW, editors. Lasers in plastic surgery and dermatology. New York: Thieme Medical Publishers, Inc; 1992. p. 1–10.

4. Silfvast WT. Laser fundamentals. Cambridge, UK: Cambridge University Press; 1996.

5. Fisher JC. The power density of a surgical laser beam: its meaning and measurement. Lasers Surg Med 1983;2:301–15.

6. Wolbarsht ML. Laser surgery: CO_2 or HF. IEEE J Quantum Elec 1984;20:1427–32.

7. Boulnois JL. Photophysical processes in recent medical laser developments: a review. Lasers Surg Med 1986;1:47–66.

8. van Gemert MJC, Welch AJ. Time constants in thermal laser medicine. Lasers Surg Med 1989;9:405–21.

9. Jacques SL. Role of tissue optics and pulse duration on tissue effects during high-power laser irradiation. Appl Opt 1993;32:2447–52.

10. Venugopalan V, Nishioka N, Mikic BB. The effect of laser parameters on the zone of thermal injury produced by laser ablation of biological tissue. J Biomech Eng 1994;116:62–70.

11. Niemz MH. Laser-tissue interactions fundamentals and applications. Berlin: Springer-Verlag; 1996.

12. White JM, Gekelman D, Shin K-B, et al. Laser interaction with dental soft tissues: What do we know from our years of applied scientific research? In: Rechmann P, Fried D, Hennig T, editors. Lasers in dentistry VIII, Proceedings SPIE 2002; 4610:39–48.

13. Welch AJ, Gardner C. Optical and thermal response of tissue to laser radiation. In: Waynant RW, editor. Lasers in medicine. Boca Raton, FL: CRC Press; 2002. p. 27–45.

Table 9.1 Recipient vessels

Location for flap	Recipient artery	Recipient vein
Hard palate	Infraorbital artery Major palatine artery	Infraorbital vein Major palatine vein
Soft palate	Lingual artery Minor palatine artery	Lingual vein Minor palatine vein
Maxillofacial	Infraorbital artery	Infraorbital vein Facial vein
Dorsum of head	Caudal auricular artery	Caudal auricular vein

Table 9.2 Essential instruments and equipment for microvascular anastomosis

Instruments and equipment	Comments
Operating microscope	twin heads with 200 mm focal length objective lens; foot-operated control for magnification, focusing, and x–y axis
Jeweler's forceps #3	both straight and angled (45°)
Needle holders	round handle, ratchetless
Vessel dilator	inserted into vessel to dilate the lumen
Dissecting scissors	for removing surrounding tissues form vessels
Adventitial scissors	for removing adventitia from the end of the vessels
Vessel approximation clamps	flat jaw, non-crushing clamp that holds the ends of the vessels together for the anastomosis
Bipolar cautery	
Hemoclips	for vessel ligation
Suture material	10–0 monofilament, taper point with round body, needle sizes range from 70–100 microns

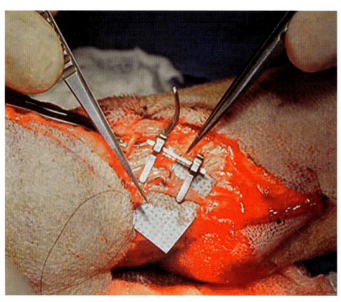

Fig. 9.1 An end-to-end artery and vein anastomosis using microvascular instruments, operating microscope, and 10–0 suture. The matching ends of the vessels are held together for suturing with an approximation clamp.

Patient positioning

The patient should be positioned on the operating table so that the surgeons have access to both the recipient and donor sites. This can allow two surgical teams to work simultaneously, which reduces procedural time. The recipient site must also be in a position to allow for comfortable access for the microvascular anastomosis with the operating microscope between two surgeons in opposite seats.

Donor tissue

When choosing the type of flap necessary for wound reconstruction it is important to first decide on the type or types of tissue needed. Deciding on skin, muscle, bone or a combination will determine which donor site will best fill the need. For example, the trapezius osteomusculocutaneous free flap provides all three tissues. Choosing a donor site that will have minimal morbidity for the patient (excessive tension of skin and reduced limb function) is also important.

ANESTHETIC CONSIDERATIONS

Maintaining the patient's body temperature, ventilation, and systemic blood pressure are critical for overall procedural success. Low blood pressure during the procedure may compromise the vasculature within the flap. Clot formation within the flap and at the anastomosis site is a major concern both during and after the surgery. A colloid solution such as dextran can be given to the patient intravenously at 10 mL/kg/h 45 minutes prior to the vessel anastomosis to in an attempt to reduce the risk of vessel thrombosis.

INSTRUMENTATION AND EQUIPMENT

Microvascular free tissue transfer is a technique dependent surgical procedure that requires delicate handling of the vascular pedicle. Trauma to the vessels will increase the risk of vessel anastomosis and flap failure. The instruments and equipment essential for performing microvascular vessel anastomosis are listed in Table 9.2.

SURGICAL TECHNIQUES

Transversus abdominis myoperitoneal free flap

A transversus abdominis myoperitoneal free flap may be used for reconstruction of intraoral defects such as oronasal fistula, congenital cleft palate, or defects created by oncologic surgery resections. This flap heals by primary intention and will develop a protective layer of squamous epithelium over its surface. The dominant vascular pedicles for this flap are the cranial abdominal artery and vein, which supplies the cranial half of the transversus abdominis muscle and the overlying peritoneum. The flap is harvested by incising the dorsal hypaxial muscle attachments and the myotendinous junction attachments ventrally. The dorsal and ventral incisions are connected by two parallel incisions. The cranial incision is made 20 mm caudal to the thirteenth rib. The caudal incision is made 75 mm caudal to the thirteenth rib. The donor site is closed primarily. The vessel anastomosis is performed and the flap secured to the surrounding tissue.

Trapezius osteomusculocutanoues free flap

The trapezius osteomusculocutanoues free flap is a versatile flap for both oral and maxillofacial reconstruction because it provides a combination of tissues: skin, muscle and bone.[3] The dominant vascular pedicles are the superficial cervical artery and vein. The superficial cervical artery provides blood supply to the cervical portion of the trapezius muscle, the overlying skin, and the scapular spine (provided that the trapezius muscle maintains its bony attachment). The strength of the scapular spine is questionable for mandibular reconstruction but it can be used for maxillary defects.

The trapezius is a thin, triangular muscle that is separated into cervical and thoracic parts (Fig. 9.2). It originates from the raphe of the neck and supraspinous ligament from the level of the third vertebra to the ninth thoracic vertebra and inserts on the scapular spine. The graft is harvested by incising the trapezius from its origin dorsally. The cleidocervicalis and omotransversarius musculature is dissected away cranially. Care is taken to preserve the prescapular branch of the superficial cervical vascular pedicle if the overlying skin is to be harvested with the muscle. Caudal attachments to the scapular spine can be incised if a bone graft is not needed. The flap is placed into the defect, the vascular anastomosis performed and the flap is secured with suture. The donor site is closed primarily with a Penrose or closed suction drain to reduce chances of seroma formation.

Medial saphenous fasciocutaneous free flap

The medial saphenous fasciocutaneous free flap may be used to reconstruct full-thickness skin defects in the maxillofacial region.[2] The dominant vascular pedicles are the medial saphenous artery and vein. It is the cutaneous branches of the saphenous artery that provides blood supply to the skin of the medial aspect of the femorotibial region of the hind limb. The section of skin available with this flap can extend from the inguinal region to the distal tibia. This entire length is usually not needed and it is advised to harvest skin proximal to the stifle to avoid closure of the donor site over the high motion area of the stifle. The width of the flap is dictated by the amount of tissue needed; however, the ability to close the donor site with minimal tension must also be considered.

Flap dissection starts with mapping out the flap of skin with a marking pen (Fig. 9.3). The skin is incised circumferentially and elevated. The medial saphenous artery and vein are identified as they branch off of the femoral artery and vein. Care is taken not to traumatize the cutaneous vessels as they branch off of the major pedicle.

Muscular branches entering the sartorius and gracilis muscles are ligated. The medial saphenous artery and vein at the distal edge of the skin flap are ligated. The proximal vascular pedicle is also incised, being sure that the surgeon has distinguished between the artery and vein. The flap is placed into the defect and the anastomosis is performed. The donor site is closed primarily with a double-layer closure.

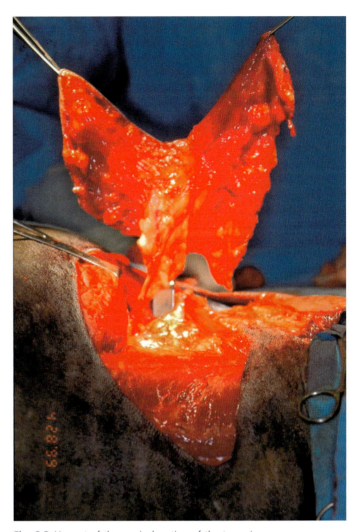

Fig. 9.2 Harvest of the cervical section of the trapezius osteomusculocutaneous free flap. The dominant vascular pedicle, superficial cervical artery and vein remain intact at the base of the flap until the tissue is needed.

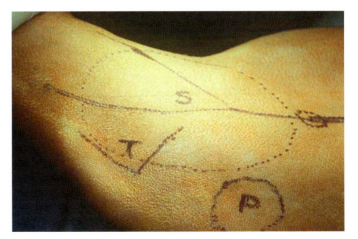

Fig. 9.3 Landmarks on the medial aspect of the thigh in the dog for the medial saphenous fasciocutaneous free flap. The circumferential borders of the flap are drawn on the skin. Identification of the patella (*P*), tibial plateau (*T*) and the medial saphenous artery and vein (*S*) aid in the flap harvest.

Free vascularized medial tibial bone graft

A free vascularized medial tibial bone graft may be used to reconstruct mandibular defects due to fracture, osteomyelitis, non-union, and post-tumor resection. The medial saphenous artery and vein are the dominant vascular pedicles for this bone graft.[7] These vessels give rise to multiple perforating periosteal branches along the medial aspect of the tibia. For graft harvest, a medial approach is made to the medial aspect of the tibia. The medial saphenous artery and vein are located and dissected along the length of the bone graft needed. Care is taken not to disrupt the soft tissue attachments between the dominant vascular pedicle and the bone, because this is where the vascular supply to periosteal perforators resides. The skin along the medial aspect of the thigh receives its blood supply from the same dominant pedicle so a section of skin may be harvested with the bone to serve as a sentinel to monitor graft viability. Approximately one-third of the circumference of the medial tibial cortex can be harvested. The graft is secured into the mandibular defect and secured with a type 1 external fixator or a bone plate and the vascular anastomosis is performed. The donor site is supported with a type 1 external fixator for 4–8 weeks to prevent postoperative tibial fracture.

POSTOPERATIVE ASSESSMENT AND COMPLICATIONS

Monitoring flap viability closely for the first 72 hours after surgery is critical, because early intervention is necessary to salvage a flap that is compromised. Compression, kinking, and thrombosis of the vascular pedicles may all lead to flap failure. During the first 72 hours a viable flap should be warm to the touch, have a bruised appearance, and be mildly edematous. The edges of the flap should readily bleed when pricked with a needle. The edema and discoloration should resolve within 7 days and the flap should appear as normal skin by 2 weeks (including hair growth). Bone graft incorporation can be monitored with serial radiographs.

Self-trauma is a problem with the veterinary patient during the postoperative healing phase. Elizabethan collars should be used to protect maxillofacial reconstructive sites for up to 2 weeks or until the flap edges are healed. Oral sites are protected with a moldable protective plate attached to the palate to prevent trauma from the tongue.

When monitoring the free flap, venous congestion will manifest with swelling, hypothermia (cool to the touch), and discoloration (blue) of the transplanted tissue. If arterial occlusion of the flap occurs it will not be swollen but will be cool to the touch and appear pale in color. When pricked with a needle, the flap will not bleed if the arterial blood supply has been occluded. Occlusion of the arterial blood supply to the flap requires surgical exploration of the anastomosis site and possible re-suturing of the pedicles. Should it occur, venous congestion within the flap may in some cases be alleviated by applying medical grade leeches (*Hirudo medicinalis*). Leeches will not only remove pooled blood from the flap tissue but, while feeding, anticoagulant within their saliva will be deposited into the flap. This may help to salvage the flap.

REFERENCES

1. Miller CW, Chang P, Bowen V. Identification and transfer of free cutaneous flaps by microvascular anastomosis in the dog. Vet Surg 1986;2:199–204.

2. Degner DA, Walshaw R, Lang OI, et al. The medial saphenous fasciocutaneous and myocutaneous free flaps in the dog. Vet Surg 1996;25:105–13.

3. Philibert D, Fowler JD. The trapezius osteomusculocutaneous flap in dogs. Vet Surg 1993;22:444–50.

4. Nicoll SA, Fowler JD, Remedios AM, et al. Development of a free latissimus dorsi muscle flap in cats. Vet Surg 1996;25:40–8.

5. Szentimrey D, Fowler JD. The anatomic basis of a free vascularized bone graft in the canine distal ulna. Vet Surg 1994;23:529–33.

6. Degner DA, Lanz OI, Walshaw R. Myoperitoneal microvascular free flaps in dogs: An anatomical study and a clinical case report. Vet Surg 1996;25:463–70.

7. Bebchuck TN, Degner CA, Walshaw R, et al. Evaluation of a free vascularized medial tibial bone graft in dogs. Vet Surg 2000;29:128–44.

8. Colfee EF, Lanz OI, Degner DA, et al. Microvascular free tissue transfer of the rectus abdominis muscle in dogs. Vet Surg 2002;31:32–43.

Chapter | 10 |

Use of the dog and cat in experimental maxillofacial surgery

M. Anthony Pogrel & Xudong Wang

The use of dogs and cats as animal models for human research has a long history which is often arbitrary, and not always based on science. In fact, the use of animal models in general has a somewhat checkered history, both scientifically and emotionally. At the present time, attempts are being made to move away from live animal models as much as possible, and to move to the use of simulation, biomimetics and tissue cultures, etc. Where animal models need to be used, an attempt has been made to move to smaller animals, including rodents, for studies where size is not an important part of the study.

However, instances still remain where it is required to use an animal that is large enough to render simulation as realistic as possible to obtain realistic results. Primates have always been felt to be the most realistic animal models for human research, but costs have increased such as to make them unusable for anything but the largest studies. Dogs and cats have been used extensively, but their use is decreasing because of noted differences in size, biology and physiology between dogs and cats and humans, and also cost issues and psychological issues related to the use of animals which are also domestic pets. Animals such as pigs,[1–3] sheep[4–6] and goats[7–9] are becoming more frequently used as animal models, in part because of the larger and more realistic size, biological similarities to humans,[3,10–12] and also because there may be less emotion attached to their use.

DOGS

In the maxillofacial region, dogs have a long history of use as an animal model, usually for hard tissue (bone and teeth) research, but also for soft tissue studies. The rationale often given for the use of dogs is that their size makes them large enough for realistic surgical procedures to be carried out. In fact, studies have shown that in some respects they are about the smallest animal that can be used for some realistic studies of human maxillofacial procedures. Their teeth are also of similar size and pulpal pattern to those of humans, and they have similar periodontal ligament attachments as human teeth.[13,14] The bony architecture of the mandible and maxilla is also similar to humans with Haversian systems (unlike rats), and they are the smallest animals with a similar pattern of bone remodeling to humans.[15,16] Growth, remodeling, structural and chemical properties, and mineralization of bone is similar to that of humans. Age-related bony changes are also similar to humans.[17] They are cooperative animals, and there is often no need for general anesthesia for relatively simple procedures such as obtaining photographs, making measurements, and even procedures such as cleaning teeth, or adjusting dental appliances or braces. This can be a considerable advantage in some studies.

Bone turnover

It is generally agreed that the bone turnover time in dogs is faster than that in humans, and that fractures heal more rapidly in dogs than humans.[18] However the process of fracture healing in dogs is essentially similar to that in humans.[18] Bone turnover time is normally expressed as sigma, which is one complete bone turnover cycle, including both a resorptive phase and an appositional phase.[19–23] This time for the beagle is felt to be two to three times that of a human,[23–28] though other studies have suggested it is around 1.5 times as great.[29] Variations are possible for a number of reasons. It is known that variations occur within the same species of dogs, and certainly there are variations between species of dogs. There is also a variation depending on age. It must be remembered that most animal experiments involving dogs are carried out on fairly young dogs, usually for financial reasons, whilst equivalent human operations may be carried out on more mature humans. Bone turnover is obviously going to be more rapid in younger animals. There are also variations in bone turnover time for cortical bone versus medullary bone, and this should be taken into account when studies are compared. Studies carried out on animals may not therefore be directly transferred to humans,[15] or even to clinical veterinary practice. The critical size defect has been established for the canine cranium at around 20 mm, and for the canine mandible it is at 15 mm if the periosteum is removed and 50 mm if it is intact.[30,31] A critical size defect is one which, if created, will not heal spontaneously. Critical size defects are used for research on bone grafting and reconstruction techniques involving a variety of osteoconductive and osteoinductive agents.[32,33]

© 2012 Elsevier Ltd
DOI: 10.1016/B978-0-7020-4618-6.00010-5

Facial growth

As we move away from the use of primates in maxillofacial studies, dogs have been examined for their use in a number of studies of facial growth. Losken et al. determined that the mandibular growth pattern of the dog shows similar relative percentage changes in different regions in juvenile through adult stages, as do those of the human being, and suggested that dogs may be an acceptable, inexpensive alternative to primates in certain maxillofacial growth situations.[34] Similarly, dogs have also been studied for their ability to be used as spontaneous animal models of human disease. For example, many dogs suffer from maxillary brachygnathism as a natural phenomenon. In fact, it is even a requirement in the official standards established for certain breeds, including the English toy spaniel, French bulldog, English bulldog and boxers.[35] Brachycephaly in dogs is a regional manifestation of achondroplasia, and occurs naturally in some breeds.[35] Hereditary multiple exostosis has also been recognized to occur in several breeds including the West Highland white terrier, cairn and Boston terriers, Great Danes and Labrador retrievers.[36] Data suggest that these animals may make suitable models for investigation of the etiology and treatment of infantile cortical hyperostosis in human infants.[36,37] Dogs have also been used in studies involving orthognathic surgery and tooth viability.[13]

Periodontal disease

The beagle suffers naturally from periodontal disease and periodontal degeneration, and has been widely used in studies of periodontal disease and in evaluations of a variety of surgical and nonsurgical treatments of periodontal disease.[14,38] More recently, the beagle has been used in studies utilizing membrane technology as a method of treating periodontal disease in humans.[39,40]

Postoperative infection rates are extremely low in dogs, and this may also need to be taken into account in studies of healing following certain procedures. Single genomic beagle models have recently been developed which should lead to more standardization of research data. Soft tissue studies on dogs have included grafting materials for vestibuloplasty (increasing the amount of gingiva for dentures to rest on).[41]

Implants

Dogs have also been used extensively in studies on various aspects of osteointegrated dental implants for tooth replacement, including osteointegration time, degree of osteointegration, effects of early and late loading, and the effects of orthodontic forces.[42-50] Some of these studies have been combined with the use of growth factors.[39,43] Although these studies have been valuable, it does need to be borne in mind that the bone turnover time is more rapid in dogs than in humans, and thus the studies may not be directly transferrable to the human situation or even to clinical veterinary practice.

Despite the possible dissimilarities between bone healing in dogs and humans, the canine model has become popular for investigating the management of periodontal disease, both around natural teeth and around implants, and the concept of a barrier membrane to encourage new bone growth. This has led to the concept of a critical-size supra-alveolar periodontal defect and the related critical-size supra-alveolar peri-implant defect in the canine animal model. In the beagle dog model, this critical size defect is around 5 mm all around a natural tooth or implant.[44,45]

Distraction

Dogs have also been used to look at various aspects of distraction osteogenesis, which is a more recent technique for slowly moving facial bones by means of gradual distraction following an initial osteotomy.[51-54] Again, many of the parameters utilized in humans have been established from animal research utilizing dogs. However, it needs to be emphasized that the bone turnover rate is faster in dogs than in humans.

CATS

The use of cats as experimental animals in oral and maxillofacial surgery is not found as frequently as dogs, possibly because they are smaller animals and therefore may not be quite as realistic a model, and also because they are not as cooperative as dogs, and therefore may need anesthetizing more often for procedures to be carried out. Nevertheless, cats have been used for a variety of hard and soft tissue studies. They have been widely used for orthodontic studies involving tooth movement because the crown to root ratio and periodontal ligaments are similar to that of humans and therefore it is felt that the tooth movement obtained orthodontically on a cat may be realistically transferred to the human.[55-58] Studies have shown that the cat may be the most realistic nonprimate model for nasal growth studies to simulate results in humans.[59] In the soft tissues, studies involving the temporalis muscle have been carried out on cats, and this appears to be related to the fact that cats have a prominent temporalis muscle which is particularly amenable to surgical procedures.[60-62]

Nerve studies

The cat has also been used for studies on the lingual and inferior alveolar nerves, with particular reference to the response of this nerve to injury, and spontaneous and surgically induced regeneration, and also the value of a number of nerve growth factors which may aid reconstruction and regrowth of the branches of the trigeminal nerve.[63-70] The rationale for utilizing the cat for these studies appears to be that there is a long history of its use, and the cat appears to lend itself to carrying out single neuron studies on the branches of the trigeminal nerve, which can be extremely valuable in a number of physiological studies. Injury to the inferior alveolar and lingual nerves occurs in humans as a result of trauma and a variety of surgical procedures including wisdom tooth removal.[71,72] Loss of sensation, or dysesthesia, causes considerable morbidity and hence the necessity for a reliable animal model.[73]

REFERENCES

1. Terheyden H, Knak C, Jepsen S, et al. Mandibular reconstruction with a prefabricated vascularized bone graft using recombinant human osteogenic protein-1: an experimental study in miniature pigs. Part I: Prefabrication. Int J Oral Maxillofac Surg 2001;30:373–9.
2. Henkel KO, Ma L, Lenz JH, et al. Closure of vertical alveolar bone defects with guided horizontal distraction osteogenesis: an experimental study in pigs and first clinical results. J Craniomaxillofac Surg 2001;29:249–53.
3. Troulis MJ, Glowacki J, Perrott DH, et al. Effects of latency and rate on bone

formation in a porcine mandibular distraction model. J Oral Maxillofac Surg 2000;58:507–13; discussion 514.

4. Uckan S, Schwimmer A, Kummer F, et al. Effect of the angle of the screw on the stability of the mandibular sagittal split ramus osteotomy: a study in sheep mandibles. Br J Oral Maxillofac Surg 2001;39:266–8.

5. Matsuura H, Miyamoto H, Ishimaru JI, et al. Costochondral grafts in reconstruction of the temporomandibular joint after condylectomy: an experimental study in sheep. Br J Oral Maxillofac Surg 2001;39:189–95.

6. Gaggl A, Schultes G, Regauer S, et al. Healing process after alveolar ridge distraction in sheep. Oral Surg Oral Med Oral Pathol Oral Radiol Endod 2000; 90:420–9.

7. Hu J, Tang Z, Wang D, et al. Changes in the inferior alveolar nerve after mandibular lengthening with different rates of distraction. J Oral Maxillofac Surg 2001;59:1041–5; discussion 1046.

8. Denissen H, Montanari C, Martinetti R, et al. Alveolar bone response to submerged bisphosphonate-complexed hydroxyapatite implants. J Periodontol 2000;71:279–86.

9. Bravetti P, Membre H, Marchal L, et al. Histologic changes in the sinus membrane after maxillary sinus augmentation in goats. J Oral Maxillofac Surg 1998;56:1170–6; discussion 1177.

10. Fukuta K, Har-Shai Y, Collares MV, et al. The viability of revascularized calvarial bone graft in a pig model. Ann Plast Surg 1992;29:136–42.

11. Gerard D, Gotcher JE, McKay H, et al. Is RAP responsible for higher bone activity around implants? J Dent Res 1992;71:1466.

12. Rose EH, Vistnes LM, Ksander GA. The panniculus carnosus in the domestic pig. Plast Reconstr Surg 1977;59:94–7.

13. Zisser G, Gattinger B. Histologic investigation of pulpal changes following maxillary and mandibular alveolar osteotomies in the dog. J Oral Maxillofac Surg 1982;40:332–9.

14. Haney JM, Zimmerman GJ, Wikesjo UM. Periodontal repair in dogs: evaluation of the natural disease model. J Clin Periodontol 1995;22:208–13.

15. Nunamaker DM. Experimental models of fracture repair. Clin Orthop Relat Res 1998:S56–65.

16. Meller Y, Kestenbaum RS, Mozes M, et al. Mineral and endocrine metabolism during fracture healing in dogs. Clin Orthop Relat Res 1984:289–95.

17. Martin RK, Albright JP, Jee WS, et al. Bone loss in the beagle tibia: influence of age, weight, and sex. Calcif Tissue Int 1981; 33:233–8.

18. Frost HM. Tetracycline-based histological analysis of bone remodeling. Calcif Tissue Res 1969;3:211–37.

19. Parfitt AM. The actions of parathyroid hormone on bone: relation to bone remodeling and turnover, calcium homeostasis, and metabolic bone disease. Part I of IV parts: mechanisms of calcium transfer between blood and bone and their cellular basis: morphological and kinetic approaches to bone turnover. Metabolism 1976;25:809–44.

20. Parfitt AM. The actions of parathyroid hormone on bone: relation to bone remodeling and turnover, calcium homeostasis, and metabolic bone diseases. II. PTH and bone cells: bone turnover and plasma calcium regulation. Metabolism 1976;25:909–55.

21. Parfitt AM. The actions of parathyroid hormone on bone: relation to bone remodeling and turnover, calcium homeostasis, and metabolic bone disease. Part III of IV parts; PTH and osteoblasts, the relationship between bone turnover and bone loss, and the state of the bones in primary hyperparathyroidism. Metabolism 1976;25:1033–69.

22. Parfitt AM. The actions of parathyroid hormone on bone: relation to bone remodeling and turnover, calcium homeostasis, and metabolic bone disease. Part IV of IV parts: The state of the bones in uremic hyperaparathyroidism – the mechanisms of skeletal resistance to PTH in renal failure and pseudohypoparathyroidism and the role of PTH in osteoporosis, osteopetrosis, and osteofluorosis. Metabolism 1976;25:1157–88.

23. Kimmel DB, Jee WS. A quantitative histologic study of bone turnover in young adult beagles. Anat Rec 1982;203:31–45.

24. High WB, Capen CC, Black HE. Histomorphometric evaluation of the effects of intermittent 1,25-dihydroxycholecalciferol administration on cortical bone remodeling in adult dogs. Am J Pathol 1981;104:41–9.

25. Anderson C, Danylchuk KD. Appositional bone formation rates in the Beagle. Am J Vet Res 1979;40:907–10.

26. Anderson C, Danylchuk KD. Age-related variations in cortical bone-remodeling measurements in male Beagles 10 to 26 months of age. Am J Vet Res 1979; 40:869–72.

27. Snow GR, Karambolova KK, Anderson C. Bone remodeling in the lumbar vertebrae of young adult beagles. Am J Vet Res 1986;47:1275–7.

28. Snow GR, Anderson C. The effects of continuous estradiol therapy on cortical bone remodeling activity in the spayed beagle. Calcif Tissue Int 1985;37:437–40.

29. Kim SG, Kim YU, Park JC, et al. Effects of presurgical and post-surgical irradiation on the healing process of Medpor in dogs. Int J Oral Maxillofac Surg 2001;30:438–42.

30. Schmitz JP, Hollinger JO. The critical size defect as an experimental model for craniomandibulofacial nonunions. Clin Orthop Relat Res 1986:299–308.

31. Huh JY, Choi BH, Kim BY, et al. Critical size defect in the canine mandible. Oral Surg Oral Med Oral Pathol Oral Radiol Endod 2005;100:296–301.

32. Sherris DA, Murakami CS, Larrabee WF Jr, et al. Mandibular reconstruction with transforming growth factor-beta1. Laryngoscope 1998;108:368–72.

33. Yudell RM, Block MS. Bone gap healing in the dog using recombinant human bone morphogenetic protein-2. J Oral Maxillofac Surg 2000;58:761–6.

34. Losken A, Mooney MP, Siegel MI. A comparative study of mandibular growth patterns in seven animal models. J Oral Maxillofac Surg 1992;50:490–5.

35. Andrews E, Ward B, Altman N. Spontaneous animal models of human disease. Vol II. New York: Academic Press; 1979. p. 222.

36. Andrews E, Ward B, Altman N. Spontaneous animal models of human disease. Vol II. New York: Academic Press; 1979. p. 223.

37. Thornburg LP. Infantile cortical hyperostosis (Caffey-Silverman syndrome). Animal model: craniomandibular osteopathy in the canine. Am J Pathol 1979;95:575–8.

38. Giannobile WV, Finkelman RD, Lynch SE. Comparison of canine and non-human primate animal models for periodontal regenerative therapy: results following a single administration of PDGF/IGF-I. J Periodontol 1994;65:1158–68.

39. Ruskin JD, Hardwick R, Buser D, et al. Alveolar ridge repair in a canine model using rhTGF-beta 1 with barrier membranes. Clin Oral Implants Res 2000;11:107–15.

40. Dongieux JW, Block MS, Morris G, et al. The effect of different membranes on onlay bone graft success in the dog mandible. Oral Surg Oral Med Oral Pathol Oral Radiol Endod 1998;86:145–51.

41. Rosner TM, Stern K, Doku HC. Autogenous dermal grafting vestibuloplasty in dogs. J Oral Maxillofac Surg 1982;40:9–12.

42. Gotfredsen K, Berglundh T, Lindhe J. Bone reactions adjacent to titanium implants subjected to static load of different duration. A study in the dog (III). Clin Oral Implants Res 2001;12:552–8.

43. Becker W, Lynch SE, Lekholm U, et al. A comparison of ePTFE membranes alone or in combination with platelet-derived growth factors and insulin-like growth factor-I or demineralized freeze-dried bone in promoting bone formation around immediate extraction socket implants. J Periodontol 1992;63:929–40.

44. Wikesjo UM, Nilveus R. Periodontal repair in dogs. Healing patterns in large

circumferential periodontal defects. J Clin Periodontol 1991;18:49–59.

45. Lee J, Decker JF, Polimeni G, et al. Evaluation of implants coated with rhBMP-2 using two different coating strategies: a critical-size supraalveolar peri-implant defect study in dogs. J Clin Periodontol 2010;37:582–90.

46. Block MS, Almerico B, Crawford C, et al. Bone response to functioning implants in dog mandibular alveolar ridges augmented with distraction osteogenesis. Int J Oral Maxillofac Implants 1998;13:342–51.

47. Block MS, Gardiner D, Almerico B, et al. Loaded hydroxylapatite-coated implants and uncoated titanium-threaded implants in distracted dog alveolar ridges. Oral Surg Oral Med Oral Pathol Oral Radiol Endod 2000;89:676–85.

48. Redlich M, Reichenberg E, Harari D, et al. The effect of mechanical force on mRNA levels of collagenase, collagen type I, and tissue inhibitors of metalloproteinases in gingivae of dogs. J Dent Res 2001;80: 2080–4.

49. Ohmae M, Saito S, Morohashi T, et al. A clinical and histological evaluation of titanium mini-implants as anchors for orthodontic intrusion in the beagle dog. Am J Orthod Dentofacial Orthop 2001;119:489–97.

50. Liou EJ, Figueroa AA, Polley JW. Rapid orthodontic tooth movement into newly distracted bone after mandibular distraction osteogenesis in a canine model. Am J Orthod Dentofacial Orthop 2000;117:391–8.

51. Cho BC, Seo MS, Baik BS. Distraction osteogenesis after membranous bone onlay grafting in a dog model. J Oral Maxillofac Surg 2001;59:1025–33.

52. Hollis BJ, Block MS, Gardiner D, et al. An experimental study of mandibular arch widening in the dog using distraction osteogenesis. J Oral Maxillofac Surg 1998;56:330–8.

53. Block MS, Chang A, Crawford C. Mandibular alveolar ridge augmentation

in the dog using distraction osteogenesis. J Oral Maxillofac Surg 1996;54:309–14.

54. Klotch DW, Ganey TM, Slater-Haase A, et al. Assessment of bone formation during osteoneogenesis: a canine model. Otolaryngol Head Neck Surg 1995;112: 291–302.

55. Guajardo G, Okamoto Y, Gogen H, et al. Immunohistochemical localization of epidermal growth factor in cat paradental tissues during tooth movement. Am J Orthod Dentofacial Orthop 2000;118: 210–19.

56. Burrow SJ, Sammon PJ, Tuncay OC. Effects of diazepam on orthodontic tooth movement and alveolar bone cAMP levels in cats. Am J Orthod Dentofacial Orthop 1986;90:102–5.

57. Long A, Loescher AR, Robinson PP. A histological study on the effect of different periods of orthodontic force on the innervation and dimensions of the cat periodontal ligament. Arch Oral Biol 1996;41:799–808.

58. Long A, Loescher AR, Robinson PP. A quantitative study on the myelinated fiber innervation of the periodontal ligament of cat canine teeth. J Dent Res 1995;74: 1310–17.

59. Losken A, Mooney MP, Siegel MI. Comparative cephalometric study of nasal cavity growth patterns in seven animal models. Cleft Palate Craniofac J 1994;31: 17–23.

60. Cheung LK. Microvascular network of the healing surface over the temporalis flap in maxillary reconstruction. Int J Oral Maxillofac Surg 1999;28:469–74.

61. Cheung LK. The epithelialization process in the healing temporalis myofascial flap in oral reconstruction. Int J Oral Maxillofac Surg 1997;26:303–9.

62. Cheung LK. An animal model for maxillary reconstruction using a temporalis muscle flap. J Oral Maxillofac Surg 1996;54:1439–45.

63. Holland GR, Robinson PP, Smith KG, et al. A quantitative morphological study

of the recovery of cat lingual nerves after transection or crushing. J Anat 1996; 188(Pt 2):289–97.

64. Smith KG, Robinson PP. An experimental study on the recovery of the lingual nerve after injury with or without repair. Int J Oral Maxillofac Surg 1995;24: 372–9.

65. Smith KG, Robinson PP. The effect of delayed nerve repair on the properties of regenerated fibres in the chorda tympani. Brain Res 1995;691:142–52.

66. Smith KG, Robinson PP. An experimental study of three methods of lingual nerve defect repair. J Oral Maxillofac Surg 1995;53:1052–62.

67. Smith KG, Robinson PP. An experimental study of lingual nerve repair using epineurial sutures or entubulation. Br J Oral Maxillofac Surg 1995;33: 211–19.

68. Smith KG, Robinson PP. The reinnervation of the tongue and salivary glands after two methods of lingual nerve repair in the cat. Arch Oral Biol 1995;40: 373–83.

69. Smith KG, Robinson PP. The re-innervation of the tongue and salivary glands after lingual nerve repair by stretch, sural nerve graft or frozen muscle graft. J Dent Res 1995;74:1850–60.

70. Holland GR, Robinson PP. Axon populations in cat lingual and chorda tympani nerves. J Dent Res 1992; 71:1468–72.

71. Pogrel MA, Thamby S. The etiology of altered sensation in the inferior alveolar, lingual, and mental nerves as a result of dental treatment. J Calif Dent Assoc 1999;27:531, 534–8.

72. Pogrel MA, Kaban LB. Injuries to the inferior alveolar and lingual nerves. J Calif Dent Assoc 1993;21:50–4.

73. Gregg JM. Studies of traumatic neuralgias in the maxillofacial region: surgical pathology and neural mechanisms. J Oral Maxillofac Surg 1990;48:228–37; discussion 238–9.

| 11 |

Chapter

Principles of exodontics

Milinda J. Lommer

DEFINITIONS

Simple extraction: an extraction not requiring a gingival incision (other than within the sulcus) or sectioning of the tooth. Also called a closed, uncomplicated, or nonsurgical extraction

Surgical extraction: an extraction which requires a gingival incision, bone removal, and/or sectioning of the tooth. Also referred to as an open or complicated extraction

Elevation: the process by which the periodontal ligament is fatigued or torn and alveolar bone is expanded to facilitate removal of the tooth from the alveolus. Using an elevator as a lever, the tooth is lifted (elevated) from its socket

Luxation: the process by which the periodontal ligament is cut or severed to loosen teeth from the surrounding alveolar bone

INDICATIONS FOR EXTRACTION

Periodontitis

Periodontal disease is frequently cited as the most common health problem affecting dogs and cats.[1-5] Because 'periodontal disease' includes both gingivitis (inflammation of soft tissue) and periodontitis (destruction of bone and soft tissue), and large-scale health surveys typically have included only visual inspection of the oral cavity with no probing or dental radiographs, it is difficult to interpret the relevance of these data with regards to the prevalence of periodontal bone loss. However, in one study of 162 dogs randomly selected for oral radiography at necropsy, more than 70% of all dogs (aged 7 months to 14 years) were found to have alveolar bone loss.[6] Both incidence and severity of periodontitis appear to increase with age in dogs:[1,6] while less than half of dogs aged 7 months to 5 years demonstrated alveolar bone loss, more than 80% of dogs older than 6 years and 95% of dogs aged 12–14 years were affected.[6] Among cats presented for dental treatment, 72% were found to have periodontitis; this percentage did not vary significantly among age groups.[7]

Two distinct patterns of bone loss have been described in both dogs[6] and cats[7]: horizontal bone loss (decreased height of interradicular and interdental alveolar bone; Fig. 11.1A) and vertical bone loss (in which the deepest portion of the pocket is apical to the alveolar margin;[8] Fig. 11.1B). Vertical defects often affect a single root or single tooth, and may not be detectable without radiography or probing, while horizontal bone loss frequently exposes furcations of multirooted teeth and is often accompanied by gingival recession.[6,7]

Extraction is the treatment of choice for teeth with significant clinical mobility or greater than 50% attachment loss. However, even in cases with less than 50% bone loss, if the furcation of a multirooted tooth is exposed (stage-3 furcation lesion), plaque retention will result in rapid progression of periodontitis at that location.[8] In human patients receiving treatment for periodontitis, furcation involvement is predictive of tooth loss.[9] Therefore, unless the clients are committed to performing meticulous home care, teeth with through-and-through furcation lesions should be extracted.[10] In selected cases and with dedicated clients, advanced techniques such as periodontal surgery and guided tissue regeneration, or hemisection and endodontic therapy, may allow preservation of periodontally compromised teeth.[11-14]

Pulp necrosis

Pulp necrosis may result from direct pulp exposure (e.g., complicated crown fractures), indirect pulp exposure (e.g., uncomplicated crown fractures, attrition, or abrasion), irreversible pulpitis in an otherwise intact tooth (e.g., gray–discolored, intact canine teeth), secondary to malformations, or as a result of severe periodontitis.[15-19] The inevitable sequela of untreated pulp necrosis is inflammation in the tissues surrounding the apex, which can result in destruction of the periapical bone and soft tissues.[20] Therefore, teeth with necrotic pulp should be treated, either by endodontic therapy (root canal treatment) or extraction.

Dental fractures

Fractured teeth may be found in approximately 27% of dogs[21] and nearly 10% of cats presented for veterinary care (231 out of 2431 cats radiographed in the Dentistry and Oral Surgery Service at the

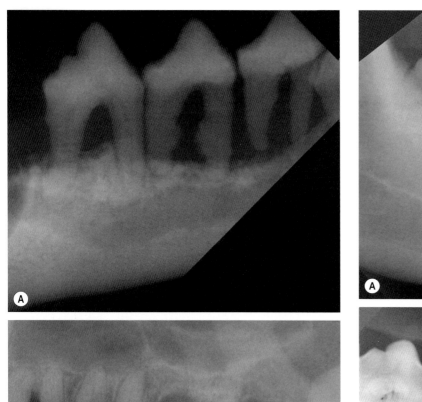

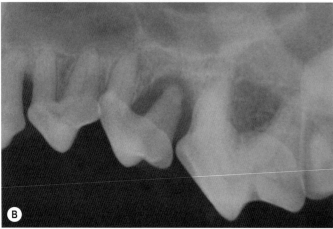

Fig. 11.1 (**A**) Horizontal bone loss affecting the mandibular premolar teeth of a small dog: the alveolar margin remains perpendicular to the long axis of the roots, but is displaced apically. (**B**) Vertical bone loss affecting the distal root of a maxillary third premolar tooth: the alveolar margin is no longer perpendicular to the long axis of the root. The result is an infrabony pocket.

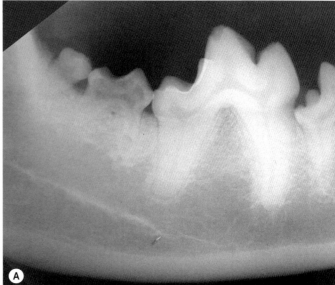

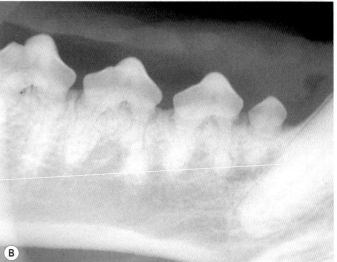

Fig. 11.2 (**A**) Intraoral radiograph of idiopathic tooth resorption of the right mandibular second molar tooth in a dog. (**B**) Intraoral radiograph of age-related external replacement root resorption of the right mandibular premolar teeth in a dog.

University of California – Davis Veterinary Medical Teaching Hospital from 1994–2008 had complicated crown fractures).[1] Advances in endodontic therapy for dogs and cats make this a realistic treatment option for many fractured teeth. However, endodontic therapy is not always feasible or advisable for every patient. Deep crown-root fractures extending apical to the alveolar margin will predispose the site to vertical bone loss, and extraction is therefore recommended for these teeth.[22] In addition, the need for additional anesthetic episodes for radiographic follow-up of root canal treatment[23] may preclude endodontic treatment in medically compromised patients, and extraction is advised for teeth with pulp necrosis in this population of patients.

Tooth resorption

Idiopathic tooth resorption is seen in up to two-thirds of domestic cats and increases in frequency with age.[24–27] Because lesions are painful and progressive regardless of attempts to treat conservatively[28],

extraction is the currently recommended treatment for teeth affected by resorption. Specific extraction techniques for teeth with intact roots and those with end-stage root resorption are discussed in Chapter 15.

While less common in dogs, resorption involving both crowns and roots has also been reported (Fig. 11.2A).[29,30] Age-related root resorption, seen in up to 43% of dogs aged 12–14 years,[6] does not affect the crowns, and extraction is generally not indicated for teeth with root resorption in the absence of coronal lesions (Fig. 11.2B).

Chronic gingivostomatitis

Gingivostomatitis consists of a number of syndromes with the common presenting clinical symptom of severe inflammation of the gingiva and oral mucosa. Although reported to affect less than 1% of domestic cats, gingivostomatitis is painful, debilitating, and sometimes results in euthanasia.[31] The initiating cause is usually not identified, and may differ from case to case. Although less common in dogs than in cats, plaque-contact ulcerative stomatitis also occurs in dogs.[32,33]

Medical management has focused on reducing plaque bacteria (by means of professional dental scaling, home care, and antibiotic therapy) and minimizing the immune response (with corticosteroids and other immunomodulatory agents).[34,35] If these measures are not effective in reducing signs of stomatitis, extractions should be considered. Up to 80% of cats[36] and nearly all dogs with gingivostomatitis will improve significantly after extractions.

Fractured deciduous teeth

Because deciduous teeth are long and narrow, and puppies are often very active chewers, fractured deciduous teeth are fairly common in dogs. As with permanent teeth, exposure of the pulp leads to bacterial infection, pulp necrosis and extension of the infection through the apex and into the surrounding bone. The permanent tooth buds are located in close proximity to the apices of the deciduous teeth, and periapical inflammation from a fractured deciduous tooth may cause enamel hypoplasia or crown malformation in the successor tooth.[22,37] In dogs, the recommended treatment for fractured deciduous teeth is extraction, which when performed carefully is unlikely to cause iatrogenic trauma to the developing permanent tooth.[38] To prevent periapical inflammation and subsequent damage to the permanent tooth, a fractured deciduous tooth should be extracted as soon as it is detected.[38]

Persistent deciduous teeth

Persistent deciduous teeth are most common in small-breed dogs, but are also seen in cats and large dogs.[38,39] The presence of a persistent deciduous tooth can force the permanent tooth to erupt in an abnormal location, causing malocclusion.[38,40] With time, the close proximity of the permanent and deciduous crowns will lead to rapid plaque accumulation and premature periodontitis. It is recommended that persistent deciduous teeth be extracted as soon as the crowns of the permanent successors are visible above the gingival margin.[38,40] Specific techniques for extraction of deciduous canine teeth are described in Chapter 13.

Malocclusion

Malocclusions can be skeletal (e.g., mandibular brachygnathism, maxillary brachygnathism, wry bite) or dental (e.g., linguoverted mandibular canines, rostral crossbite, rotated teeth). Both skeletal and dental malocclusions can result in abnormal contact of teeth onto other teeth or soft tissue, which can cause periodontal bone loss, pulp necrosis, root resorption, and oronasal fistula.[38] For malpositioned, structurally and functionally important teeth, such as linguoverted mandibular canine teeth, orthodontic treatment or crown amputation with partial coronal pulpectomy would be preferred to extraction. Because it typically requires multiple anesthetic episodes, orthodontic treatment is neither feasible nor desirable for every patient with a malocclusion. To help prevent long-term problems, extraction should be considered for crowded teeth, rotated teeth, and teeth causing occlusal trauma (Fig. 11.3).

Supernumerary teeth

Supernumerary teeth are reportedly present in 11% of dogs.[41] In dolichocephalic breeds, such as greyhounds (in which there is a reported 36% incidence of supernumerary teeth[42]), no intervention is required. However, in brachycephalic breeds, or whenever a supernumerary

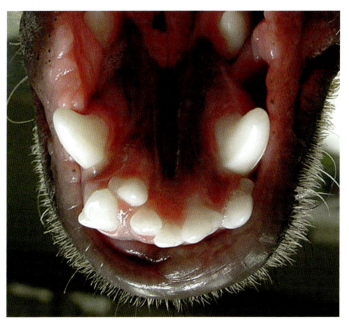

Fig. 11.3 Crowded incisor teeth in a dog; the right mandibular second incisor tooth is displaced lingually and should be extracted.

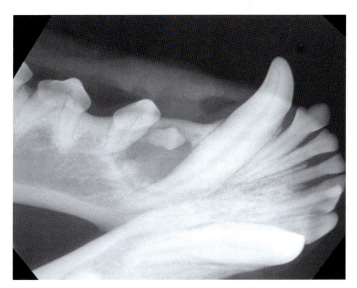

Fig. 11.4 Dentigerous cyst surrounding an unerupted mandibular first premolar tooth.

tooth causes crowding and/or displacement of other teeth, the supernumerary tooth should be extracted as soon as it is discovered. Failure to do so may lead to plaque retention and premature periodontitis, ultimately resulting in the loss of adjacent teeth in addition to the supernumerary tooth.[38]

Unerupted teeth

Embedded or impacted teeth are frequently associated with dentigerous cyst formation (Fig. 11.4).[43-48] Canine teeth and mandibular first premolar teeth appear to be the most commonly affected teeth. The reduced enamel epithelium, which normally would form the junctional epithelium of an erupted tooth, produces fluid, which accumulates between the epithelium and the unerupted crown, causing expansion of the cyst and destruction of the surrounding bone.[49] Extraction of the embedded tooth and enucleation of the entire cyst lining must be performed to prevent recurrence of dentigerous cysts.

Teeth associated with pathologic lesions

In patients with nonresectable oral tumors, teeth with significant periodontal bone loss, evidence of pulp necrosis, or surrounded by neoplastic tissue should be extracted prior to radiation therapy, in order to minimize the risk of osteoradionecrosis.[10,50]

Teeth involved in jaw fractures

Severely fractured teeth or periodontally compromised teeth in a mandibular or maxillary fracture line should be extracted to reduce the risk of infection at the fracture site. However, periodontally sound teeth should be retained, as they may contribute to stabilization of the fracture, and manipulation of the fracture fragment during extraction attempts could cause further damage.[10]

Failed endodontic treatment

Recheck radiographs are required to evaluate whether endodontic treatment has been successful in preventing or resolving periapical inflammation.[23] Although the reported failure rate of root canal treatment in dogs is relatively low at 6%,[23] when endodontic failure does occur extraction must be presented as the definitive treatment option, alongside conservative therapies such as retreatment or surgical endodontic treatment (apicoectomy).

CONTRAINDICATIONS FOR EXTRACTION

General contraindications

If a client has not been informed that extractions might be necessary, every attempt should be made to contact the client for approval prior to extracting teeth. It is prudent to include a paragraph on the anesthesia release form (Fig. 11.5) granting permission to extract teeth in the event that the client cannot be reached.

It should be noted that extracted teeth, unlike other tissues removed from a patient, remain the legal property of the client. It is advisable to clean the extracted teeth (by soaking in hydrogen peroxide or bleach), place them in gauze inside an envelope or plastic vial labeled with the patient's identity and date, and to offer them to the client at the time of discharge.

Other legal aspects to consider include the role of veterinary technicians in performing dental extractions. The American Veterinary Dental College 'considers the extraction of teeth to be included in the practice of veterinary dentistry. Decision making is the responsibility of the veterinarian, with the consent of the pet owner, when electing to extract teeth. Only veterinarians shall determine which teeth are to be extracted and perform extraction procedures.'[51] Many states and provinces specifically prohibit the performance of dental extractions by veterinary technicians.[52,53] In other states, licensed veterinary technicians may be allowed to perform only nonsurgical extractions (i.e., those extractions not requiring creating a flap, removal of bone or sectioning of teeth).[54] There are also states with less well-defined laws, allowing registered veterinary technicians to perform 'dental extractions' under the direct supervision of a licensed veterinarian, but

prohibiting technicians from performing 'surgery.'[55] In any case, the legal responsibility for the welfare of the patient is the veterinarian's alone, and the supervising clinician should ensure that veterinary technicians performing dental procedures are properly trained.

Similarly, extractions should not be performed when proper instruments, appropriate equipment (e.g., for creating flaps, removing alveolar bone and sectioning multirooted teeth), and adequate lighting are not available. The armamentarium for oral surgery is discussed in Chapter 6.

On occasion, veterinarians are asked to extract the canine teeth of an aggressive animal. However, extraction of the canine teeth does not render the animal harmless, and significant damage can be inflicted by premolar and molar teeth. In order to successfully manage an aggressive patient and prevent injury to family members or other animals, the underlying behavior issue must be addressed through behavior modification and, when indicated, medical management.

Systemic contraindications

Many patients presented for dental care will have systemic disorders, such as renal disease, mitral valve insufficiency, diabetes, hyper- or hypothyroidism, or hyperadrenocorticism. As long as the disease process is well controlled, general anesthesia and oral surgery are not contraindicated. However, treatment should be deferred in patients with congestive heart failure, uremia, uncontrolled endocrine disorders, severe coagulopathies, or untreated leukemia or lymphoma.[56]

Local contraindications

Extraction of teeth in the field of previous radiation treatment may lead to osteoradionecrosis and should be avoided. Whenever possible, periodontally compromised or fractured teeth should be removed prior to radiation therapy.[56]

It has been suggested that extraction of teeth within a malignant neoplasm may disseminate tumor cells into the bloodstream and hasten metastasis;[56] therefore, teeth embedded in suspected tumors should ideally not be extracted at the time of biopsy, but rather should be removed along with the surrounding tumor at the time of definitive surgical treatment once a diagnosis has been made.[56]

CLINICAL EVALUATION OF TEETH FOR EXTRACTION

Mobility

The mobility of each tooth should be evaluated preoperatively as part of the oral health assessment and charting. Increased mobility may be associated with extensive bone loss, which facilitates extraction and reduces the need for a surgical approach.[10,56] In the absence of significant periodontitis, increased mobility is likely due to a root fracture, which may necessitate a surgical approach, and should be verified radiographically before proceeding.

Condition of crown

Teeth with extensive coronal resorption are likely to fracture during extraction attempts. A surgical approach to extraction and placement of extraction forceps as far apically as possible are advised for teeth with destruction of large portions of the crown.[56]

PRACTICE NAME HERE

CONSENT FOR ANESTHESIA AND TREATMENT

Client's Name: _____ Pet's Name: _____

Date: _____ Telephone number where I can be reached today: _____

Anesthetic safety information:

✓ **Pre-surgical assessment:** Pre-surgical blood tests and physical examination enable us to assess and minimize the risk of anesthesia for your pet.

✓ **Monitoring:** We further minimize anesthetic risk by monitoring heart rate and rhythm, respiration rate and quality, body temperature, blood oxygenation, and blood pressure throughout the procedure.

✓ **IV Catheterization:** For most procedures requiring anesthesia, an intravenous catheter is placed to provide us with an easy route to administer medications and fluid (which support blood pressure and kidney function) during the procedure.

✓ **Pain Management:** We will pro-actively manage pain associated with any oral surgical procedure by administering pain medications before and/or after the procedure, in addition to use of local anesthetics (similar to Novacaine). As with any drug, side effects may be associated with administration of pain medications and local anesthetic agents.

Authorization for anesthesia and treatment:

I certify that I am the owner of the above-named animal or am responsible for it and have authority to execute this consent. I authorize the performance of the following procedures:

_____

_____

at an estimated cost of: _____

I authorize the use of such anesthetics as deemed advisable by the Doctor in the performance of these surgical, diagnostic, or therapeutic procedures. I realize that the administration of any anesthetic agents and the performance of any surgical procedure carries with it a small but realistic possibility of complications, which can include death. Any questions I have regarding these risks have been answered to my satisfaction.

I recognize that unexpected problems may be detected on dental radiographs or examination under anesthesia. I authorize the Doctor to provide such treatment as may be indicated, including extraction of teeth.

I am aware of the nature of the procedures being performed, and I acknowledge that no guarantee has been made as to the results that may be obtained.

Signature: _____ Date: _____

Fig. 11.5 Sample anesthesia release form, with a paragraph authorizing extraction of teeth in the event that the client cannot be reached during the procedure.

RADIOGRAPHIC EVALUATION OF TEETH FOR EXTRACTION

Pre-extraction radiographs are a vital part of treatment planning. It is important to determine the configuration of the roots, proximity to adjacent teeth and other structures, and the condition of the surrounding bone.[56]

Configuration of the roots

In a survey of 226 dogs, 23.0% were found to have fused roots, 21.7% had root resorption or ankylosis, 12.8% had hypercementosis, 10.7% had supernumerary roots, 3.5% had root dilacerations (Fig. 11.6) and

3.1% had root fractures.[41] In cats, root resorption was identified in 35.6%.[57] Each of these factors could complicate extraction attempts, and knowledge about root status before extraction planning will facilitate uncomplicated completion of the procedure.

Proximity to adjacent teeth and other important structures

The relationship of the tooth to be extracted to adjacent erupted or unerupted teeth should be determined radiographically.[56] When bone removal is necessary, it is important to use caution to preserve the attachment of adjacent teeth. When extracting deciduous teeth, gentle technique must be employed to avoid damaging the underlying permanent tooth buds. On the maxilla, the infraorbital artery, vein and

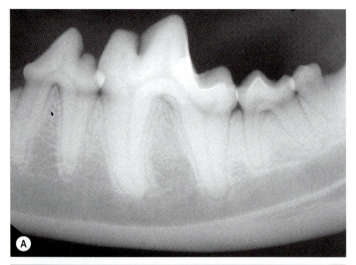

Fig. 11.6 Dilacerated roots of the right mandibular fourth premolar and first molar teeth.

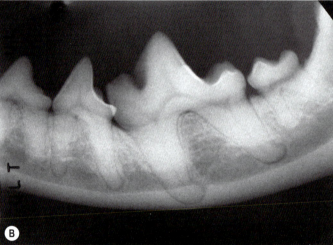

Fig. 11.7 Intraoral radiographs of the mandibular premolar and molar teeth of a large (**A**) and small (**B**) dog. Notice the location of the apices of the roots of the first molar tooth in relation to the ventral border of the mandible.

nerve exit the infraorbital foramen dorsal to the distal root of the maxillary third premolar tooth.[58] On the caudal palate, the major palatine artery exits the major palatine foramen (located medial to the fourth premolar tooth) and runs rostrally to the palatine fissure, where it anastomoses with branches of the infraorbital and nasal vessels. The parotid salivary duct opens into the oral cavity through a papilla at the rostral end of a ridge of mucosa dorsal to the distal root of the maxillary fourth premolar tooth.[58] The zygomatic papilla, through which the major duct from the zygomatic salivary gland exits, is located about 10 mm caudal to the parotid papilla, dorsal to the maxillary first molar.[58] It is possible to damage any of these important structures during attempts to extract the maxillary premolars and molars. Significant differences exist among breeds, making radiographs of each patient imperative prior to commencing extractions.

The maxillary recess is a lateral diverticulum of the nasal cavity, the opening of which lies in a transverse plane through the mesial roots of the maxillary fourth premolar tooth.[58] It is possible to dislodge a root into this recess if excessive force is used during extraction attempts. In brachycephalic breeds, the orbit lies directly dorsal to the maxillary fourth premolar, first molar and second molar teeth. Orbital penetration has been reported during attempts to extract these teeth.[59]

The mandibular canal, containing the inferior alveolar artery, vein and nerve, is located on the ventral aspect of each mandible. A root or root fragment may be inadvertently displaced into the mandibular canal if inappropriate force is applied during attempts to remove the root.

Condition of the surrounding bone

The density of the bone surrounding the tooth to be extracted may be assessed radiographically; bone that is more radiolucent may be less dense, making extraction easier, while bone with increased opacity may make extraction more difficult.[56] In addition, periapical lucencies may be present around roots of nonvital teeth, and the associated granulomas or cysts should be debrided following removal of the roots.[56]

The proportion of the mandible occupied by the teeth varies with breed; small dogs have proportionally larger mandibular first molar teeth relative to the height of the mandible when compared with small dogs (Fig. 11.7).[60] It is possible to cause iatrogenic fracture of the mandible during attempts to extract mandibular canines or first molars if excessive force is applied or if extensive bone loss is present.

The more information the operator has before initiating surgery, the less likely the patient is to suffer such complications, which underscores the importance of preoperative radiographs.

PATIENT AND SURGEON PREPARATION

Patient positioning is a matter of operator preference. Lateral recumbency is preferred by most veterinarians, allowing drainage of fluids and good visibility of the buccal surfaces of the uppermost teeth, but providing limited visibility and restricted access to the teeth on the opposite quadrant.[10] The patient must therefore be turned during the procedure to access teeth on the opposite side. Dorsal recumbency allows excellent visualization of all teeth, which is particularly helpful when sectioning the maxillary fourth premolar and first molar teeth, and allows the patient to remain in one position throughout the procedure. To prevent fluid accumulation in the mouth of a patient in dorsal recumbency, a sandbag, 'pool noodle' (Fig. 11.8), or rolled towel placed under the neck will help tilt the nose downward. Use of

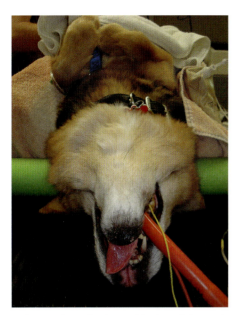

Fig. 11.8 Use of a 'pool noodle' for positioning of the patient's neck while in dorsal recumbency.

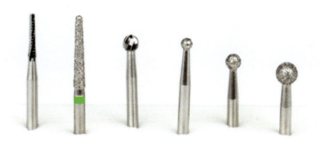

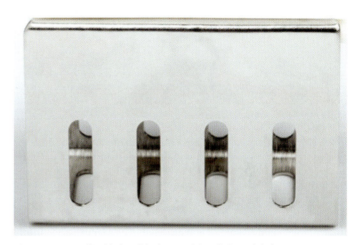

Fig. 11.9 A sterilizable bur block containing (left to right) a cross-cut fissure carbide bur, tapered diamond bur, ½-round carbide bur, and small, medium and large round diamond burs.

a pharyngeal pack, cuffed endotracheal tube and suction are also recommended when working with a patient in dorsal recumbency.[10]

The use of a pharyngeal gauze pack is recommended regardless of patient positioning to prevent teeth or fragments of teeth from entering the oropharynx, where they could be aspirated or swallowed during recovery.[56]

Removal of calculus prior to extractions will allow more accurate assessment of the tooth structure and provides a cleaner environment for surgery. Rinsing the oral cavity with a 0.05% chlorhexidine gluconate solution prior to the procedure will reduce bacteremia and aerosolized bacteria.[10,61] Although it is impossible to render the oral cavity a 'sterile' environment, aseptic technique should be used for surgical extractions. Instruments should be sterilized prior to use, and the use of drapes is recommended to prevent calculus, hair, and other debris from contaminating the surgical field.[10]

To prevent contact with aerosolized bacteria and fluid particles, the operator should wear a mask, gloves, and protective eyewear. Because occasionally a fragment of tooth or a fractured dental bur will become airborne, hard plastic goggles are recommended instead of simple splash-proof face shields, which may not protect against ocular injury.[10] Long hair should be tied back or preferably covered with a surgical cap.[56]

INSTRUMENTS AND MATERIALS

Instruments for creating mucogingival flaps

A #15 blade is typically used to incise the gingiva and mucosa. The round scalpel handle no. 5 (see Fig. 6.1B) is easier to hold in a modified pen grip (see Fig. 6.2) than is a flat scalpel handle. The round handle allows it to be rotated, which facilitates following the contour of the tooth when making a sulcular incision. A periosteal elevator such as a #24G (see Figs 6.7B & 6.8) or Molt #9 (see Fig. 6.7A) is employed to reflect the gingiva or mucosa from the bone as a single layer with the underlying periosteum.

Tissue retractors

Once a mucoperiosteal flap is elevated and bone is exposed, the flap is reflected or retracted using a periosteal elevator, in order to protect it during osseous surgery or sectioning of a tooth. The same periosteal elevator used for elevating the flap can be used for this purpose. Some retractors, such as the Cawood–Minnesota retractor (see Fig. 6.8B), are specifically made for keeping tongue, lips and cheeks away from the surgical site.

Instruments for sectioning teeth and removing alveolar bone

Air-driven dental handpieces are common in veterinary practice, and use of high-speed handpieces with either carbide or diamond burs has largely replaced other methods for sectioning teeth and removing bone. Cross-cut fissure carbide or tapered diamond burs are useful for sectioning multirooted teeth, while round diamond burs are ideal for removal of alveolar bone (Fig. 11.9). Dental handpieces should be held with a modified pen grasp (Fig. 11.10).

Dental elevators

One of the most commonly used instruments in dental extractions is the elevator (e.g., Seldin #304W (Hu-Friedy Mfg. Co., Chicago, IL 60618)), which is used to loosen teeth prior to application of the

103

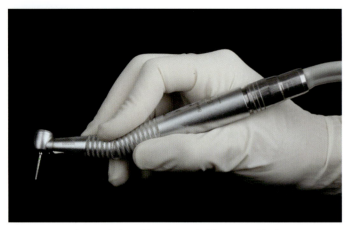

Fig. 11.10 High-speed dental handpiece held in a modified pen grip.

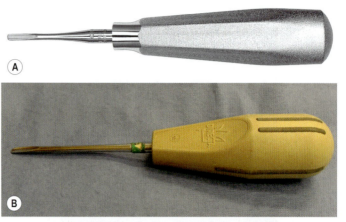

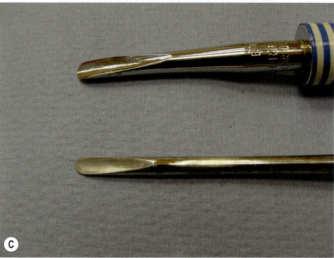

Fig. 11.11 (**A**) Seldin #304W elevator. (**B**) Luxator. (**C**) Close-up of blades of elevator (*top*) and luxator (*bottom*). The flat blade of the luxator is designed to enter the periodontal space in order to cut the periodontal ligament fibers, while the semicircular shape of the elevator blade is better for leveraging against the tooth to fatigue and tear the periodontal ligament fibers. (**A**, *Courtesy of Hu-Friedy, Chicago, IL*)

extraction forceps. The elevator is used as a lever, transmitting rotational force from the handle to the blade, to tear Sharpey's fibers and to lift the tooth from its alveolus.

Elevators consist of three components: a handle, a shank, and a blade (Fig. 11.11A). The handle is typically made of steel and is of a substantial size, so it may be comfortably held in the palm of the hand and used to apply controlled force. The steel shank connects the handle to the blade, and must be strong enough to transmit the force from the handle to the blade. The blade is the working end of the elevator, which is used to transmit force to the tooth or alveolar bone. Its width may vary from 2 to 4 mm. The blade is made of strong steel and has a concave surface on its working side, so that it may be used in the same manner as a shoehorn.[62]

Some elevator blades have sharp tips, which may be used in a similar manner as luxators, to cut the periodontal ligament rather than fatigue it. When using elevators in this fashion, the blade is placed parallel to the long axis of the root and advanced apically.

Elevators are available with a straight shank and blade, or with the blade offset at an angle from the shank. The angled elevators are designed to facilitate access to the caudal areas of the mouth but must be used with care, as the forces applied to the handle do change direction with the angle of the blade.

Triangular-shaped elevators, such as Cryer elevators (Hu-Friedy Mfg. Co., Chicago, IL 60618), come in pairs (left and right), and are designed for use with a 'wheel-and-axle' motion. The tip of the elevator is placed into the alveolus, with the shank on the buccal alveolar bone perpendicular to the root. The sharp tip of the elevator is used to engage the cementum of the root surface, the handle is turned, and the root is thus elevated from the alveolus.[62]

Winged elevators have recently become popular in veterinary dentistry. These elevators have a short shaft and large-diameter handles for improved control and more comfortable use by clinicians with smaller hands.[63] The winged blades, available in 1.5-, 2.5-, 3.5- and 4.5-mm widths, conform to roots of various circumferences, achieving better purchase on the tooth surface. However, if too much torque is placed on small teeth, root fracture may occur, so care must be employed.

Luxators

The luxator is a sharp instrument with a less concave blade than an elevator (Fig. 11.11B, C). It is used to cut or sever Sharpey's fibers within the periodontal ligament and loosen the tooth prior to extraction. The shank and blade are placed parallel to the root surface of

the tooth, and the tip of the luxator is pushed into the alveolar socket. Because the luxator is not used as a first-class or wheel-and-axle lever, the handle does not need to transmit rotational forces, and is usually made of plastic rather than steel. The shank and blade are made of softer steel than that of an elevator. The thin blade is designed to be resharpened frequently.[64] Luxators (e.g., Ericsson luxators (JS Dental Manufacturing, Inc., Ridgefield, CT 06877)) are available in widths of 1–5 mm, and with a straight or angled blade. The gouge (e.g., Coupland gouge) is related to the luxator. It has sharp straight-edged blades and is semitubular in shape. Luxators should be held in the palm with the index finger extended towards the tip of the blade (Fig. 11.12). This will minimize trauma to the patient in the event of instrument slippage.

Root tip picks

There are two types of root tip picks: the apical elevator (Fig. 11.13A) and the root tip 'teaser' (Fig. 11.13B). The apical elevator has a handle, shank and blade similar to a standard dental elevator, but with a smaller-diameter handle and a sharper, narrower blade. It may be used

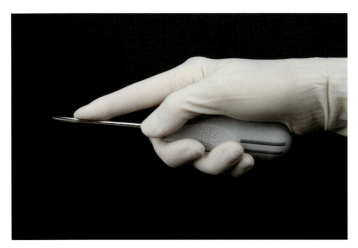

Fig. 11.12 Proper grasp of a luxator. The index finger is extended along the shaft towards the tip of the blade in order to minimize trauma to the patient should the instrument slip during extraction.

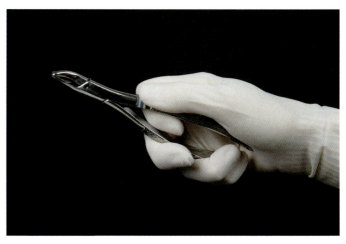

Fig. 11.14 Proper grasp of extraction forceps. The index finger is placed between the handles to prevent generation of excessive force, which can lead to crushing of the tooth.

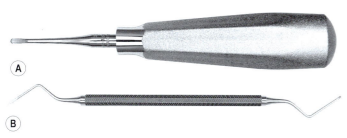

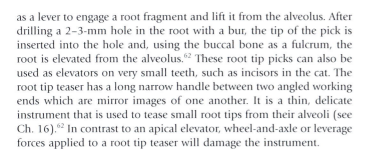

Fig. 11.13 (**A**) Apexo #301 apical elevator. (**B**) Root tip teaser. *(Courtesy of Hu-Friedy, Chicago, IL)*

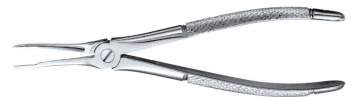

Fig. 11.15 FX-49 forceps. *(Courtesy of Hu-Friedy, Chicago, IL)*

as a lever to engage a root fragment and lift it from the alveolus. After drilling a 2–3-mm hole in the root with a bur, the tip of the pick is inserted into the hole and, using the buccal bone as a fulcrum, the root is elevated from the alveolus.[62] These root tip picks can also be used as elevators on very small teeth, such as incisors in the cat. The root tip teaser has a long narrow handle between two angled working ends which are mirror images of one another. It is a thin, delicate instrument that is used to tease small root tips from their alveoli (see Ch. 16).[62] In contrast to an apical elevator, wheel-and-axle or leverage forces applied to a root tip teaser will damage the instrument.

Extraction forceps

Extraction forceps are used after elevation or luxation to grasp the loosened tooth and remove it from the alveolus.[62] The three components of extraction forceps are the handle, hinge and beak. The handles should be of sufficient size to grasp comfortably; they are usually serrated to prevent slippage, and may be straight or curved. The hinge transfers the force applied to the handles to the beak. The beak is designed to adapt to the tooth root at the cemento-enamel junction, and should be placed parallel to the long axis of the tooth. It is not designed to grasp the crown of the tooth. Narrow beaks should be used for smaller teeth, wider beaks for larger teeth. The more closely the forceps' beaks adapt to the tooth roots, the more efficient will be the extraction.[62] The chance for root fracture increases if the beaks are not properly adapted to the root surface. Extraction forceps should be grasped in the palm, with the index finger between the handles (Fig. 11.14) to avoid generating excessive pressure, which might crush the tooth.

In human dentistry, specific extraction forceps have been designed for each kind of tooth. Many of these forceps are unsuitable for use in the dog and cat. Sharply curved forceps, such as the so-called 'lower molar forceps,' and forceps with sharp triangular tips are most likely to cause root fractures. Extraction forceps designed for veterinary use are available, but several extraction forceps designed for use in human patients can be successfully used in veterinary practice. For example, so-called 'upper anterior forceps' (such as the pedodontic Cryer # 150S (Hu-Friedy Mfg. Co., Chicago, IL 60618)) have been found to be suitable for use in the dog and cat.[65,66] These forceps have a slightly conical grip and fit most teeth, in spite of the great variation that exists in the size and shape of teeth in dogs and cats. Root forceps, such as the #X49 forceps (Hu-Friedy Mfg. Co., Chicago, IL 60618) (Fig. 11.15), differ from conventional extraction forceps in that they have long, narrow beaks which close completely, making them particularly useful for grasping small root fragments.

Instruments for suturing flaps

Fine suture material with small swaged-on needles is generally used in oral surgery (see Ch. 7). The needle holders indicated in oral surgery are therefore delicate to match the size of the needles. The Halsey needle holder (see Fig. 6.11A) is a very versatile needle holder well suited for most intraoral procedures. Similarly, the delicate Adson 1X2 tissue forceps (see Fig. 6.5A) is used most commonly in oral surgery for gentle tissue handling. Choice of suture scissors is based on operator preference. Some surgeons working without assistants prefer a needle holder with built-in scissors such as the Olson-Hegar needle holder (see Fig. 6.11D).

TREATMENT PLANNING

Simple versus surgical extraction

Also called a closed, uncomplicated or nonsurgical extraction, a simple extraction is performed without incising the gingiva (other than within the gingival sulcus) or sectioning the tooth. An extraction which requires a gingival incision, bone removal, and/or sectioning of the tooth is a surgical extraction, also known as an open or complicated extraction.

Small, single-rooted teeth are typically extracted nonsurgically. Maxillary second molars in the dog often have three partly fused roots, so these teeth are also usually extracted in a nonsurgical manner. In some cases of severe periodontitis, extensive bone loss may enable nonsurgical extraction of a multirooted tooth, but a surgical approach is recommended for most multirooted teeth. Canine teeth should also be extracted surgically in most cases; nonsurgical extraction of a periodontally compromised maxillary canine tooth can lead to formation of a permanent oronasal fistula. Surgical extraction should also be considered for smaller, single-rooted teeth which are ankylosed or which have undergone root resorption (e.g., severely abraded incisor teeth with pulp exposure in dogs with a history of frequent chewing).

When determining whether to perform surgical or nonsurgical extraction, the clinician must consider clinical findings, such as mobility, and radiographic findings, including root morphology and clinical attachment level. Significant bone loss and the resulting increase in mobility associated with periodontal disease usually leads to uncomplicated tooth extraction. On the other hand, if a tooth is being extracted due to fracture or some cause other than periodontal disease, and is periodontally healthy, normal mobility is expected, and considerable resistance to extraction may be encountered. Similarly, if radiographs reveal dilaceration or other abnormalities in root morphology, electing a surgical approach initially will save time compared with the effort required to extract a root fragment following an unsuccessful attempt at a simple extraction. Regardless of whether a simple or surgical extraction is elected, the tissues should be handled with care, the alveoli flushed gently to remove debris, and, for all but the smallest simple extraction sites, the gingiva sutured to allow primary-intention healing.

PRINCIPLES OF FLAP DESIGN, DEVELOPMENT AND MANAGEMENT

Local flaps are employed for surgical extractions; the term 'local flap' refers to a section of soft tissue (gingiva and/or mucosa and periosteum), which is outlined by a surgical incision, contains its own blood supply, allows access to underlying tissues, can be replaced in its original position, and is expected to heal after being sutured in place.[67] Proper extraction technique requires that the operator have a clear understanding of the principles of design and management of local flaps.

Design parameters for soft tissue flaps

When designing a flap, several goals must be achieved: the flap must be of sufficient size to allow adequate exposure of the surgical area, the base of the flap must be as wide as or broader than the free margin in order to preserve its blood supply, and the edges of the flap must lie over intact bone at the conclusion of the procedure.[67] If the

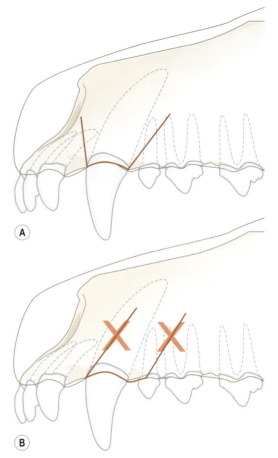

Fig. 11.16 (**A**) Correct placement of releasing incisions at mesiobuccal and distobuccal line angles. Incisions are oblique to allow a wide-based flap. (**B**) These two incisions are made incorrectly: (1) crosses the area of bone removal, leaving the incision over an empty space, (2) crosses the attached gingiva directly over the buccal aspect of the adjacent tooth, which will likely result in a gingival defect.

incisions are unsupported by sound bone, the flap tends to collapse into the bony defect, which can lead to delayed healing and wound dehiscence.[67]

When designing the flap, it is important to consider adjacent vital structures, such as the infraorbital artery, vein and nerve on the maxilla and the middle mental neurovascular bundle exiting the middle mental foramen on the mandible.

In order to minimize tension on the suture line and prevent a defect in the attached gingiva following healing, vertical releasing incisions should be made at line angles of adjacent teeth rather than directly on the buccal aspect of a tooth (Fig. 11.16).

Sulcular Incision versus excision of the free gingiva and sulcus epithelium

The purpose of making a sulcular incision is to free the gingival attachment from the tooth to provide increased visualization of and access to the underlying alveolar bone and periodontal ligament space. In cases of periodontitis, the sulcular epithelium is diseased 'pocket epithelium', with macrophages, PMNs, and lymphocytes creating increased distances between epithelial cells and disrupting epithelial basal lamina.[68] Some surgeons prefer to excise the free gingiva (i.e., the 1–2-mm section of gingiva that is not attached to the tooth surface) and the pocket epithelium rather than simply incising the sulcus.[69] While there are no published studies demonstrating that excising the pocket epithelium and free gingiva leads to more rapid healing of extraction sites in dogs or cats with periodontitis, bone regeneration may occur more rapidly in the absence of diseased epithelium. In one study of human dental patients, alveoli of teeth extracted due to advanced periodontitis contained mostly connective tissue for 14 weeks after extraction, with >50% new bone fill noted after 16 weeks, while alveoli of teeth extracted for nonperiodontal reasons showed >50% new bone fill after 8 weeks.[70] Although bone regeneration occurred more slowly in diseased extraction sites than disease-free sites, no long-term differences were observed.

Types of gingival and mucogingival flaps

An envelope flap is a gingival flap (i.e., not extending apical to the mucogingival junction) created by making a sulcular incision and elevating some of the attached gingiva on the lingual and buccal aspects, with minimal extension interproximally, and no vertical releasing incisions (Fig. 11.17A). An extended envelope flap is useful for extraction of several adjacent teeth. When more exposure is required or a single tooth is being extracted, a triangle flap is useful.

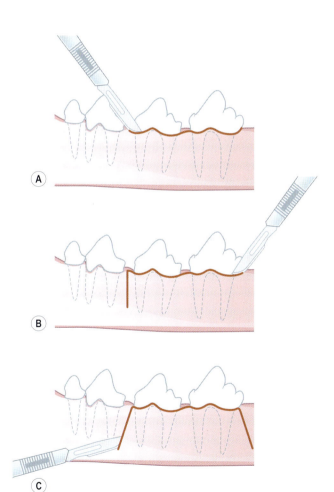

Fig. 11.17 (A) Envelope flap: a single incision is made in the gingival sulcus. To excise pocket epithelium, an internal bevel incision can be made. (B) Triangle (three-cornered) flap: a sulcular incision is made, followed by a single vertical releasing incision; (C) Pedicle (four-cornered) flap: two vertical releasing incisions are created, providing maximum exposure of the alveolar bone.

The triangle flap and pedicle flap are mucogingival flaps, i.e., extending apical to the mucogingival junction. Flaps used for extraction procedures are full-thickness flaps that also include the periosteum. A triangle flap is a mucogingival flap consisting of a sulcular incision and one vertical releasing incision, creating a three-cornered flap with corners at the distal extent of the sulcular incision, the coronal aspect of the vertical releasing incision (at the mesial end of the envelope incision) and the apical extent of the vertical releasing incision (Fig. 11.17B).[67] A pedicle flap is a sulcular incision with two vertical releasing incisions, creating a four-cornered flap (Fig. 11.17C); this flap provides the best exposure for removal of buccal alveolar bone for a challenging extraction or retrieval of a fractured root fragment.

Technique for developing a mucogingival flap

In order to provide proper exposure of the alveolar bone supporting the teeth to be extracted, gingiva, mucosa and periosteum must be reflected. First, the gingiva is incised, using a #15 blade on a scalpel handle held in a pen grasp, inserted into the gingival sulcus and drawn with a continuous, smooth motion.[67] Excising the free gingiva of teeth affected by periodontitis and creating an internal bevel incision to eliminate the pocket epithelium will allow primary-intention healing of healthy gingiva and may allow more rapid bone regeneration in the alveolus.[70] Next, if a vertical releasing incision is to be made, the opposite hand is used to tense the alveolar mucosa and the blade is drawn, beginning at the mesiobuccal line angle of the tooth, in an apical and slightly mesial direction through the mucogingival junction and extending several millimeters into the alveolar mucosa. If desired, a second vertical releasing incision is made beginning at the distobuccal line angle of the tooth and extending apically and slightly distally. Alternatively, this incision may be made interproximally, or at the mesiobuccal line angle of the adjacent tooth. The scalpel blade will dull when pressed against bone, so multiple blades should be employed for patients with multiple extractions.[67] Incisions should extend apical to the mucogingival junction, so that the flap is as long as the root(s) of the tooth. Once the incisions are created, a periosteal elevator is introduced into the sulcus at the mesial aspect, and may be turned laterally to pry the gingiva from the underlying bone. The periosteal elevator is then used with pushing and rotating strokes apically and distally to reflect the mucosa and periosteum from the bone (see Ch. 6).[67] After reflection of the flap, the periosteal elevator, a Seldin elevator, or a Cawood–Minnesota retractor (Fig. 11.18) may be used to prevent trauma to the flap during the remainder of the extraction.

Bone removal (alveolotomy or partial alveolectomy)

After reflection of the flap, removal of the buccal alveolar bone may be performed. Using a round diamond (or carbide) bur in fine, sweeping motions, the buccal alveolar bone is removed beginning at the alveolar margin and moving as far apically as desired. While minimal alveolectomy is required for teeth affected by periodontitis, removal of up to 75% of the buccal alveolar bone will facilitate extraction of teeth with little to no bone loss, or ankylosed teeth.

Alveoloplasty

The sharp bone edges present after luxation and/or elevation will delay healing of the gingival flap and may lead to considerable postoperative discomfort. Alveoloplasty (the removal of these sharp bone

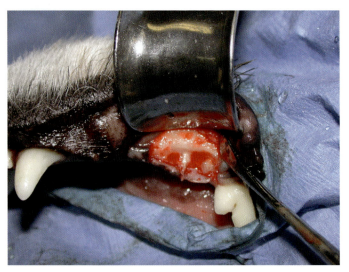

Fig. 11.18 Use of a Cawood–Minnesota retractor to retract the lip and a periosteal elevator to retract the mucogingival flap during location of a fractured root.

edges) is performed with a round diamond bur on a high-speed handpiece, bone rongeurs or a small file.

Management of the alveolus

Following alveoloplasty, the empty alveolus is cleared of debris.[69] In cases of advanced periodontitis, gentle curettage of the alveolus should be performed to remove pocket epithelium and any remnants of subgingival calculus. Overzealous curettage should be avoided, because disruption of the blood clot within the alveolus will delay healing.[71–73]

Placement of bone grafting materials in the alveolus is advocated by some practitioners as a way to prevent 'collapse' of the alveolar margin following extraction of large teeth such as canine teeth and mandibular first molar teeth.[74,75] *Autogenous grafts*, i.e., those collected directly from the patient, have historically been the 'gold standard' bone replacement material,[76] and they are the only truly osteogenic graft option. Collection of a free 'crescent graft' from the mandibular ramus has been proposed for immediate use in human extraction sites, with minimal postoperative morbidity.[77] This approach may be adapted for use in dogs (harvesting bone just caudal to the mandibular molars) but may be less suitable for cats, where collection of an adequate sample size may not be feasible.

When a graft is desired but an autogenous graft is not practical, an *allograft* (typically freeze-dried or frozen cancellous and/or cortical bone) is an excellent option. In addition to osteoconductive properties, demineralized freeze-dried bone allografts contain bone morphogenetic proteins (BMPs), which reportedly stimulate new bone production (osteoinduction). Numerous clinical studies in human patients[78–82] and experimental studies in dogs[83,84] have shown production of new bone following placement of freeze-dried bone allografts. Demineralization of the freeze-dried bone exposes the collagen fibrils and associated components of bone matrix including bone morphogenetic proteins; therefore, demineralized freeze-dried bone (DFDB) is considered osteoinductive, while non-demineralized freeze-dried bone (FDB) is considered osteoconductive only.[85] Both canine and feline freeze-dried bone are commercially available in a mixture of demineralized bone matrix and cancellous chips <0.7 mm in diameter, specifically designed for oral and periodontal use (OsteoAllograft® Perio Mix, Veterinary Transplant Services, Inc. Kent, WA 98032).

Alloplasts are synthetic or naturally occurring inert materials which serve primarily to maintain space. As such, they are osteoconductive only. Bioactive ceramics, also called bioglass materials, generally contain oxides of calcium, sodium, phosphorous and silicone, which reportedly stimulate collagen synthesis and new bone formation. Bioactive ceramics have a broad antimicrobial effect on microorganisms on teeth and implants.[86–88] One bioactive glass (Consil®: Nutramax Laboratories, Inc., Edgewood, MD 21040), available in both particulate and putty forms, is marketed specifically for veterinary use; it has been used in extraction site alveolar margin maintenance.[89] While there are no clinical studies in dogs, experimental evidence suggests that bioactive glass is less effective than demineralized freeze-dried bone allograft in inducing new bone formation in intrabony pockets adjacent to implants in dogs.[84]

It is important to note that placement of any material in the alveolus may result in postoperative complications, and should be performed in selected cases only after appropriate discussion with clients.

Principles of suturing

Following completion of the surgical procedure, the extraction sites should be gently lavaged with sterile saline and the flap edges should be apposed without tension. The sharper the incision and the less trauma the wound edges have sustained, the more likely the site is to heal by primary intention. Sutures not only hold the flap edges in place over the underlying bone, they also aid in maintenance of the blood clot, which plays an important role in healing.[90] If appropriate suture techniques are not employed, the flap may retract away from the bone or the clot may be dislodged, both of which will result in delayed healing of the extraction site.[67]

The armamentarium for extraction site closure includes a needle holder, tissue forceps, and suture material. A small needle holder, such as a 5-inch Mayo-Hegar or Halsey (see Fig. 6.11), is ideal for cats and small dogs. The needle holder should be held with the thumb and ring finger through the rings and the index finger extended along the length to provide stability and control.[67] The suture needle should be a small diameter, $\frac{3}{8}$ to $\frac{1}{2}$ circle with a reverse cutting edge, which facilitates passage through the mucoperiosteal and gingival tissue.[67] Selection of suture material is discussed in Chapter 7.

The needle should enter the mucosa at a right angle, to make the smallest possible hole in the tissue; if the needle passes through the mucosa obliquely, the suture will tear through the superficial layers of the flap when the knot is tied, which results in greater injury to the soft tissues.[67] Similarly, if an inadequate bite of tissue is taken, the suture may tear through the edge of the flap. There should be approximately 3 mm of tissue between the suture and the edge of the flap.[67] The needle holder should be turned rather than pushed so it passes easily through the tissue at right angles, minimizing trauma (Fig. 11.19).

When replacing a triangle or pedicle flap, in general it is helpful to suture the mucogingival junctions first, in order to restore the tissue to its presurgical location. The needle should be passed through the flap mucosa first, regrasped with the needle holder, then passed through the attached mucosa. If the two margins of the incision are close together, an experienced surgeon may be able to insert the needle through both sides of the incision in a single pass. However, this can result in tearing of the gingiva or mucosa, so two passes are recommended for most extraction sites.[67]

Once the sutures are passed through both the mobile flap and the immobile mucosa, they are tied with an instrument tie in a simple interrupted pattern, with approximately 2–3 mm between sutures. A simple continuous pattern may be employed for long incisions or in situations where multiple, plaque-retentive knots are undesirable, as in patients with plaque-reactive stomatitis.

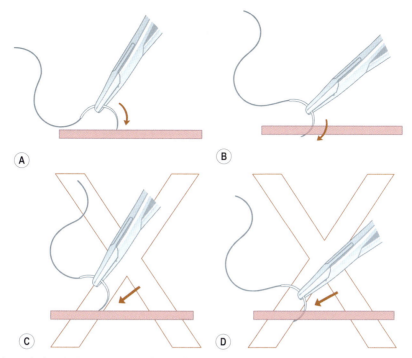

Fig. 11.19 (A) When passing through the gingiva or mucosa, the needle should enter the tissue at a 90° angle. **(B)** The needle holder should be rotated so the needle passes easily through the tissue. **(C)** If the needle enters the gingiva or mucosa at an acute angle and is pushed (rather than rotated) through the tissue, **(D)** tearing of the tissue is likely to occur.

MECHANICAL PRINCIPLES INVOLVED IN TOOTH EXTRACTION

The removal of tooth roots from their alveoli employs the use of the following mechanical principles: the wedge principle, wheel-and-axle motion, leverage, rotation, and traction. Inserting a luxator into the periodontal ligament space acts as a wedge to expand the alveolar bone while severing the periodontal ligament fibers (Fig. 11.20A). Wheel-and-axle motion is employed when an elevator is inserted perpendicular to and between two roots (allowing the side of the elevator blade to contact a purchase point on one of the roots) and the handle is turned, acting as an axle, while the blade of the elevator acts as a wheel, engaging the root and lifting (elevating) it from the alveolus (Fig. 11.20B).[56] Levers employ a long lever arm and a short effector arm to transmit moderate forces into small movements against significant resistance.[56] Elevators may occasionally be used as levers, engaging the blade in a purchase point on the root and directing the handle downward to lift the tooth from its alveolus. Following luxation or elevation, the beaks of the extraction forceps are placed as apically as possible on the tooth, parallel to the long axis of the root. It is important not to move the forceps side-to-side to 'rock' the tooth, as this will create shearing forces near the root apex and will lead to root fracture (Fig. 11.21A). Rather, the beaks of the extraction forceps are placed on the root of the tooth and the tooth is rotated gently to fatigue the remaining periodontal ligament fibers (Fig. 11.21B). Finally, after the periodontal ligament fibers have been fatigued or severed and significant mobility is achieved following luxation, elevation and rotation, minimal tractional force is applied with extraction forceps to gently deliver a tooth from its alveolus.

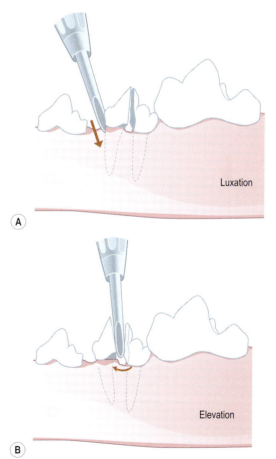

Fig. 11.20 (A) Use of a straight luxator as a wedge to displace the root from the alveolar bone. **(B)** Use of an elevator as a wheel-and-axle machine.

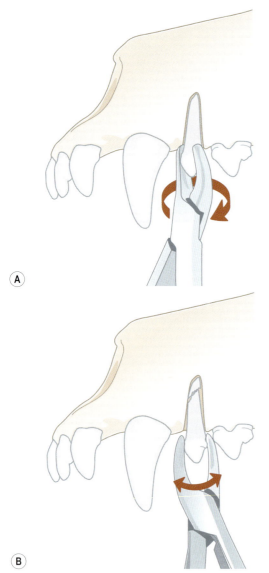

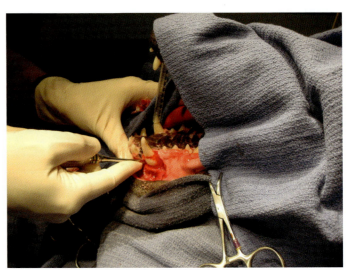

Fig. 11.22 Use of the nondominant hand to stabilize the tooth during extraction. This provides tactile feedback regarding mobility of the tooth and readiness for application of extraction forceps.

Fig. 11.21 (A) Rotational forces are applied with the beaks of extraction forceps placed as far apically on the tooth as possible. (B) If the tooth is 'rocked' or moved side-to-side rather than rotated, root fracture results.

PRINCIPLES AND TECHNIQUES FOR TOOTH EXTRACTION

A surgical approach to extraction should not be reserved for extreme situations such as a periodontally sound, fractured tooth in an older dog, or considered a salvage procedure for a unsuccessful simple extraction. When correctly performed, a surgical extraction technique may be more conservative, cause less morbidity, and take less time than a nonsurgical extraction. Nonsurgical extractions requiring application of great force may result in damage to the adjacent soft tissues and removal of large amounts of associated bone, causing significantly more morbidity than a controlled surgical technique.[67]

Whether surgical or nonsurgical extraction is elected, the three fundamental requirements for a satisfactory procedure remain constant: (1) adequate visualization of the tooth to be extracted, (2) an unimpeded pathway for the removal of the tooth, and (3) use of controlled force to luxate or elevate, and remove the tooth.[56] Proper patient positioning, good lighting, irrigation and suction will improve visibility and make extraction less challenging. Similarly, appropriate sectioning of multirooted teeth and use of well-maintained instruments will allow easier achievement of the stated goals.[10]

For a tooth to be removed from its alveolus, the soft tissue attachment to the crown must be disrupted, the alveolar bone must be expanded (or removed), and the periodontal ligament fibers must be severed or torn.[56] This is achieved by incising the gingival attachment, removing some alveolar bone with a bur when necessary, and introducing a luxator or elevator into the periodontal ligament space.

In order to prevent damage to adjacent tissues caused by slippage of the elevator or luxator, it is helpful to extend the index finger along the shaft. In addition, the operator's nondominant hand should be used to stabilize the jaw and the tooth being extracted (Fig. 11.22), relaying tactile information about the tooth's mobility as luxation or elevation proceeds, which helps indicate readiness for placement of extraction forceps and delivery of the tooth from its alveolus.[56] If all of the periodontal ligament fibers are severed, extraction forceps may not even be required to remove the tooth.[10] Techniques for extraction of specific teeth are discussed in detail in subsequent chapters.

Removal of root fragments

If a fracture occurs in the coronal half of a root, the remaining fragment should be visible without additional bone removal, and use of a small (1- or 2-mm) luxator will usually allow delivery of the remaining root. However, if the fracture occurs in the apical third of the root, enlargement of the mucoperiosteal flap and removal of additional buccal bone will most likely be required for successful retrieval of the fragment. This is particularly true for dilacerated roots, or bulbous roots with hypercementosis.[67] Excellent light and suction will be required for proper visualization and successful removal of a fractured root fragment. Once the fragment is visualized, a root tip pick or 1-mm luxator is inserted into the periodontal ligament space around the root until the fragment is mobilized and can be teased from the alveolus. When using the luxator or root tip pick, it is important not

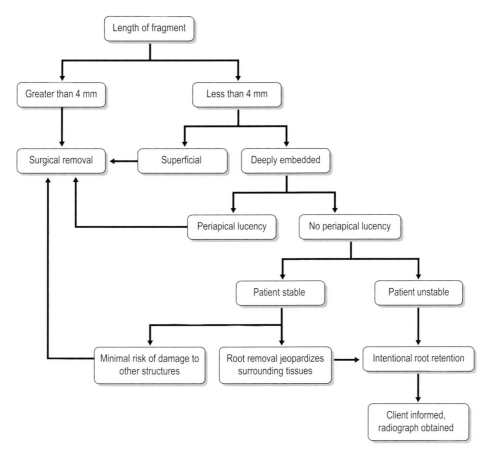

Fig. 11.23 Flow chart for decision-making for fractured roots.

to apply excessive apical force, which could displace the fragment into other anatomic locations such as the nasal cavity or mandibular canal.[67] A technique has also been described in which a thin, tapered diamond bur is used to create space around the root, allowing introduction of an instrument for removal of the root fragment.[91]

Intentional root retention

Except in cases of end-stage resorption in which the roots have been almost entirely replaced by bone-like material, the goal of any extraction should always be to extract the entire tooth. However, when a root tip has fractured and when attempts to remove it have been unsuccessful, the surgeon may consider leaving the root in place. In some situations the risks of additional surgery to remove a small root fragment may outweigh the benefits (Fig. 11.23).

Three conditions must be met for a tooth root to be left in the alveolus.[67] First, the root fragment must be small, no more than 3–4 mm in length. Second, the root must be deeply embedded in bone and not superficial, to prevent any subsequent bone resorption from exposing the tooth root. Third, the tooth involved must not be infected, and there must be no periapical radiolucency. If these three conditions exist, and if the risk of further surgery is considered to be greater than the benefit, the surgeon may consider leaving the fragment.

The risk of further surgery is considered greater than the benefit in the following situations: (1) removal of the root will require significant destruction of adjacent tissue or extreme removal of surrounding bone; (2) removal of the root jeopardizes vital structures, such as the inferior alveolar nerve; and (3) the patient is not stable under anesthesia, and prolongation of the procedure could be life-threatening.

If the decision has been made to intentionally leave a root fragment in the alveolus, a strict protocol must be observed.[67] First, radiographic documentation of the root tip's presence and position must be obtained and recorded in the patient's record. Second, the client must be informed that, in the surgeon's judgment, leaving the root in place will do less harm to the patient than further surgery. The client should also be instructed to contact the veterinarian immediately if problems develop in the area of the retained root, such as swelling or a draining tract. Finally, the patient should be re-radiographed at regular intervals in the future to determine whether evidence of inflammation is present around the root, or to document absence of such evidence.

Intentional root retention for teeth with end-stage resorption is discussed further in Chapter 15.

POSTOPERATIVE CARE AND ASSESSMENT

Pain management

Whenever extractions are anticipated, preemptive analgesia should be attained. This may be accomplished by the use of opioids, nonsteroidal antiinflammatory agents, and/or alpha-2 agonists as premedicants, and local anesthetics delivered prior to beginning the extractions.

Postoperative analgesia may include nonsteroidal antiinflammatory drugs, non-narcotic opioids such as tramadol, or a combination of the two, which may provide better antiinflammatory activity than either agent alone.[92] For patients in whom multiple extractions are expected, placement of a fentanyl transdermal delivery system may be a better choice than oral medications for at-home use. If possible, the patch should be placed 12–24 hours prior to the procedure in order for adequate blood levels to be reached by the time extractions have commenced. However, even with patch placement 12 hours prior to induction, additional opioids may need to be administered for acute postoperative pain.[93]

Nutritional support

Following surgical extraction of multirooted teeth, soft food should be offered for 3–5 days. In addition, chew toys and hard treats should be avoided for 7–10 days in order to prevent disruption of the sutures. A feeding tube may be considered for patients undergoing full-mouth or near-full-mouth extractions, but this is rarely necessary.

Oral hygiene

Keeping the teeth and oral cavity clean following extraction results in more rapid healing of surgical wounds.[94] Oral rinses or gels containing known antiseptics such as chlorhexidine gluconate may be used twice daily following meals for the first postoperative week, and may result in more rapid healing in veterinary patients with compromised oral hygiene. By the third or fourth day post surgery, it is acceptable for clients to resume gentle brushing of their dog's teeth, avoiding the areas immediately adjacent to the extraction sites until the end of the first postoperative week.

Postoperative assessment

The client should be instructed to observe the patient for lethargy, inappetence, or halitosis, and the patient should be examined 1–2 weeks following the procedure to evaluate healing. For patients who have not had home care previously performed, this postoperative visit provides an opportunity to instruct the client in tooth-brushing techniques and to discuss other home care measures.

REFERENCES

1. Harvey CE, Shofer FS, Laster L. Association of age and body weight with periodontal disease in North American dogs [published erratum appears in J Vet Dent 1994 Dec;11(4):133]. J Vet Dent 1994; 11:94–105.

2. Lund EM, Armstrong PJ, Kirk CA, et al. Health status and population characteristics of dogs and cats examined at private veterinary practices in the United States. J Am Vet Med Assoc 1999; 214:1336–41.

3. Isogai H, Isogai E, Okamoto H, et al. Epidemiological study on periodontal diseases and some other dental disorders in dogs. Jap J Vet Sci 1989;51:1151–62.

4. Klein T. Predisposing factors and gross examination findings in periodontal disease. Clin Tech Small Anim Pract 2000;15:189–96.

5. Harvey CE. Periodontal disease in dogs. Etiopathogenesis, prevalence, and significance. Vet Clin North Am Small Anim Pract 1998;28:1111–28.

6. Hamp SE, Hamp M, Olsson SE, et al. Radiography of spontaneous periodontitis in dogs. J Periodontal Res 1997;32: 589–97.

7. Lommer MJ, Verstraete FJ. Radiographic patterns of periodontitis in cats: 147 cases (1998–1999). J Am Vet Med Assoc 2001; 218:230–4.

8. Wolf HF, Rateitschak EM, Rateitschak KH, et al. Color atlas of dental medicine: periodontology. 3rd ed. Stuttgart: Georg Thieme Verlag; 2005.

9. McGuire MK, Nunn ME. Prognosis versus actual outcome. III. The effectiveness of clinical parameters in accurately predicting tooth survival. J Periodontol 1996;67: 666–74.

10. Verstraete FJM. Exodontics. In: Slatter DH, editor. Textbook of small animal surgery. 3rd ed. Philadelphia: WB Saunders Co; 2003. p. 2696–709.

11. Reiter AM, Lewis JR, Rawlinson JE, et al. Hemisection and partial retention of carnassial teeth in client-owned dogs. J Vet Dent 2005;22:216–26.

12. Kim CS, Choi SH, Cho KS, et al. Periodontal healing in one-wall intra-bony defects in dogs following implantation of autogenous bone or a coral-derived biomaterial. J Clin Periodontol 2005; 32:583–9.

13. Koo KT, Polimeni G, Qahash M, et al. Periodontal repair in dogs: guided tissue regeneration enhances bone formation in sites implanted with a coral-derived calcium carbonate biomaterial. J Clin Periodontol 2005;32:104–10.

14. Beckman BW. Treatment of an infrabony pocket in an American Eskimo dog. J Vet Dent 2004;21:159–63.

15. Verstraete FJM. Oral pathology. In: Slatter DH, editor. Textbook of small animal surgery. 3rd ed. Philadelphia: WB Saunders Co; 2003. p. 2638–51.

16. Hale FA. Localized intrinsic staining of teeth due to pulpitis and pulp necrosis in dogs. J Vet Dent 2001;18:14–20.

17. Rossman LE, Garber DA, Harvey CE. Disorders of teeth. In: Harvey CE, editor. Veterinary dentistry. 1st ed. Philadelphia: W.B. Saunders; 1985. p. 79–105.

18. Stein KE, Marretta SM, Eurell JA. Dens invaginatus of the mandibular first molars in a dog. J Vet Dent 2005;22:21–5.

19. Ammons WIHG. The periodontic-endodontic continuum. In: Newman MG, Takei HH, Klokkevold PR et al, editors. Carranza's Clinical periodontology. 10th ed. St.Louis: Saunders Elsevier; 2006. p. 871–80.

20. Nair PNR. Pathobiology of primary apical periodontitis. In: Cohen S, Hargreaves KM, editor. Pathways of the pulp. 9th ed. St. Louis: Mosby; 2006. p. 541–79.

21. Golden AL, Stoller N, Harvey CE. A survey of oral and dental diseases in dogs anesthetized at a veterinary hospital. J Am Anim Hosp Assoc 1982;18:891–9.

22. Andreasen JO, Andreasen FM. Textbook and color atlas of traumatic injuries to the teeth. 3rd ed. Copenhagen: Munksgaard; 1994.

23. Kuntsi-Vaattovaara H, Verstraete FJM, Kass PH. Results of root canal treatment in dogs: 127 cases (1995–2000). J Am Vet Med Assoc 2002;220:775–80.

24. Ingham KE, Gorrel C, Blackburn J, et al. Prevalence of odontoclastic resorptive lesions in a population of clinically healthy cats. J Small Anim Pract 2001;42:439–43.

25. Lommer MJ, Verstraete FJ. Prevalence of odontoclastic resorption lesions and periapical radiographic lucencies in cats: 265 cases (1995–1998). J Am Vet Med Assoc 2000;217:1866–9.

26. Coles S. The prevalence of buccal cervical root resorptions in Australian cats. J Vet Dent 1990;7:15–6.

27. Lund EM, Bohacek LK, Dahlke JL, et al. Prevalence and risk factors for odontoclastic resorptive lesions in cats. J Am Vet Med Assoc 1998;212:392–5.

28. Lyon KF. Subgingival odontoclastic resorptive lesions. Classification, treatment, and results in 58 cats. Vet Clin North Am Small Anim Pract 1992;22:1417–32.

29. Yoshikawa H, Watanabe K, Ozawa T. Odontoclastic resorptive lesions in a dog. J Vet Med Sci 2008;70:103–5.

30. Sarkiala-Kessel E. Diagnostic imaging in veterinary dental practice. Diagnostic imaging findings and interpretation. J Am Vet Med Assoc 2008;233:389–91.

31. Healey KA, Dawson S, Burrow R, et al. Prevalence of feline chronic gingivo-stomatitis in first opinion veterinary practice. J Feline Med Surg 2007;9: 373–81.

32. Greene RT, Harling DE, Dillman RC. Fiberglass-induced pyogranulomatous stomatitis in a dog. J Am Anim Hosp Assoc 1987;23:401–4.

33. McKeever PJ, Klausner JS. Plant awn, candidal, nocardial, and necrotizing ulcerative stomatitis in the dog. J Am Anim Hosp Assoc 1986;22:17–24.

34. Lyon KF. Gingivostomatitis. Vet Clin North Am Small Anim Pract 2005;35:891–911.

35. Sato R, Inanami O, Tanaka Y, et al. Oral administration of bovine lactoferrin for treatment of intractable stomatitis in feline immunodeficiency virus (FIV)-positive and FIV-negative cats. Am J Vet Res 1996;57:1443–6.

36. Hennet P. Chronic gingivo-stomatitis in cats: long-term follow-up of 30 cases treated by dental extractions. J Vet Dent 1997;14:15–21.

37. Flores MT, Malmgren B, Andersson L, et al. Guidelines for the management of traumatic dental injuries. III. Primary teeth. Dent Traumatol 2007;23:196–202.

38. Hale FA. Juvenile veterinary dentistry. Vet Clin North Am Small Anim Pract 2005; 35:789–817.

39. Verstraete FJM, van Aarde RJ, Nieuwoudt BA, et al. The dental pathology of feral cats on Marion Island, part I: congenital, developmental and traumatic abnormalities. J Comp Pathol 1996; 115:265–82.

40. Legendre LF. Dentistry on deciduous teeth: what, when, and how. Can Vet J 1994; 35:793–794.

41. Verstraete FJM, Kass PH, Terpak CH. Diagnostic value of full-mouth radiography in dogs. Am J Vet Res 1998;59:686–91.

42. Dole RS, Spurgeon TL. Frequency of supernumerary teeth in a dolichocephalic canine breed, the greyhound. Am J Vet Res 1998;59:16–7.

43. Baxter CJ. Bilateral mandibular dentigerous cysts in a dog. J Small Anim Pract 2004;45:210–12.

44. Gardner DG. Dentigerous cysts in animals. Oral Surg Oral Med Oral Pathol 1993;75:348–52.

45. Lemmons MS, Gengler WR, Beebe DE. Diagnostic imaging in veterinary dental practice. Unerupted tooth resulting in a dentigerous cyst causing resorption of bone. J Am Vet Med Assoc 2006;228: 1023–4.

46. Lobprise HB, Wiggs RB. Dentigerous cyst in a dog. J Vet Dent 1992;9:13–5.

47. Sitzman C. Dentigerous cyst in a dog. J Vet Dent 1999;16:186–7.

48. Rashmir-Raven A, Cash WC, DeBowes RM, et al. Dentigerous cysts. Compend Cont Educ Pract Vet 1990;12:1120–6.

49. Regezi JA, Sciubba JJ, Jordan RC. Oral pathology – clinical pathologic correlations. 4th ed. Philadelphia: WB Saunders Co; 2003.

50. Bath M, Perhavec JC. Basic exodontia. In: Fonseca RJ, editor. Oral and maxillofacial surgery. 1st ed. Philadelphia: W.B. Saunders; 2000. p. 207–28.

51. Anonymous. American Veterinary Dental College Position Statement on Veterinary Dental Health Care Providers. 2006.

52. Anonymous. Idaho Statutes, Title 54: Professions, Vocations and Businesses; Chapter 21: Veterinarians. *http://www.legislature.idaho.gov/idstat/Title54/T54CH21SECT54-2103.htm; accessed 10/19/09.*

53. Anonymous. College of Veterinarians of Ontario Position Statement on Veterinary Dentistry. *http://www.cvo.org/uploadattachments/dentistry.pdf accessed 10/19/09.*

54. Anonymous. Georgia Veterinary Medical Board: Scope of Practice for Veterinary Technicians. *http://sos.georgia.gov/plb/veterinary/minutes/20060614.pdf accessed 10/19/09.*

55. Anonymous. California Veterinary Medical Board Laws and Regulations Section 2036: Animal Health Care Tasks for R.V.T. *http://www.vmb.ca.gov/laws_regs/rvttasks.shtml accessed 10/19/09.*

56. Peterson L. Principles of uncomplicated exodontia. In: Peterson LJ, Ellis III E, Hupp J et al, editors. Contemporary oral and maxillofacial surgery. 4th ed. St. Louis: Mosby; 2007. p. 113–55.

57. Verstraete FJM, Kass PH, Terpak CH. Diagnostic value of full-mouth radiography in cats. Am J Vet Res 1998;59:692–5.

58. Evans HE. Miller's anatomy of the dog. 3rd ed. Philadelphia: WB Saunders Co; 1993.

59. Smith MM, Smith EM, La Croix N, et al. Orbital penetration associated with tooth extraction. J Vet Dent 2003;20:8–17.

60. Gioso MA, Shofer F, Barros PS, et al. Mandible and mandibular first molar tooth measurements in dogs: relationship of radiographic height to body weight. J Vet Dent 2001;18:65–8.

61. Bowersock TL, Wu CC, Inskeep GA, et al. Prevention of bacteremia in dogs undergoing dental scaling by prior administration of oral clindamycin or chlorhexidine oral rinse. J Vet Dent 2000;17:11–6.

62. Peterson LJ. Armamentarium for basic oral surgery. In: Peterson LJ, Ellis E, Hupp HR et al, editors. Contemporary oral and maxillofacial surgery. 4th ed. St. Louis: Mosby; 2003. p. 76–112.

63. Holmstrom SE, Frost P, Eisner ER. Exodontics. In: Holmstrom SE, Frost P, Eisner ER, editors. Veterinary dental techniques for the small animal practitioner. 3rd ed. Philadelphia: WB Saunders; 2004. p. 291–338.

64. Harvey CE, Emily PP. Oral surgery. In: Harvey CE, Emily PP, editors. Small animal dentistry. St. Louis: Mosby; 1993. p. 312–77.

65. Dorn AS. Dental extractions and complications. In: Slatter DG, editor. Textbook of small animal surgery. 2nd ed. Philadelphia: WB Saunders; 1993. p. 2326–32.

66. Verstraete FJ. Instrumentation and technique of removal of permanent teeth in the dog. J S Afr Vet Assoc 1983;54:231–8.

67. Peterson L. Principles of complicated exodontia. In: Peterson LJ, Ellis III E, Hupp J et al, editors. Contemporary oral and maxillofacial surgery. 4th ed. St. Louis: Mosby; 2007. p. 156–83.

68. Shafik SS, Ramzi F. Inflammatory cells and pocket epithelium in periodontitis cases. Transmission and scanning electron microscopic study. Egypt Dent J 1990; 36:219–33.

69. Verstraete FJ. Exodontics. In: Slatter DG, editor. Textbook of small animal surgery. 3rd ed. Philadelphia: WB Saunders; 2003. p. 2696–709.

70. Ahn JJ, Shin HI. Bone tissue formation in extraction sockets from sites with advanced periodontal disease: a histomorphometric study in humans. Int J Oral Maxillofac Implants 2008;23: 1133–8.

71. Okamoto T, Okamoto R, Alves Rezende MC, et al. Interference of the blood clot on granulation tissue formation after tooth extraction. Histomorphological study in rats. Braz Dent J 1994;5:85–92.

72. Houston JP, McCollum J, Pietz D, et al. Alveolar osteitis: a review of its etiology, prevention, and treatment modalities. Gen Dent 2002;50:457–63.

73. Devlin H, Sloan P. Early bone healing events in the human extraction socket. Int J Oral Maxillofac Surg 2002;31:641–5.

74. DeForge DH. Evaluation of Bioglass/PerioGlas (Consil) synthetic bone graft particulate in the dog and cat. J Vet Dent 1997;14:141–5.

75. Wiggs RB, Lobprise HB, Mitchell PQ. Oral and periodontal tissue: maintenance, augmentation, rejuvenation and regeneration. Veterinary Clinics of North America: Small Animal Practice 1998; 28:1165–88.

76. Bashutski JD, Wang HL. Periodontal and endodontic regeneration. J Endod 2009; 35:321–8.

77. Hassani A, Motamedi MH, Tabeshfar S, et al. The 'crescent' graft: a new design for bone reconstruction in implant dentistry. J Oral Maxillofac Surg 2009;67:1735–8.

78. Mellonig JT. Decalcified freeze-dried bone allograft as an implant material in human

periodontal defects. Int J Periodontics Restorative Dent 1984;4:40–55.

79. Mellonig JT. Freeze-dried bone allografts in periodontal reconstructive surgery. Dent Clin North Am 1991;35: 505–20.

80. Quintero G, Mellonig JT, Gambill VM, et al. A six-month clinical evaluation of decalcified freeze-dried bone allografts in periodontal osseous defects. J Periodontol 1982;53:726–30.

81. Rummelhart JM, Mellonig JT, Gray JL, et al. A comparison of freeze-dried bone allograft and demineralized freeze-dried bone allograft in human periodontal osseous defects. J Periodontol 1989; 60:655–63.

82. Bowers GM, Chadroff B, Carnevale R, et al. Histologic evaluation of new attachment apparatus formation in humans. Part II. J Periodontol 1989; 60:675–82.

83. von AT, Cochran DL, Hermann JS, et al. Lateral ridge augmentation and implant placement: an experimental study evaluating implant osseointegration in different augmentation materials in the canine mandible. Int J Oral Maxillofac Implants 2001;16:343–54.

84. Hall EE, Meffert RM, Hermann JS, et al. Comparison of bioactive glass to demineralized freeze-dried bone allograft in the treatment of intrabony defects around implants in the canine mandible. J Periodontol 1999;70:526–35.

85. Carranza FA, Takei HH, Cochran DL. Reconstructive periodontal surgery. In: Newman MG, Takei HH, Klokkevold PR et al, editors. Carranza's Clinical periodontology. St. Louis: Elsevier; 2006. p. 968–90.

86. Allan I, Newman H, Wilson M. Antibacterial activity of particulate bioglass against supra- and subgingival bacteria. Biomaterials 2001;22:1683–7.

87. Allan I, Newman H, Wilson M. Particulate bioglass reduces the viability of bacterial biofilms formed on its surface in an in vitro model. Clin Oral Implants Res 2002;13:53–8.

88. Stoor P, Soderling E, Salonen JI. Antibacterial effects of a bioactive glass paste on oral microorganisms. Acta Odontol Scand 1998;56:161–5.

89. DeForge DH. Evaluation of Bioglass/ PerioGlas (Consil) synthetic bone graft particulate in the dog and cat. J Vet Dent 1997;14:141–5.

90. Amler M, Johnson P, Salman I. Histological and histochemical investigation of human alveolar socket healing in undisturbed extraction wounds. J Am Dent Assoc 1960;61:32–44.

91. Woodward TM. Extraction of fractured tooth roots. J Vet Dent 2006;23:126–9.

92. El-Sharrawy E, El-Hakim I, Sameeh E. Attenuation of C-reactive protein increases after exodontia by tramadol and ibuprofen. Anesth Prog 2006;53:78–82.

93. Egger C, Glerum L, Michelle HK, et al. Efficacy and cost-effectiveness of transdermal fentanyl patches for the relief of post-operative pain in dogs after anterior cruciate ligament and pelvic limb repair. Vet Anaesth Analg 2007;34: 200–8.

94. Peterson LJ. Postoperative patient management. In: Peterson LJ, Ellis III E, Hupp JR et al, editors. Contemporary oral and maxillofacial surgery. 4th ed. St. Louis: Mosby; 2003. p. 214–20.

Chapter 12

Simple extraction of single-rooted teeth

Milinda J. Lommer & Frank J.M. Verstraete

PREOPERATIVE CONCERNS

General health status

For patients with pre-existing medical conditions, special precautions may be required to prevent infection, minimize hemorrhage, and prevent exacerbation of the patient's disease state. As discussed in Chapter 3, patients on immunosuppressive drugs or with an immune disorder should receive intravenous antibiotics at the time of the procedure and oral antibiotics afterwards. Gentle tissue handling is especially important in diabetic patients, who may experience delayed wound healing, whether extractions are surgical or nonsurgical. Although simple extraction of single-rooted teeth is relatively atraumatic, patients with severe thrombocytopenia or clotting factor deficiencies should receive blood or plasma transfusions prior to or during the procedure, as even a nonsurgical extraction can lead to excessive hemorrhage in these patients.

Periodontal status

Prior to initiating exodontic treatment, the mobility of the tooth to be extracted should be evaluated. If a tooth is being extracted due to fracture or some cause other than periodontal disease, and is periodontally healthy, normal mobility is expected, and considerable resistance to extraction may be encountered. Severe periodontal disease, conversely, typically results in greater-than-normal mobility and a relatively easy tooth extraction. Periodontal disease of individual incisor teeth is relatively uncommon; it is more common to see horizontal bone loss affecting all or most incisors, particularly mandibular incisor teeth.[1,2] Toy breeds may have mobile mandibular incisor teeth with horizontal bone loss but relatively healthy gingiva.

If a tooth has less-than-normal mobility or radiographs suggest ankylosis or root resorption, a nonsurgical approach to extraction is likely to result in root fracture, and a surgical approach should be considered. This is typically the case for severely abraded incisor teeth with pulp exposure in aggressively chewing dogs.

Extraction of incisor teeth may significantly change the appearance of the patient, and clients should be informed of this prior to the procedure.

It is occasionally necessary to extract a small tooth of lesser functional significance in order to preserve a more important, adjacent tooth. For example, extraction of a periodontally compromised mandibular third molar tooth will allow better access to the second molar tooth, improving the success of home care.

SURGICAL ANATOMY

All teeth in dogs and cats are structurally similar, consisting of a pulp cavity surrounded by dentin, which is covered by cementum (on the root) or enamel (on the crown). The crown and root meet at the cemento-enamel junction (CEJ), also known as the 'neck' of the tooth. The pulp cavity communicates with the tissues in the periapical region via an apical delta. The tooth-supporting structures include cementum, alveolar bone, gingiva, and periodontal ligament. The periodontal ligament consists primarily of Sharpey's fibers (type I collagen) which insert into cementum and bone to secure the tooth in the alveolus.

Permanent teeth

Incisor teeth

Although upper incisor teeth are rooted in the incisive rather than maxillary bones, the term 'maxillary incisor teeth' will be used to differentiate these teeth from the mandibular incisor teeth. Located in the rostral portion of the mouth between the canine teeth, incisors are typically slender, slightly curved, and laterally compressed, so that they are slightly flattened mesiodistally. This is most prominent in the mandibular incisors of the dog (Fig. 12.1A), which are often in very close proximity to one another, with only a thin section of alveolar bone between them. Maxillary and mandibular incisor teeth in the cat are also closely juxtaposed (Fig. 12.1B). It may be difficult to extract one incisor without injuring the adjacent teeth.

Because the incisor teeth appear small compared to other teeth, it is often assumed that extraction will be uncomplicated. However, the crown:root ratio of incisor teeth in the dog is approximately 1:3; the roots are considerably longer than might be expected. This can make

DOI: 10.1016/B978-0-7020-4618-6.00012-9

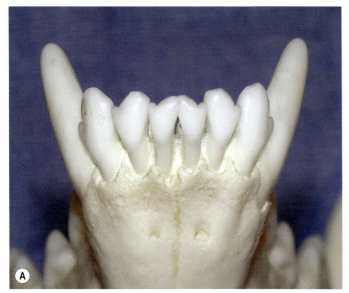

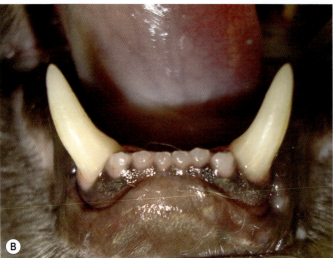

Fig. 12.1 (**A**) Mandibular incisor teeth in the skull of a dog. (**B**) Mandibular incisor teeth in the cat are in close proximity to one another.

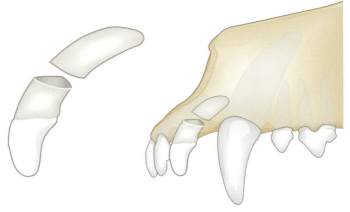

Fig. 12.2 Maxillary third incisor tooth in the dog. Note the triangular cross-section and curved root.

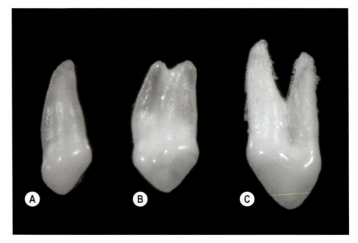

Fig. 12.3 Anatomical variations in the root structure of the maxillary second premolar tooth in the cat: (**A**) single root. (**B**) dichotomous root. (**C**) Two roots. *(From Verstraete FJ, Terpak CH. Anatomical variations in the dentition of the domestic cat. J Vet Dent 1997;14:137–140.)*

extraction more difficult than originally anticipated, particularly if the teeth are being extracted for reasons other than periodontal disease.

The root of the maxillary third incisor tooth in the dog (Fig. 12.2) has a triangular cross-section, is usually quite curved, and may be of substantial length, often making it the most challenging of the single-rooted teeth to extract (except for canine teeth). The maxillary incisor teeth are separated from the nasal cavity by a relatively thin plate of the incisive bone, and it is possible to penetrate into the nasal cavity during attempts to extract these teeth. In the dog and cat, the incisor crowns have visible tubercles, and on the palatal surface of each maxillary incisor tooth is a ridge known as the cingulum, upon which rest the mandibular incisor teeth.[3]

First premolar teeth in the dog

These teeth are in close proximity to the canine teeth. They have a pointed crown and a short, conical, tapered root. The mandibular first premolar teeth are often embedded, and may give rise to dentigerous cysts (see Fig. 11.4).

Maxillary second premolar teeth in the cat

Similar to the first premolar teeth in the dog, a cat's maxillary second premolar tooth has a pointed crown and a short, conical, tapered root. Anatomical variations in the root structure are common; in one study, the frequencies of a single root, a dichotomous root and two roots were found to be 27.7%, 55.1% and 9.2%, respectively (Fig. 12.3).[4]

Maxillary first molar teeth in the cat

Although often classified as two-rooted, the maxillary first molar tooth of the cat may also have a single root or two fused roots. In one study, this tooth was found to have a single root in 35.0% of cases and dichotomous roots in 34.7%; only 28.0% of molars had two fully formed roots (Fig. 12.4).[4] Regardless of the conformation, they are typically extracted in a closed fashion without sectioning. The maxillary first molar tooth, rooted in the maxillary bone, is located immediately ventral to the orbit; care must be taken not to penetrate through the bone into the orbit during extraction.

Mandibular third molar teeth in the dog

These teeth have a flattened crown and a short, conical, tapered root.

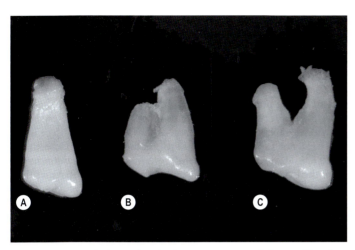

Fig. 12.4 Anatomical variations in the root structure of the maxillary first molar tooth in the cat: (**A**) single root. (**B**) dichotomous root. (**C**) Two roots. *(From Verstraete FJ, Terpak CH. Anatomical variations in the dentition of the domestic cat. J Vet Dent 1997;14:137–140.)*

Deciduous teeth

Deciduous incisor and canine teeth are smaller and more slender than their permanent counterparts; the roots are typically long and narrow, with a wide pulp cavity and very thin dentin walls. The molar teeth and first premolar teeth do not have deciduous precursors.

THERAPEUTIC DECISION-MAKING

Simple versus surgical extraction

Preoperative radiographs are essential to provide the surgeon with accurate information about the tooth to be extracted, its root(s), adjacent teeth, and surrounding tissues. Even a single-rooted tooth may have a dilaceration (abrupt curve or hook at the root apex), which might complicate a nonsurgical extraction. Presence of other anatomical variations, such as dichotomous roots (commonly affecting incisor teeth in dogs), may also affect the decision to perform a nonsurgical extraction. External root resorption and ankylosis, common in dogs with severely abraded incisor teeth, is indication for a surgical extraction; a wide mucogingival flap exposing the alveolar bone over all six teeth facilitates surgical extraction. (Extensive root resorption, seen with odontoclastic resorption lesions, is discussed in Chapter 15.) Previous root canal treatment may result in a more brittle tooth root, and ankylosis may be present; therefore, surgical extraction may be indicated for endodontically treated teeth.[5] Because of their short, conical roots, first premolars and mandibular third molars in the dog rarely require surgical extraction. Conversely, the root of the maxillary third incisor tooth in the dog has a triangular cross-section and is often dramatically curved, making this tooth more suitable for surgical extraction in many cases.

Suturing

Although a simple extraction wound may be left unsutured, placing 1–2 sutures to approximate the gingival wound edges and secure the blood clot present in the vacated alveolus will allow more rapid healing, by first rather than second intention. In addition, the expanded alveolar bone plates and overlying soft tissues can be approximated by digital compression. The socket should only be debrided if necessary. Debris, calculus, tooth or bone fragments in the alveolus should be removed with gentle curettage or suction. If a periapical lesion is visible on preoperative radiographs but there was no granuloma attached to the apex upon tooth removal, the alveolus should be gently curetted to remove the granuloma or cyst. In the absence of debris or periapical lesions, the alveolus should not be curetted, as the remnants of the periodontal ligament and the bleeding bony walls are in optimum condition to promote rapid healing.[5]

If multiple teeth were extracted and if the gingiva can be apposed without tension, several absorbable sutures should be placed in a simple interrupted pattern. Wound closure is also indicated when the gingiva is inadvertently lacerated. Also, for patients where delayed wound healing might be expected or a hemostatic disorder might be present, even a single simple extraction site should be sutured. Suturing may prevent accumulation of debris in the alveolus, and may therefore facilitate healing. However, oral soft tissues heal rapidly, and many suture materials remain in the mouth long after healing has occurred. This may be a source of discomfort or irritation to the patient. To avoid this, the smallest-sized suture material should be selected which will be appropriate for the location. In veterinary dentistry, sizes 4–0 and 5–0 are sufficient to maintain apposition and are less likely to cause irritation to the patient than size 3–0 or larger. Suture material selection is discussed in Chapter 7.

SIMPLE EXTRACTION TECHNIQUE

Prior to attempting extraction, calculus should be removed from the tooth to be extracted and adjacent teeth. This allows better adaptation of the instruments to the tooth, and prevents contamination of the alveolus with calculus after the extraction. The mouth should be rinsed with 0.05–0.12% chlorhexidine gluconate to decrease oral bacterial contamination and reduce the incidence of postoperative infection.[5] Mask, gloves, and eye protection should be worn by the surgeon to prevent injury. When using the elevator, luxator or extraction forceps, the nondominant hand should be used to stabilize the jaw.

Elevation technique

Elevators are used mainly as levers.[5] There are three types of leverage typically employed. A first-class lever involves a fulcrum (typically alveolar bone) between the resistance (tooth) and the applied force (elevator). An elevator or luxator inserted into the periodontal ligament space parallel to the long axis of the root acts as a wedge lever (see Fig. 11.13A). Finally, wheel-and-axle levers are employed when an elevator, after gaining purchase on the tooth surface and positioned perpendicular to the long axis of the root, is rotated such that the force on the tooth is directed outward from the alveolus (see Fig. 11.13B).[6]

There are two primary techniques for using an elevator to nonsurgically extract a single-rooted tooth. The gingival attachment to the tooth should be severed with a scalpel blade prior to using the elevator. The first technique involves placement of the elevator blade into the periodontal space, parallel to the long axis of the tooth, with the concave surface of the blade against the root. Gentle rotational forces are employed to push the root away from the elevator, tearing the periodontal ligament while expanding the alveolar bone slightly. The rotational movements should be slow and steady; the operator may hold the elevator in the rotated position for several seconds to fatigue the periodontal ligament. In the second technique, the elevator blade is placed at the level of the alveolar margin, perpendicular to the long axis of the tooth, and rotated with the concave surface against the tooth. This is performed with gradually increasing pressure, in several locations around the circumference of the tooth, until the periodontal

periodontal ligament prior to application of traction to deliver the tooth.

Maxillary first molar teeth of the cat

Although these teeth may have two divergent or fused roots, they may be extracted in the same manner as a single-rooted tooth. They are typically flat on the mesial and distal surfaces, where a luxator may be introduced parallel to the long axis of the tooth. Care must be taken not to penetrate too deeply, as the orbit is immediately dorsal to the alveolus of the first molar tooth in most cats. After luxation, extraction forceps are used to apply traction in an occlusal direction for completion of the extraction process. Alternatively, an elevator may be placed perpendicular to the long axis of the tooth between the fourth premolar and the first molar teeth, and gentle leverage applied to lift the first molar tooth from its alveolus.

Deciduous teeth

In some instances, when the normal root resorption process has taken place, deciduous teeth may be easier to extract than permanent teeth. However, if it is necessary to remove deciduous teeth before substantial root resorption has occurred, extraction must be approached cautiously. The roots of deciduous teeth are very long and delicate, and fracture easily. After incising the soft tissue attachment at the gingival margin, a luxator with a narrow (2-mm) blade should be employed to gently penetrate the periodontal ligament space and sever the Sharpey's fibers. Alternatively, special, curved elevators with narrow blades have been developed (Fahrenkrug elevator (Shipp's Dental and Specialty Products, Inc., Marana, AZ 85658)) for use with curved-rooted teeth such as canines. With either a luxator or an elevator, the tip must always be directed towards the root surface of the deciduous tooth.[6] Because damage to the permanent tooth may occur, leverage against the permanent tooth should not be used, and the elevator or luxator should not be allowed to penetrate deeply on the lingual surface of the deciduous tooth (in the direction of the permanent tooth). Rotational movements should be minimal, to avoid fracturing the fragile roots. Finally, tractional forces should not be applied until substantial mobility has been achieved, and traction should be very gentle. Surgical extraction of deciduous canine teeth is addressed in Chapter 13.

Postextraction care of the alveolus

If severe periodontitis is present, rinsing the alveolus with a 0.05–0.12% chlorhexidine gluconate solution is advised to reduce bacterial contamination and delayed healing. The alveolus should be debrided if there is obvious debris such as calculus, bone fragments, or tooth fragments in the alveolus, or if a periapical granuloma, abscess, or cyst was present. If there was no periapical lesion and there is no debris, curetting the alveolus may cause injury and delay healing. The blood clot should not be disrupted, as it will provide the best conditions for rapid healing.[5] Any expanded alveolar bony plates should be compressed and repositioned to their original position. Suturing may or may not be performed.

POSTOPERATIVE CARE AND ASSESSMENT

Use of oral rinses

Rinsing with an antibacterial solution is not necessary following routine extraction of a small number of single-rooted teeth in an otherwise healthy patient. In patients with medical conditions where infection or delayed healing might be anticipated, use of a 0.05–0.12% chlorhexidine gluconate solution once or twice daily for 3–5 days following the procedure should be considered.

Dietary change

Most patients will prefer a soft food diet for 2–4 days following dental extractions. For cats, commercial canned food is readily available. For dogs normally on a dry food diet, changing to canned food may cause gastrointestinal upset, so it is generally recommended to soak the dry food in warm water prior to feeding in order to soften its consistency.

Recheck examination

A postoperative visit is not required following uncomplicated nonsurgical extractions. However, recheck examination provides an opportunity to discuss future oral health recommendations, and is an ideal time to instruct the client on oral home care techniques.

Anticipating delayed wound healing

In patients with underlying medical conditions resulting in immune deficiencies, or where severe periodontitis is present preoperatively, extraction sites may not heal as rapidly as in a healthy patient. In these situations, use of a broad-spectrum systemic antibiotic and antimicrobial oral rinses, together with a soft food diet for 7–10 days, should be considered. The client should be instructed to observe the patient for lethargy, inappetence, or halitosis, and the patient should be assessed at 5-day intervals following the procedure to evaluate healing.

REFERENCES

1. Harvey CE, Shofer FS, Laster L. Association of age and body weight with periodontal disease in North American dogs. J Vet Dent 1994;11:94–105.
2. DuPont G. Tooth splinting for severely mobile mandibular incisor teeth in a dog. J Vet Dent 1995;12:93–5.
3. Evans HE. The digestive apparatus and abdomen. In: Evans HE, editor. Miller's anatomy of the dog. 3rd ed. Philadelphia: WB Saunders; 1993. p. 385–462.
4. Verstraete FJ, Terpak CH. Anatomical variations in the dentition of the domestic cat. J Vet Dent 1997;14:137–40.
5. Peterson L. Principles of uncomplicated exodontia. In: Peterson LJ, Ellis E III, Hupp J et al, editors. Contemporary oral and maxillofacial surgery. 4th ed. St. Louis: Mosby; 2007. p. 113–55.
6. Holmstrom SE, Frost P, Eisner ER. Exodontics. In: Holmstrom SE, Frost P, Eisner ER, editors. Veterinary dental techniques for the small animal practitioner. 3rd ed. Philadelphia: WB Saunders; 2004. p. 291–338.
7. Dorn AS. Dental extractions and complications. In: Slatter DG, editor. Textbook of small animal surgery. 2nd ed. Philadelphia: WB Saunders; 1993. p. 2326–32.
8. Gorrel C. Tooth extraction. In: Gorrel C, editor. Veterinary dentistry for the general practitioner. Edinburgh: WB Saunders; 2004. p. 157–74.

Chapter 13

Extraction of canine teeth in dogs

Anson J. Tsugawa, Milinda J. Lommer & Frank J.M. Verstraete

INDICATIONS FOR EXTRACTION

The canine teeth are the longest teeth in the dog with large roots nearly three times as long as their crowns.[1] For the dog, not only are they an important functional component of mastication, but structurally, they occupy a large portion of the jaws. As a result of their structural and functional importance, extraction should not be taken lightly or performed without careful consideration of alternative treatments. Iatrogenic mandibular jaw fracture and oronasal fistula are the most deleterious complications associated with extraction of these teeth; more minor complications include glossoptosis and maxillary lip entrapment.

Extraction should be performed for medical reasons only. A procedure commonly referred to as 'disarming,' in which the canine teeth of an aggressive animal are extracted with the goal of minimizing trauma to humans or other animals, is not an acceptable indication for extraction. Surgical intervention should not be viewed as an alternative to behavioral modification and medical management by a trained animal behaviorist.[2]

Perhaps the most common indication for extraction of canine teeth is severe periodontitis, where the severity of alveolar bone loss has resulted in a mobile tooth, or oronasal fistula formation.

Teeth with complicated crown fractures and discolored, intact teeth are likely to have nonvital pulp,[3] and are candidates for extraction if root canal treatment is not elected. Deep crown–root fractures extending apical to the alveolar margin that are not manageable by advanced periodontal surgery are also an indication for extraction.

Embedded or impacted canine teeth associated with odontogenic cysts should be extracted in the process of enucleating the cyst and its lining.

In puppies with mandibular brachygnathism, extraction of deciduous canine teeth may be indicated prior to eruption of the permanent canine teeth, particularly if the deciduous mandibular canine teeth are located distal to the deciduous maxillary canine teeth when the mouth is closed, causing a 'dental interlock' and preventing independent growth of the maxilla and mandible.[4] Extraction of deciduous teeth to prevent malocclusion of the permanent dentition is referred to as 'interceptive orthodontics.'[4,5]

Once the permanent teeth begin to erupt, the deciduous predecessors should exfoliate. Failure of a deciduous tooth to exfoliate, resulting in a persistent deciduous tooth, may cause malocclusion of the permanent teeth and often results in food entrapment, with subsequent periodontal disease.[6] Therefore, extraction of persistent deciduous teeth should be performed as soon as the condition is diagnosed.[6]

In certain traumatic dental and skeletal malocclusions, or to treat mandibular drift following a mandibulectomy, extraction of the permanent mandibular canine teeth is a therapeutic option.

In reference to jaw fractures with canine teeth in the fracture line, unless severely compromised such that they would interfere with healing, the canine teeth should be preserved, as they are a common anchorage surface for many maxillofacial fracture repair techniques.

The indications for extraction of canine teeth are numerous and are not limited to the aforementioned list. Due to the structural and functional importance of the canine teeth in the dog, the clinician is reminded to consider alternatives to extractions whenever possible.

SURGICAL ANATOMY

Functionally, the canine teeth (*dentes canini*) are designed for piercing/holding prey, and as slashing/tearing weapons in fighting. The canine teeth have roots measuring upwards of 50–60 mm in large-breed dogs.[7] The roots of the canine teeth curve caudally so the apices extend as far as the second premolar teeth.[8] They are pointed at their coronal and apical ends and have a wider midportion at the level of the cemento-enamel junction.[1] In cross-section, canine teeth are linguobuccally compressed and oval in shape.[1]

Maxillary canine tooth

Since the widest section of the canine tooth is usually within the alveolus, a surgical approach to extraction including a full-thickness mucoperiosteal flap is often necessary. Avoidance of local vital structures in the flap design is encouraged, and in the region of the maxillary canine tooth, two structures of importance should be mentioned as sources of hemorrhage if transected: the lateral nasal branches of

DOI: 10.1016/B978-0-7020-4618-6.00013-0

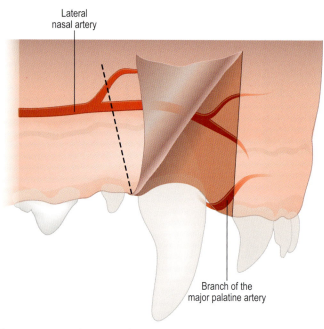

Fig. 13.1 Potential sources of hemorrhage encountered during development of a mucoperiosteal pedicle flap for surgical extraction of a maxillary canine tooth: lateral nasal artery; major palatine artery; and location for a distal vertical releasing incision (*dotted line*).

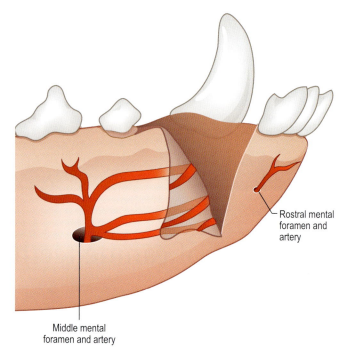

Fig. 13.2 The mental neurovascular structures exiting from the middle mental foramen are avoided with a vertical releasing incision on the mesial aspect of the canine tooth.

the infraorbital artery, and its anastomosis with the branches of the major palatine artery that runs between the maxillary canine and third incisor teeth. The former is typically transected when a vertical releasing incision is created. In general, if a full-thickness flap design is employed, blunt reflection of the flap down to bone usually carries the majority of large vessels within the reflected flap. If a vertical releasing incision is created mesial to the maxillary canine tooth, it is placed at a level 2–3 mm mesial to the mesial line angle of the tooth to allow the incision line to rest over solid bone upon closure of the flap (see Ch. 11). In the process of creating this interproximal incision, it is likely that a small branch of the major palatine artery that passes through the interdental space between the canine tooth and the third incisor will be transected (Fig. 13.1). Hemorrhage may be brisk, but is also well controlled with tamponade and when the flap is sutured closed. Often, the attached gingiva at the mesial corner of the flap, where the palpable jugum slopes down into the interproximal space between the maxillary third incisor and canine teeth, is toughest to pry away; a combination of sharp dissection, making sure the incision is complete, and use of the sharp end of the periosteal elevator, facilitates this initial reflection. Once the flap has been reflected to the desired extent to provide the necessary visualization and access to the area, the prominent jugum overlying the maxillary canine will be clearly visible and accessible for alveolectomy.

Mandibular canine tooth

As mentioned above, appropriately planned flaps should avoid local vital structures, and for the mandible, the mental neurovascular structures that exit from the middle mental foramen are readily avoidable with an appropriately planned vertical releasing incision on the mesial aspect (Fig. 13.2). The interproximal space between the mandibular canine and third incisor teeth is minimal compared to the maxilla, and the incision for the vertical release must be carefully placed at line angles to avoid tension upon apposition of the flap, flap dehiscence

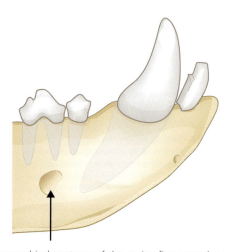

Fig. 13.3 Topographical anatomy of the canine first premolar and second premolar teeth showing the proximity of mandibular canine root to the middle mental foramen (*arrow*), first premolar tooth and mesial root of the second premolar tooth.

and damage to the gingiva of the third incisor tooth. The mandibular canine root is also located lingual and ventral to the mandibular first and second premolar tooth roots, and aggressive alveolectomy or extraction technique may risk damage to these teeth (Fig. 13.3). Contrary to extractions performed elsewhere on the mandible, there is little risk of laceration or damage to the inferior alveolar artery at the level of the mandibular canine alveolus. Anatomically, the root of the mandibular canine tooth does occupy a significant portion of the rostral mandible; conservative alveolectomy is recommended for extraction to avoid excessive weakening of the mandible, or worse, fracture of the mandible through the lingual wall of the alveolus.

Deciduous canine teeth

The roots of deciduous canine teeth are long and slender, and lie close to the developing crown of the permanent tooth.[5] The deciduous maxillary canine teeth are located distal to their permanent successors, while the deciduous mandibular canines are typically buccal to the permanent canines.

THERAPEUTIC DECISION-MAKING

Simple or surgical extraction technique

Canine teeth have long and curved roots that are generally difficult to extract by simple (nonsurgical or closed) extraction technique. Unless a canine tooth is severely mobile, surgical (open) technique is indicated. The deleterious sequelae of forcibly extracting a canine tooth are numerous and include jaw fracture and oronasal communication. Complications such as iatrogenic mandibular fracture typically occur when nonsurgical exodontic techniques are used when severe periodontal disease is apparent.[9] For deciduous canine teeth, whose roots are slender and may not be entirely resorbed, a surgical technique may be the safest approach to avoid damage to the developing permanent tooth. Even severely mobile canine teeth, which can be delivered with gloved fingers or by simple extraction, must be addressed with surgical flap closure, especially the maxillary canine teeth, where oronasal communication is a concern.

Selection of flap design

Unless there is significant gingival recession and/or axial mobility associated with a canine tooth, an envelope flap will probably not provide the exposure and access necessary for the atraumatic extraction of a canine tooth. Therefore, the use of at least one or two vertical releasing incisions, creating three- (triangle) and four-cornered (pedicle) mucoperiosteal flaps, respectively, is recommended.

Maxillary canine tooth

The epithelial attachment to the maxillary canine tooth is severed by introducing a #15 scalpel blade down the gingival sulcus and along the entire circumference of the tooth. As an alternative to the sulcular incision, approximately 1 mm of the free gingival margin can be excised before the flap is elevated.[10] In cases where the gingiva is severely inflamed, closure will be simplified by removing the most friable edges of gingiva at the time of the initial incision. The sulcular incision is extended interproximally for 2–3 mm on the mesial and distal aspects. On the buccal side of the tooth, with tension applied to the alveolar mucosa so that the incision can be made cleanly through it, two divergent incisions are made in the gingiva extending into the alveolar mucosa (Fig. 13.4A). The flap should be of sufficient width to allow for the suture line to rest over solid bone and not the vacated alveolus. Since the root of the maxillary canine tooth arcs caudally as far as the maxillary second premolar tooth, some clinicians advocate placement of the distal vertical releasing incision at the distal line angle of the maxillary second premolar tooth (Fig. 13.4B).[11] Alternatively, a single vertical releasing incision can be made, either mesial or distal to the canine tooth, creating a three-cornered or triangle flap (Fig. 13.4C). If an envelope flap is converted into a three-cornered flap, it is preferable to place the vertical releasing incision at the mesial end of the envelope flap.[12] The mucoperiosteal pedicle flap is reflected using blunt dissection with a periosteal elevator. The sharp end of the periosteal elevator is introduced under the free gingival end of the flap

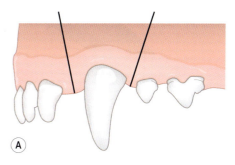

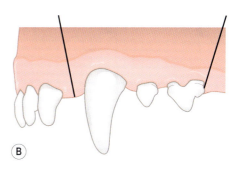

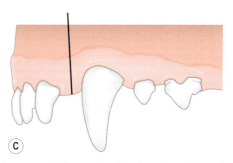

Fig. 13.4 Diagrammatic illustrations showing the position of releasing incisions for the various full-thickness mucoperiosteal flap designs for surgical extraction of a maxillary canine tooth: (**A**) pedicle flap; (**B**) pedicle flap with distal vertical releasing incision at the distal line angle of the maxillary second premolar tooth; (**C**) triangle flap.

and is used to separate the attached gingiva from the underlying bone. Once the free edge of the flap has been raised, the broad end of the periosteal elevator can be used to reflect the flap to the desired amount. A size 4 or 6 round bur mounted on a high-speed handpiece is commonly used to perform the buccal alveolectomy, although a bone chisel or rongeurs may also be used. Continuous irrigation should be used when performing the alveolectomy. Regarding the amount of buccal bone that needs to be removed to facilitate extraction, generally only one-third to one-half of the root length with a width approximately the same as the mesiodistal dimensions of the tooth is usually all that is necessary.[12] Some clinicians advocate the creation of small grooves in the margins of the tooth, or channels in the bone along the mesial and distal margins of the root with a round diamond bur to facilitate placement of the elevator or luxator between the periodontal ligament and bone (Fig. 13.5).[7,13,14] This allows the dental elevator or luxator to be inserted more deeply into the periodontal ligament space. During alveolectomy, a Seldin retractor (see Fig. 6.9A) or Minnesota retractor (see Fig. 6.9B) with pressure applied perpendicular to bone can be used to hold the flap in place without pulling

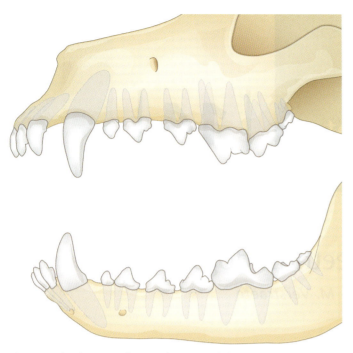

Fig. 14.2 The dentition of a typical mesaticephalic dog.

smaller than the first, and the roots are relatively short and somewhat fused; as a result, this tooth is typically extracted without sectioning. The first molar tooth is a large tooth with a short crown: the palatal root is short, conical and wide relative to the two long and slender buccal roots. The maxillary fourth premolar tooth is a large three-rooted tooth with a pointed crown. The distal root typically has a triangular shape with a broad base at the cemento-enamel junction. The mesiobuccal and palatal roots are usually narrow and slender, with a less triangular shape.[7]

Mandibular premolar and molar teeth

The mandibular second, third, and fourth premolar and first and second molar teeth each have two roots. Fused roots are relatively common, usually affecting the second premolar teeth.[6] The roots of the large premolars and molars may have a distinct radicular sulcus, corresponding with an interradicular septum crest or intra-aveolar crest: in particular, the mesial root of the mandibular first molar tooth has a prominent radicular sulcus.[2,8]

Adjacent structures

On the maxilla, the infraorbital artery, vein and nerve exit the infraorbital foramen dorsal to the distal root of the maxillary third premolar tooth.[9] On the caudal palate, the major palatine artery exits the major palatine foramen (located medial to the fourth premolar tooth) and runs rostrally to the palatine fissure, where it anastomoses with infraorbital and nasal vessels. The parotid salivary duct opens into the oral cavity through a papilla at the rostral end of a fold of mucosa dorsal to the distal root of the maxillary fourth premolar tooth.[9] The zygomatic salivary gland sends one major duct and two to four minor ducts to the caudal oral cavity. The zygomatic papilla, through which the major duct exits, is located about 10 mm caudal to the parotid papilla in a medium-sized dog, dorsal to the maxillary first molar tooth.[9] The maxillary recess (*recessus maxillaris*) is a lateral diverticulum of the nasal cavity, the opening of which lies in a transverse plane

through the mesial roots of the maxillary fourth premolar tooth.[9] It is possible to dislodge a root into this recess if excessive force is used during extraction attempts. In brachycephalic breeds, the orbit lies directly dorsal to the maxillary fourth premolar, first molar and second molar teeth. Orbital penetration has been reported during attempts to extract these teeth.[10]

On the ventral aspect of each mandible is located the mandibular canal, containing the inferior alveolar artery, vein and nerve. These structures exit the canal through three mental foramina on the rostral mandible. The largest of these is the middle mental foramen, located ventral to the second premolar tooth. When creating mucogingival flaps, care must be taken to avoid inadvertently transecting the mental neurovascular bundle. The proportion of the mandible occupied by the teeth varies with breed; small dogs have proportionally larger mandibular first molar teeth relative to the height of the mandible when compared with small dogs (see Fig. 11.7).[11] It is possible to cause iatrogenic fracture of the mandible during attempts to extract mandibular first molar teeth if excessive force is applied.

THERAPEUTIC DECISION-MAKING

Pre-extraction radiographs of teeth to be removed should be obtained. This will allow confirmation of the diagnosis, visualization of root morphology, identification of root resorption or root ankylosis, and evaluation of the quality of the supporting jaw bone.[2]

Surgical or simple (nonsurgical) extraction

While a severely mobile multirooted tooth may be a candidate for simple extraction, most multirooted teeth will require surgical extraction, which involves sectioning the tooth, with or without creation of a gingival or mucogingival flap and removal of alveolar bone.

Flap design

The three primary gingival and mucogingival–periosteal flap designs (envelope, triangle and pedicle – see Ch. 11) are used for surgical extractions of multirooted teeth in dogs. An envelope flap (which is a gingival flap, as the alveolar mucosa is typically not included) may be used for sectioning of mobile multirooted teeth where removal of alveolar bone is not required. Flap design will be discussed in further detail with the description of technique for each tooth type.

SURGICAL TECHNIQUE

Extraction of maxillary second and third premolar, and mandibular second, third and fourth premolar teeth

For extraction of a single premolar tooth, a triangle mucoperiosteal flap, with a vertical releasing incision at the mesial interproximal space or line angle of the mesial adjacent tooth, is most useful. When two or more adjacent teeth are being extracted, an envelope flap typically provides adequate visualization and exposure of the buccal alveolar bone (Fig. 14.3A, B). If necessary, 1–3 mm of bone may be removed from the alveolar margin to expose the furcations and visualize the roots prior to sectioning (Fig. 14.3C). A tapered bur on a high-speed handpiece is used to section the teeth, beginning at the furcation and progressing coronally, so each root may be separately extracted

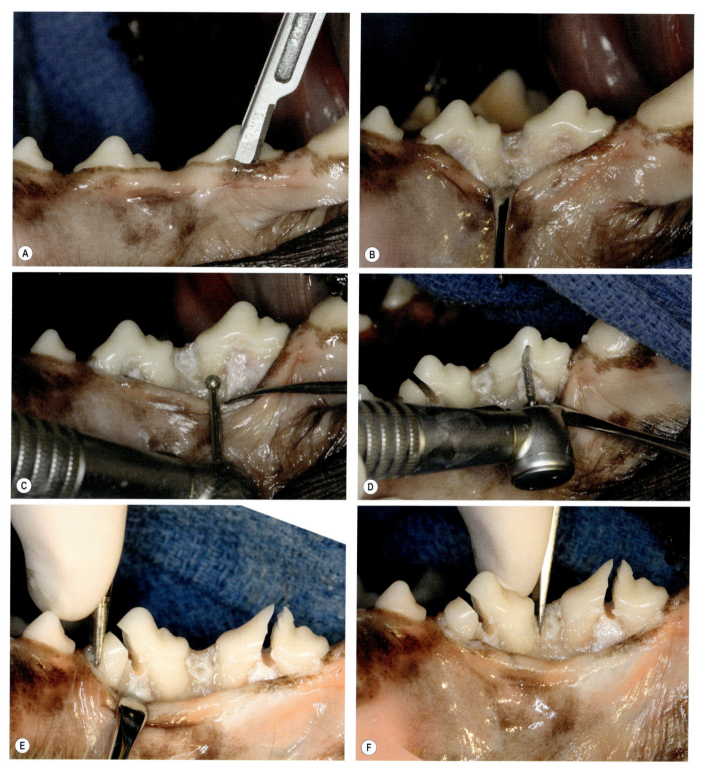

Fig. 14.3 Extraction of a maxillary second and third premolar teeth in a dog. The patient is in dorsal recumbency. (**A**) An envelope flap is created and reflected (**B**) to expose the alveolar bone. (**C**) A round diamond bur on a high-speed handpiece is utilized to remove a small amount of buccal alveolar bone. (**D**) Then a tapered diamond bur is used to section the roots. This may be performed directly through the center of the crown (as was done at P3) or at an angle to minimize the amount of crown the bur travels through (as at P2). Luxation on the mesial (**E**) and distal (**F**) aspects of each root is performed to sever the periodontal ligament fibers.

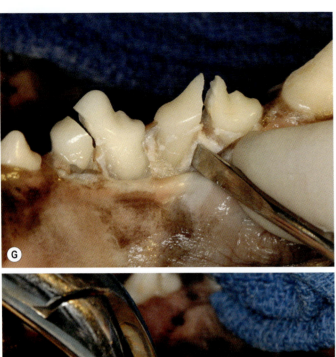

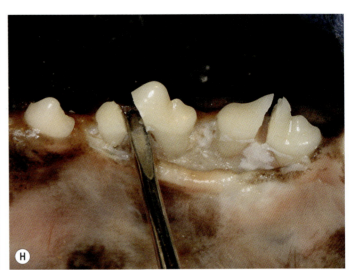

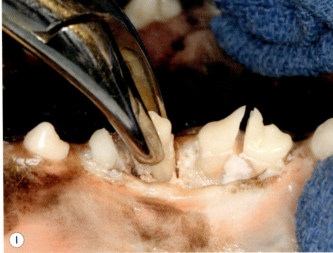

Fig. 14.3, cont'd. (**G**) The luxator may also be used perpendicular to the long axis of the root. (**H**) Elevation may be employed as an alternative or adjunct to luxation. (**I**) Finally, extraction forceps are placed on each root and rotated gently to free any remaining attachment.

(Fig. 14.3D). A luxator is introduced on the mesial (Fig. 14.3E) and distal (Fig. 14.3F) aspects of each root, using gentle pressure and small axial rotations (5–10°) to direct the blade apically in the periodontal space, cutting the periodontal attachment.[2] Alternatively, the luxator may be placed in the periodontal ligament space at a 90° angle to the root in order to sever periodontal ligament fibers (Fig. 14.3G). Once some mobility has been achieved, an elevator may be placed between sectioned roots, and gentle rotational pressure applied to fatigue the periodontal ligament and lift the root from the alveolus (Fig. 14.3H). When using the elevation technique, care must be employed to avoid generating excessive force, or root fracture will occur. Once each root has demonstrated significant mobility, extraction forceps are placed as far apically as possible. Applying gentle rotational forces and minimal traction with the extraction forceps, each root is delivered from its alveolus (Fig. 14.3I). Premature application of extraction forceps, or use of excessive force with extraction forceps, may result in root fracture.

If a root fracture occurs, it is important to have good lighting and visibility before attempting removal of the remaining fragment. If fracture occurred close to the cemento-enamel junction and the remaining fragment is large, a 2-mm dental luxator or small elevator may be sufficient to loosen and remove it. Small root tips may be mobilized using 1- or 2-mm luxators, root tip picks or root tip elevators and then removed with root tip forceps. It may be necessary to extend the mucogingival flap and remove more alveolar bone in order to obtain access to a small root fragment. Drilling out root tips ('pulverization,' 'atomization') can result in damage to the infraorbital or inferior alveolar arteries and nerves, fatal air embolism or other iatrogenic trauma, and is not advisable.[12]

After all roots and root fragments are removed, any expanded alveolar bone is gently compressed back into position, and sharp bony edges are reduced with a round bur. The empty alveoli are flushed with sterile saline solution, and the mucogingival flap is repositioned and sutured without tension.[2]

Extraction of maxillary fourth premolar teeth

Dorsal recumbency allows much better visualization of the three roots of the caudal maxillary teeth, and is therefore preferred to lateral recumbency for extraction of these teeth. A pedicle flap provides optimum visibility for extraction of the maxillary fourth premolar tooth, but a triangle flap may be sufficient for cases where extensive alveolectomy is not required and avoids the salivary papillae. As previously mentioned, the infraorbital blood vessels and nerve exit the infraorbital foramen dorsal to the distal root of the maxillary third premolar tooth. Therefore, when making a vertical releasing incision mesial to the maxillary fourth premolar tooth, care must be taken not to incise through the infraorbital neurovascular bundle. A perpendicular rather than divergent incision is less likely to damage the infraorbital vessels and nerve (Fig. 14.4). If a pedicle flap is selected, the incision at the distal aspect of the tooth should be extended 2–3 mm into the sulcus of the first molar and a vertical incision made, being careful to avoid the parotid and zygomatic papillae.[2] After the incisions are made, the full-thickness mucogingival flap is elevated and reflected to expose the buccal alveolar bone (Fig. 14.5A). Partial alveolectomy may be performed to facilitate exposure of the furcation between the mesiobuccal and distal roots. To facilitate extraction, particularly if the tooth is periodontally healthy or if ankylosis is evident on preoperative radiographs, additional alveolectomy may be performed along the root surfaces (Fig. 14.5B). Following alveolectomy, a tapered diamond or cylindrical carbide bur on a high-speed handpiece is introduced horizontally into the furcation, and moved coronally to separate the distal from the mesial root (Fig. 14.5C). After reflecting the gingiva on the mesial aspect of the tooth to better visualize the furcation between the mesiobuccal and palatal roots, the bur is held at a 30° angle to the vertical axis of the tooth, and moved through the furcation from mesial to distal (Fig. 14.5D, E). Once the tooth has been sectioned into three parts, a luxator may be introduced on the distal and mesial aspects of the two buccal roots (Fig. 14.5F, G, H). Placement of the luxator on the buccal aspect of the tooth should be avoided, as it is easy to slip out of the periodontal ligament space and across the surface of the alveolar bone, damaging the soft tissues. Horizontal leverage with an elevator placed between the distal and mesiobuccal roots may be employed after luxation has severed some of the periodontal ligament and the roots are somewhat mobile (Fig. 14.5I). It is important not to use excessive force when elevating, as the mesiobuccal root is more slender than the distal root and likely to fracture if excessive torque is generated.

After the distal and mesiobuccal roots have been removed using extraction forceps (Fig. 14.5J), the palatal root is more easily visualized. Removal of some bone from the furcation region between the mesiobuccal and palatal roots will further improve visibility for placement of the luxator. The luxator should be introduced into the periodontal ligament space on the mesial and distal aspects of the root, and at a 60° angle to the hard palate (Fig. 14.5K).[2] Elevation is not recommended for this long, slender tooth root because fracture is likely. Once the luxators have been advanced apically and the root is mobile, extraction forceps are employed, with minimal rotational and tractional forces, to deliver the root from the alveolus.

Following removal of all three roots, any rough bony edges are smoothed with a round diamond bur on a high-speed handpiece (Fig. 14.5L) and the alveoli are flushed with saline. The mucogingival flap may be undermined further, and the periosteum may be incised if necessary, to ensure closure without tension. It may be preferable to suture the flap back in its original location (i.e., align the mucogingival junction of the flap with the mucogingival junction of the third premolar tooth, even though this may leave a small space at the palatal root alveolus; Fig. 14.5M) rather than attempting to suture the corner of the flap to the palatal mucosa. This ensures the presence of attached gingiva (rather than mucosa) at the distal aspect of the third premolar tooth.

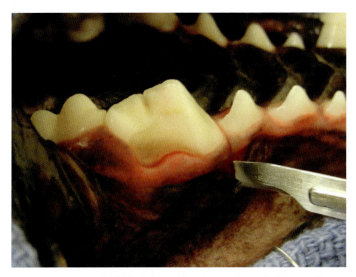

Fig. 14.4 A #15 scalpel blade is employed to make an incision at the mesial–buccal line angle of the left maxillary fourth premolar tooth for creation of a triangle flap.

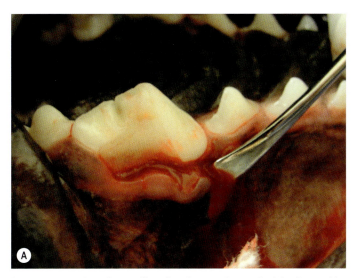
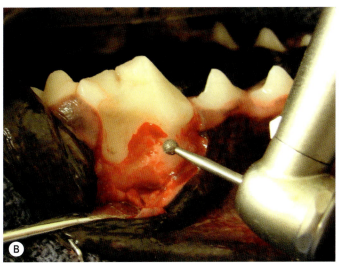

Fig. 14.5 Extraction of a maxillary fourth premolar tooth. (**A**) After making the incision, a triangle mucogingival flap is elevated. (**B**) Partial alveolectomy is performed using a round diamond bur.

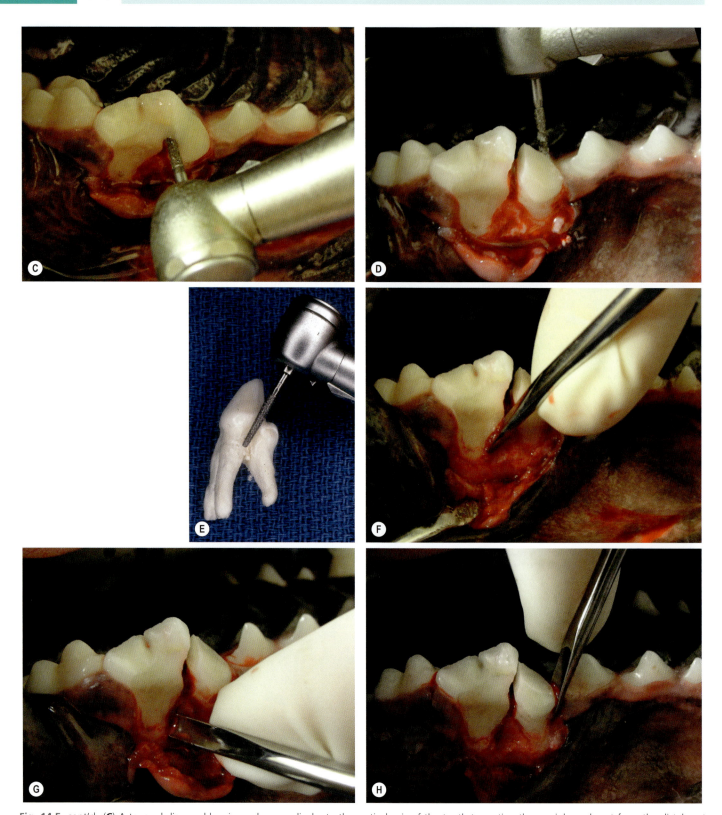

Fig. 14.5, cont'd. (**C**) A tapered diamond bur is used perpendicular to the vertical axis of the tooth to section the mesiobuccal root from the distal root and (**D**) at a 30° to the vertical axis of the tooth to section the palatal from the mesiobuccal root. (**E**) This anatomic specimen demonstrates the angle at which the handpiece should be held for optimum sectioning of the palatal from the mesiobuccal root. Although the luxator may be placed parallel to the long axis of the root, (**F**) it may also be helpful to use the luxator in a perpendicular manner, (**G**) to sever the periodontal ligament fibers. After the luxator has been introduced on the mesial and distal aspects of the distal and mesiobuccal roots, (**H**) careful elevation may be performed between the mesiobuccal and distal roots.

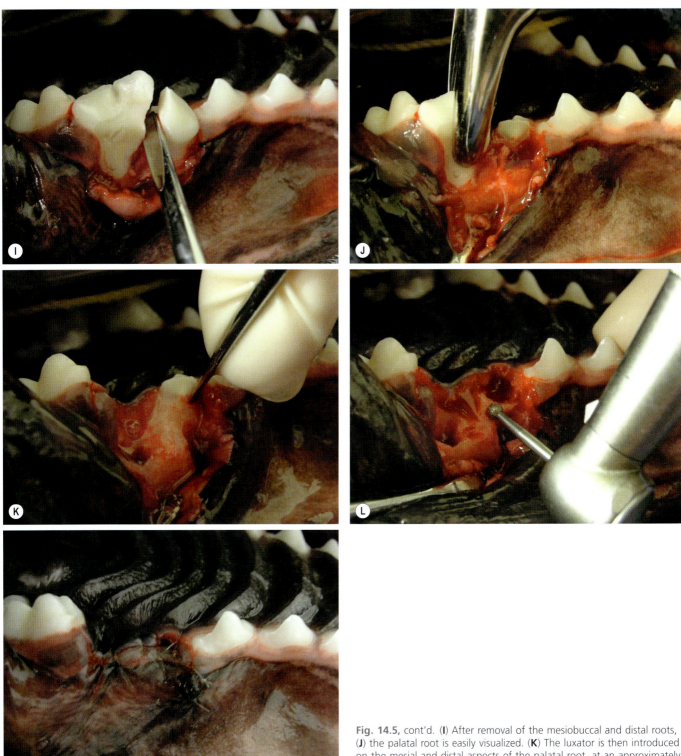

Fig. 14.5, cont'd. (**I**) After removal of the mesiobuccal and distal roots, (**J**) the palatal root is easily visualized. (**K**) The luxator is then introduced on the mesial and distal aspects of the palatal root, at an approximately 60° angle to the hard palate. (**L**) Alveoloplasty, or removal of sharp bone edges, is performed prior to (**M**) suturing the flap.

Extraction of maxillary first molar teeth

Even in the presence of significant periodontal disease, it is advisable to extract the maxillary first molar tooth surgically. The two buccal roots are long and slender when compared with the palatal root, and are therefore easily fractured.

With the patient in dorsal recumbency, a sulcular incision is made and extended 1–2 mm mesially. Taking care not to damage the zygomatic papilla, a vertical releasing incision can be made into the mucosa, creating a triangle flap, if necessary. After reflecting the gingiva from the mesial aspect of the tooth, a tapered bur is held vertically and moved from mesial to distal in order to section the palatal root from the two buccal roots (Fig. 14.6). The palatal root may be extracted first; it is shorter and more conical, making its extraction less challenging. Frequently, this root can be extracted with extraction forceps alone. If an elevation technique is employed using the two mesial roots for leverage, the mesial roots may fracture. Therefore, if extraction forceps alone are insufficient to remove this root, use of luxators rather than elevators is recommended. The buccal roots are separated from one another using a tapered bur. Removal of buccal alveolar bone may facilitate extraction of the two long, narrow buccal roots. Tissue retractors (e.g., Cawood–Minnesota retractor) should be employed to prevent damage to the cheeks from the bur during partial alveolectomy and sectioning of this tooth. Following sectioning and partial alveolectomy, a luxator is introduced on the mesial and distal aspects of each of the buccal roots, taking care not to penetrate into the orbit. An elevator may be carefully employed once luxation has resulted in significant mobility of the two buccal roots. Minimal tractional and rotational forces should be applied with extraction forceps for final delivery of each buccal root.

If a vertical releasing incision was made, it should be sutured. Otherwise, tension-free closure of the gingiva may not be possible without extensive flap development, and the site may be left to heal by second intention.

Extraction of maxillary second molar teeth

The three roots of the maxillary second molar tooth are often fused, making sectioning unnecessary for extraction of the resulting short, conical tooth. In this case, the tooth may be removed intact with an elevator. If the roots are not fused, they may be curved and therefore fracture easily.[2] If visibility allows, the tooth may be sectioned as described for the maxillary first molar tooth, and each root removed separately. If root fracture occurs, fragments may be retrieved with a 1-mm luxator or a root tip elevator. Luxators and elevators must be used with extreme caution, as there is often a minimal amount of bone distal to this tooth, and inadvertent dorsal slippage of a luxator can easily lead to orbital trauma or laceration of the maxillary artery.

Extraction of mandibular first molar teeth

This is a very large tooth, the roots of which are often adjacent to the mandibular canal. Extraction of a periodontally sound mandibular first molar tooth is difficult, and may result in iatrogenic fracture. In addition, dilacerated roots may make extraction even more challenging, with an increased risk of root or mandibular fracture (see Fig. 11.6). When possible, conservative therapy (endodontic treatment for a fractured tooth, or periodontal surgery and guided tissue regeneration for periodontally compromised teeth) should be offered as an alternative to extraction. If extraction is elected, creation of a triangle mucogingival–periosteal flap and removal of 50–75% of the buccal alveolar bone will greatly facilitate extraction. When sectioning this tooth, it is suggested to start at the furcation and proceed in a distal–coronal direction, creating an oblique line between the distal and mesial roots which avoids cutting through the tall central cusp (Fig. 14.7). A combination of luxators and elevators may be employed for extraction of the two large roots. Luxators should be placed on the distal and mesial aspects of each root to avoid soft tissue trauma due to slippage on the buccal or lingual aspects. After luxators have severed substantial periodontal ligament fibers such that the roots are somewhat mobile, an elevator can be introduced between the two roots, rotated 5–10°, and held for several seconds to fatigue the remaining periodontal ligament and lift the roots from their alveoli. Extraction forceps may then be used with gentle traction to deliver the roots. If the alveolar bone has been expanded during the extraction, it should be compressed into its original position. Any sharp bony edges should be removed with a round diamond bur on a high-speed handpiece and the alveoli should be flushed with saline prior to apposition and suturing of the mucogingival flap.

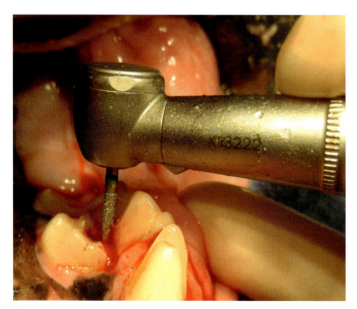

Fig. 14.6 A tapered diamond bur is used to section the palatal root from the more slender buccal roots of a maxillary first molar tooth.

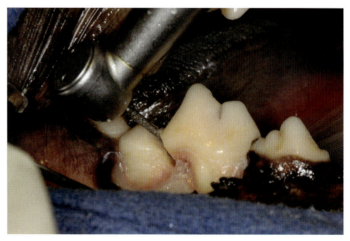

Fig. 14.7 A tapered diamond bur is used to section the roots of a mandibular first molar tooth.

COMPLICATIONS

Complications of extractions are discussed in Chapter 16. Root fracture is the most common complication when extracting multirooted teeth. As previously discussed, removal of root fragments is most easily achieved following additional removal of alveolar bone and with excellent visibility. Magnification loupes, adequate lighting, availability of suction, and the use of 1- and 2-mm luxators will greatly facilitate removal of fractured root fragments.

Less common complications include iatrogenic mandibular fracture when extracting mandibular first molar teeth in small-breed dogs, and orbital penetration during extraction of maxillary fourth premolar or first molar teeth.[10] Proper preoperative assessment, including intraoral radiographs, and careful technique will help prevent these catastrophic complications.

REFERENCES

1. Wolf HF, Rateitschak EM, Rateitschak KH, et al. Color atlas of dental medicine: periodontology. 3rd ed. Stuttgart: Georg Thieme Verlag; 2005.
2. Verstraete FJM. Exodontics. In: Slatter DH, editor. Textbook of small animal surgery. 3rd ed. Philadelphia: WB Saunders Co; 2003. p. 2696–709.
3. Beckman BW. Treatment of an infrabony pocket in an American Eskimo dog. J Vet Dent 2004;21:159–63.
4. Reiter AM, Lewis JR, Rawlinson JE, et al. Hemisection and partial retention of carnassial teeth in client-owned dogs. J Vet Dent 2005;22:216–26.
5. Peterson LJ. Prevention and management of surgical complications. In: Peterson LJ, Ellis III E, Hupp HR et al, editors. Contemporary oral and maxillofacial surgery. 4th ed. St. Louis: Mosby; 2003. p. 221–35.
6. Verstraete FJM, Kass PH, Terpak CH. Diagnostic value of full-mouth radiography in dogs. Am J Vet Res 1998;59:686–91.
7. Evans H. The digestive apparatus and abdomen. In: Evans H, editor. Miller's anatomy of the dog. 3rd ed. Philadelphia: WB Saunders; 1993. p. 385–462.
8. Bodingbauer J. Die Wurzelseptumleiste (Crista septi interradicularis, s. intraalveolaris) und die Wurzelrinnen (Sulci radiculares) – eine zusätzliche Anlage des Zahnhalteapparates bei Fleischfressern. II. Mitteilung [The root septum crests (Crista septi interradicularis, s. intraalveolaris) and the root sulci (Sulci radiculares) – an additional feature of the tooth holding apparatus in carnivores]. Säugetierkundl Mitt 1955;3:5–10.
9. Evans HE. Miller's anatomy of the dog. 3rd ed. Philadelphia: WB Saunders Co; 1993.
10. Smith MM, Smith EM, La Croix N, et al. Orbital penetration associated with tooth extraction. J Vet Dent 2003; 20:8–17.
11. Gioso MA, Shofer F, Barros PS, et al. Mandible and mandibular first molar tooth measurements in dogs: relationship of radiographic height to body weight. J Vet Dent 2001;18:65–8.
12. Grossman LI, Oliet S, del Rio CE. Endodontic surgery. In: Grossman LI, Oliet S, del Rio CE, editors. Endodontic practice. 11th ed. Philadelphia: Lea & Febiger; 1988. p. 289–312.

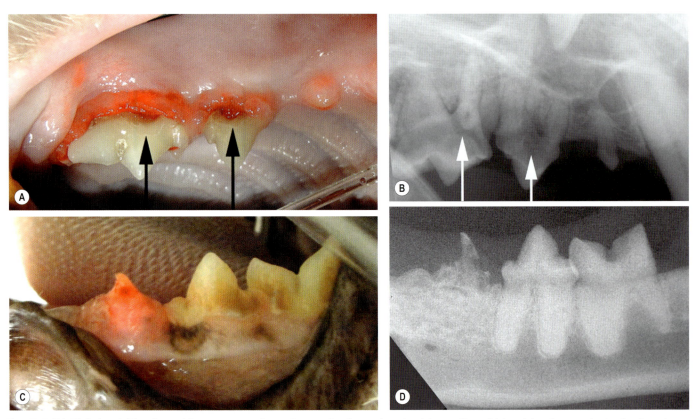

Fig. 15.1 (**A**) Clinical and (**B**) radiographic appearance of type-1 resorption (*arrows*) at the right maxillary third and fourth premolar teeth of a cat. Note also the third root on the third premolar tooth. These teeth should be extracted in toto. (**C**) Clinical and (**D**) radiographic appearance of type-2 resorption at the left mandibular third premolar tooth. This tooth is a good candidate for coronectomy.

blunt apex. The incisors are very slender and fragile. The maxillary second premolar tooth is the only single-rooted premolar. However, anatomical variations in the root structure are common: in one study, the frequencies of a single root, a dichotomous root and two roots were found to be 27.7%, 55.1% and 9.2%, respectively.[10] The maxillary third premolar tooth is two-rooted, although a third root is present in approximately 10% of cases (Fig. 15.3).[10]

The maxillary fourth premolar tooth has three roots. The distal root is much larger than the mesiobuccal and palatal roots, and the furcation is located more mesially rather than in the middle of the tooth. Although often classified as two-rooted, the maxillary first molar tooth of the cat may also have a single root or two fused roots. This tooth was found to have a single root in 35.0% of cases and dichotomous roots in 34.7%; only 28.0% of molar teeth had two fully formed roots.[10] The mandibular third and fourth premolar teeth are similar in shape and size, and each has two slightly divergent roots. The mandibular first molar tooth has two divergent roots, with the distal root typically much more slender than the mesial root.

The maxillary teeth are separated from the nasal cavity by a relatively thin plate of bone, and it is possible to penetrate into the nasal cavity during attempts to extract maxillary canine and premolar teeth, particularly the palatal root of the fourth premolar tooth. In addition, the maxillary first molar tooth is located immediately ventral to the orbit; care must be taken not to penetrate through the bone into the orbit during extraction.[11]

The roots of the mandibular premolar and molar teeth terminate just dorsal to the mandibular canal, which contains the inferior alveolar artery, vein and nerve. If excessive force is applied during extraction, it is possible for an instrument or a root fragment to penetrate into the mandibular canal, which may result in severe hemorrhage.

SPECIAL INSTRUMENTS AND MATERIALS

Instruments suitable for feline exodontics

The examples listed in Table 15.1 represent the author's personal preference; many suitable alternatives are available.

THERAPEUTIC DECISION-MAKING

Pre-extraction radiographs of teeth to be removed should be obtained. This will allow evaluation of supporting bone levels or extent of periodontal bone loss, identification of root resorption or ankylosis, and assessment of root morphology.[2,12] As previously mentioned, anatomical variations are common in cats and, when present, will affect the extraction technique. Furthermore, radiography is particularly important when deciding whether to extract a tooth affected by resorption *in toto* or by coronectomy. The classification system outlined in Tables 15.2 and 15.3 has been developed by the American Veterinary Dental College and is helpful in determining the appropriate extraction technique.[13]

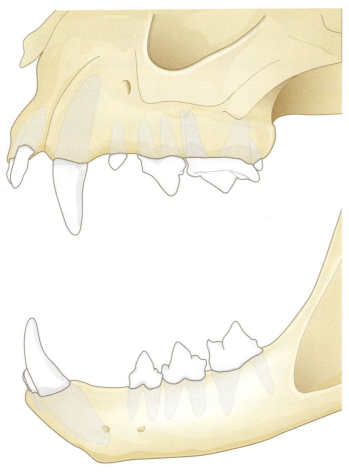

Fig. 15.2 Dentition of the cat.

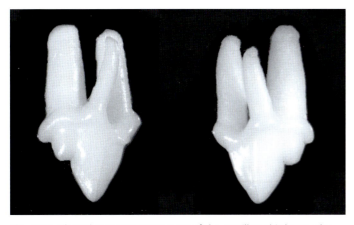

Fig. 15.3 Bilateral supernumerary roots of the maxillary third premolar tooth. *(From Verstraete FJ, Terpak CH. Anatomical variations in the dentition of the domestic cat. J Vet Dent 1997;14:137–140.)*

Extraction versus coronectomy (crown amputation with intentional root retention) for tooth resorption

Variable stages of root resorption result in a high risk of root fracture, making extraction of resorbing teeth especially difficult. Root fractures with retention of the apical fragment may result in persistent pain and

complications such as osteomyelitis of the alveolar bone.[2] However, teeth affected by resorption only, in the absence of periodontal disease or pre-existing fractures, do not appear to be associated with pulpal necrosis or periapical pathology.[4,14] Therefore, coronectomy appears to be an acceptable alternative to extraction in selected cases.[4,6,7] Pre-extraction radiographs are crucial in case selection: only teeth with advanced root resorption, but without periodontal or endodontal lesions, are good candidates for coronectomy.[2,7]

This technique is especially useful for teeth with extensive resorption where the patient has a high risk of anesthetic complications and expeditious treatment is desirable. Coronectomy should not be performed on fractured teeth or teeth with significant periodontitis, and is not recommended in cats with gingivitis/stomatitis, except where extensive root resorption (stage 4c) is confirmed radiographically.

Postextraction radiographs are indicated in these cases, to document how much root structure was left behind and confirm the smoothness of the alveolar margin.

Simple versus surgical extraction

The decision to extract a tooth surgically or nonsurgically should be based on clinical and radiographic findings prior to beginning the extraction procedure (see Ch. 11). Unlike a surgical extraction, a simple extraction does not involve sectioning the tooth, creating a mucogingival flap, or removing alveolar bone.[12] A tooth with significant bone loss and clinical mobility is a good candidate for simple extraction, while a fractured canine tooth with normal alveolar bone levels would be an indication for surgical extraction.

The buccal alveolar bone at the canine teeth is normally up to 2 mm thick. Although the exact mechanism by which this occurs has not been elucidated, increased width of this bone (referred to as buccal bone expansion) is associated with vertical bone loss.[15] The presence of buccal bone expansion may make a nonsurgical extraction of a canine tooth possible;[15] however, raising a flap, partial alveolectomy, debridement and alveoloplasty are indicated to allow soft tissue closure over a flat, smooth surface. Following removal of expanded buccal alveolar bone, the ipsilateral mandibular canine tooth may occlude onto the lip.[2] It may therefore be indicated to perform odontoplasty and application of a light-cured dentinal sealer to reduce the height and sharpness of the cusp tip of the ipsilateral mandibular canine tooth to prevent occlusal trauma to the lip following extraction of a maxillary canine tooth.

Flap design

The three primary mucoperiosteal flap designs (envelope, triangle and pedicle – see Ch. 11) are used for surgical extractions in cats. An envelope flap, which is a gingival flap, as the alveolar mucosa is typically not included, is used for coronectomy. An extended envelope flap, which does include some alveolar mucosa, may be used for the extraction of all premolar and molar teeth in one quadrant.

Full-mouth and premolar–molar extractions

When extensive extractions are planned for treatment of chronic gingivostomatitis, several factors must be taken into consideration. In many cases, the inflammation is less severe at the incisor and canine teeth, so premolar–molar extractions may be elected, with planned conservation of the incisor and canine teeth. Survey dental radiographs prior to extraction are indicated for the reasons mentioned above; they are also useful for determining whether the incisor and canine teeth require extraction for reasons not related to the gingival and mucosal inflammation (e.g., the presence of significant

Table 15.1 Instruments suitable for feline exodontics

Instruments and suture material	Comments
Periosteal elevator	The rounded end of a P24G periosteal elevator (P24G, Hu-Friedy Mfg. Co., Chicago, IL) (see Fig. 6.8) is ideal for gently elevating mucogingival-periosteal flaps without tearing the tissues.
Bur	A very narrow, taper diamond bur (Maxima Diamond 850–010 C, Henry Schein, Inc. Melville, NY) is well suited to sectioning cat premolar teeth.
Luxators	Luxators (JS Dental Mfg. Co., Ridgefield, CT) (see Fig. 12.4B, C) with 1-, 2- or 3-mm wide blades, straight handles, and sharp blades are used for luxation.
Elevators	An elevator (LTXS 2S and LTXS 3S, Cislak Manufacturing, Inc. Niles, IL) with a narrow tip and a shorter handle is better suited to cats than a large-handled, large-bladed elevator, which can generate excessive rotational force and result in root fracture.
Pedodontic extraction forceps	Small, straight-beaked forceps, such as a Cryer #150S or #150K (F150S and F150K, Hu-Friedy Mfg. Co., Chicago, IL) (see Fig. 12.5) are suitable for most extractions.
Root tip elevators	Root tip elevators such as the Davis #11 root tip elevator (ED11, Hu-Friedy Mfg. Co., Chicago, IL) are useful for teasing mobile root fragments from their alveoli; because the end is rounded, it is less likely to cause trauma or penetrate through the alveolus.
Root tip forceps	Root tip forceps, such as FX-49 forceps (FX49, Hu-Friedy Mfg. Co., Chicago, IL) (see Fig. 12.6), with long, narrow beaks are excellent for retrieving fractured roots.
Small needle holders	Small (4.5" or 5") needle holders, such as a Halsey needle holder (NH-5036, Hu-Friedy Mfg. Co., Chicago, IL) (see Fig. 6.11A), are much easier to maneuver in the small mouth of a cat than the more common 6", 7" or 8" needle holders.
Small surgical curette	A curette, such as a Miller #10 (CM10, Hu-Friedy Mfg. Co., Chicago, IL) (see Fig. 6.14), is used for removing debris from the alveolus after extraction.
Suture material	Absorbable monofilament suture material (Monocryl, Ethicon, Inc., Somerville, NJ) on a small, reverse-cutting needle, size 5–0, is suitable for cats.

Table 15.2 Classification of tooth resorption based on clinical stage[13]

Stage	Definition
TR1	Mild dental hard tissue loss (cementum or cementum and enamel).
TR2	Moderate dental hard tissue loss (cementum or cementum and enamel with loss of dentin that does not extend to the pulp cavity).
TR3	Deep dental hard tissue loss (cementum or cementum and enamel with loss of dentin that extends to the pulp cavity); most of the tooth retains its integrity.
TR4	Extensive dental hard tissue loss (cementum or cementum and enamel with loss of dentin that extends to the pulp cavity); most of the tooth has lost its integrity. **TR4a**: Crown and root are equally affected. **TR4b**: Crown is more severely affected than the root. **TR4c**: Root is more severely affected than the crown.
TR5	Remnants of dental hard tissue are visible only as irregular radiopacities, and gingival covering is complete.

Table 15.3 Classification of tooth resorption based on radiographic appearance[13]

Type	Definition
Type 1	Focal or multifocal radiolucency in a tooth with otherwise normal radiopacity and normal periodontal ligament space.
Type 2	Narrowing or disappearing of the periodontal ligament space in at least some areas, and decreased radiopacity of part of the tooth.
Type 3	Features of both type 1 and type 2 are present in the same tooth. A tooth with this appearance has areas of normal periodontal ligament space and areas of narrow or lost periodontal ligament space. There is focal or multifocal radiolucency in some areas of the tooth and decreased radiopacity in other areas.

periodontal bone loss or tooth resorption). For cases with severe generalized stomatitis, full-mouth extractions may be indicated. In these situations, it may be desirable to stage the procedure, extracting all teeth on one side of the mouth under one anesthetic episode, then completing extractions of the remaining two quadrants 2–3 weeks later. All root fragments must be removed.[17] Pain management for patients undergoing full-mouth or premolar–molar extractions is imperative.[2,16] In addition, nutritional support via a feeding tube (nasoesophageal, pharyngostomy, esophagostomy or percutaneous gastrostomy tube) should be considered prior to surgery, particularly for patients who are debilitated (see Chs 4 and 5).[2,16]

SURGICAL TECHNIQUE

Extraction of incisor teeth

After incising the gingival epithelial attachment by inserting a scalpel blade into the gingival sulcus circumferentially around the tooth, a 1- or 2-mm luxator is gently inserted into the periodontal space on the mesial side of the incisor tooth. The luxator is advanced using gentle pressure, cutting the periodontal fibers to within two-thirds of the length of the root. The luxator is then applied in a similar fashion to the distal aspect of the root. The tooth should now be dislodged but, if necessary, the process may be repeated on the lingual side or until the entire root circumference is loosened from its periodontal attachment. Completely severing the periodontal attachment minimizes the risk of root fracture and often allows the tooth to be delivered out of the alveolus without the use of forceps.[2] If this is not the case, a root tip elevator, rather than forceps, should be used to elevate the loosened tooth from the alveolus. Unlike the elevation technique, the luxation technique does not use the adjacent alveolar bone or tooth as a fulcrum to lever out the tooth, an important factor considering the proximity of the incisors to one another and the potential for

damage to an adjacent tooth during extraction. Suturing is rarely required unless a number of adjacent incisor teeth have been extracted.

Extraction of maxillary canine teeth

After incising the gingival epithelial attachment circumferentially around the tooth and extending the incisions 2–3 mm interproximally, diverging vertical releasing incisions are made through the buccal gingiva and alveolar mucosa at the mesial and distal aspects of the tooth (Fig. 15.4A). A full-thickness mucogingival pedicle flap is elevated (Fig. 15.4B, C). The flap should be of sufficient width to allow for the suture line to rest over solid bone and not the vacated alveolus. A round bur on a high-speed dental handpiece is used to remove buccal alveolar bone if needed (Fig. 15.4D). A 2- or 3-mm luxator (Fig. 15.4E) is introduced on the mesial and distal aspects of the tooth, using firm pressure and small axial rotational movements to direct the blade apically in the periodontal space, severing the periodontal ligament fibers to within about two-thirds the length of the root.[2] Avoid placing the blade on the buccal or palatal aspects of the tooth, as slippage may easily occur, resulting in laceration of the soft tissues or penetration into the nasal cavity. After sufficient mobility has been achieved, extraction forceps are placed as far apically as

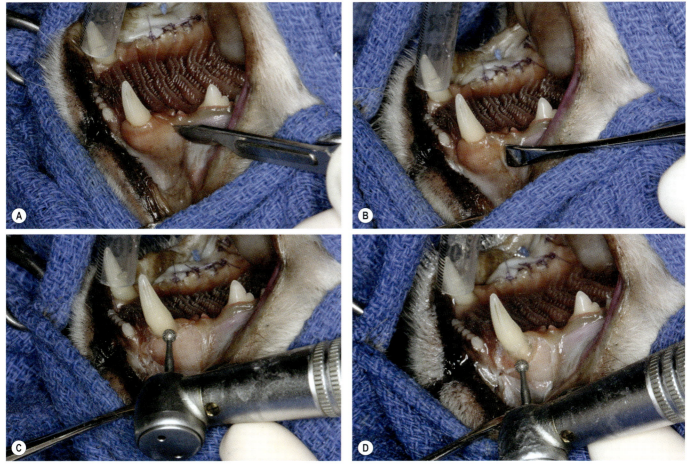

Fig. 15.4 Technique for extraction of a maxillary canine tooth, demonstrated on a cadaver specimen. (**A**) A pedicle flap is created with a #15 scalpel blade and (**B**) elevated with a periosteal elevator (**C**) to expose the buccal alveolar bone. (**D**) Buccal alveolectomy is performed using a round diamond bur on a high-speed handpiece.

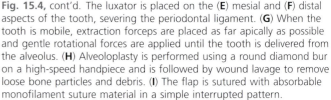

Fig. 15.4, cont'd. The luxator is placed on the (**E**) mesial and (**F**) distal aspects of the tooth, severing the periodontal ligament. (**G**) When the tooth is mobile, extraction forceps are placed as far apically as possible and gentle rotational forces are applied until the tooth is delivered from the alveolus. (**H**) Alveoloplasty is performed using a round diamond bur on a high-speed handpiece and is followed by wound lavage to remove loose bone particles and debris. (**I**) The flap is sutured with absorbable monofilament suture material in a simple interrupted pattern.

possible on the root (Fig. 15.4F), and gentle rotational and tractional forces are applied to deliver the tooth from the alveolus. If indicated, the alveolus is cleaned of debris with a small surgical curette and flushed. The alveolar margin should be smoothed with a round bur on a high-speed handpiece (Fig. 15.4G), and, if buccal bone expansion is present, additional alveolectomy may be required in order to suture the gingiva without tension (Fig. 15.4H).

After extraction of a maxillary canine tooth, it is important to verify whether a communication with the nasal cavity is present, either due to severe periodontal bone loss or avulsion of part of the alveolar process during extraction.[2] If a communication is present, special care must be taken to ensure complete closure of the extraction site. This may require removal of additional buccal bone, particularly if buccal bone expansion is present. Following removal of buccal bone and extraction of a maxillary canine tooth, entrapment of the upper lip by the ipsilateral mandibular canine tooth may occur.[2] To minimize lip trauma, odontoplasty and application of a light-cured dentinal sealer may be performed to reduce the crown height of the mandibular canine tooth by 1–2 mm. Preoperative occlusal and lateral radiographs are helpful in determining the location of the pulp cavity in relation to the cusp tip; care must be taken not to expose the pulp during odontoplasty.

Extraction of mandibular canine teeth

After incising the gingival epithelial attachment circumferentially around the tooth, the incision is extended 2–3 mm mesially and a vertical releasing incision is created at the mesial–buccal line angle of the canine tooth. Rather than creating a distal vertical releasing incision, which would transect the frenulum, an interproximal incision is made on the alveolar margin up to the mesial aspect of the third premolar tooth; this flap design keeps the lower lip frenulum intact (see Ch. 13). Partial buccal alveolectomy is performed as needed, then a 2- or 3-mm luxator is introduced on the mesial and distal aspects of the tooth. Using firm pressure and small axial rotational movements, the blade of the luxator is directed apically in the periodontal space, severing the periodontal ligament fibers to within about two-thirds the length of the root.[2] Placement of the blade on the buccal or lingual aspects of the tooth should be avoided, as this can easily result in instrument slippage and subsequent damage to the buccal or sublingual soft tissues. As with maxillary canine teeth, extraction forceps are placed as far apically as possible on the root after sufficient mobility has been achieved through luxation. Premature application of extraction forceps and excessive rotational forces may lead to fracture through the alveolar process on the lingual aspect of the tooth (see Fig. 16.5), resulting in instability between the mandible and the mandibular symphysis. Therefore, it is prudent to continue using a luxation technique and not to apply the extraction forceps until the canine tooth is mobile enough to remove with only mild tractional forces and minimal rotational forces.

Extensive removal of buccal alveolar bone may facilitate extraction of a canine tooth with evidence of ankylosis. A lingual approach for extraction of mandibular canine teeth has also been described, but was considered less applicable for cats than dogs, based on anatomical differences.[17]

Extraction of premolar and molar teeth

The maxillary second premolar and first molar teeth are usually extracted in a nonsurgical fashion, using the luxation technique described above. Because the remaining premolar teeth and the mandibular molar teeth are multirooted, a surgical approach is typically indicated, unless severe alveolar bone loss is present, in which case the tooth may be removed intact after its remaining periodontal ligament has been severed. For extraction of a single two- or three-rooted premolar tooth or the mandibular molar tooth, a triangle mucogingival flap, with a vertical releasing incision at the mesial interproximal space, is most useful. When multiple adjacent teeth are being extracted, an envelope flap typically provides adequate visualization and exposure of the buccal alveolar bone. If necessary, 1–3 mm of bone may be removed from the alveolar margin to expose the furcations prior to sectioning. A narrow, tapered bur on a high-speed handpiece is used to section the teeth, beginning at the furcation and progressing coronally, so each root may be separately extracted.

A 2- or 3-mm luxator or luxating elevator is introduced on the mesial and distal aspects of each root, using gentle pressure and small axial rotations (5–10°) to direct the blade apically in the periodontal space, cutting the periodontal attachment.[2] If desired, once some mobility has been achieved, the elevator may be placed horizontally between sectioned roots and gentle rotational pressure applied to fatigue the periodontal ligament and lift the root from the alveolus. When using the elevation technique, root fracture will occur unless extreme caution is exercised to avoid generating excessive force.

For the maxillary fourth premolar tooth, a narrow, tapered diamond bur is used perpendicular to the vertical axis of the tooth, beginning at the furcation and moving coronally, to separate the distal root from the mesiobuccal root. Some veterinarians prefer to then remove the distal root to provide better visualization when sectioning the mesiobuccal root from the palatal root, which is achieved by inserting a narrow, tapered diamond bur into the mesial furcation, at an approximately 30° angle to the vertical axis of the tooth (see Fig 14.5C). A 2-mm luxator is introduced into the periodontal ligament space on the mesial and distal aspects of the mesiobuccal root, and, if needed, extraction forceps are employed to remove the root after sufficient mobility has been achieved. Following extraction of the mesiobuccal and distal roots, the palatal root is more easily visualized, allowing access with a luxator or elevator. Additional alveolectomy may be required for optimum access to the palatal root.

For the mandibular first molar tooth, the proximity of the fourth premolar tooth may prevent adequate access to the mesial aspect of the mesial root. The luxator may be inserted into the periodontal ligament space along the mesial aspect of the mesial root in a horizontal rather than vertical manner to minimize risk of damaging the fourth premolar tooth.

Premolar–molar and full-mouth extractions

When extracting all premolar and molar teeth in a quadrant, an extended envelope flap provides sufficient exposure for good visualization of the underlying teeth and alveolar bone (Fig. 15.5A, B).[2] If indicated, some of the bone at the alveolar margin may be removed, using a round bur on a high-speed handpiece, to expose the furcation region of multirooted teeth (Fig. 15.5C). A tapered bur is then used to section multirooted teeth into single roots (Fig. 15.5D, E), each of which subsequently may be more easily removed using a combination of luxation and elevation on the mesial and distal aspects of each root (Fig. 15.5F, G). The luxator may be placed vertically (F) or horizontally (G) into the periodontal ligament space to sever the periodontal ligament fibers. However, if an elevator is placed between the sectioned fragments of a multirooted tooth (i.e., in the furcation), excessive rotational forces will result in root fracture. When using horizontal leverage, very gentle forces should be applied. Once each root is sufficiently mobile, extraction forceps are placed as far apically on the root as possible, and very gentle rotational and tractional forces are applied (Fig. 15.5G). The palatal root of the maxillary fourth premolar tooth is more easily visualized after the mesiobuccal and distal roots have been removed. If necessary, additional alveolectomy may be performed to improve visibility of the palatal root and allow proper placement of the luxator blade into the periodontal ligament space (Fig 15.5H). Following removal, each root tip should be carefully inspected. An intact root tip is rounded and usually has soft tissue attached to it at the apex. If there is any doubt as to whether the entire root has been removed, a radiograph should be made to ascertain whether a fragment remains. Unless end-stage root resorption is present, all root fragments must be removed, or recurrent inflammation may occur.[18]

If a root fracture has occurred, it is important to have good lighting and visibility before attempting removal of the remaining fragment. If fracture occurred close to the cemento-enamel junction and the remaining fragment is large, a 1- or 2-mm dental luxator or small elevator may be sufficient to loosen and remove it. Small root tips may be mobilized using root tip picks or root tip elevators, then removed with root tip forceps. It may be necessary to extend the mucogingival flap and remove more alveolar bone in order to obtain access to a small root fragment. Attempting to drill out root tips (sometimes referred to as 'pulverization' or 'atomization') can result in damage to the infraorbital or inferior alveolar arteries and nerves,

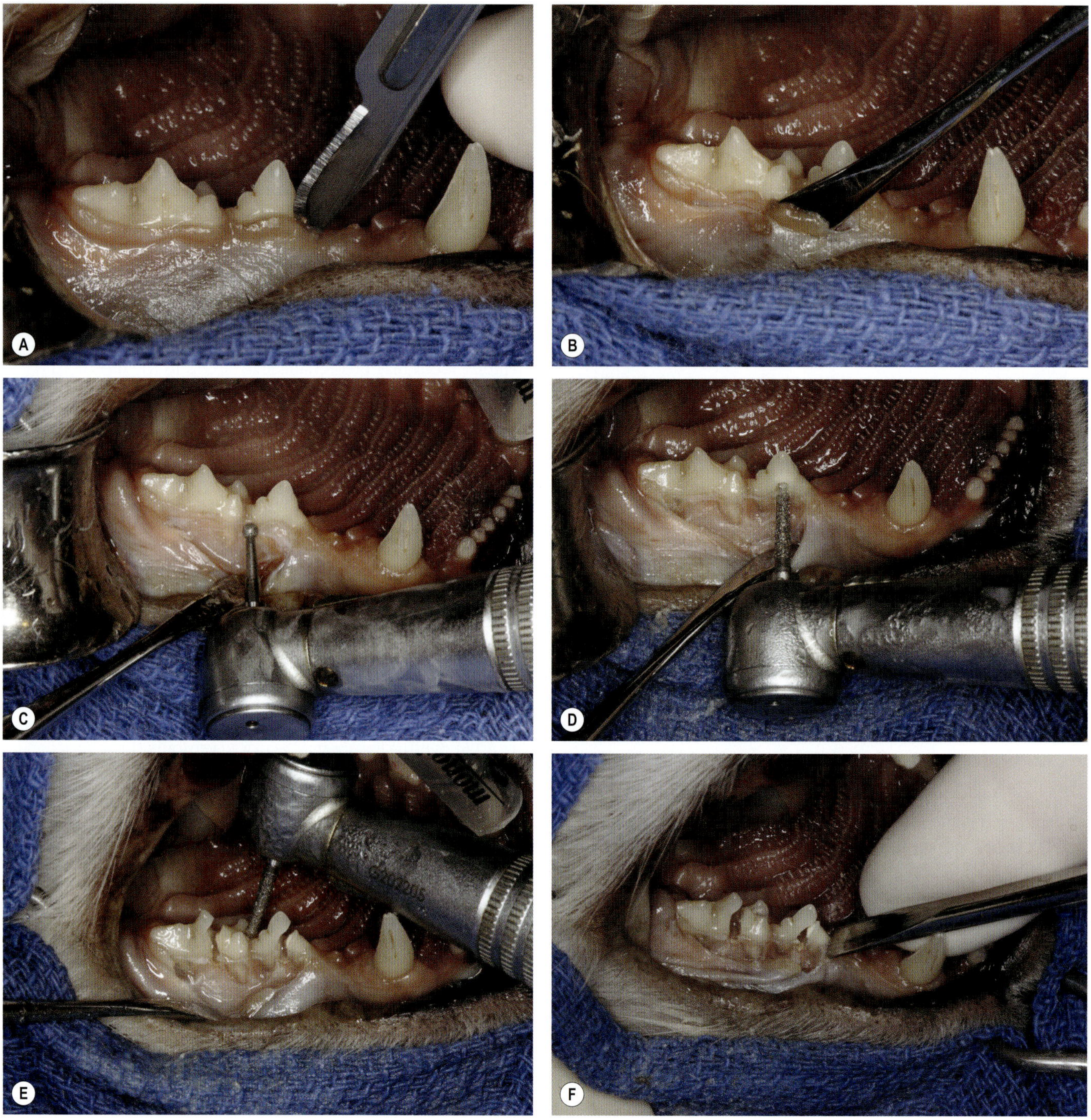

Fig. 15.5 Technique for extraction of the left maxillary third and fourth premolar teeth demonstrated on a cadaver specimen: (**A**) An envelope flap is created by inserting the blade into the gingival sulcus, beginning mesial to P3 and extending distally to P4, (**B**) A periosteal elevator is employed to elevate the full-thickness mucogingival flap from the underlying bone. (**C**) Alveolectomy is performed using a round diamond bur on a high-speed handpiece. (**D**) The teeth are sectioned using a tapered diamond bur on a high-speed handpiece. (**E**) The palatal root is separated from the mesiobuccal root using the same tapered diamond bur held almost vertically, at 30° angle to the palatal root. (**F, G**) Luxators are placed on the mesial and distal aspects of each root to sever the periodontal ligament. Luxators may be used either parallel (**F**) or perpendicular (**G**) to the root. (**H**) Extraction forceps are placed as far apically as possible on the roots, and gentle tractional and rotation forces are applied until each root is delivered from its alveolus. (**I**) The palatal root of the fourth premolar tooth is more easily visualized following removal of the mesiobuccal and distal roots. Additional alveolectomy will allow optimum visualization for proper placement of the luxator into the periodontal ligament space around the palatal root. (**J**) After all roots have been removed, alveoloplasty is performed with a round diamond bur on a high-speed handpiece to remove any sharp bony edges. (**K**) When suturing the flap, the needle should be passed entirely through the buccal gingiva prior to entering the palatal gingiva. This will minimize tearing of the gingiva. (**L**) The envelope flap has been closed without tension using absorbable monofilament suture material in a simple interrupted pattern.

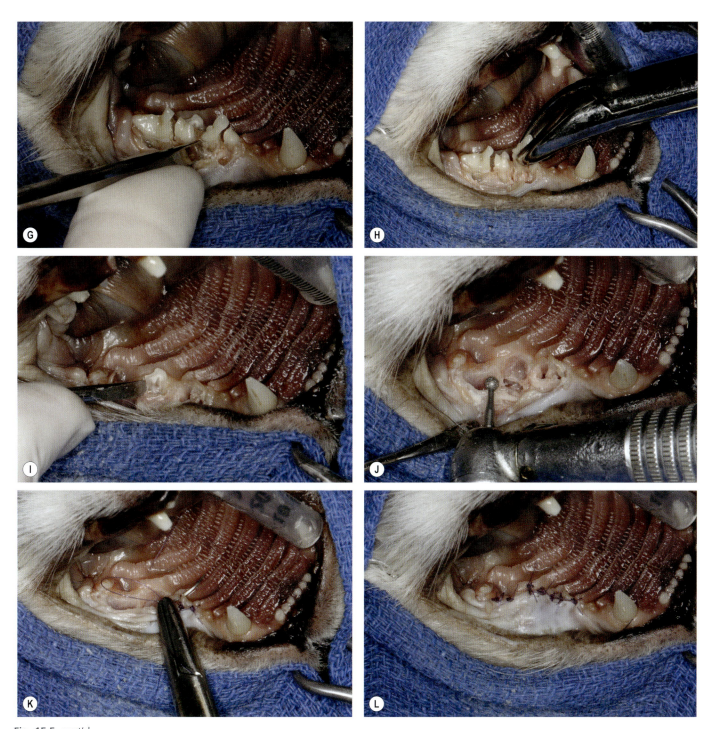

Fig. 15.5, cont'd.

fatal air embolism[19] or other iatrogenic trauma, and this technique is not recommended.

After all roots and root fragments are removed, any expanded alveolar bone is gently compressed back into position, and sharp bony edges are reduced with a round bur (Fig. 15.5I). The empty alveoli are lavaged, and the mucogingival flap is repositioned and sutured without tension (Fig. 15.5J, K).[2] Feline gingiva and mucosa may be quite friable; use of fine suture material and gentle tissue handling are recommended.

Coronectomy (crown amputation with intentional root retention)

Preoperative radiographs (Fig. 15.6A) are essential in determining whether a tooth is a good candidate for coronectomy. A gingival or mucogingival flap is elevated (Fig. 15.6B); for premolar and molar teeth, a small envelope flap is suitable. To achieve tension-free closure following coronectomy of a canine tooth, a triangle flap is indicated. Amputation of the crown is performed at the level of the alveolar

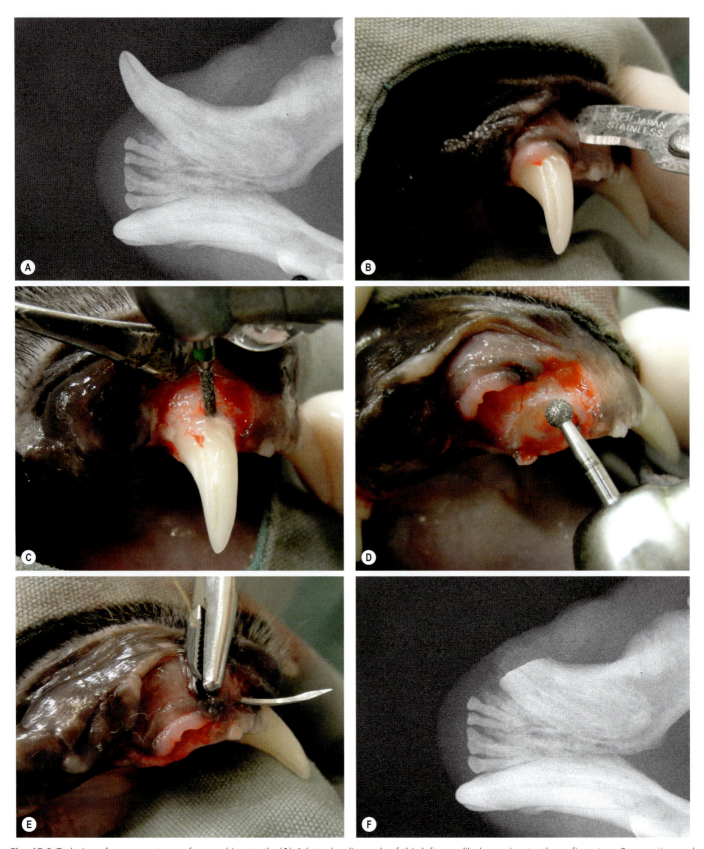

Fig. 15.6 Technique for coronectomy of a resorbing tooth. (**A**) A lateral radiograph of this left mandibular canine tooth confirms type-2 resorption and no evidence of periodontitis or endodontic disease, making this tooth a good candidate for coronectomy. (**B**) With the patient in dorsal recumbency, a triangle flap is created and elevated. (**C**) Using a tissue retractor to prevent trauma to the flap, a tapered diamond bur is used to amputate the crown at the level of the alveolar margin. (**D**) A small round diamond bur is used to perform alveoloplasty. (**E**) Closure with absorbable monofilament suture material in a simple interrupted pattern. (**F**) A postoperative radiograph confirms that there are no sharp edges of the tooth and documents the condition of the root following the procedure.

margin, using a taper or round bur on a high-speed handpiece (Fig. 15.6C). Any sharp bony edges are removed with a round bur on a high-speed handpiece (Fig. 15.6D), the surgical site is irrigated, and the gingiva is sutured over the remaining roots (Fig. 15.6E).[7] Postextraction radiographs (Fig. 15.6F) should routinely be obtained in these cases.

POSTOPERATIVE CARE AND ASSESSMENT

Pain management

Preemptive analgesia, with use of a balanced anesthesia technique and local or regional anesthesia, will help ensure a more comfortable postoperative period for patients undergoing extractions (see Ch. 4). For pain management at home following routine extractions, buprenorphine may be dispensed. Oral mucosal administration of buprenorphine is easy for clients to perform, well tolerated by cats, and results in similar plasma concentrations as intramuscular or intravenous injection of buprenorphine.[20]

Although at this time there are no nonsteroidal antiinflammatory drugs (NSAIDs) approved for oral use in cats by the Food and Drug Administration, short-term use of NSAIDs may be beneficial following extractions, particularly when significant inflammation is present. However, because NSAIDs impair renal autoregulation under conditions of hypotension, these drugs should be avoided in patients with pre-existing renal insufficiency or those who have had perioperative hypotensive episodes.[21] For cats undergoing full-mouth or premolar–molar extractions, if a fentanyl patch is to be employed, it should be placed either prior to or during surgery. Because adequate blood levels of fentanyl are not achieved until 12–24 hours after placement, injectable opioids (pure agonists rather than mixed agonist–antagonists) should be administered postoperatively if the patch is placed at the time of surgery (see Ch. 4).

Nutritional support

Most cats will eat readily following dental extractions, provided excessive tissue trauma has not occurred and analgesia has been adequate. For debilitated patients with severe oral inflammation and multiple anticipated extractions, a feeding tube (nasoesophageal, pharyngostomy, esophagostomy or percutaneous gastrostomy tube) should be placed at the time of the procedure to ensure sufficient caloric intake following surgery (see Ch. 5).

Postoperative assessment

The client should be instructed to observe the patient for lethargy, inappetence, or halitosis, and the patient should be examined 1–2 weeks following the procedure to evaluate healing. For long-term assessment of resorbing teeth on which coronectomy was performed, radiographs should be obtained when the patient is anesthetized for future dental care.

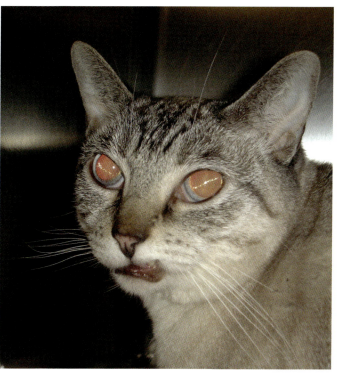

Fig. 15.7 Entrapment of the upper lip by the left mandibular canine tooth following extraction of the left maxillary canine tooth.

COMPLICATIONS

Complications for extractions are discussed in Chapter 16. Common complications in the cat include root fractures and trauma to adjacent tissues. If extraction forceps are employed prematurely or with excessive force, sections of the buccal or lingual alveolar bone may be inadvertently removed with the extracted tooth. If this occurs when extracting a maxillary canine tooth, a communication between the nasal and oral cavities results, which can lead to permanent oronasal fistula formation if proper flap closure is not achieved. Less common complications include dislodging root fragments into the mandibular canal or nasal passages, fracture through the lingual alveolus of a mandibular canine resulting in mandibular symphyseal instability and orbital penetration.[11] Most complications can be avoided with proper instrumentation and careful technique.

A common postoperative complication is maxillary lip entrapment by the mandibular canine tooth following removal of expansile buccal bone to facilitate closure of a maxillary canine tooth extraction site (Fig. 15.7). As previously mentioned, this can be prevented by removing 1–2 mm of the cusp tip of the mandibular canine tooth.

REFERENCES

1. Wolf HF, Rateitschak EM, Rateitschak KH, et al. Furcation involvement – furcation treatment. In: Wolf HF, Rateitschak EM, Rateitschak KH, et al, editors. Color atlas of dental medicine: periodontology. 3rd ed. Stuttgart: Thieme Verlag; 2005. p. 381–96.

2. Verstraete FJ. Exodontics. In: Slatter DG, editor. Textbook of small animal surgery. 3rd ed. Philadelphia: WB Saunders; 2003. p. 2696–709.

3. Reiter AM, Mendoza KA. Feline odontoclastic resorptive lesions an unsolved enigma in veterinary dentistry. Vet Clin North Am Small Anim Pract 2002;32:791–837.

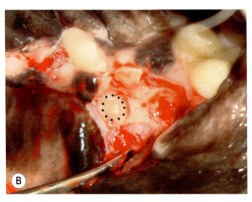
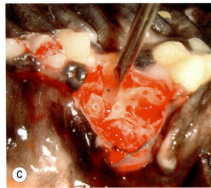

Fig. 16.1 (**A**) Following removal of buccal alveolar bone, (**B**) a tapered diamond bur is employed to create a 'trough' around the fractured mesiobuccal root fragment (*dotted line*) of the right maxillary fourth premolar tooth of a dog. (**C**) This provides room for placement of a narrow-bladed luxator to facilitate removal of the root fragment.

based on auditory and tactile stimuli: a cracking sound is typically heard, and, when the tooth is removed, the root end is sharp and jagged rather than smooth and rounded.[6] If the fracture occurs towards the coronal aspect of the root, visibility may be sufficient to insert a 1.3-mm 'luxating elevator' (Cislak Manufacturing, Inc., Niles, IL 60714) or 2-mm (JS Dental Manufacturing, Inc., Ridgefield, CT 06877) luxator into the periodontal ligament space and continue the extraction attempt. However, if the root fractures deep within the alveolus, visibility and the ability to place an instrument into the periodontal ligament space are significantly diminished. In these situations, radiography is very helpful in determining the location, size, and morphology of the root fragment. 'Blind' attempts to extract a root fragment which cannot be visualized will cause significant damage to the surrounding bone, and may result in dislodgement of the root fragment into the mandibular canal, nasal cavity, or maxillary sinus. Instead, additional bone removal should be performed; the combination of alveolectomy and judicious use of the air–water syringe will greatly improve visibility and access.[7] The use of magnification loupes is also extremely helpful in recognizing the root–bone interface. Once the root is visualized, a very small luxator such as a 1.3-mm 'luxating elevator' (Cislak Manufacturing, Inc., Niles, IL 60714), 1- and 2-mm luxators (JS Dental Manufacturing, Inc., Ridgefield, CT 06877) may be inserted into the periodontal ligament space to sever the remaining attachment and allow retrieval of the fragment. For more difficult cases, such as ankylosed roots, in which it is impossible to insert a luxator into the periodontal ligament space, a small round diamond bur (#1/2) or a tapered diamond bur may be used to create space around the root fragment for placement of the instrument (Fig. 16.1).[7]

Failure to remove root fragments, particularly those from teeth with pre-existing endodontic disease, will lead to continued inflammation in the surrounding tissues, which may result in osteomyelitis, draining tracts and chronic pain.[8,9] If attempts to remove root fragments are unsuccessful, radiographs should be obtained to document the location and size of the fragments, the client should be informed, and referral to a veterinary dentist should be offered in the interest of providing the best care for the patient.

Displacement of a root or root tip into the mandibular canal, nasal cavity or maxillary recess

This complication arises when the periapical bone is compromised, or when excessive apical force is employed during an extraction attempt (Fig. 16.2). In order to avoid displacing a root through its alveolus into the mandibular canal, nasal cavity or maxillary recess,

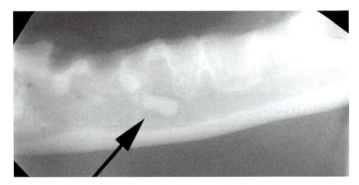

Fig. 16.2 The mesial root (*arrow*) of the mandibular fourth premolar tooth in a cat has been displaced into the mandibular canal during attempts to extract it.

the operator should carefully plan each extraction based on radiographic and clinical evaluation. Elevation of a mucogingival flap and adequate bone removal will facilitate extraction and prevent this complication. If a root fragment is displaced but still visible or accessible through the surgical site, the fragment should be carefully removed using a plain Adson forceps or a narrow-beaked extraction forceps (FX-49 forceps, Hu-Friedy, Chicago, IL 60618).

If the root tip cannot be removed with the surgical technique immediately after the complication arises, attempts to find the fragment with various instruments must be avoided as damage to nearby vessels and nerves would be more detrimental than leaving the root in place.[1,2] Radiographs should be obtained to document the root's location, and the client should be informed of the complication. If the pet demonstrates signs of pain or paresthesia such as pawing at or rubbing the face following the procedure, referral to an experienced veterinary oral surgeon should be offered.

The client should be advised to observe the patient for nasal discharge, and to report persistent sneezing or nasal discharge promptly. Although rare, a root tip in the nasal cavity may become a sequestrum (Fig. 16.3), in which case rhinotomy should be performed to remove the root fragment.

Soft tissue injuries

The most common soft tissue injury is tearing of the mucogingival flap during surgical extraction. This usually results from an attempt to be conservative with the flap size, and the flap is retracted beyond

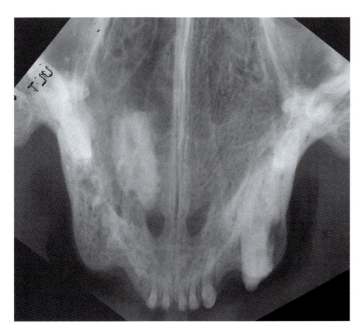

Fig. 16.3 The root of this cat's right maxillary canine tooth had been dislodged into the nasal cavity during an attempt to extract the tooth 2 years previously. Following rhinotomy to remove the root, the cat's chronic mucopurulent nasal discharge resolved.

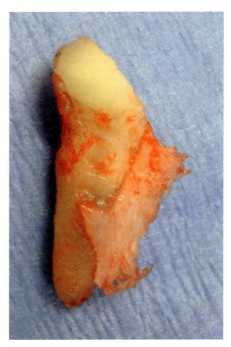

Fig. 16.4 This extracted mesiobuccal root of a maxillary fourth premolar tooth has a significant amount of buccal bone attached, indicating that the extraction forceps were applied too early in the process and excessive force was used to free the tooth.

the tissue's ability to stretch.[1] It may also occur if the tissues are friable and gentle technique is not employed. This complication can largely be avoided by the creation of a large enough mucogingival flap and careful elevation beginning at the attached gingiva. If a tear does occur, the flap should be gently repositioned following the surgery. In most cases, suturing the tear will result in adequate but delayed healing.[1]

Trauma to the cheeks and lips from a bur may occur if these tissues are not adequately retracted prior to introduction of the high-speed handpiece into the oral cavity. These injuries can largely be avoided with the help of an assistant and tissue retractors such as a Cawood–Minnesota retractor.

Puncture wounds of the soft tissues may occur if excessive force is employed during extraction attempts and the luxator or elevator slips. Commonly injured areas are the ventral mandible (e.g., when the luxator slips over the buccal bone during attempts to extract a mandibular canine tooth) and the palate (when attempting to extract the palatal root of the maxillary fourth premolar tooth). The most severe puncture injuries involve orbital penetration during extraction of maxillary molar teeth, resulting in severe ocular infection and necessitating enucleation.[10,11] This can be avoided by careful positioning of the luxator or elevator between the tooth and bone on the mesial and distal (rather than buccal and lingual) aspects of the tooth, and use of finesse rather than force during extractions.

Fracture of the alveolar process

This complication may occur if extraction movements are abrupt and awkward, if extraction forceps are used prematurely, or if there is ankylosis, and part of the alveolar bone (usually buccal) is removed together with the tooth (Fig. 16.4). When the fragment of bone is attached to and removed with the tooth, the remaining bone edges of the empty alveolus are smoothed with a round diamond bur prior to suturing the flap. If the fractured portion of the alveolar bone is separated from the tooth but remains attached to the periosteum, it can

be repositioned with the flap and should be stable after the flap is sutured.[2]

Prevention of this complication is achieved by adequate assessment of the tooth and its alveolus via intraoral radiographs, and by controlled removal of alveolar bone (using a round diamond bur on a dental handpiece with continuous irrigation) prior to luxation or elevation, and avoiding use of extraction forceps prior to sufficient loosening of the tooth by luxation and/or elevation.[1]

Fracture of an instrument in the tissues

Instrument fracture is uncommon, but may result from excessive force during luxation or elevation, incorrect use of luxators as elevators, and use of burs for multiple procedures. If the fractured metal fragments are visible, they are carefully removed from the tissues. Radiographs are obtained to confirm complete removal or to identify additional fragments. After radiographic localization, the broken pieces are removed surgically at the same time as the remaining roots.[2]

Fracture of the crown of an adjacent tooth

If adjacent teeth are used as a fulcrum during elevation attempts, fracture of these teeth may occur. If the fracture is superficial and does not involve pulp, the fracture edges are smoothed (odontoplasty) and a light-cured dentinal sealer is applied. If pulp is exposed, the affected tooth must be treated endodontically (with vital pulp therapy or root canal treatment) or extracted. This complication can be avoided by not using adjacent teeth for leverage during extraction attempts.

Mandibular fracture

Anecdotal information suggests that fracture of the mandible during attempts to extract a mandibular canine or first molar tooth is a fairly common occurrence in veterinary practice. At the mandibular

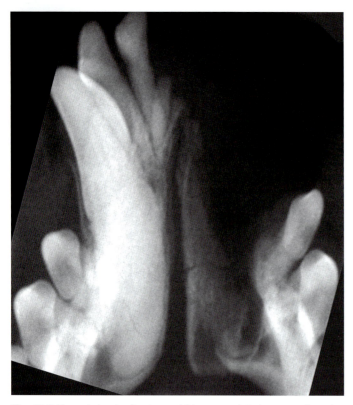

Fig. 16.5 Lingual alveolar fracture, which occurred during extraction of the left mandibular canine tooth.

canine of small dogs and cats, the lingual alveolar bone is often no more than 2–3 mm thick, and premature use of extraction forceps in a twisting manner results in fracture through the lingual alveolus (Fig. 16.5). The operator is typically aware of the fracture, because following removal of the tooth, there appears to be significant instability of the mandibular symphysis. In actuality, the symphysis is intact, but the fractured lingual alveolar bone just caudal to the symphysis results in a similar feeling of independent movement of both mandibles. Stability can be achieved with a circumferential wire around the rostral mandibles, much like that used for symphyseal separation, but at the level of the mesial aspect of the third premolar tooth (being careful not to injury the sublingual and mandibular salivary ducts when tightening the wire). If sufficient teeth are present, the use of an intraoral composite splint may be considered. Placement of a bone graft is not mandatory but may help speed the healing process.

When significant periodontal bone loss exists at the mandibular first molar teeth, fracture of the mandibular body may occur during extraction attempts. Preoperative radiographs will help identify patients at risk of this complication, and alternatives to extraction, such as periodontal surgery and guided bone regeneration[12] or hemisection and root canal treatment of the remaining root,[13] should be considered. If a fracture occurs, the extraction should be completed and a muzzle applied postoperatively. Once tissues have healed, further fracture treatment planning can be performed. Use of internal fixation techniques and placement of a bone graft (OsteoAllograft, Veterinary Transplant Services, Inc., Kent, WA 98032) may allow healing, but the clients should be informed that the severe preexisting periodontal disease in this location may delay healing. If nonunion occurs, additional extractions and the placement of a plate may be required to achieve stability.

Nerve damage

The branches of the trigeminal nerve, including the inferior alveolar nerve, mental nerves, lingual nerve, and infraorbital nerve, are the structures most likely to be damaged during extraction attempts.[1] Nerve injury may occur secondary to local anesthesia, during creation of an incision that extends to the region of the mental or infraorbital foramen, when bone near a nerve is heated excessively due to inadequate irrigation during burring, or during removal of root fragments in or near the mandibular canal. Damage may consist of temporary interruption of nerve conduction (neuropraxia), degeneration of nerve axons (axonotmesis), or permanent interruption of nerve conduction (neurotmesis).[2] Signs of neuropraxia (sensory disturbances such as burning sensation, pins and needles, or numbness) usually resolve within a few days to weeks. Signs of axonotmesis are similar but of longer duration, lasting 6–8 weeks, with the potential for permanent sensory deficits. The most serious nerve damage, neurotmesis, can be produced by ischemia due to prolonged compression, excessive traction on the associated soft tissues, or severance of the nerve fibers, and may result in permanent paresthesia or anesthesia.[2]

If patients exhibit signs of persistent pain postoperatively (hiding, pawing at the face, difficulty prehending or masticating food, or reluctance to groom for more than 1 week after surgery) the extraction site should be examined clinically and radiographically. If there are no root fragments and the soft tissues have healed uneventfully, neuropathic pain should be considered. Although not FDA approved for use in dogs or cats, gabapentin has been used successfully for the management of neuropathic pain in dogs[14] and there is anecdotal information supporting its use in cats.[15]

Air embolism

The use of air–water syringes and air-driven dental handpieces, while facilitating sectioning of teeth and removal of alveolar bone and allowing continuous fluid irrigation of the tissues, presents the possibility of introducing air into blood vessels,[16–18] which can be fatal.[19–21] Therefore, caution must be exercised when using the air–water syringe or high-speed handpieces, particularly in close proximity to vessels whose integrity may have been compromised by trauma from the extraction procedure.

POSTOPERATIVE COMPLICATIONS

Swelling

Postoperative swelling (Fig. 16.6) may occur secondary to traumatic extraction techniques or excessive compression of tissues resulting in obstruction of lymph vessels.[2] When patient compliance permits, cold compresses may be applied for 10–15 minutes every half hour for the first 4–6 hours after surgery.[2] Administration of nonsteroidal antiinflammatory medications (if not contraindicated based on the patient's medical history and/or perioperative anesthetic complications) may help minimize the severity of the swelling and its associated discomfort.

Pain

All patients undergoing oral surgery should receive analgesics. As discussed in Chapter 4, administration of analgesics and the use of local anesthetics prior to beginning extractions will help prevent 'wind-up' and will decrease the incidence and severity of postoperative pain. In addition, gentle tissue handling, complete tooth extraction,

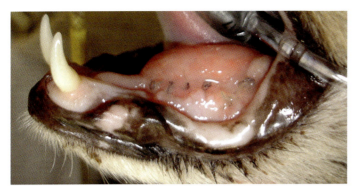

Fig. 16.6 Sublingual swelling following extraction of mandibular premolar and molar teeth in a cat.

and smoothing of the alveolar bone (alveoloplasty) prior to suturing the gingiva will result in a more comfortable patient than one who has tooth fragments protruding through gingiva, rough bone edges, and extraction sites left open to heal by second intention.

When postoperative pain is evident (demonstrated by inactivity, hiding, pawing at the face, reluctance to groom, difficulty eating and/ or reluctance to eat), it must be addressed. Coadministration of opioids and nonsteroidal antiinflammatory medications should be considered. The use of liquid medications or those which do not require manipulation of the oral cavity (such as transdermal fentanyl patches) may facilitate administration and improve compliance. In severe cases, placement of an esophagostomy tube may be required to allow delivery of medications and to ensure adequate nutrition.

Infection

Infection of extraction sites may result from failure to sufficiently reduce oral bacteria by cleaning the teeth before commencing extractions, use of improperly sterilized instruments,[2] and failure to remove debris from surgical sites prior to closure.[1] Patients with severe periodontal disease, active periapical infections or systemic diseases likely to cause immunosuppression should receive antibiotics intravenously at the time of surgery and, in some cases, postoperatively (by oral administration). The use of antibiotics and antiseptics is discussed in Chapter 3.

Delayed healing or wound dehiscence

There are a number of factors influencing healing of an extraction site. Systemic factors causing delayed healing include diabetes mellitus, hyperadrenocorticism, and chronic corticosteroid administration. Local factors such as presence of infection, sharp alveolar bone edges or protruding root remnants may also delay or prevent healing. In addition, tension on the gingival flap, caused by insufficient elevation of the periosteum, will lead to dehiscence.[1,2]

Although it has a reported incidence of up to 4% following routine dental extractions in humans,[22] 'dry socket,' or alveolar osteitis, appears to occur very rarely in dogs[23] and has never been reported in cats. In humans, the suspected etiology is loss of the clot in the alveolus due to increased fibrinolysis (which may result from trauma during the extraction), and estrogens may play a role.[22,24] Although alveolar osteitis is an unlikely complication after extraction, overzealous curettage of the postextraction alveolus should be avoided, and a clot should remain prior to closure of extraction sites.

As mentioned in Chapter 15, the presence of buccal bone expansion may complicate extraction of canine teeth in cats. Expansion of the

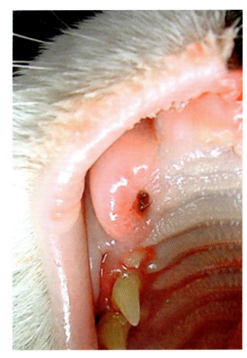

Fig. 16.7 Nonsurgical extraction of this cat's right maxillary canine tooth, with expansion of the buccal alveolar bone due to periodontitis resulted in delayed healing.

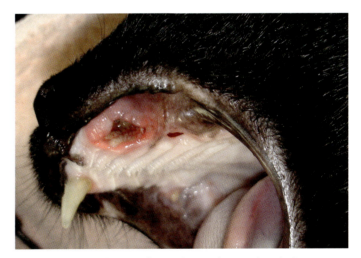

Fig. 16.8 A nonhealing maxillary canine tooth extraction site in a cat, which was diagnosed as squamous cell carcinoma following biopsy of the soft tissues surrounding the site.

buccal alveolar bone is typically associated with vertical bone loss[25] and, if nonsurgical extraction of affected canine teeth is performed, healing may be delayed (Fig 16.7). Unless a flap is elevated, the expanded buccal bone removed, and the alveolus debrided of diseased epithelium, the extraction site will heal by second intention, which may take several weeks.

A common cause of nonhealing extraction sites in cats is neoplasia (Fig. 16.8). Often, teeth found to be 'loose' at the time of routine dental cleaning are extracted without preoperative radiographs or dental charting to determine the underlying cause of the increased mobility. When the patient returns with a painful, nonhealing extraction site 1–2 weeks after surgery, biopsy may reveal the true cause of the mobile teeth, which is most often squamous cell carcinoma. Any nonhealing extraction site should be radiographed and biopsied prior to attempts to resuture the wound.

Occlusal trauma

Particularly in cats, entrapment of the upper lip by the mandibular canine tooth may occur following extraction of a maxillary canine tooth (see Fig. 15.8).[26] This can largely be prevented by reducing the crown height of the ipsilateral mandibular canine tooth, as discussed in Chapter 15. Crown height reduction of the mandibular premolars and molar teeth may also be indicated to reduce occlusal trauma to the maxillary soft tissues following extraction of all maxillary premolar and molar teeth in the cat.

Oronasal communication and fistula

Small, dolichocephalic breeds, such as toy and miniature poodles and miniature dachshunds, appear to be predisposed to develop severe vertical bone loss at the palatal aspects of the maxillary canine teeth. A connection between the oral and nasal cavities may result, with the pocket epithelium on the palatal aspect of the maxillary canine tooth becoming continuous with the palatal mucosa on one side of the maxillary bone and the nasal mucosa on the other. If the maxillary canine teeth are nonsurgically extracted, or if the surgical extraction does not include removal of the palatal pocket epithelium, an oronasal fistula will become evident within a few weeks after the procedure (Fig. 16.9). Sneezing after eating or drinking, nasal discharge, and face rubbing may be observed. Chronic exposure of the nasal cavity to oral bacteria will lead to rhinitis, destruction of nasal turbinates, and may result in pneumonia. Therefore, oronasal fistulas should be addressed as soon as possible after diagnosis. For small fistulae, single-flap repair[27] may be sufficient for closure. For larger fistulae, double-flap repair[28] or use of an auricular cartilage graft[29] should be considered.

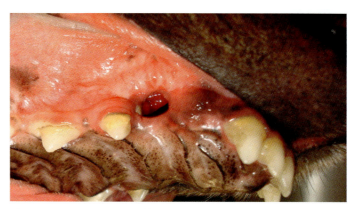

Fig. 16.9 Persistent oronasal fistula after extraction of the right maxillary canine tooth from a miniature dachshund several months previously.

Alveolar margin recession

Following extraction of large teeth such as canine teeth and mandibular first molar teeth, atrophy of the maxilla or mandible may occur. Bone grafting techniques may prevent or reduce the severity of recession of the alveolar margin.[30,31] Selection of appropriate materials for placement in the alveolus following extraction is discussed in Chapter 11.

SUMMARY

Most peri- and postoperative complications can be prevented by careful surgical planning, which includes a thorough review of the patient's medical history, complete physical examination and comprehensive oral evaluation including preoperative intraoral radiographs. When complications do arise, honest communication with the client and immediate attempts to remedy the situation will allow the continued delivery of optimum patient care.

REFERENCES

1. Peterson LJ. Prevention and management of surgical complications. In: Peterson LJ, Ellis III E, Hupp HR, et al, editors. Contemporary oral and maxillofacial surgery. 4th ed. St. Louis: Mosby; 2003. p. 221–35.

2. Fragiskos FD. Perioperative and postoperative complications. In: Fragiskos FD, editor. Oral surgery. Berlin & Heidelberg: Springer-Verlag; 2007. p. 181–203.

3. Boudreaux MK, Reinhart GA, Vaughn DM, et al. The effects of varying dietary n-6 to n-3 fatty acid ratios on platelet reactivity, coagulation screening assays, and antithrombin III activity in dogs. J Am Anim Hosp Assoc 1997;33: 235–43.

4. Casali RE, Hale JA, LeNarz L, et al. Improved graft patency associated with altered platelet function induced by marine fatty acids in dogs. J Surg Res 1986;40:6–12.

5. Cerbone AM, Cirillo F, Coppola A, et al. Persistent impairment of platelet aggregation following cessation of a short-course dietary supplementation of moderate amounts of N-3 fatty acid ethyl esters. Thromb Haemost 1999;82: 128–33.

6. DeBowes LJ. Simple and surgical exodontia. Vet Clin North Am Small Anim Pract 2005;35:963–84.

7. Woodward TM. Extraction of fractured tooth roots. J Vet Dent 2006;23:126–9.

8. Yeoh SC, MacMahon S, Schifter M. Chronic suppurative osteomyelitis of the mandible: case report. Aust Dent J 2005; 50:200–3.

9. Bowles WH, Daniel RE. Reevaluation of submerged vital roots. J Am Dent Assoc 1983;107:429–32.

10. Smith MM, Smith EM, La CN, et al. Orbital penetration associated with tooth extraction. J Vet Dent 2003;20:8–17.

11. Ramsey DT, Marretta SM, Hamor RE, et al. Ophthalmic manifestations and complications of dental disease in dogs and cats. J Am Anim Hosp Assoc 1996; 32:215–24.

12. Beckman BW. Treatment of an infrabony pocket in an American Eskimo dog. J Vet Dent 2004;21:159–63.

13. Reiter AM, Lewis JR, Rawlinson JE, et al. Hemisection and partial retention of carnassial teeth in client-owned dogs. J Vet Dent 2005;22:216–26.

14. Cashmore RG, Harcourt-Brown TR, Freeman PM, et al. Clinical diagnosis and treatment of suspected neuropathic pain in three dogs. Aust Vet J 2009;87: 45–50.

15. Robertson SA. Managing pain in feline patients. Vet Clin North Am Small Anim Pract 2008;38:1267–90, vi.

16. Burrowes P, Wallace C, Davies JM, et al. Pulmonary edema as a radiologic

manifestation of venous air embolism secondary to dental implant surgery. Chest 1992;101:561–2.

17. Davies JM, Campbell LA. Fatal air embolism during dental implant surgery: a report of three cases. Can J Anaesth 1990;37:112–21.

18. Magni G, Imperiale C, Rosa G, et al. Nonfatal cerebral air embolism after dental surgery. Anesth Analg 2008;106: 249–51.

19. Gunew M, Marshall R, Lui M, et al. Fatal venous air embolism in a cat undergoing dental extractions. J Small Anim Pract 2008;49:601–4.

20. Ober CP, Spotswood TC, Hancock R. Fatal venous air embolism in a cat with a retropharyngeal diverticulum. Vet Radiol Ultrasound 2006;47:153–8.

21. Thayer GW, Carrig CB, Evans AT. Fatal venous air embolism associated with pneumocystography in a cat. J Am Vet Med Assoc 1980;176:643–5.

22. Noroozi AR, Philbert RF. Modern concepts in understanding and management of the 'dry socket' syndrome: comprehensive review of the literature. Oral Surg Oral Med Oral Pathol Oral Radiol Endod 2009;107:30–5.

23. Van Cauwelaert de WS. Alveolar osteitis (dry socket) in a dog: a case report. J Vet Dent 1998;15:85–7.

24. Houston JP, McCollum J, Pietz D, et al. Alveolar osteitis: a review of its etiology, prevention, and treatment modalities. Gen Dent 2002;50:457–63.

25. Lommer MJ, Verstraete FJ. Radiographic patterns of periodontitis in cats: 147 cases (1998–1999). J Am Vet Med Assoc 2001; 218:230–4.

26. Verstraete FJ. Exodontics. In: Slatter DG, editor. Textbook of small animal surgery. 3rd ed. Philadelphia: WB Saunders; 2003. p. 2696–709.

27. Marretta SM, Smith MM. Single mucoperiosteal flap for oronasal fistula repair. J Vet Dent 2005;22:200–5.

28. van de Wetering A. Repair of an oronasal fistula using a double flap technique. J Vet Dent 2005;22:243–5.

29. Soukup JW, Snyder CJ, Gengler WR. Free auricular cartilage autograft for repair of an oronasal fistula in a dog. J Vet Dent 2009;26:86–95.

30. DeForge DH. Evaluation of Bioglass/ PerioGlas (Consil) synthetic bone graft particulate in the dog and cat. J Vet Dent 1997;14:141–5.

31. Wiggs RB, Lobprise HB, Mitchell PQ. Oral and periodontal tissue: maintenance, augmentation, rejuvenation and regeneration. Vet Clin North Am Small Anim Prac 1998;28:1165–88.

Chapter | 17 |

Principles of periodontal surgery

Cecilia E. Gorrel & Fraser A. Hale

DEFINITIONS

Attached gingiva: the portion of the gingiva that is apical to the gingival sulcus – this is the gingiva that is physically attached to the cementum and alveolar bone by means of the junctional epithelium and the connective tissue attachment[1]

Biologic width: the physiologic dimension of the junctional epithelium and connective tissue attachment (see surgical anatomy and Fig. 21.1)[3,4]

Cause-related periodontal therapy: therapy targeting the cause of periodontal disease, i.e., plaque, and consisting of professional periodontal therapy (removal of dental deposits) and establishing proper home care techniques, followed by regular professional maintenance therapy

Connective tissue attachment: apical (toward the root tip) to the junctional epithelium and ending at the margin of the alveolar bone, connective tissue fibers from the gingiva insert directly into the cementum of the supra-alveolar root to form the connective tissue attachment[1–3]

Free gingiva: the most coronal portion of the gingiva that is not attached to the tooth and that makes up the soft tissue wall of the gingival sulcus (Fig. 17.1)

Gingival recession: the gradual loss of gingival tissue as the free gingival margin migrates apically while the mucogingival junction remains unmoved[6]

Gingival sulcus: shallow potential space or groove surrounding each tooth, lined by tooth structure on one side and sulcular epithelium on the other side – normal sulcus depth is 0.5–1 mm in small dogs, 1–3 mm in medium and large dogs, and 0.5–1 mm in cats

Gingivitis: plaque-induced inflammation limited to the gingiva

Infrabony pocket: periodontal pocket whose base (level of epithelial attachment) is apical to the alveolar margin, and which occurs in conjunction with vertical bone loss

Junctional epithelium: the unkeratinized, highly permeable epithelium at the bottom of the sulcus, which forms the epithelial attachment to the tooth surface[1]

New attachment: formation of new cementum with inserting collagen fibers on a root surface deprived of its periodontal ligament tissue[7,8]

Periodontal pocket: increased probing depth due to the apical (towards the root apex) migration of the level of epithelial attachment

Periodontal probing depth: distance from the free gingival margin to the base of the sulcus or periodontal pocket, measured with a graduated periodontal probe[5]

Periodontal surgery; surgical techniques aimed at removing the predisposing factors and inciting causes of periodontitis, and preserving or regenerating the periodontium

Periodontitis: plaque-induced inflammation of the periodontium, resulting in various combinations of progressive gingival recession, destruction of periodontal ligament and alveolar bone (attachment loss)

Periodontium: the attachment apparatus of the tooth, consisting of gingiva, periodontal ligament, cementum and alveolar bone

Pseudopocket: increased probing depth due to the coronal (toward the crown tip) migration of the free gingival margin due to gingival enlargement

Reattachment: the reunion of surrounding soft tissue and a root surface with preserved periodontal ligament tissue[7,8]

Regeneration: reformation of cementum, periodontal ligament and alveolar bone[8]

Suprabony pocket: periodontal pocket whose base (level of epithelial attachment) is coronal to the alveolar margin, and which occurs in conjunction with horizontal bone loss

PREOPERATIVE CONCERNS

Treatment planning in the management of periodontal disease requires careful consideration of many factors.[6,9,10] These factors can be divided into three broad categories, namely, the client, the patient and the environment.[10]

© 2012 Elsevier Ltd
DOI: 10.1016/B978-0-7020-4618-6.00017-8

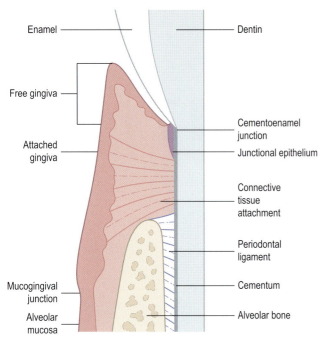

Fig. 17.1 Cross-sectional depiction of the periodontal tissues near the junction of the crown and root of the tooth.

Enamel

Free gingiva

Attached gingiva

Mucogingival junction

Alveolar mucosa

Dentin

Cementoenamel junction

Junctional epithelium

Connective tissue attachment

Periodontal ligament

Cementum

Alveolar bone

Client

Regardless of the condition presented, it is the client who must present the animal for initial treatment and for follow-up care, provide all postsurgical care and daily home care, and pay for the professional services provided. While the surgeon might have a desire to perform advanced procedures to save periodontally compromised teeth, the client's wishes, expectations, capabilities and limitations must be considered. If there are any barriers (financial, physical, motivational) that would stand in the way of the postsurgical care necessary for the long-term success of a surgical plan, then an alternate plan, such as extraction, is indicated.[6,10]

Some clients will request that no extractions be performed regardless of the level of disease. The surgeon must ensure that whatever treatment is performed is in the best *medical* interest of the patient. To perform advanced periodontal surgery on a nonsalvageable tooth, or failure to extract teeth with a hopeless prognosis in order to please the client is not in the patient's best interest and should be considered unethical. It is the surgeon's responsibility to help the client understand the realities of periodontal disease and to obtain informed consent to perform those procedures that will maximize the patient's periodontal health, even if that means extraction.

Patient – health status

Periodontal evaluation, surgery and maintenance therapy all require general anesthesia. If there is reason to suspect that the patient's health will be declining or the anesthetic risk increasing significantly or rapidly, then developing a plan that relies for its success on repeated anesthetics for maintenance therapy would be inappropriate.

Systemic or metabolic disease that would interfere with the long-term success of the treatment plan is also a contraindication for periodontal surgery. There is a negative synergy between periodontal disease and diabetes mellitus in that diabetic patients have a higher risk for the development of periodontal disease, and the stress on the body imposed by chronic periodontal disease makes it harder to regulate a diabetic patient.[11–13] There are several other metabolic diseases that have a negative impact on the periodontal prognosis either on their own or because of the medications required to manage them, and these must be carefully considered.

Anatomical factors such as severe dental crowding may have a negative impact on the periodontal prognosis; some of these factors can be ameliorated to improve the prognosis, e.g., by selective extraction.[14]

The animal's attitude toward being handled and manipulated is another important factor. Some animals can be quickly trained to accept and enjoy daily tooth brushing. Other animals will not tolerate this. If the animal is not likely to be compliant for home care, extraction would be more appropriate than periodontal surgery.[10]

While several diets and treats have been shown to aid in the control of plaque,[15] tooth brushing must be considered the mainstay of any home care program. This is especially important for patients with dietary or nutritional issues that prevent the use of dentally beneficial diets and treats.

Environment

In some cases, periodontal surgery is performed by a veterinary dental specialist to whom the client and patient have been referred by their primary care veterinarian. In a multidoctor general practice, sometimes periodontal surgery is performed by the veterinarian with the greatest interest and skill in the field of dentistry but who is not the patient's primary care practitioner. In either case, the patient and client will likely have future contact with someone other than the person who performed the surgery. The primary care veterinarian must offer the necessary support in the long term, and encourage the client to return to the specialist for necessary follow-up assessments and maintenance therapy.

To treat or extract?

The primary objective for the veterinary dental patient is to achieve and maintain a mouth free from pain and infection.[10] While it can be very rewarding for the oral surgeon to return a periodontally diseased tooth to health, the likelihood of achieving and maintaining that objective is often too remote to justify the attempt. Domestic dogs and cats can live very happily in an edentulous state, and are far better off with no teeth than with diseased teeth.[10]

In summary, the surgeon must consider the following prior to undertaking advanced periodontal surgery:[9,10]

- What is the nature and extent of disease?
- What is the duration of disease? In periodontal disease, rapid onset carries a poorer prognosis.
- Is the condition localized or generalized? The prognosis for a patient with generalized periodontal disease is not as good as for a patient with overall good periodontal health who has one foreign-body-induced lesion, for example.
- What are the causative factors? Are they purely local or are there systemic factors that may be uncontrollable, such as FIV infection in a cat?
- How old is the patient? If the dog is 13 years old, we may need only manage the tooth for a few more years, but if the dog is only 2 years old, we will need to manage the problem for many years.
- To what degree are the roots and furcations involved? Furcation involvement makes both the initial treatment and home care more challenging.[16,17]

- Are there occlusal factors to consider? Overcrowding and rotation of teeth make management of periodontal disease more difficult.
- Generally, advanced periodontal treatment takes longer than extraction, therefore it costs more and increases the risk of anesthetic complications.[18]
- Generally, periodontal surgery is technically more challenging than extraction.
- Is the tooth strategically important enough to justify the investment in time, effort and money?
- Visualize what the mouth would be like without the tooth, remembering that loss of a tooth leads to resorption of the supporting alveolar bone. Preserving the mandibular canine tooth in a working dog is a higher priority than preserving the maxillary first premolar tooth in a pet dog.
- Does the surgeon have the appropriate equipment and training to treat the tooth properly?

Once the surgeon has completed an assessment of the above issues, a rational, achievable and medically appropriate treatment plan can be developed. In human patients, periodontal surgery is not the first-line treatment for periodontitis. Cause-related therapy, i.e., removal of dental deposits and establishing proper homecare techniques, is performed first, and the need for surgery is evaluated after a reasonable time to allow for healing and improvement in tissue health. If the human patient cannot maintain good oral hygiene, there is no indication for periodontal surgery. Periodontal surgery is a possible adjunct to cause-related therapy, but only if plaque control is optimal.

The need for general anesthesia in veterinary patients often means that the veterinary dentist is required to obtain a diagnosis, provide cause-related therapy and perform periodontal surgery in one session. Veterinary patients with periodontal disease will often have oral sensitivity and pain, with the result that clients are unable to establish an effective home care program preoperatively.[6] This means that we must sometimes make treatment decisions based on untested assumptions regarding the patient's ability to respond to treatment and the client's ability to establish an effective plaque-control program. Clients must therefore be made aware, and be willing to accept, that the prognosis is based on these assumptions and if reality falls short of expectation, so will the results.

THERAPEUTIC-DECISION MAKING

Objectives of periodontal surgery

Historically, 'pocket elimination' has been the main objective of periodontal surgery.[19] However, increased probing depth does not necessarily indicate periodontal destruction. True periodontal pockets (due to destruction of epithelial and connective tissue attachments, periodontal ligament and alveolar bone) need to be differentiated from pseudopockets (due to proliferation of the gingiva, e.g., gingival hyperplasia). Moreover, there is no established correlation between probing depth and the presence or absence of active disease.[19] This means that signs other than increased probing depth need to be present to justify surgical therapy. These include clinical signs of inflammation (especially exudation and bleeding on probing to the bottom of the pocket), as well as aberrations of gingival morphology. Finally, since proper plaque control (home care) is a decisive factor for good prognosis, this must be considered prior to surgery.[20,21]

The main objective of periodontal surgery is to contribute to the long-term preservation of the periodontium by facilitating plaque removal and plaque control.[8] Periodontal surgery can serve this purpose by: (1) creating accessibility for professional scaling and root planing, and (2) establishing a gingival morphology which facilitates home care. In addition, periodontal surgery may aim to regenerate lost periodontal attachment.

Selection of surgical technique

Many of the technical problems experienced in periodontal surgery stem from the difficulties in accurately assessing prior to anesthesia and surgery the degree and type of periodontal breakdown that has occurred. At the time of surgery, previously undiagnosed defects may be identified, or some defects may be more complex than anticipated. Consequently, a combination of techniques may be required at the same site. As a general rule, techniques that preserve or induce the formation of periodontal tissue should be preferred over those that remove tissue.

Infrabony pockets are described by depth and by the extent of the bony circumference involved (Fig. 17.2). The surrounding alveolar

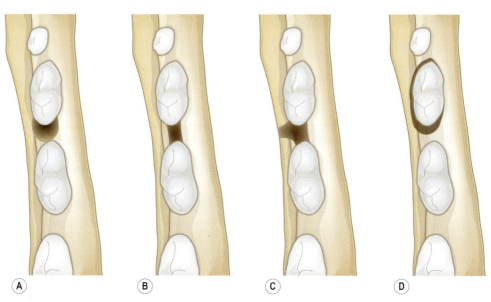

Fig. 17.2 Occlusal views of the right mandible of a dog showing: (**A**) a three-walled bony defect, (**B**) a two-walled bony defect, (**C**) a one-walled bony defect and (**D**) a cup defect. *(From Tsugawa AJ, Verstraete FJM. How to obtain and interpret periodontal radiographs in dogs.* Clin Tech Small Anim Pract *2000;15:204–210.)*

bone is thought of as forming four walls (mesial, buccal, distal, palatal/lingual). When bone is present around the entire circumference of the pocket, a four-wall defect is present. When bone is missing on one face, a three-wall defect is present. Two- and one-wall defects have two and three surfaces of the tooth root without bony support, respectively.[22–24] In general, the more bony walls there are surrounding an infrabony pocket, the greater the potential for the regeneration of lost periodontal tissues following complete removal of all irritants and inflamed soft tissues from the defect.

Gingivectomy/gingivoplasty

Gingivectomy is the excision of gingival tissue, usually to remove the diseased wall of a periodontal pocket (true pocket or pseudopocket).[25] Gingivoplasty is the recontouring of the gingiva to its proper anatomical form without the reduction of periodontal pocket depth (see Ch. 18).[25] This is typically a combined procedure, which can be used in isolation or together with other surgical procedures such as flap surgery.[26] The main indication for gingivectomy or gingivoplasty in veterinary dentistry is in the management of gingival enlargements. Gingivectomy may also be used for type 1 surgical crown lengthening (see Ch. 21).

Flap operations with or without osseous surgery

Flap procedures can be used in all cases where surgical treatment of periodontal disease is indicated. These procedures can be performed with or without osseous surgery (see Chs 19 and 20). Flap procedures are particularly useful where periodontal pockets extend beyond the mucogingival junction, the furcation is involved and/or recontouring of bony lesions is required. The advantages of flap operations include: (1) existing keratinized gingiva is preserved; (2) the operator has increased visualization of the defect and can ensure thorough debridement of dental deposits and inflamed soft tissues; (3) the marginal bone is exposed, whereby the morphology of bony defects can be identified and the proper treatment rendered; (4) the flap can either be replaced at its original position or shifted apically or coronally, thereby making it possible to adjust the gingival margin to the local conditions; and (5) the flap procedure preserves the oral epithelium.

Healing processes for commonly used techniques

In order to understand what periodontal surgery aims to achieve, it is necessary to understand the patterns of wound healing that occur in the periodontium. All wounds heal in three phases: an inflammatory phase, followed by a proliferation phase and then a maturation/remodeling phase (see Ch. 1). The wounds caused by periodontal surgery follow this pattern, with specific variations for each of the commonly used methods (gingivectomy/gingivoplasty vs. flap techniques).

Gingivectomy/gingivoplasty

The healing of a gingivectomy/gingivoplasty wound is similar to that of a simple soft tissue wound, except that there is a tooth in the center of the wound. Following incision with a scalpel blade or gingivectomy knife, the wound is covered by a fibrin clot and the underlying tissue becomes acutely inflamed with some necrosis.[25] The clot is replaced by granulation tissue, and after 12–24 hours epithelial cells at the margin of the wound begin to migrate across the granulation tissue bed.[26] The epithelial activity reaches its peak by 24–36 hours post incision. Surface epithelialization is generally complete after 5–14 days, but complete epithelial repair and keratinization may take a month.[25] Complete repair of the underlying connective tissue takes about 7 weeks.[25]

Wound healing following electrosurgery/radiosurgery can be affected by various factors such as the frequency of the signal produced by the instrument, the wave form utilized, the power setting utilized and technique.[27–32] Use of a high-frequency radiosurgical unit (3.0–4.0 MHz) and a fully filtered wave form at an appropriate power setting results in tissue damage and healing similar to cold steel incision.[25,32] Lower-frequency electrosurgical units and other wave forms will result in greater thermal necrosis of the wound and delayed healing. Slow passage of the electrode through the tissues and excessive power settings also increase lateral heat dissipation into tissues, resulting in collateral damage and delayed healing. Electrosurgery is contraindicated in close proximity to bone as it can result in greater gingival recession, bone necrosis and loss of bone height.[25]

Healing following laser surgery is delayed compared to that with cold steel.[25,33] The risk of collateral damage to the surrounding hard tissues (enamel, cementum and bone) is also of concern.[33,34]

Flap techniques

The pattern of healing in the absence of vertical bone loss is as follows. There is no open wound after suturing the flap in place. The soft tissue collar around the tooth consists of keratinized gingival epithelium on the oral surface of the flap with its underlying connective tissue in contact with the alveolar bone and root surface. The junctional epithelial attachment and gingival sulcus have been removed during the procedure. Immediately postoperatively, there is a blood clot between the tooth and the flap. The fibrin in the clot functions as a glue between the tooth and flap.[35] As healing starts, both the connective tissue and epithelium are activated. The gingival epithelium will start to grow down between the tooth and the flap to form a new junctional epithelial attachment. Simultaneously, new connective tissue will grow into the fibrin clot trying to gain attachment to the root surface. The situation is now a race between the junctional epithelium growing apically to cover the exposed connective tissue at the root surface, and the connective tissue gaining new attachment to the root surface. The result of the race will determine at which level the junctional epithelium's apical attachment will be after healing. Usually, the connective tissue will have time to form some attachment to the root surface coronal to the level of the alveolar bone before the junctional epithelium has grown down. The final stage of the healing process is the reformation of the normal junctional epithelial attachment and gingival sulcus. At 2 weeks, the union of the flap to the tooth is still weak due to the immaturity of the collagen fibers. One month following surgery, the gingival sulcus is fully epithelialized, and a well-defined junctional epithelial attachment is present.[35] Following full-thickness flap surgery, which temporarily denudes bone, there will be superficial bone necrosis resulting in bone loss of about 1 mm (more if the bone is thin).[35]

When vertical bone loss is present, the pattern of healing differs in that first a blood clot forms between the root and the alveolar bone. The blood clot starts to be replaced by connective tissue as fibroblasts become activated, reproduce and synthesize collagen. New cementum may form on the root surface. Collagen fibers from the periodontal membrane become embedded in the newly formed cementum, forming a new periodontal ligament. Osteoblasts are activated and start laying down bone in the vertical wall of the bony pocket.

The above sequence, i.e., the formation of normal bone and normal periodontal ligament, takes months to occur. The threat to the above events occurring successfully is the apically-directed growth of the junctional epithelium trying to cover the 'wound' between the tooth and the connective tissue. Various techniques, e.g., guided tissue regeneration, have been advocated to encourage new attachment by preventing epithelial downgrowth.[36,37] Other outcomes, such as external root resorption and ankylosis, are also possible.[8] A more extensive discussion of guided tissue regeneration follows in Chapter 20.

POSTOPERATIVE CARE AND ASSESSMENT

With a carefully performed procedure (gentle handling of tissues, ensuring that exposed bone is kept moist, ensuring complete coverage of the alveolar bone when suturing flaps), most patients experience only minimal postoperative discomfort. The pain experienced is limited to the first few days and can be adequately controlled with analgesic drugs (see Ch. 4).

Feeding soft food is recommended during the early phase of healing (10–14 days) in order to reduce discomfort and maintain good wound stability. Postoperative plaque control is the most important variable in determining the long-term result of periodontal surgery. Disease recurrence is inevitable, regardless of surgical technique used, if postoperative plaque control is suboptimal.[20,21,38,39] In the immediate postoperative period (10–14 days), plaque formation may be retarded by chemical, rather than mechanical, methods.[40] Ideally, twice-daily rinsing with 0.1–0.2% chlorhexidine gluconate solution should be performed. However, it is also important that the clients not disturb the surgical site, as this would not only cause pain for the patient but could also disrupt healing. Therefore, they must be instructed to handle the mouth very gently, taking care to avoid putting pressure or tension across any suture lines. The immediate postsurgical application of a wax-polymer barrier product (Ora-Vet, Merial Ltd. Duluth, GA) to the crowns of the teeth may also help inhibit bacterial colonization of the tooth surfaces during the healing phase.[41]

Administration of systemic antibiotics following periodontal surgery appears to be beneficial, resulting in increased attachment levels when compared with periodontal surgery alone, with administration of tetracycline or metronidazole proving to be more beneficial than other antibiotic regimens.[42]

It is important to return to and maintain good mechanical oral hygiene measures as soon as the tissues have healed sufficiently that brushing will not cause pain or disrupt healing, especially since rinsing with chlorhexidine does not prevent subgingival recolonization of plaque.

The initial healing should be evaluated after 10–14 days. Following this examination, the client should start gentle brushing of the operated areas using a soft-bristled, nylon toothbrush that has been softened in hot water. Adjunctive continued use of chlorhexidine rinses may be advised, as may continued used of the wax barrier product. Diets and treats shown to help reduce plaque accumulation should be considered if there are no medical or dietary contraindications for the patient.[15] Recheck appointments for conscious examination are scheduled at 2-week intervals to closely monitor plaque control. During this postoperative maintenance phase, adjustments of the methods for optimal home care are made depending on the healing status of the tissues. Depending on compliance, the time interval between visits for supportive care may gradually be increased. The next full periodontal assessment and professional maintenance therapy may be scheduled for between 3 and 12 months postoperatively, depending on a variety of factors. Since complete periodontal healing and regeneration of periodontal tissues takes months, assessing prior to 3 months may underestimate the final result. Conversely, waiting too long before reassessing risks allows time for the reestablishment of the disease process and loss of all gains achieved.

PROGNOSIS

The prognosis for the outcome of periodontal surgery is affected by many factors including: (1) the skill of the surgeon; (2) the habits and diet of the patient; (3) the level of home care (plaque control); and (4) the patient's susceptibility/resistance to periodontal disease. With so many variables, the prognosis is always somewhat uncertain, and the clients must be aware of and willing to accept this prior to undertaking the procedure. With careful case selection and treatment planning, followed by establishment and maintenance of proper postoperative plaque-control measures, most surgical treatment techniques will result in conditions that favor the maintenance of a healthy periodontium.

REFERENCES

1. Wolf HF, Rateitschak EM, Rateitschak KH, et al. Structural biology. In: Rateitschak KH, Wolf HF, editors. Color atlas of dental medicine: periodontology. 3rd ed. Stuttgart, Germany: Thieme; 2005. p. 7–20.
2. Schroeder HE. Marginal periodontium. In: Oral structural biology. New York: Thieme Medical Publishing; 1991. p. 230–64.
3. Melnick PR. Preparation of the periodontium for restorative dentistry. In: Newman MG, Takei HH, Klokkevold PR, et al, editors. Clinical periodontology. 10th ed. Philadelphia, PA: WB Saunders; 2006. p. 1039–49.
4. Wolf HF, Rateitschak EM, Rateitschak KH, et al. Perio-prosthetics 2, supplemental measures, esthetics. In: Rateitschak KH, Wolf HF, editors. Color atlas of dental medicine: periodontology. 3rd ed. Stuttgart, Germany: Thieme; 2005. p. 489–509.
5. Wolf HF, Rateitschak EM, Rateitschak KH, et al. Data collection – diagnosis – prognosis. In: Rateitschak KH, Wolf HF, editors. Color atlas of dental medicine: periodontology. 3rd ed. Stuttgart, Germany: Thieme; 2005. p. 165–77.
6. Harvey CE. Management of periodontal disease: understanding the options. Vet Clin North Am Small Anim Pract 2005; 35:819–36.
7. Isidor F, Karring T, Nyman S, et al. New attachment-reattachment following reconstructive periodontal surgery. J Clin Periodontol 1985;12:728–35.
8. Wolf HF, Rateitschak EM, Rateitschak KH, et al. Treatment of inflammatory periodontal disease. In: Rateitschak KH, Wolf HF, editors. Color atlas of dental medicine: periodontology. 3rd ed. Stuttgart, Germany: Thieme; 2005. p. 201–10.
9. Hale FA. Treatment planning in veterinary dentistry. In: Understanding veterinary dentistry. Guelph, Canada: Published by the author; 2004. p. 9–13.
10. Hale FA. The owner-animal-environment triad in the treatment of canine periodontal disease. J Vet Dent 2003;20:118–22.
11. Klokkevold PR, Mealey BL. Influence of systemic disorders and stress on the periodontium. In: Newman MG, Takei HH, Klokkevold PR, et al, editors. Clinical periodontology. 10th ed. Philadelphia, PA: WB Saunders; 2006. p. 284–311.
12. Mealey BL, Klokkevold PR. Periodontal medicine: impact of periodontal infection on systemic health. In: Newman MG, Takei HH, Klokkevold PR, et al, editors. Clinical periodontology. 10th ed. Philadelphia, PA: WB Saunders; 2006. p. 312–29.

13. Wolf HF, Rateitschak EM, Rateitschak KH, et al. Systemic pre-phase. In: Rateitschak KH, Wolf HF, editors. Color atlas of dental medicine: periodontology. 3rd ed. Stuttgart, Germany: Thieme; 2005. p. 211–6.

14. Hale FA. Juvenile veterinary dentistry. Vet Clin North Am Small Anim Pract 2005;35:789–817.

15. Anonymous. Veterinary Oral Health Council. http://www.avdc.org/vohc.html, accessed 12 Nov 2007.

16. Novak KF, Goodman SF, Takei HH. Determination of prognosis. In: Newman MG, Takei HH, Klokkevold PR, et al, editors. Clinical periodontology. 10th ed. Philadelphia, PA: WB Saunders; 2006. p. 614–25.

17. Ammons WF, Harrington GW. Furcation: involvement and treatment. In: Newman MG, Takei HH, Klokkevold PR, et al, editors. Clinical periodontology. 10th ed. Philadelphia, PA: WB Saunders; 2006. p. 991–1004.

18. Lagasse RS. Anesthesia safety: model or myth? A review of the published literature and analysis of current original data. Anesthesiology 2002;97:1335–7.

19. Carranza FA, Takei HH. Phase II periodontal therapy. In: Newman MG, Takei HH, Klokkevold PR, et al, editors. Clinical periodontology. 10th ed. Philadelphia, PA: WB Saunders; 2006. p. 881–6.

20. Nyman S, Lindhe J, Rosling B. Periodontal surgery in plaque-infected dentitions. J Clin Periodontol 1977;4:240–9.

21. Axelsson P, Lindhe J. The significance of maintenance care in the treatment of periodontal disease. J Clin Periodontol 1981;8:281–94.

22. Wiggs RB, Lobprise HB. Veterinary dentistry, principles and practice. Philadelphia, PA: Raven-Lippincott; 1997. p. 186–231.

23. Carranza FA, Takei HH. Bone loss and patterns of bone destruction. In: Newman MG, Takei HH, Klokkevold PR, et al, editors. Clinical periodontology. 10th ed. Philadelphia, PA: WB Saunders; 2006. p. 452–66.

24. Wolf HF, Rateitschak EM, Rateitschak KH, et al. Periodontitis. In: Rateitschak KH, Wolf HF, editors. Color atlas of dental medicine: periodontology. 3rd ed. Stuttgart, Germany: Thieme; 2005. p. 95–118.

25. Takei HH, Carranza FA. Gingival surgical techniques. In: Newman MG, Takei HH, Klokkevold PR, et al, editors. Clinical periodontology. 10th ed. Philadelphia, PA: WB Saunders; 2006. p. 909–17

26. Wolf HF, Rateitschak EM, Rateitschak KH, et al. Gingivectomy and gingivoplasty. In: Rateitschak KH, Wolf HF, editors. Color atlas of dental medicine: periodontology. 3rd ed. Stuttgart, Germany: Thieme; 2005. p. 367–80.

27. Sherman JA. Principles and theory of radiosurgery. In: Oral surgery. 2nd ed. London: Martin Dunitz; 1997. p. 1–8.

28. Sherman JA. Waveform types and properties. In: Oral surgery. 2nd ed. London: Martin Dunitz; 1997. p. 9–14.

29. Sherman JA. Radiosurgical techniques. In: Oral surgery. 2nd ed. London: Martin Dunitz; 1997. p. 45–154.

30. Miller WW. Using high-frequency radio wave technology in veterinary surgery. Vet Med 2004;99:796–802.

31. Elkin AD. Optimizing the use of radiosurgery and all its varieties. Vet Forum 1998 (April):50–6.

32. Turner RJ, Cohen RA, Voet RL, et al. Analysis of tissue margins of cone biopsy specimens obtained with 'cold knife' CO_2 and Nd:YAG lasers and a a radiofrequency surgical unit. J Repro Med 1992;37:607–10.

33. Lewis JR, Reiter AM. Management of generalized gingival enlargement in a dog – case report and literature review. J Vet Dent 2005;22:160–9.

34. Ishikawa I, Aoki A. Lasers in periodontics. In: Newman MG, Takei HH, Klokkevold PR, et al, editors. Clinical periodontology. 10th ed. Philadelphia, PA: WB Saunders; 2006. p. 1035–7.

35. Takei HH, Carranza FA. The periodontal flap. In: Newman MG, Takei HH, Klokkevold PR, et al, editors. Clinical periodontology. 10th ed. Philadelphia, PA: WB Saunders; 2006. p. 926–36.

36. Carranza FA. Reconstructive periodontal surgery. In: Newman MG, Takei HH, Klokkevold PR, et al, editors. Clinical periodontology. 10th ed. Philadelphia, PA: WB Saunders; 2006. p. 968–90.

37. Wolf HF, Rateitschak EM, Rateitschak KH, et al. Regenerative methods. In: Rateitschak KH, Wolf HF, editors. Color atlas of dental medicine: periodontology. 3rd ed. Stuttgart, Germany: Thieme; 2005. p. 323–54.

38. Rosling B, Nyman S, Lindhe J, et al. The healing potential of the periodontal tissue following different techniques of periodontal surgery in plaque-free dentitions. J Clin Periodontol 1976;3:233–55.

39. Lindhe J, Westfelt E, Nyman S, et al. Long-term effect of surgical/non-surgical treatment of periodontal disease. J Clin Periodontol 1984; 11:448–58.

40. Hamp SE, Rosling B, Lindhe J. Effect of chlorhexidine on gingival wound healing in the dog. A histometric study. J Clin Periodontol 1975;2:143–52.

41. Gengler WR, Kunkle BN, Romano D, et al. Evaluation of a barrier sealant in dogs. J Vet Dent 2005;22:157–9.

42. Haffajee AD, Socransky SS, Gunsolley JC. Systemic anti-infective periodontal therapy. A systematic review. Ann Periodontol 2003;8:115–81.

Chapter | **18** |

Gingivectomy and gingivoplasty

Cecilia E. Gorrel & Fraser A. Hale

DEFINITIONS

Gingivectomy refers to the surgical excision of gingival tissue and is performed to reduce the depth of a suprabony periodontal pocket by removing a portion of the gingival wall of that pocket. *Gingivoplasty* refers to the reshaping of the gingiva to create anatomically normal and physiologically beneficial gingival contours.[1] The two techniques are typically combined.

PREOPERATIVE CONCERNS

As the gingival tissues have a rich vascular supply, gingivectomy/gingivoplasty tends to result in considerable intraoperative bleeding. If a clotting profile and platelet count have not already been performed, then a *buccal mucosal bleeding time* (BMBT) test can quickly be done in the anesthetized patient prior to the first incision. This test is performed by employing a BMBT device (Simplate, Organon Teknika, Durham, NC) or by making a stab incision into the buccal mucosa with a # 11 scalpel blade and recording the time it takes for the wound to stop bleeding. Mucosal bleeding times of less than 3–5 minutes are considered normal.[2]

There are several drugs that may predispose to the development of gingival enlargement (see Ch. 42) and so the patient history should be reviewed to see if any of these medications have been administered to the patient.[3] If it is determined that the gingival enlargements are likely drug-induced then efforts to cease administration of that drug should be made. Often, this will result in dramatic improvement and may even make surgery unnecessary. If the patient absolutely requires the causative drug and no substitute can be found, the client must be made aware that the gingival enlargement will almost certainly reoccur following surgery. Maintaining excellent plaque control may reduce or retard the recurrence as it is felt that, while the drug increases the likelihood of developing enlargements, inflammation is still necessary for its development.[3]

Vitamin C deficiency has been reported to cause gingival enlargement. Degeneration of the gingival collagen and alterations in the gingival defenses against plaque result in edema, inflammation and gingival enlargement.[4]

The literature contains at least one report of a localized gingival enlargement due to disseminated cryptococcosis in a Siamese cat.[5]

SURGICAL ANATOMY

The gingiva surrounds the teeth and the marginal parts of the alveolar bone, forming a cuff around each tooth (see Fig. 17.1). It can be divided into the free gingiva, which is closely adapted to, but not attached to, the tooth surface, and the attached gingiva that is attached to the suprabony cementum and the underlying periosteum of the alveolar bone. The attached gingiva is delineated from the oral mucosa by the mucogingival junction (Fig. 18.1), except on the palatal aspect of the maxillary teeth, where it blends imperceptibly with the palatal mucosa (Fig. 18.2).[6,7]

The gingival tissues in the spaces between the closely spaced teeth (the interproximal spaces) form a gingival papilla (Fig. 18.3).[7,8] This triangularly shaped structure is important in excluding food, hair and

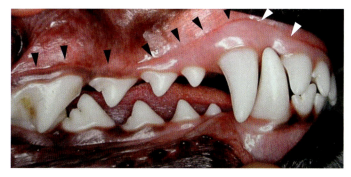

Fig. 18.1 Healthy gingiva in a dog showing the mucogingival junction (*arrowheads*). Regardless of where the free gingival margin may go (coronally with enlargement or apically with recession), the mucogingival junction remains unmoved. It is apparent in this photo that the width of the attached gingiva varies considerably throughout the mouth.

© 2012 Elsevier Ltd
DOI: 10.1016/B978-0-7020-4618-6.00018-X

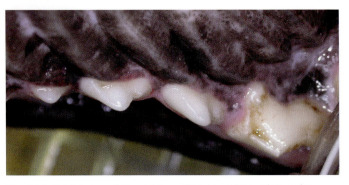

Fig. 18.2 Palatal view of the right maxillary premolar teeth in a dog showing how the gingiva blends imperceptibly with the palatal mucosa. Note the crown fracture of the fourth premolar necessitating endodontic treatment or extraction.

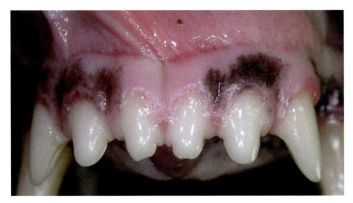

Fig. 18.3 Maxillary incisor teeth of a dog depicting the gingival papillae.

other foreign material from becoming trapped in the interproximal space.[8] Between the facial and lingual/palatal gingival papillae, there may be a valley-like architecture known as the gingival col.[7,8]

As the free gingiva is not attached to the tooth, there is a shallow potential space between the free gingiva and the tooth known as the gingival sulcus (see Fig. 17.1). The depth of the sulcus can be assessed by gently inserting a graduated periodontal probe until resistance is encountered. This resistance is taken to be the base of the sulcus. The depth from the free gingival margin to the base of the sulcus can thus be measured.

In the periodontally healthy individual, the sulcus depth is 0.5–1 mm in small dogs, 1–3 mm in medium and large dogs, and 0.5–1 mm in cats. In the healthy situation, where the band of gingival tissue is wider, the sulcus will often be deeper and where the band of gingiva is narrower, the sulcus will be shallower. For example, the distance from the free gingival margin to the mucogingival junction on the buccal aspect of the maxillary canine tooth in a large dog may be as much as 15 mm and there a probing depth of 3 mm would be acceptable. On the other hand, the distance from the free gingival margin to the mucogingival junction over the maxillary fourth premolar tooth in a cat would be approximately 1.5 mm and there a probing depth over 0.5 mm would be considered abnormal (Fig. 18.1).

The oral surface of the gingival epithelium contains the four layers typical of epithelia elsewhere, namely the stratum basale, stratum spinosum, stratum granulosum and stratum corneum.[7,9,10] The stratum corneum may be orthokeratinized or parakeratinized.[7,9,10] Local irritation interferes with keratinization, and healthy gingiva is more keratinized than diseased, irritated gingiva.[7] Nonepithelial cells are also present in the oral gingival epithelium. These include melanocytes,

and Langerhans cells in the stratum spinosum.[9] The Langerhans cells participate in the local immune response by presenting antigen to and participating in the activation of T-helper lymphocytes.[9]

The gingival sulcus is lined by the oral sulcular epithelium, which is nonkeratinized.[7,10] The sulcular epithelium has the potential to keratinize if the sulcular microflora is totally eliminated or if the epithelium is reflected and exposed to the oral cavity. On the other hand, the outer gingival epithelium will lose its keratinization if brought into contact with the tooth. This is one basis for the theory that local irritants, such as bacterial toxins, may prevent sulcular and oral epithelial keratinization.[7]

Apical to the gingival sulcus is a band of highly permeable epithelium called the junctional epithelium, which forms the epithelial attachment to the tooth.[7] The junctional epithelium is a nonkeratinized stratified squamous epithelium which is derived from remnants of the reduced enamel epithelium during eruption of the tooth. Unlike other oral epithelia, it has only two layers (stratum basale and stratum suprabasale).[11] The junctional epithelium also contains a few leukocytes.[11]

Apical to the junctional epithelium is the connective tissue attachment. Here, fiber bundles of the gingival connective tissue insert into the supra-alveolar cementum.[11] The gingival connective tissue is also firmly attached to the periosteum of the alveolar bone.

Biologic width is defined as the dimensional width of the junctional epithelium and connective tissue attachment (see Fig. 21.1).[12] In human patients, biologic width is typically 2–3 mm. The dimensions in veterinary patients will be quite variable and in proportion to the size of the tooth and its periodontal tissues. Biologic width is commonly discussed in reference to the distance that must be maintained between the alveolar margin and any restoration on a tooth to leave sufficient room for each of the elements of the gingival attachment and a gingival sulcus (the dentogingival complex). When considering gingivectomy/gingivoplasty, biologic width must be respected. If the gingivectomy incision approaches too close to the bone, there will be insufficient room for the establishment of all the elements of the dentogingival complex. The result will be inflammatory resorption of alveolar bone and gradual reestablishment of biologic width in a more apical location.[12]

INSTRUMENTATION AND EQUIPMENT

Gingivectomy/gingivoplasty can be performed with cold steel (scalpel blade, gingivectomy knives, scissors) (Fig. 18.4), diamond or fluted carbide burs (on a high-speed dental handpiece) (Fig. 18.5), electrosurgery, radio wave radiosurgery (Fig. 18.6) or laser surgery. Each modality has its advantages and disadvantages.[1,13–15] Often the choice of modality is directed by availability. For example, veterinarians who have invested in laser are inclined to use it for gingivectomy/gingivoplasty; those with a radiosurgical unit are inclined to use that; those with neither or with surgical training are inclined to use cold steel. Used properly and within their limitations, all will perform adequately. Used inappropriately or beyond their limitations, all can cause great harm to the patient. Therefore, it is essential that surgeons be very familiar with the technical aspects of the modality they intend to utilize.

Cold steel

Cold steel incision is, in many ways, the preferred modality for gingivectomy/gingivoplasty, being listed first in virtually all references of note.[1,4,13–17] It can provide a clean and neat incision with no collateral tissue damage and rapid healing (see Ch. 17). It is inexpensive and readily accessible. However, as the gingival tissues are highly vascular, cold steel incision does result in considerable intraoperative bleeding, often obscuring the field of view and requiring frequent swabbing by an assistant. Also, gingival enlargements are often highly fibrous and may contain osseous metaplasia. This can force the surgeon to apply considerable pressure to incise the tissues, resulting in less control of the cut and the potential to slip and make accidental incisions. Also, cold blades dull quickly when cutting through such tissues and when contacting the underlying dental enamel and so scalpel blades need to be replaced and gingivectomy knives and scissors need to be sharpened frequently during the procedure.

Diamond or fluted carbide bur

While few references make mention of the use of carbide or diamond dental burs in a high-speed handpiece, it is an option to be considered.[4,18] In this technique, diamond or fluted carbide dental burs (in a high-speed handpiece) are used to create the desired incision and bevel (Fig. 18.5).[4] The burs permit good contouring and produce less hemorrhage than cold steel. Accidental damage of the tooth surface with the bur is a risk when using this technique. Protecting the tooth surface (e.g., with a plastic spatula) is recommended if possible. Ample irrigation is used to prevent thermal damage. The time spent cutting the gingiva around a tooth should be as short as possible.

Electrosurgery and radiosurgery

While these two modalities are often discussed together and even interchangeably, there are significant and important differences between them and they are not interchangeable.

Electrosurgery uses relatively low-frequency electrical energy (0.5–2.9 MHz).[19] It creates heat in the tissue due to the resistance of the tissues to the passing of electrical current through the patient between two points of contact (typically the active handpiece electrode and a grounding plate which must be in direct physical contact with the patient).[19,20] Since the separation of tissues is achieved through generation of heat at the electrode contact point, there is lateral dissipation of heat into the tissues beyond the incision line.

Radiosurgery is achieved by passing high-frequency radio wave energy (3.0–4.0 MHz) through the patient between the active electrode and a passive antenna, which need only be in proximity to the patient, not in direct physical contact. The units depicted in the photographs operate at 3.8 and 4.0 MHz respectively (Fig. 18.6). Tissue resistance to the passage of the radio waves causes ionic agitation in the cells at the active electrode tip. This causes molecular friction and heating of the tissue. The heat comes from molecular friction in the cells, not from the electrode tip itself.[20]

Various studies have demonstrated that high-frequency radio wave radiosurgery, when used properly, results in a smaller zone of thermal

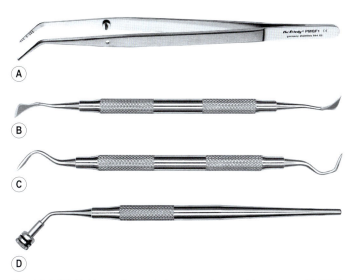

Fig. 18.4 (**A**) Goldman–Fox periodontal pocket marking forceps (PMGF1). (**B**) Kirkland gingivectomy knife (KK15/16). (**C**) Orban gingivectomy knife (KO1/2). (**D**) Universal 360° scalpel handle (K360). *(Courtesy of Hu-Friedy Mfg. Inc., Chicago, IL)*

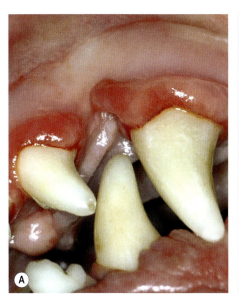
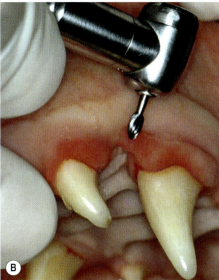
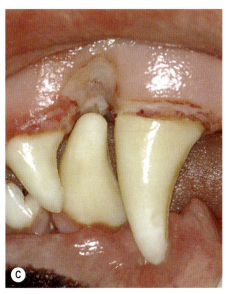

Fig. 18.5 (**A**) Gingival enlargement at the left maxillary third incisor and canine teeth in a dog. (**B**) An egg-shaped, 12-fluted bur in a high-speed handpiece is used to remove the gingival enlargement and sculpt the gingiva to physiologic height and contour. (**C**) Postoperative appearance. *(From Lewis JR, Reiter AM. Management of generalized gingival enlargement in a dog – case report and literature review. J Vet Dent 2005;22:160–169. With permission.)*

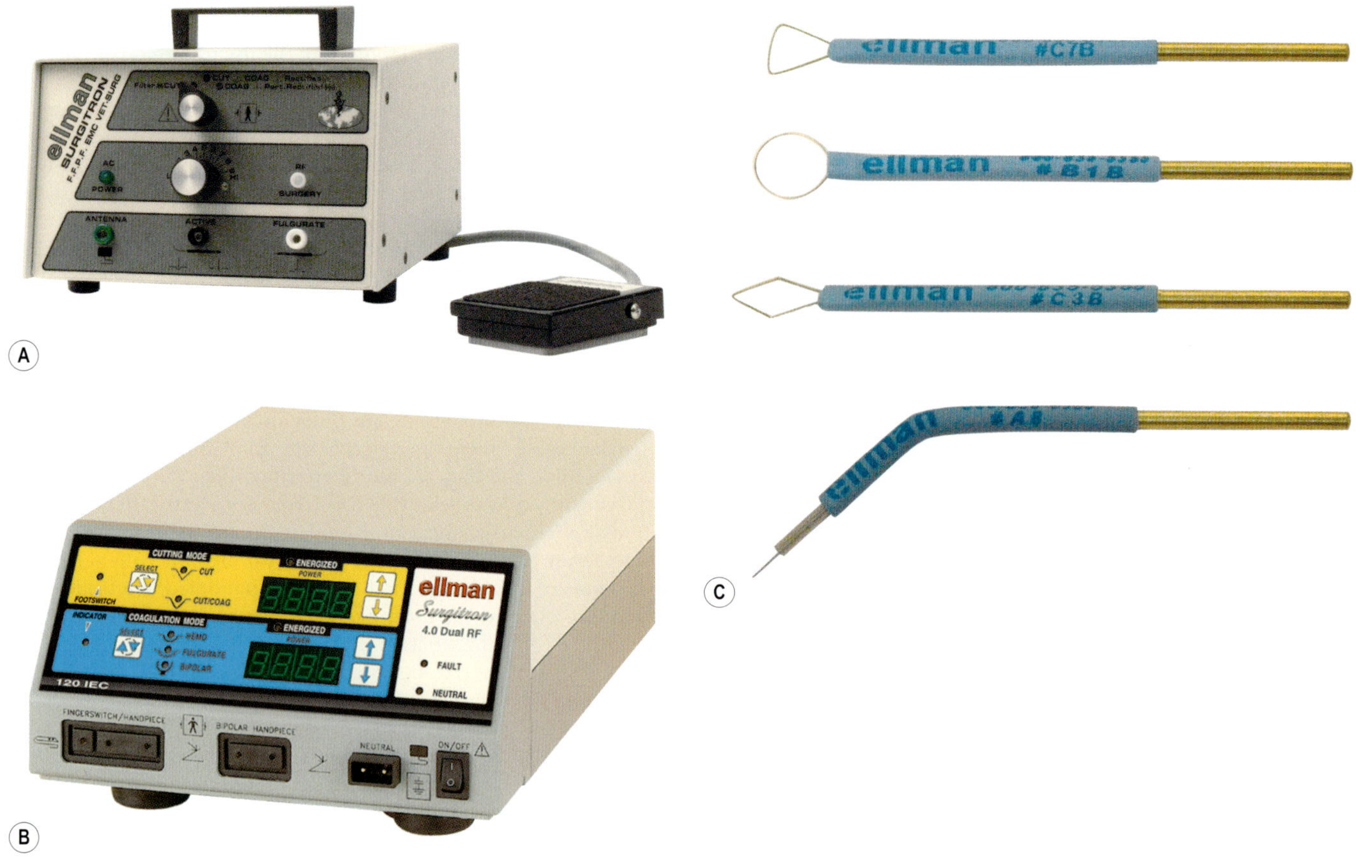

Fig. 18.6 (**A**) Ellman Surgitron EMC, 3.8 MHz radiosurgical unit. (**B**) Ellman Surgitron RF 4.0 MHz unit. (**C**) Electrode tips for use with the Ellman units, from top, C7B triangle loop, B1B round loop, C3B diamond loop and A8B wire tip. (*Courtesy of Ellman International Inc., Oceanside, NY*)

necrosis at the incision compared to electrosurgery at lower frequencies and laser.[20–22]

Electrosurgical and radiosurgical units can be configured to produce four different waveforms, though not all units offer all waveform options. The fully filtered waveform provides a pure, continuous flow of current and offers the smoothest incision with the least amount of thermal necrosis and tissue shrinkage, and healing is very similar to a cold incision.[23] Due to the minimal lateral heat transfer of the fully filtered waveform, it can be used in relatively close proximity to bone. It does not provide significant hemostasis (coagulation of small vessels).[24,25]

The fully rectified waveform offers simultaneous cutting and hemostasis by coagulating small vessels. The cost of this hemostasis is a slightly wider zone of thermal damage and more tissue shrinkage. Therefore, this waveform should not be used in close proximity to bone or dental hard tissues. It is a suitable waveform for bulk removal of excess gingival tissue, provided the electrode can be kept a few millimeters from bone and tooth.[24,25]

The partially rectified waveform provides an intermittent flow of energy that provides effective hemostasis by coagulating vessels up to 1/16″ (1.6 mm) in diameter while causing more thermal necrosis and tissue shrinkage. This waveform is not suitable for gingivectomy/gingivoplasty.

The fulguration, or spark-gap waveform is the most destructive of the four waves, causing considerable thermal necrosis, tissue shrinkage and scarring. It has no application in gingivectomy/gingivoplasty.[24,25]

In summary, high-frequency radio wave surgery using a fully filtered waveform at an appropriate power setting and with a suitably shaped electrode (Fig. 18.6C) provides a very smooth, pressure-free incision allowing the surgeon to easily sculpt the tissues to a desirable height and contour, even when approaching very close to the bone. The fully rectified waveform also offers simultaneous hemostasis but, due to a slight increase in lateral heat transfer, should not be used in close proximity to bone. Since one imperative in gingivectomy/gingivoplasty is to ensure the preservation of sufficient gingival tissues (both in height and thickness) to support the periodontal health of the tooth, the incision should not approach the bone and so the fully rectified waveform is quite acceptable.

Lasers

Laser technology is evolving at a rapid pace, as are the attitudes towards its suitability for various dental applications. One respected human dental textbook has changed its outlook on the subject considerably from one edition to the next.[26,27] The most common laser in veterinary practice at the time of writing is the CO_2 laser. Compared to cold steel and radio surgery, laser incisions have more thermal necrosis and take longer to heal (see Ch. 17).[4,20–22,24] Laser should not be used close to bone. There are safety concerns regarding reflected or misdirected beams and risk of damage to surrounding tissues such as enamel and cementum.[14] These factors aside, some surgeons familiar with and skilled in the use of laser technology have used it successfully for gingivectomy/gingivoplasty (see Ch. 8).

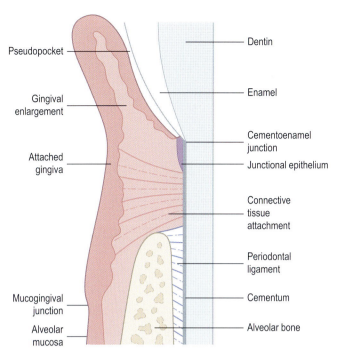

Pseudopocket

Gingival enlargement

Attached gingiva

Mucogingival junction

Alveolar mucosa

Dentin

Enamel

Cementoenamel junction

Junctional epithelium

Connective tissue attachment

Periodontal ligament

Cementum

Alveolar bone

Fig. 18.7 Cross-sectional anatomy of a pseudopocket resulting from gingival enlargement with no periodontal attachment loss.

THERAPEUTIC DECISION-MAKING

Gingivectomy/gingivoplasty is used for reduction of suprabony periodontal pocket depth and reshaping abnormal gingival contours.

In dogs and cats, the main indication for the technique is in the treatment of gingival enlargements such as idiopathic gingival hyperplasia and drug-induced gingival overgrowth, both of which can be either focal or generalized. In these cases, excess gingival tissue results in the development of periodontal pseudopockets and abnormal gingival contours (see Chs 17 and 42) (Fig. 18.7). The aim is to remove the gingival wall of the pseudopockets and restore normal gingival architecture. In cases of drug-induced gingival overgrowth, withdrawal of the offending drug will often result in dramatic improvement and surgery may not be required. On the other hand, some residual enlargement may persist and so gingivectomy/gingivoplasty may still be indicated.

When attempting to reduce the depth of a true periodontal pocket gingivectomy/gingivoplasty must be applied cautiously if at all. The goal of periodontal surgery is the long-term preservation of the periodontal tissues.[1,13,15] The periodontal health and future of a tooth relies on the maintenance of a collar of attached gingiva (minimum of 2 mm) around the entire circumference of the tooth.[13] Periodontal disease can result in the loss of gingival tissues through gingival recession. To excise gingiva further reduces the amount of gingiva available to support and protect the tooth. Reduction of the depth of true periodontal pockets should be attained through modalities intended to increase the level of attachment of the gingiva to the tooth (see Ch. 19). Gingivectomy/gingivoplasty should be limited to removing only small amounts of gingiva where an abundance of gingival tissue will remain after the incision, and healing and biologic width will not be compromised and furcations not exposed by the incision.

A third indication for gingivectomy/gingivoplasty is in type 1 surgical crown-lengthening as outlined in Chapter 21. Again, this should be limited to the removal of only minor amounts of gingival tissue

where an abundance will remain postoperatively and where the objectives of the surgery can be met without compromising biologic width or exposing furcations.[12,28]

In some circumstances, clinical and historical findings may make the histologic diagnosis seem obvious. For example, in a boxer dog with generalized gingival enlargements surrounding all teeth symmetrically, a diagnosis of idiopathic fibrous gingival hyperplasia seems very likely. However, as one case report highlighted, making such assumptions can be dangerous. In the boxer dog presented, the tissues submitted for histologic examination reveal three separate diagnoses, namely fibrous gingival hyperplasia, fibrous epulis with osseous metaplasia and mast cell tumor.[29] Therefore, it is important to submit tissues for histopathology.[4,29]

SURGICAL TECHNIQUES

Regardless of the modality employed, the surgeon must plan the line of incision carefully. A method often described in the literature is as follows.[1,4,16] Pocket depths are measured with a graduated periodontal probe. The probe is withdrawn from the pocket and held against the outer surface of the gingiva to show the depth of the pocket. The tip of the probe is then turned horizontally and driven into the gingiva to produce a bleeding point at the level of the bottom of the pocket (Fig. 18.8). Alternatively, pocket-marking forceps (see Fig. 18.4) may be used such that the probing beak of the instrument is placed parallel to the long axis of the tooth and inserted into the pocket. When the bottom of the pocket has been reached, the forceps are closed to pierce the gingiva on the oral surface, thus producing a bleeding point. The process is repeated along the whole circumference of the pocket producing bleeding points at several points around each tooth. The surgeon now has a dotted line (Fig. 18.8).

The above methods are applicable when dealing with uncomplicated pseudopockets and relatively shallow periodontal pockets in areas with abundant attached gingiva. However, when a pseudopocket is combined with a significant true periodontal pocket, the resultant line of bleeding points may be too close to or even apical to the mucogingival junction as well as apical to the furcations of multirooted teeth. To use these bleeding points as a guide for the line of excision would result in removal of excess gingival tissue and periodontal compromise of the tooth. In such instances, the surgeon should endeavor to keep the newly created free gingival margin 1–2 mm in dogs and coronal to the cementoenamel junction of each tooth (Fig. 18.9). Any clinically significant true pocket that persists is then managed with conservative or regenerative periodontal therapies.

When bleeding points are used as the guide, the primary incision, whether by blade, bur or electrode, is made joining the bleeding points and recreating the scalloped edge of the normal gingival anatomy (see Figs 18.1 & 18.3).[1,15] The initial, debulking incision starts with the blade or electrode entering the tissue on the oral side of the gingiva at or just apical to the bleeding points with the instrument angled coronally as it penetrates the tissues to create a beveled incision. The goal is to re-establish the normal gingival cross-sectional profile (Fig. 18.9). Once the primary incision is completed on the buccal and lingual aspects of the teeth, the interproximal soft tissue is separated from the interdental gingiva by a secondary incision using a gingivectomy knife.[4,15] The incised tissues are carefully removed by means of a periodontal curette or a scaler. Remaining tissue tags are removed with a curette or a pair of scissors.[15] Further sculpting of the gingival profile may be accomplished with cold steel, dental burs, laser or radiosurgery (Fig. 18.10 and see Figs 18.5, 8.8 & 8.9). Hemorrhage is controlled with gauze swabs and digital pressure. The crown and any exposed root surfaces are carefully scaled and polished.

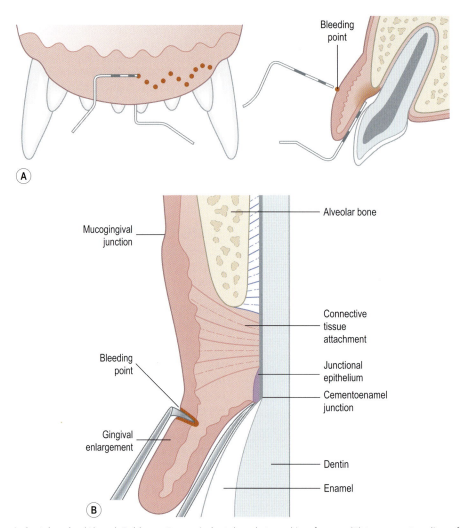

Fig. 18.8 The use of a periodontal probe (**A**) and Goldman–Fox periodontal pocket-marking forceps (**B**) to generate a line of bleeding points as a visual reference to guide the surgeon's initial incision.

When the incisions are made with a radiosurgery unit, the electrode should be activated at the minimal effective power setting in fully filter (cutting) mode and stroked across the gingiva at the required angle. The incision should be placed approximately 1 mm coronal to the desired final result to allow for the postoperative tissue shrinkage that may occur with this technique. The cut surface should be pink and not bleeding if the setting is correct (Fig. 18.11). Blanched tissue indicates that the setting is too high and should be reduced.[30]

In veterinary dentistry, gingivectomy/gingivoplasty is usually performed using a combination of the methods. For example, gross debulking of generalized gingival hyperplasia may be done by cold-blade excision, while creating a physiological contour with the correct bevel may be done with a round diamond bur on a high-speed handpiece.

Periodontal dressings to protect the wound surface during healing are not generally used in veterinary practice as dogs and cats are disinclined to tolerate them. However, the open wounds can be painted with several coats of tincture of myrrh and benzoin (Tincture of myrrh and benzoin, Ellman International Inc., Oceanside, NY) as a topical anodyne.[4] The crowns of the teeth can also be coated with a wax-polymer barrier (Ora-Vet, Merial Ltd., Duluth, GA) to inhibit bacterial recolonization of the teeth during the healing period.[31]

POSTOPERATIVE CARE AND ASSESSMENT

The postoperative phase is uncomfortable and analgesics are indicated for the first few days. It is crucial that plaque not be allowed to form on the tooth surfaces, as this will interfere with healing. Animals that have undergone this procedure are unlikely to accept tooth brushing immediately postoperatively, so chemical plaque control is indicated. Moreover, it has been shown that twice-daily applications of a 0.2% aqueous solution of chlorhexidine gluconate optimize healing of gingivectomy wounds.[32]

The healing of a gingivectomy/gingivoplasty wound is similar to that of a simple, open soft tissue wound except that there is a tooth in the center of the wound. During the inflammatory phase of healing, the underlying alveolar bone is slightly resorbed. Superficially, healing is complete when the epithelium reaches the tooth. Epithelialization is generally complete within 14 days after surgery. This epithelium, however, is initially thin and nonkeratinized, with keratinization taking up to a month.[1] The normal gingival anatomy (epithelial attachment, gingival sulcus, keratinized gingival epithelium) slowly reforms and the connective tissue matures. Complete healing generally takes 7 weeks.[1] However, on clinical examination, the surface of

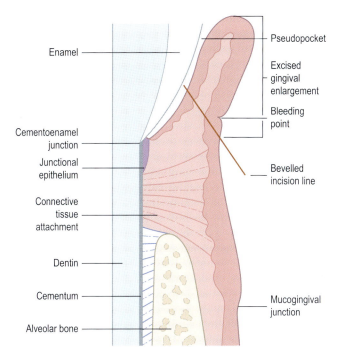

Fig. 18.9 The correct angle and placement of the initial incision. The instrument enters the tissue at or slightly apical to the bleeding points and is angled coronally to meet the tooth coronal to the cemento-enamel junction. In this way, the dentogingival complex is preserved, biologic width is not compromised and the cross-sectional profile of the gingival tissues is returned to normal.

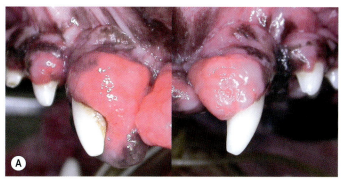

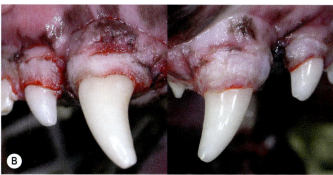

Fig. 18.11 (**A**) Preoperative photographs of the left and right maxillary canine and third incisor teeth of a 7-year-old, spayed female boxer dog showing conspicuous gingival enlargements with pseudopocket formation. (**B**) Immediate postoperative photographs of these same teeth following radiosurgical gingivectomy/gingivoplasty using a fully filtered wave form and a C7B triangular loop electrode (see Fig. 18.6, *top*). Note the desirable anatomic form (height and profile), the relative lack of hemorrhage and the lack of a visible char layer.

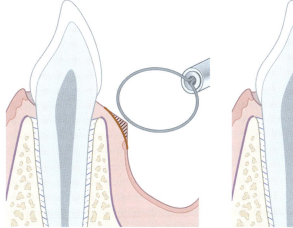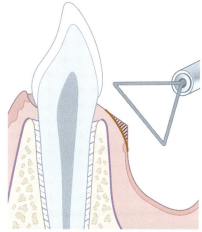

Fig. 18.10 Following the initial incision, some final sculpting of contours and anatomy may be achieved by cold steel or by careful use of 'hot' technique as shown here as a triangle loop in a radiosurgical unit is used to plane the surface to the desired shape.

the gingiva may already appear healed after 13–15 days.[33] Optimal plaque control is required for healing. Regeneration of the lost bone does not usually occur during the maturation phase.

Meticulous plaque control by means of daily tooth brushing (possibly augmented by the weekly application of a wax-polymer barrier and feeding diets and treats known to aid in the reduction of plaque) is necessary to prevent or at least delay recurrence.[1,4,15,34] Regularly scheduled professional periodontal maintenance therapy should be part of the long-term plan.

COMPLICATIONS

With cold incision, complications may include excessive hemorrhage. This may be controlled by the application of direct pressure with saline-soaked gauze or the application of a topical hemostatic agent. Improper planning of the line of incision that infringes on the biologic width or exposes bone directly will result in undesirable tissue loss during healing.

Thermal injury to the teeth and adjacent structures can occur if the gingival resection is performed using electrosurgery, radiosurgery, laser or high-speed burs.[1,4,24,27] This may result in sloughing of soft tissues and exposure of underlying bone. Use of excessive power with 'hot' modalities can result in excessive soft tissue necrosis as well as damage to bone, and so postoperative sloughing and bone sequestration are further potential complications with 'hot' incisions. Thermal damage and necrosis of the dental pulp is also possible with careless use of laser, radiosurgery and electrosurgery.

Use of diamond and carbide burs can result in physical damage to the crowns and roots of the teeth if these cutting burs come in contact with the dental hard tissues.

PROGNOSIS

Optimal home care is decisive for the long-term prognosis. In the absence of meticulous plaque control, rapid recurrence is common.

REFERENCES

1. Takei HH, Carranza FA. Gingival surgical techniques. In: Newman MG, Takei HH, Klokkevold PR, et al, editors. Carranza's clinical periodontology. 10th ed. Philadelphia, PA: WB Saunders; 2006. p. 909–17.

2. Marks SL. The buccal mucosal bleeding time. J Am Anim Hosp Assoc 2000;36: 289–90.

3. Carranza FA, Hogan EL. Gingival enlargements. In: Newman MG, Takei HH, Klokkevold PR, et al, editors. Carranza's clinical periodontology. 10th ed. Philadelphia, PA: WB Saunders; 2006. p. 373–90.

4. Lewis JR, Reiter AM. Management of generalized gingival enlargement in a dog – case report and literature review. J Vet Dent 2005;22:160–9.

5. Odom T, Anderson JG. Proliferative gingival lesion in a cat with disseminated cryptococcosis. J Vet Dent 2000;17: 177–81.

6. Gracis M. Orodental anatomy and physiology. In: Tutt C, Deeprose J, Crossley D, editors. BSAVA manual of canine and feline dentistry. 3rd ed. Gloucester, UK: British Small Animal Veterinary Association; 2007. p. 1–21.

7. Fiorellini JP, Kim DM, Ishikawa SO. The gingiva. In: Newman MG, Takei HH, Klokkevold PR, et al, editors. Carranza's clinical periodontology. 10th ed. Philadelphia, PA: WB Saunders; 2006. p. 46–67.

8. Wiggs RB, Lobprise HB. Oral anatomy and physiology. In: Veterinary dentistry, principles and practice. Philadelphia, PA: Raven-Lippincott; 1997. p. 55–86.

9 Schroeder HE. Oral mucosa. In: Oral structural biology. New York: Thieme Medical Publishing; 1991. p. 350–91.

10. Stern IB. Oral mucous membrane. In: Bhaskar SN, editor. Orban's oral histology and embryology. 11th ed. St. Louis, MO: Mosby Year Book; 1991. p. 260–336.

11. Schroeder HE. Marginal periodontium. In: Oral structural biology. New York: Thieme Medical Publishing; 1991. p. 230–64.

12. Melnick PR. Preparation of the periodontium for restorative dentistry. In: Newman MG, Takei HH, Klokkevold PR,

et al, editors. Carranza's clinical periodontology. 10th ed. Philadelphia, PA: WB Saunders; 2006. p. 1039–49.

13. Bellows J. Periodontal equipment, materials and techniques. In: Small animal dental equipment, materials and techniques. Ames, IA: Blackwell; 2004. p. 115–73.

14. Holmstrom SE, Frost Fitch P, Eisner ER. Periodontal therapy and surgery. In: Veterinary Dental Techniques. 3rd ed. Philadelphia, PA: WB Saunders; 2004. p. 233–90.

15. Wolf HF, Rateitschak EM, Rateitschak KH, et al. Gingivectomy and gingivoplasty. In: Rateitschak KH, Wolf HF, editors. Color atlas of dental medicine: periodontology. 3rd ed. Stuttgart, Germany: Thieme; 2004. p. 367–80.

16. Goldman HM. Gingivectomy. Oral Surg Oral Med Oral Pathol 1951:4: 1136–57.

17. Ostermeier S. Other oral and dental conditions. In: Tutt C, Deeprose J, Crossley D, editors. BSAVA manual of canine and feline dentistry. 3rd ed. Gloucester, UK: British Small Animal Veterinary Association; 2007. p. 160–77.

18. Strahan JD, Waite IM. The gingivectomy procedure. In: A colour atlas of periodontology. 1st ed. London: Wolfe Medical Publications; 1978. p. 58–62.

19. Sherman JA. Principles and theory of radiosurgery. In: Oral surgery. 2nd ed. London: Martin Dunitz; 1997. p. 1–8.

20. Silverman EB, Read RW, Boyle CR, et al. Histologic comparison of canine skin biopsies collected using monopolar electrosurgery, CO_2 laser, radio wave radiosurgery, skin biopsy punch and scalpel. Vet Surg 2007;36:50–6.

21. Olivar AC, Forouhar FA, Gillies CG, et al. Transmission electron microscopy; evaluation of damage to human oviducts caused by different surgical instruments. Ann Clin Lab Sci 1999:29;281–5.

22. Turner RJ, Cohen RA, Voet RL, et al. Analysis of tissue margins of cone biopsy specimens obtained with 'cold knife' CO_2 and Nd:YAG lasers and a a radiofrequency surgical unit. J Reprod Med 1992;37: 607–10.

23. Elkin AD. Optimizing the use of radiosurgery and all its varieties. Vet Forum April 1998:50–6.

24. Sherman JA. Waveform types and properties. In: Oral surgery. 2nd ed. London: Martin Dunitz; 1997. p. 9–14.

25. Miller WW. Using high-frequency radio wave technology in veterinary surgery. Vet Med 2004;99:796–802.

26. Carranza FA. Gingivectomy technique. In: Newman MG, Takei HH, Carranza FA, editors. Carranza's clinical periodontology. 9th ed. Philadelphia, PA: WB Saunders; 2002. p. 749–53.

27. Ishikawa I, Aoki A. Lasers in Periodontics. In: Newman MG, Takei HH, Klokkevold PR, et al, editors. Carranza's clinical periodontology. 10th ed. Philadelphia, PA: WB Saunders; 2006. p. 1035–7.

28. Wolf HF, Rateitschak EM, Rateitschak KH, et al. Perio-prosthetics 2, supplemental measures, esthetics. In: Rateitschak KH, Wolf HF, editors. Color atlas of dental medicine: periodontology. 3rd ed. Stuttgart, Germany: Thieme; 2004. p. 489–509.

29. Sitzman C. Simultaneous hyperplasia, metaplasia and neoplasia in an 8-year-old boxer dog; a case report. J Vet Dent 2000: 17:27–30.

30. Sherman JA. Radiosurgical techniques. In: Oral surgery. 2nd ed. London: Martin Dunitz; 1997. p. 45–154.

31. Gengler WR, Kunkle BN, Romano D, et al. Evaluation of a barrier sealant in dogs. J Vet Dent 2005;22:157–9.

32. Hamp SE, Rosling B, Lindhe J. Effect of chlorhexidine on gingival wound healing in the dog. A histometric study. J Clin Periodontol 1975;2:143–52.

33. Ramfjord SP, Engler WO, Hiniker JJ. A radioautographic study of healing following simple gingivectomy. II. The connective tissue. J Periodontol 1966; 37:179–89.

34. Wolf HF, Rateitschak EM, Rateitschak KH, et al. Oral pathological alterations of gingiva and periodontium. In: Rateitschak KH, Wolf HF, editors. Color atlas of dental medicine: periodontology. 3rd ed. Stuttgart, Germany: Thieme; 2004. p. 119–38.

Chapter | 19 |

Periodontal flaps and mucogingival surgery

Barry B. Staley & Patricia Frost Fitch

DEFINITIONS

Dehiscence: an area of tooth root denuded of bone, extending through the alveolar margin

Envelope flap: a full- or split-thickness flap used to access the root surface without vertical releasing incisions and replaced in its original position

Fenestration: an area of tooth root denuded of bone with an intact alveolar margin

Free gingival graft: a split-thickness graft of an area of keratinized gingiva (often from the buccal surface of the maxillary canine) transplanted to another site where a bed is prepared and the periosteum, connective tissue and blood supply left at the donor site is left to heal by second intention

Full-thickness flap: a mucoperiosteal flap reflected from the alveolar bone, including the periosteum

Pedicle (sliding or lateral) flap: a periodontal (often split-thickness) flap that is moved in an apical, coronal, mesial or distal direction

Periodontal flap: a section of gingiva and/or mucosa that is surgically separated from the underlying tissue and that retains at least one vascular attachment to the donor site

Reverse (or internal) bevel incision: an incision made at the crest of the free gingival margin down through the connective tissue to the periosteum covering the alveolar margin

Split/partial-thickness flap: a flap reflected from the alveolar bone that contains epithelium and a layer of connective tissue, leaving the periosteum on the bony surface

Subepithelial connective tissue graft (palate): a layer of connective tissue harvested from underneath the palatal epithelium and transplanted to another site where a connective tissue bed is prepared

Sulcular (or crevicular) incision: an incision made within the periodontal pocket between the cementum and the epithelial lining of the sulcus, extending through the epithelial attachment to the crest of periodontal ligament–bone interface

PREOPERATIVE CONSIDERATIONS

Periodontal flap

The design of the periodontal flap will depend on the type of pocket: suprabony versus infrabony, and the types of infrabony defects (one-, two-, or three-wall defects).

The gold standard in diagnosis of the periodontal pocket is the periodontal probe and the use of conventional dental radiographs. Therefore full-mouth probing of at least six measurements on each tooth (distobuccal, buccal, mesiobuccal, distolingual, lingual, mesiolingual) and horizontal probing for furcation lesions combined with a full-mouth series of radiographs are necessary to make an accurate diagnosis. In a classic study that documented the diagnostic yield of full-mouth radiographs in dogs, it was found that the extent of periodontal disease and bone loss was greater than what was clinically diagnosed or expected in 26.2% of dogs.[1]

The goal is to identify any pockets over 4 mm because clinical studies have shown that scaling and root planing do not remove all of the subgingival plaque and the long-term maintenance is therefore compromised.[2] The removal of plaque and of all the factors that favor its accumulation is therefore the primary consideration in therapy.[3]

Mucogingival surgery

Mucogingival lesions may be defined as developmental and acquired aberrations in the morphology, position and/or amount of gingiva surrounding teeth. When considering mucogingival surgery and surgical methods, problems related to the band of keratinized attached gingiva, osseous defects or dehiscence, periodontal pockets beyond the mucogingival junction, thickness of the alveolar process, tooth position in the dental arch, root protrusion, and gingival thickness must be taken into account.

The evaluation and diagnosis of these issues will be via the use of the periodontal probe and dental radiographs, with special attention to the mucogingival zone around the tooth and bone. The normal amount of keratinized attached gingiva in the dog is 2–5 mm and in the cat 1–2 mm.[4] Any width smaller than this would be considered inadequate, and surgical correction may be an option. It is important

© 2012 Elsevier Ltd
DOI: 10.1016/B978-0-7020-4618-6.00019-1

to note that the concern is about attached keratinized tissue and not the total volume of keratinized tissue. The total volume of keratinized tissue is comprised of free gingiva plus attached gingiva. When assessing the periodontal pocket with the periodontal probe one must estimate the amount of keratinized attached gingiva by subtracting the pocket depth from the total keratinized tissue observed clinically.

SURGICAL ANATOMY

Periodontal flap and mucogingival surgery

Landmarks

The key landmarks are: cementum, sulcular epithelium, epithelial attachment, gingival connective tissue, free gingival margin, keratinized attached gingiva, mucogingival junction, alveolar mucosa, alveolar bone, periodontal ligament (PDL) and periosteum.

Differences between dogs and cats

There are several differences in dog and cat anatomy. The normal gingival sulcus for a cat is 0.5–1 mm but for the dog it is 2–3 mm. The cat also has less keratinized attached gingiva with a somewhat thinner alveolar mucosa. The cat oral soft tissues are thinner and more delicate; therefore smaller surgical instruments will be indicated.

SPECIAL INSTRUMENTS

A selection of instruments for periodontal surgery suitable for use in dogs and cats is listed in Table 19.1. In addition to these hand instruments, an ultrasonic scaler designed for periodontal debridement and subgingival use is indicated.

Specialized instruments for cats are the small beaver blades and round beaver blade handles (Micro Bistouri M-6700, Advanced Surgical Technologies, Sacramento, CA) and small feline scaler/curettes (P-102 and small periosteal elevators EX-19, EX-50 and EX-9, Cislak, Lakeview, IL).

THERAPEUTIC DECISION-MAKING

Periodontal flaps

There are two types of flaps in periodontal surgery based on whether the flap includes periosteum (full thickness, or mucoperiosteal) or not (split/partial thickness). A combination split/full-thickness flap also exists (Fig. 19.1).

Flaps are also classified by their placement. With the apically positioned flap, the flap is displaced apically from the original position. With the replaced (or nondisplaced) flap, the flap is returned and sutured to the original position. The apically positioned flap is used in resectional procedures while the replaced flap is used in surgical procedures for tissue regeneration.

Since the goal of periodontal therapy is the removal of plaque and of all the factors that favor its accumulation, the periodontal pocket over 4 mm is an area where subgingival plaque can accumulate and continue the inflammatory process and eventual tissue destruction. Clinical research has demonstrated that it is difficult or impossible to predictably remove the accretions on a root surface in a pocket that is deeper than 4 mm. The clinician is thus faced with three possibilities if a probing depth greater than 4 mm is present: (1) maintenance

Table 19.1 Instruments for periodontal surgery in dogs and cats

Description	Details
Periodontal probe/shepherd hook explorer combination	#23/CP-12[a]
Scalpel handle	#7K[a]; #5 (round)[a]; K360[a]
Scalpel blade	#15C[b]
Kramer–Nevins tissue pliers	TPKN[a]
Tissue forceps	Adson 1X2[a]
Curved tissue scissors	Goldman–Fox #16[a]
Double-ended Gracey curettes (extended shanks and mini blades)	#7–8; #11–12; #13–14[a]
Kramer–Nevins interproximal knife	#7, #11[a]
Kramer-Nevins surgical curettes	e.g., #3/4[a]
Curved sickle scaler (small and medium)	204S[a]
Schulger surgical file	#9/10[a]
Ochsenbein chisels	#1[a]; #2[a]
Small needle holder (tungsten carbide inserts)	Castroviejo[a]; Halsey (NH-5036)[a]
Periosteal elevator	#7 wax spatula[a]; Goldman–Fox #14[a]; #24G[a]
Tissue retractor	Cawood–Minnesota retractor CRM2[a], Seldin #23 retractor[a]
Carbide and diamond round burs	#2, 4, 6 and 8[c]

[a]Hu-Friedy, Chicago, IL
[b]BD Bard/Parker, Franklin Lakes, NJ
[c]Brasseler USA, Savannah, GA

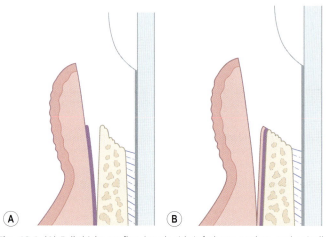

Fig. 19.1 (**A**) Full-thickness flap (used with infrabony pockets and apically positioned flaps; the periosteum is included in the reflected flap). (**B**) Split-thickness flap (used with suprabony pockets and apically positioned flaps; the periosteum is left on the bone).

as is, with poor long-term results; (2) reduction by subtraction – pocket resectional procedures; or (3) reduction by addition – regeneration of bone–PDL–cementum.[5]

Classification of the type of pocket using the periodontal probe and radiographic analysis will dictate the flap design. Suprabony pockets with hyperplastic tissue (no bone loss) can be reduced by gingivectomy (see Ch. 18). Suprabony pockets with horizontal bone loss will be approached with split/full/split-thickness flaps and osteoplasty/ostectomy.

Most of the infrabony pockets will be approached via mucoperiosteal flaps to gain access to the tooth surface and alveolar bone to perform osteoplasty and/or regeneration procedures.

One-wall and some two-wall bony defects are treated by means of a split-thickness flap and osteoplasty/ostectomy, with the flap apically positioned to the height of the new bone margin. This flap is a split/full/split-thickness flap and will be described in the surgical techniques section to follow. The goal of ostectomy is to make the interproximal bone flat mesial-to-distal and buccal-to-lingual. The interproximal bone should be occlusal to or at approximately the same level as the radicular bone. The opposite is described as reverse architecture, and will result in continued soft tissue pocketing. The treatment objective of the parabolic bony architecture will be influenced by the size of the embrasure, because it is more difficult to control soft tissue growth in a narrow interproximal site. The osteoplasty and ostectomy are performed with round burs, files and chisels.

Indications for the apically positioned flaps are: (1) eliminating pockets (suprabony, one- and some two-walled infrabony defects); (2) preserving keratinized attached gingiva and increasing its width; and (3) establishing gingival morphology to facilitate good hygiene.

Contraindications include: (1) some two- and three-walled infrabony defects (suitable for regenerative procedures); (2) severe periodontal pockets; (3) teeth with marked mobility and severe attachment loss; (4) teeth with an unfavorable clinical crown:root ratio; and (5) lack of keratinized free gingiva or attached gingiva to move apically.

Some two- and three-wall osseous defects can be treated by bone regeneration techniques (see Ch. 20). The access flap for these procedures is a full-thickness mucoperiosteal flap. Indications for a replaced flap and regeneration are: (1) some two- and three-walled defects; (2) to restore lost attachment (bone–PDL–cementum); (3) to avoid gingival recession; and (4) to decrease pocket depth.

Possible concerns include the fact that these are technically demanding procedures, which require a longer anesthetic period. Postoperative plaque control is essential and a second procedure may be required to eliminate remaining pockets.

Mucogingival surgery

Mucogingival surgical procedures correct or eliminate anatomic, developmental or traumatic lesions of the gingiva or alveolar mucosa. These are conditions associated with keratinized attached gingiva, shallow vestibules, frenulum interfering with free gingival margins, and oral tissue trauma.

Evaluating the patient for an adequate zone of keratinized attached gingiva is important because the keratinized attached gingiva has dense connective tissue fibers with less vascularization, and is therefore more able to resist the initiation and progression of the inflammatory process in periodontal disease. The loose nonkeratinized alveolar mucosa is less fibrous and more vascular than the keratinized attached gingiva. This is of particular significance because inflammation extends perivascularly.[5] In general, veterinary patients lack good consistent home care and regular 4-month recall teeth cleaning. Any area with plaque build-up in the presence of gingival recession is an area of concern and mucogingival surgery should be considered an option.

The normal dimensions of keratinized attached tissue and the ideal labial–lingual width of the alveolar process (thickness of the periodontium) have a significant effect on mucogingival problems. Therefore, inadequate keratinized attached gingiva or dehiscence (thin alveolar bone) may predispose a tooth to recession with inflammation or trauma. In the absence of disease, recession may not occur despite the predisposition. Malpositioned teeth are likely to have inadequate keratinized attached gingiva and dehiscence or fenestration of the alveolar bone. The gingivae of prominent teeth are prone to recession.[5]

Indications for mucogingival surgery are: (1) to create an adequate zone of keratinized attached gingiva; (2) to establish a strong keratinized attached gingiva to protect the mucogingival complex during mastication of hard food and objects; (3) the presence of gingival recession; and (4) to cover dehiscence and fenestration. Adequate interdental papillae and interdental alveolar bone adjacent to gingival recession and a sufficient blood supply at the donor site are prerequisites.

Contraindications include: (1) an insufficient width and thickness of keratinized tissue at the donor site; (2) gingival recession in an area that is extremely protrusive; (3) deep periodontal pockets and loss of interdental alveolar bone adjacent to the recipient site; (4) a narrow and shallow vestibule; (5) a deep and wide recession area; (6) involvement of multiple teeth; (7) uncontrolled periodontal disease; and (8) poor client/patient plaque control.

SURGICAL TECHNIQUES

Periodontal flap surgery

Apically positioned flap

Initial incision and releasing incisions

The initial incision, using a #15C scalpel blade in the dog or a beaver blade in the cat, is a reverse-bevel (split-thickness) incision starting at the crest of the free gingival margin. The incision is continued to the margin of the alveolar bone (Fig. 19.2). Vertical incisions are made one tooth mesial and one tooth distal to the defects, making sure the vertical incisions are at the line angles of these teeth. Vertical incisions are not made over furcation areas or in the middle of the

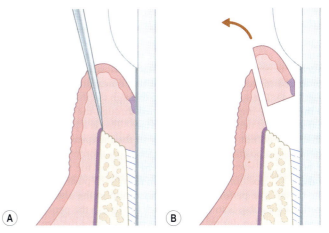

Fig. 19.2 (A) Reverse-bevel incision (used with split-thickness, apically positioned, coronally positioned, and pedicle flaps). **(B)** Removal of sulcular epithelium.

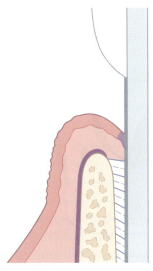

Fig. 19.5 Apically positioned flap (repositioned at the new osseous margin).

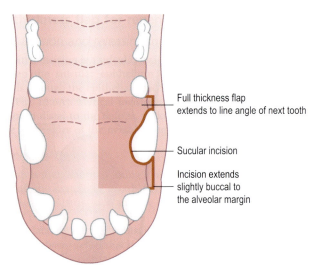

Full thickness flap extends to line angle of next tooth

Sucular incision

Incision extends slightly buccal to the alveolar margin

Fig. 19.7 Palatal flap (used with three-wall infrabony pockets and bone grafting).

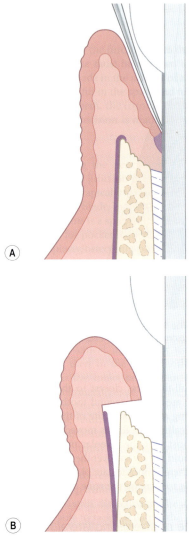

(A)

(B)

Fig. 19.6 (**A**) Sulcular incision (used with full-thickness flaps and three-wall infrabony defects). (**B**) Reflected full-thickness flap with sulcular epithelium.

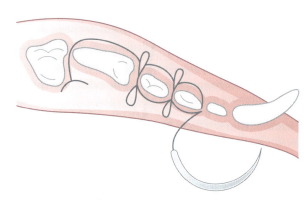

Fig. 19.8 Continuous sling suture.

apically. The mesial vertical incision is sutured (periosteal tacking) after the mesial and distal coronal interrupted sutures to the interproximal papilla have been placed. Periosteal tacking sutures are placed on the distal vertical aspect of the flap into the exposed periosteum covering the second tooth distal (Fig. 19.10C).

Free gingival graft

Preparation of the recipient site

At the area of recession that will be the recipient site, a reverse-bevel incision is made around the free gingival margin of the recession to remove the pocket epithelium (Fig. 19.11A). A horizontal incision is made 1–2 mm coronal to the mucogingival junction. Two vertical incisions are made apically and into the alveolar mucosa. A second horizontal incision is made to connect the vertical incisions. The rectangular piece of tissue thus created is removed by split-thickness dissection, leaving the periosteum covering the exposed area. The size of the defect created should be large enough to accommodate and secure the free gingival graft (Fig. 19.11B). Hemorrhage is controlled with wet gauze and pressure.

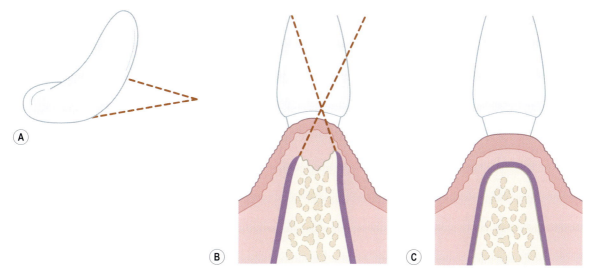

Fig. 19.9 (**A**) Mesial wedge excision. (**B**) Angled incisions to excise the wedge. (**C**) Tissue apposition following wedge excision, osteoplasty, and apically positioned flap.

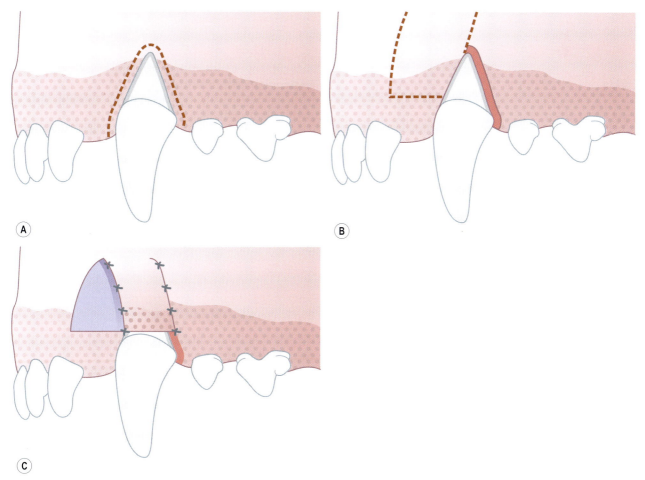

Fig. 19.10 Pedicle/sliding/lateral flap: (**A**) Excision of the sulcular epithelium. (**B**) Angled vertical incision toward the sliding direction. (**C**) Tacking sutures to the periosteum.

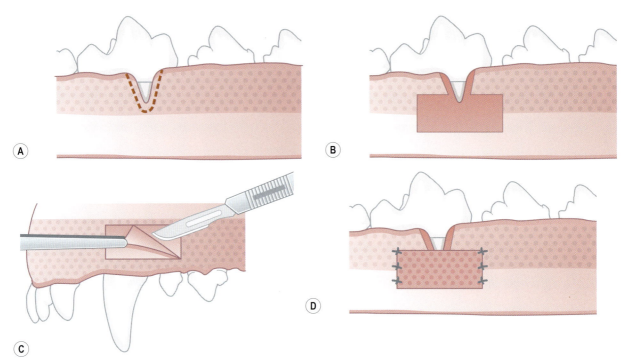

Fig. 19.11 Free gingival graft: (**A**) Excision of the sulcular epithelium. (**B**) Preparation of the recipient bed. (**C**) Preparation of the donor site. (**D**) Tacking sutures to the connective tissue bed.

Preparation of the donor site

A donor area is selected where there is sufficient keratinized attached gingiva (often the buccal aspect of the maxillary canine). The recipient site is measured and a small piece of aluminum foil template matching the size of the recipient site is made. The template is then placed on the donor site and incisions drawn around the edges of the foil through the epithelium to the periosteum of the donor area.[8] A corner of the donor epithelium is dissected with a # 15C scalpel blade and the graft removed by split-thickness dissection (Fig. 19.11C).

Suturing the free graft

The graft is sutured to the connective tissue bed using periosteal tacking sutures. The coronal mesial and distal corners are sutured first, followed by the mesial and distal sides. Hemostasis is achieved by gentle pressure using moistened gauze over the grafted area. The graft will fail if a thick blood clot is present under the graft. It is not necessary to suture the graft to the apical alveolar mucosa, as the sutures can get buried, delay healing, and are not needed to retain the graft in position (Fig. 19.11D).

Subepithelial connective tissue graft (palate)

This graft is usually used to cover root surfaces after recession. This is mainly done for cosmetic reasons in humans so its use in veterinary dentistry is limited.

Preparation of the donor site

The connective tissue is exposed by means of a split-thickness flap on the palate. The subepithelial connective tissue is harvested, leaving the periosteum and the overlying split-thickness flap. The flap is subsequently replaced on the palate ('trap door approach').

Preparation of the recipient site

The recipient site is prepared the same way as the free gingival graft except that the split-thickness alveolar mucosa is not discarded but replaced over the connective tissue graft placed over the area of recession.

Suturing the graft and overlying flap

The connective tissue graft is sutured first (coronal, mesial and distal) to the recipient periosteum and then the alveolar mucosa flap sutured to the interproximal gingiva. The vertical wound edges are also sutured to the connective tissue and periosteum.

POSTOPERATIVE CARE AND ASSESSMENT

Periodontal flap

Decreasing plaque accumulation postoperatively is best achieved by daily oral flushing with 0.05–0.2% chlorhexidine gluconate solution for 2 weeks. Alternatively, chlorhexidine patches may be used. Appropriate pain medication (see Ch. 4) is used and a soft diet instituted for two weeks. Return to routine oral hygiene will aid in the healing process.

Evaluation of the surgical site is crucial and is performed at 7–10 days. Periodontal probing and radiographic evaluation should be done after 6–12 months; this requires general anesthesia and may be combined with routine periodontal treatment.

Mucogingival surgery

Soft diet, chlorhexidine rinses or patches, and pain control are indicated. Immobility of the graft is crucial and an Elizabethan collar may be indicated to prevent the patient from dislodging the graft.

Evaluation by means of periodontal probing and measuring the width of attached gingiva is indicated after 1 year and may be combined with routine periodontal treatment.

COMPLICATIONS

Periodontal flap

Sloughing of the flap is a serious complication, which may happen if the flap is sutured under tension. A flap may move from the original sutured position; as a result, bone margins may become exposed or the flap may heal coronally to the intended position and recreate a periodontal pocket.

Mucogingival surgery

Bleeding under the graft may cause sloughing of the graft. A graft may be dislodged by the patient's paws or tongue. If placed over thin bone, resorption may occur and the graft lost.

PROGNOSIS

Periodontal flap

The correct diagnosis of pocket type and bony defect is a prerequisite for a successful outcome. Following the selection of the appropriate treatment, skillful surgical technique, including correct flap design and careful suturing, is conducive to a good prognosis. Meticulous home care is crucial and follow-up evaluations are necessary to assess the success or failure of the procedure.

Mucogingival surgery

A good prognosis is expected when treating a narrow and shallow recession, provided the correct diagnosis is made and the procedure is skillfully executed.

REFERENCES

1. Verstraete FJM, Kass PH, Terpak CH. Diagnostic value of full-mouth radiography in dogs. Am J Vet Res 1998;59:686–91.
2. Sato N. Periodontal surgery: a clinical atlas. Chicago, IL: Quintessence Publishing; 2000.
3. Newman MG, Takei HH, Carranza FA. Carranza's clinical periodontology. 9th ed. Philadelphia, PA: Saunders; 2002.
4. Wiggs RB, Lobprise HB. Veterinary dentistry principles and practice. Philadelphia, PA: Lippincott-Raven; 1997. p. 186–231.
5. Nevins M, Mellonig JT. Periodontal therapy: clinical approaches and evidence of success. Chicago, IL: Quintessence Publishing; 1998.
6. Silverstein LH. Principles of dental suturing. New Jersey: Montage Media; 1999. p. 34–69.
7. Holmstrom SE, Frost P, Eisner ER. Veterinary dental techniques – for the small animal practitioner. 2nd ed. Philadelphia, PA: Saunders; 1998. p. 167–214.
8. Cohen ES. Atlas of cosmetic and reconstructive periodontal surgery. 2nd ed. Baltimore, MD: William & Wilkins; 1999. p. 65–164.

Chapter | 20 |

Osteoconductive and osteoinductive agents in periodontal surgery

Milinda J. Lommer, Robert B. Wiggs[†], Jamie G. Anderson

DEFINITIONS

Allograft: a graft obtained from genetically dissimilar individual of the same species as the recipient; includes freeze-dried bone and demineralized freeze-dried bone; may be osteoinductive as well as osteoconductive

Alloplast: synthetic or naturally occurring inert materials implanted into host tissue to occupy space and act as a scaffold for new bone production; includes hydroxyapetite, tri-calcium phosphate, polymers and bioactive glass

Autogenous graft: obtained from a remote location in the recipient (host); the only osteogenic graft material

Guided tissue regeneration (GTR): advanced periodontal therapy using barrier membranes and/or graft materials to encourage the growth of periodontal ligament, cementum and bone cells and exclude unwanted epithelial cells from a healing periodontal pocket

Osteoconductive: materials that occupy space and act as a scaffold on which new bone can grow

Osteogenic: materials containing live cells that lay down bone matrix

Osteoinductive: materials containing growth factors or hormones that signal the host to produce new bone

Xenograft: tissue obtained from an individual of a different species than the host; processing to remove antigenicity renders most of these materials osteoconductive only

INTRODUCTION

Periodontal disease is an inflammatory response to infection within the gingival sulcus, as a result of complex interaction between bacteria, their by-products, and the response of various components of the host's own immune system. Periodontitis (loss of alveolar bone)

occurs at different rates, depending on many factors.[1,2] Optimum therapy includes management of the infection, control of the host immune response, and regeneration of diseased or lost portions of the periodontium.[3]

The outcome of periodontal therapy is highly dependent upon the type of tissue that first repopulates the root surface.[4] A healing periodontal pocket is invaded by cells from four different sources: gingival epithelium, gingival connective tissue, alveolar bone, and periodontal ligament (Fig. 20.1).[4]

Proliferation of gingival epithelial cells along the root surface before the other tissues reach the area results in a long junctional epithelium, which may be unstable and has a high chance of pocket recurrence.[5] If gingival connective tissue is first to repopulate the root surface, the fibers will be parallel to the root surface and alveolar bone will regenerate with no connection to the cementum.[6] When bone is the first repopulator, the typical response is root resorption and ankylosis. Only when periodontal ligament cells proliferate coronally can new cementum and periodontal ligament formation occur, restoring healthy attachment.[6] Unfortunately, epithelial cells migrate 10 times faster than other periodontal tissue types, so conventional periodontal therapy typically results in reparative healing by formation of long junctional epithelium rather than regenerative healing which restores the periodontal ligament, cementum, and bone.[7]

The ideal outcome of periodontal surgery is elimination of the pocket and reconstruction of the periodontal tissues.[8] Because of the aforementioned reasons, this can be achieved only after removal of junctional and pocket epithelium and prevention of their migration into the healing periodontal space after surgery. Regenerative procedures typically involve the use of bone grafting materials and/or barrier membranes to promote the growth of desired periodontal tissues while excluding unwanted cell types such as gingival epithelial cells (Fig. 20.2).[9]

GUIDED TISSUE REGENERATION

Guided tissue regeneration (GTR) is an advanced periodontal therapy which attempts to restore tissues (periodontal ligament, cementum, and alveolar bone) lost due to periodontal disease. GTR has the

---

†Deceased.

DOI: 10.1016/B978-0-7020-4618-6.00020-8

potential to save teeth that might otherwise be lost due to disease or extraction.

In periodontal GTR, a selective barrier (comprised of a barrier membrane, particulate graft, or both) is placed between a properly prepared tooth root surface and the gingival tissues, which are closed over the area with a flap.[10] The basic principles of GTR appear straightforward and simple, but failure to strictly adhere to them can result in treatment failure. Success is dependent upon correct selection of site, proper choice of materials, appropriate technique for the site and material, skill of the surgeon, and client commitment to oral hygiene for the patient.

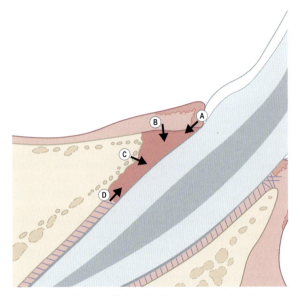

Fig. 20.1 Sources of new cells in a healing periodontal pocket. Following curettage and debridement of the pocket epithelium, cells from the following tissues enter the clot: (A) gingival epithelium (B) gingival connective tissue (C) alveolar bone (D) periodontal ligament.

Patient and client selection

General anesthesia is required both to perform the guided tissue regeneration procedure and to reevaluate the treated area(s) at regular intervals. Guided tissue regeneration is technically more challenging and often more time consuming than extraction, so the anesthetic period may be prolonged for the initial treatment. In addition, general anesthesia is required for reassessment of the treated area(s) with radiographs and probing. Therefore, patients for whom GTR is considered should be in good general health, without contraindications for repeated anesthetic episodes. The patient must be compliant for visual inspection of the surgical site 2 weeks postoperatively, and must receive daily toothbrushing at home. The client must be dedicated to the preservation of the pet's oral health, willing to perform daily home care, and comfortable with the need for follow-up radiographs under general anesthesia. Further, the client must be informed that results of GTR are unpredictable, success is not guaranteed, and the tooth or teeth in question may require extraction in the future.

Patient preparation

Following intraoral radiographs and prior to diagnostic dental charting, the oral cavity should be disinfected with an agent such as dilute chlorhexidine gluconate, with a concentration not exceeding 0.12%, because at concentrations higher than 0.12%, chlorhexidine inhibits attachment of periodontal cells to the root surface.[11] Further, chlorhexidine solutions are contraindicated for the direct treatment of the root surface and periodontal tissues within the pocket prior to surgery, for even at concentrations as low as 0.0025% chlorhexidine may have adverse affects on the growth of periodontal cells.[11] Contamination of the surgical field should be minimized by the placement of cotton rolls or rubber dams to restrict salivary or other contaminate incursion.[3] These protective barriers can also provide a degree of protection against accidents related to dental instruments.

Site selection

Guided tissue regeneration should be considered for structurally and functionally important teeth, such as canine teeth and mandibular first molar teeth, with infrabony pockets. Currently, clinical

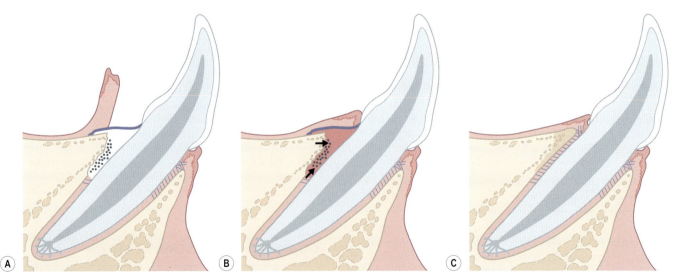

Fig. 20.2 (**A**) Guided tissue regeneration involves placement of a bone graft and/or barrier membrane to prevent migration of gingival cells into a healing periodontal pocket. (**B**) This allows the more slowly growing osteoblasts and periodontal ligament fibroblasts to repopulate the pocket, (**C**) resulting in formation of new bone and periodontal ligament attachment and elimination of the pocket.

indications include stage-2 furcation lesions, 2- or 3-walled vertical interproximal sites, and three-walled palatal defects of single-rooted teeth.[9] Areas with abundant gingival attachment are typically preferred as they facilitate good flap coverage of the barrier. Although there is limited evidence that combination GTR therapy using a membrane and bone graft material may allow some regeneration in suprabony defects,[12] areas with horizontal bone loss (suprabony defects) are generally considered poor candidates for GTR.[10]

Flap creation

Initially, a flap must be created to allow access to the pocket. In designing this flap, the ultimate closure of the site with the incorporation of the barrier must be taken into consideration. Every precaution should be taken to preserve the blood supply of the flap during its creation, elevation and replacement, as this greatly affects healing and the ultimate success of the procedure. Local anesthesia is recommended; if using a local anesthetic with epinephrine (which prolongs the anesthetic effect and reduces excess bleeding), the epinephrine should not exceed a concentration of 1 : 100 000 as it may restrict the blood flow to the flap, adversely affecting the flap's vitality.[3] Periodontal flap design is discussed in detail in Chapter 19.

Pocket preparation

Treatment of the pocket must be planned to provide a compartment of adequate dimensions for the development of the desired new bone and periodontal tissues. The pocket must be debrided of all granulation and other undesired soft tissues to expose the alveolar bone walls and root cementum. Treatment of the tooth root of the affected site includes root debridement and subgingival curettage to remove all invading soft tissues, such as epithelial, connective and granulation tissues from the pocket.[10,13,14] Once exposed, the surfaces of the tooth root may benefit from a surface conditioning treatment with either citric acid, tetracycline or EDTA preparations.[8] Root conditioners may aid in attachment of the blood clot and other tissues to the root surface and enhance healing. Citric acid, in particular, has been reported to demineralize the root surface, eliminate bacteria and endotoxins from the root surface, remove the smear layer, and expose the collagen in the cementum; fibrin linkage to the exposed collagen fibers reportedly prevents gingival epithelial cells from migrating over the roots.[8] Not all authors agree which root conditioner is best or exactly when it should be used.[3] Therefore the use of these products should be guided by the barrier manufacturers' recommendations. Osteoplasty (recontouring of the alveolar bone associated with the pocket) may also be performed to improve the site architecture for the barrier placement and flap closure.

Barrier selection

As previously mentioned, the barrier inhibits downgrowth of gingival epithelium and connective tissue into the pocket, preventing these cells from colonizing the root surface.[10] This allows time for the more slowly growing periodontal ligament, cementum and alveolar bone cells to reproduce and recreate the normal periodontal architecture. Research suggests that barriers need to be in place and reasonably intact for between 28 and 42 days to be effective in guided tissue regeneration.[10] The major decisions in barrier selection are between membrane and particulate graft material, or a combination of these.[3] Particulate graft materials have the advantages of generally being less expensive per application and being able to maintain a substantial compartment. Some particulates are mixed with saline or acquired blood from the patient while others may be placed into the socket dry and gently packed into the defect. When placed dry, the particulate is

typically saturated very quickly with blood seeping from the alveolar bone. This blood percolating from the bone is rich in bone morphogenetic proteins that can enhance bone formation. If particulate materials are used that require blood as a mixing agent, blood from the bleeding alveolar bone surrounding the pocket may be collected with a 25-gauge needle attached to a 1-mL or tuberculin syringe. If there is no free blood available at the site, either saline can be mixed with the particulate or the alveolar bone can be shallowly penetrated with a needle or sterile bur to produce the required minimal bleeding for a healthy clot formation.

Membranes are highly adaptive and can provide a compartment over root surfaces with poor collateral bone support. However, the resulting compartment may be relatively thin and not as conductive to substantial new growth. The membrane should be selected in a configuration that best fits the particular defect, or custom fitted and seated to the area by trimming with sterile scissors, if allowed by the manufacturer. Sharp corners, wrinkles, folds and overlapping of the material should be avoided when possible to provide a suitable fit for flap closure. Tucking the membrane under the periosteum and placing sutures in the membrane prior to gingival closure will help to stabilize the membrane and help prevent migration due to movement and pressures generated by mastication and tongue motion. Table 20.1 summarizes factors that influence the outcome of GTR procedures.[9]

Table 20.1 Factors influencing outcome of GTR procedures

	Positive effect on outcome	**Negative effect on outcome**
Anatomic factors	Deep (≥4 mm) infrabony defect	Shallow infrabony defect
	Narrow defect angle (<45 degrees)	Wide defect angle (>45 degrees)
	Vertical bone loss	Horizontal bone loss
	3-wall defects	1- or 2-wall defects
	Minimal furcation involvement	Deep furcation involvement
	Adequate tissue thickness (>1.1 mm)	
	Adequate keratinized gingiva (2 mm)	
Patient/ client factors	Good oral hygiene/ compliance	Poor oral hygiene/compliance
	Systemic health	Systemically compromised patient
Surgery-related factors	Passive flap tension	Excessive flap tension
	Stable wound	Early mechanical disruption
	Sterile surgery	Contamination during surgery
	Primary wound closure	Inadequate wound closure
	Short, minimally traumatic surgery	Prolonged/traumatic surgery
	Proper incision location	Poorly designed incisions
	No membrane exposure	Membrane exposure

Table 20.2 Summary of bone grafting materials and substitutes

	Autogenous	Allograft	Alloplast	Xenograft
Source	Patient	Same species	Synthetic	Different species
Properties	Osteogenic, osteoinductive, osteoconductive	Osteoinductive, osteoconductive	Osteoconductive	Osteoconductive
Examples	Cancellous bone collected from iliac crest	Demineralized freeze-dried bone and freeze-dried bone, e.g. OsteoAllograft®	Bioactive ceramics e.g. Consil®	Bovine cancellous bone e.g. Bio-Oss® (Geistlich Biomaterials, Inc., Switzerland)

GRAFT MATERIALS

Autogenous grafts, i.e., those collected directly from the patient, have historically been the 'gold standard' bone replacement material,[9] and they are the only truly osteogenic graft option. Although experimental periodontal studies in dogs have failed to show an advantage in periodontal healing when comparing autogenous bone with other materials (coral-derived biomaterial, tricalcium phosphate, or demineralized freeze-dried canine bone allograft),[15,16] periodontal regeneration (formation of new cementum and periodontal ligament in addition to new bone) reportedly occurs more predictably with autografts and demineralized freeze-dried allografts than with other materials.[17]

In addition to their osteoconductive properties, *allografts* (typically freeze-dried or frozen cancellous and/or cortical bone) may contain bone morphogenetic proteins (BMP), which stimulate new bone production (osteoinduction). Numerous clinical studies have evaluated the success of freeze-dried bone allografts in inducing new bone formation in human patients.[18-22] Experimental studies in dogs have shown production of new bone[15,23] and cementum[16,24] following placement of freeze-dried bone allografts. Demineralization of the freeze-dried bone exposes the collagen fibrils and associated components of bone matrix including bone morphogenetic proteins; therefore, demineralized freeze-dried bone (DFDB) is considered osteoinductive, while nondemineralized freeze-dried bone (FDB) is considered osteoconductive only.[8] Both canine and feline freeze-dried bone are commercially available in a mixture of demineralized bone matrix and cancellous chips < 0.7 mm in diameter, specifically designed for oral and periodontal use (OsteoAllograft® Perio Mix, Veterinary Transplant Services, Inc. Kent, WA 98032). Allografts are appealing in that there is no need for an additional surgical procedure to procure bone from a remote site on the patient.

Alloplasts are synthetic or naturally occurring inert materials which serve primarily to maintain space, and are therefore not ideal to promote periodontal regeneration.[9] Calcium sulfate (plaster of Paris) was one of the first synthetic materials used as a bone supplement and for osteoconduction.[25,26] Results in reported studies are mixed,[26-28] and resorption is inconsistent. Osteoconductive ceramics include hydroxylapatites (HA) and tricalcium phosphates (TCP). The original tricalcium phosphates resorbed quickly (within days to weeks), while hydroxylapatites resorbed slowly if at all. Currently available products have more controlled resorption rates. Hydroxylapatite (HA), a calcium phosphate mineral component of bone and coral, is available in particulate forms (Calcitite®: Calcitek®, Inc., Carlsbad, CA 92008; OsteoGen®: Impladent Ltd., Holliswood, NY 11423; OsteoGraf®: CeraMed Corp, Lakewood, CO 80228). Tricalcium phosphate (TCP) is available in particulate (SynthoGraft®, Boston, MA 02130) and putty (FormPutty®: Theken Spine, Inc. Akron, OH 44306) forms, with controlled resorption rates varying from several days up to 12 months.[29,30]

Bioactive ceramics, also called bioglass materials, generally contain oxides of calcium, sodium, phosphorous, and silicone, which stimulate collagen synthesis and new bone formation. Most bioglass materials use silicone oxide as a matrix former. The minerals are slowly released in an aqueous environment, increasing pH and osmotic pressure at the site, which may slow or prevent resorption of the bioglass. Bioactive ceramics have a broad antimicrobial effect on microorganisms on teeth and implants.[31-33] One bioactive glass (Consil®: Nutramax Laboratories, Inc., Edgewood, MD 21040), available in both particulate and putty forms, is marketed specifically for veterinary use; it has been used in extraction site alveolar margin maintenance,[34] to treat bone loss associated with lumpy jaw conditions,[35] and guided tissue regeneration procedures in dogs.[3,23,36]

While there are no veterinary clinical studies in dogs, experimental evidence suggests that bioactive glass is less effective than demineralized freeze-dried bone allograft in inducing new bone formation in infrabony pockets adjacent to implants in dogs.[23]

The most common *xenograft* is bovine cancellous bone, processed at a high temperature (1100°C) to remove all organic matter, eliminating the risk of zoonotic infection and graft rejection. This treatment, however, renders the material osteoconductive only. The resulting anorganic bone mineral has been used experimentally in extraction sites and for guided tissue regeneration in dogs.[37-43] Table 20.2 summarizes available graft materials and their sources.

MEMBRANE BARRIERS

A periodontal membrane is a selective barrier that is biocompatibile, integrates well with tissues, prevents ingrowth of cells outside the membrane, and which can be positioned to produce sufficient space for the desired new tissue to proliferate. The membrane may also act as a carrier for materials intended to enhance cellular activity or survivability. There are numerous types of membranes, both absorbable and non-absorbable (see Table 20.1). Gore-tex® (W.L. Gore & Associates, Inc., Newark, DE 19711), a nonabsorbable expanded polytetrafluoroethylene (ePTFE) membrane, was one of the first commercially available barriers. Clinical studies have shown that infrabony defects treated with ePTFE membranes can be expected to achieve 3–5 mm of bone fill and 4–7 mm of clinical attachment level gain.[44-46] However, ePTFE and other nonabsorbable membranes are impractical in veterinary patients because a second procedure is required for removal of the membrane.

The human periodontal literature describes many absorbable membranes, some of which have been shown to be effective in canine models of periodontal defects. A description of several types of absorbable membranes follows. It should be noted that none of these products are approved for clinical use in veterinary patients; therefore their use requires informed consent from the clients.

Synthetic absorbable membranes

Vicryl® (Ethicon, Inc., Somerville, NJ 08876) (polyglactin 910) membranes have been used successfully in experiments regenerating periodontal bone in ferrets[47] and in dogs.[48–50] Synthetic polylactic acid liquid membranes have been used in the treatment of experimentally created periodontal defects in dogs, with mixed results.[51–54]

Naturally-derived absorbable membranes

Sometimes called extracellular matrix scaffolds, these membranes are created from human, bovine, equine or porcine small intestinal submucosa, urinary bladder, pericardium, skin, or fascia which has been decellularized. Composed of 90% collagen, these acellular membranes also contain glycosaminoglycans and growth factors, which supports the growth and differentiation of a variety of cell types,[55] making them attractive for periodontal reconstruction applications. Over a dozen collagen membranes are commercially available, some of which have been modified by cross-linking proteins within the collagen to vary the resorption rate.[9] However, cross-linking may lead to a higher complication rate.[56] One porcine urinary bladder-derived membrane is licensed for veterinary use (ACell Vet, Jessup, MA 20794)

and is available in sheet, gel, granule and powder forms; however, there are currently no published reports of its use for oral surgical applications in veterinary patients.

PROPOSED GUIDED TISSUE REGENERATION TECHNIQUE USING ALLOGRAFT AND ABSORBABLE MEMBRANE (Fig. 20.3)

1. Elevate a periodontal flap (see Ch. 19).
2. Debride the osseous defect, removing all granulation tissue.
3. Remove all root deposits using hand and/or ultrasonic instrumentation.
4. If desired, condition the root surface with EDTA or citric acid.
5. Place the particulate allograft material in the osseous defect.
6. Trim the membrane to the approximate size of the area being treated. The apical border of the material should extend 3–4 mm apical to the margin of the defect and laterally 2–3 mm beyond the defect. The occlusal border of the membrane should lie 2 mm apical to the cemento-enamel junction.
7. Suture the membrane tightly around the tooth with a sling suture.
8. Suture the flap back in its original position or slightly coronal to it, in a simple interrupted pattern.

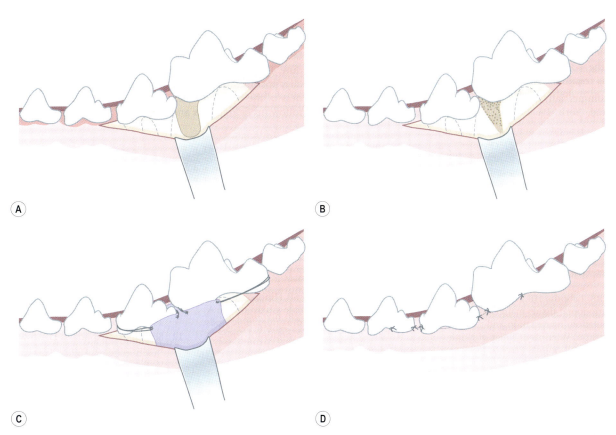

Fig. 20.3 (**A**) A periodontal flap is elevated. (**B**) After debridement of the pocket, particulate allograft material is placed in the osseous defect. (**C**) The pretrimmed membrane is placed over the graft material and, if needed, sutured with a sling suture; the apical border of the membrane should extend 3–4 mm apical to the margin of the defect and laterally 2–3 mm beyond the defect. (**D**) The flap is replaced and sutured.

material: Structure and function. Acta Biomater 2009;5:1–13.

56. Bornstein MM, Bosshardt D, Buser D. Effect of two different bioabsorbable collagen membranes on guided bone regeneration: a comparative histomorphometric study in the dog mandible. J Periodontol 2007;78: 1943–53.

57. McGuire MK, Scheyer ET, Schupbach P. Growth factor-mediated treatment of recession defects: a randomized controlled trial and histologic and microcomputed tomography examination. J Periodontol 2009;80:550–64.

58. Nakashima M, Reddi AH. The application of bone morphogenetic proteins to dental tissue engineering. Nat Biotechnol 2003; 21:1025–32.

59. Prescott RS, Alsanea R, Fayad MI, et al. In vivo generation of dental pulp-like tissue by using dental pulp stem cells, a collagen scaffold, and dentin matrix protein 1 after subcutaneous transplantation in mice. J Endod 2008;34:421–6.

60. Guzman-Martinez N, Silva-Herzog FD, Mendez GV, et al. The effect of Emdogain and 24% EDTA root conditioning on periodontal healing of replanted dog's teeth. Dent Traumatol 2009;25:43–50.

61. Iqbal MK, Bamaas N. Effect of enamel matrix derivative (EMDOGAIN) upon periodontal healing after replantation of permanent incisors in beagle dogs. Dent Traumatol 2001;17:36–45.

62. Esposito M, Coulthard P, Thomsen P, et al. Enamel matrix derivative for periodontal tissue regeneration in treatment of intrabony defects: a Cochrane systematic review. J Dent Educ 2004;68:834–44.

63. Trombelli L, Farina R. Clinical outcomes with bioactive agents alone or in combination with grafting or guided tissue regeneration. J Clin Periodontol 2008; 35:117–35.

64. Mellonig JT. Enamel matrix derivative for periodontal reconstructive surgery: technique and clinical and histologic case report. Int J Periodontics Restorative Dent 1999;19:8–19.

65. Mellonig JT, Valderrama MP, Cochran DL. Histological and clinical evaluation of recombinant human platelet-derived growth factor combined with beta tricalcium phosphate for the treatment of human Class III furcation defects. Int J Periodontics Restorative Dent 2009; 29:169–77.

66. Peng L, Cheng X, Zhuo R, et al. Novel gene-activated matrix with embedded chitosan/plasmid DNA nanoparticles encoding PDGF for periodontal tissue engineering. J Biomed Mater Res A 2009;90:564–76.

67. Simion M, Rocchietta I, Monforte M, et al. Three-dimensional alveolar bone reconstruction with a combination of recombinant human platelet-derived growth factor BB and guided bone regeneration: a case report. Int J Periodontics Restorative Dent 2008; 28:239–43.

68. Lynch SE, Wisner-Lynch L, Nevins M, et al. A new era in periodontal and periimplant regeneration: use of growth-factor enhanced matrices incorporating rhPDGF. Compend Contin Educ Dent 2006;27: 672–8.

69. Jung RE, Glauser R, Scharer P, et al. Effect of rhBMP-2 on guided bone regeneration in humans. Clin Oral Implants Res 2003; 14:556–68.

70. Palmer RM, Cortellini P. Periodontal tissue engineering and regeneration: Consensus Report of the Sixth European Workshop on Periodontology. J Clin Periodontol 2008;35:83–6.

71. Pack PD, Haber J. The incidence of clinical infection after periodontal surgery. A retrospective study. J Periodontol 1983; 54:441–3.

72. Herrera D, Alonso B, Leon R, et al. Antimicrobial therapy in periodontitis: the use of systemic antimicrobials against the subgingival biofilm. J Clin Periodontol 2008;35:45–66.

Chapter 21

Crown-lengthening

Fraser A. Hale

DEFINITIONS

Biologic width: the dimensional width of the junctional epithelium and connective tissue attachment (see Surgical Anatomy and Fig. 21.1)[1–3]

Clinical crown: that portion of the natural tooth structure exposed supragingivally

Dentogingival complex: the sum of the widths of the gingival sulcus, junctional epithelium and connective tissue attachment to root cementum[1]

Emergence profile: the anatomic shape of the tooth as it emerges through the gingiva[4]

Ostectomy: the excision of bone

Osteoplasty: the modification or change of the configuration of bone

Type-I crown-lengthening: a gingivectomy to expose more of the tooth[3,5]

Type-II crown-lengthening: an apically repositioned flap with osseous contouring to expose more of the tooth[3,5]

Type-III crown-lengthening: the forced eruption with an orthodontic device to expose more of the tooth[3,5]

PREOPERATIVE CONSIDERATIONS

Crown-lengthening refers to procedures designed to expose more tooth structure (crown and root) supragingivally. It may be done to expose lesions where they can be managed more effectively or to achieve greater clinical crown surface area for the retention of a prosthetic crown or bridge.[1,6] In the case of an under-erupted tooth, crown-lengthening can be used to expose the enamel, to which the gingiva and periodontal ligament will not firmly attach, to eradicate or reduce the periodontal pseudopocket and concomitant pericoronitis.[1,7,8]

Type-I crown-lengthening is simple gingivectomy (see Ch. 18). Type-III crown-lengthening is an orthodontic procedure (see Ch. 54).

Type-II crown-lengthening is the surgical repositioning of the alveolar margin and gingiva to expose more of the tooth while maintaining appropriate periodontal relationships, which will be the focus of this chapter.

Crown-lengthening is most easily accomplished on single-rooted teeth such as the canine teeth. For multirooted teeth, the need to avoid exposure of the furcation limits the degree to which the periodontal tissue can be moved apically.

Surgical crown-lengthening is a relatively advanced periodontal surgery, which generates both a risk of failure and a cost to the client. In deciding if the procedure is justified, the surgeon should consider the functional significance of the tooth, the animal's overall periodontal status, and the client's commitment to home care (see Ch. 17).

Indications

Coronal fractures and caries lesions may extend subgingivally. Preservation of the affected tooth depends on restoration of the defect and managing the adjacent periodontal tissues. Gingiva and periodontal ligament will only attach to bone and cementum.[9] Therefore, leaving dentin exposed or placing a restoration deeply subgingival will result in a deep periodontal pocket. To avoid this, an apically repositioned flap with apical repositioning of the alveolar margin can be used to bring the lesion/restoration supragingival (or at least suprabony).[9,10] Not only does this make restoring the defect much easier, it also improves access for home care around the restoration and improves the long-term periodontal prognosis for the tooth.[3,6,11]

The placement of a prosthetic crown requires that sufficient clinical crown be available to hold the prosthesis in place.[1,3,12] Crown fractures may result in insufficient natural tooth structure remaining above the gingiva for prosthetic retention. In such cases, crown-lengthening can provide the necessary clinical crown for prosthetic restoration.

Another method for creating additional clinical crown for prosthetic retention is through the use of a post-and-core build-up. Though this can increase the surface area for bonding without periodontal surgery, it can also weaken the tooth and predispose to cracked roots.[13] Therefore, for a tooth subject to strong forces, such as the canine tooth, surgical crown-lengthening, which does not weaken the tooth, is preferred.

© 2012 Elsevier Ltd
DOI: 10.1016/B978-0-7020-4618-6.00021-X

SURGICAL ANATOMY

Periodontium

The coronal margin of the alveolar process, where the cribriform and cortical plates meet, is the alveolar margin. The alveolar margin is typically 1–2 mm apical to the cemento-enamel junction so that there is a band of root cementum residing coronal to the alveolus.[11,14–16]

The free gingival margin is typically 1–2 mm coronal to the cemento-enamel junction in dogs and 0.5–1 mm in cats. The gingiva attaches to the cementum of the root that is coronal to the alveolar margin and to the cortical plate of the alveolar process. Immediately apical to the gingival sulcus is the junctional epithelium, which forms a relatively loose attachment to the cementum. Normally, the zone of junctional epithelium will be about 1–2 mm wide. Apical to the junctional epithelium is the more firmly attached connective tissue attachment to root cementum and to the cortical plate. This zone would also typically be 1–2 mm wide.[14,15,17]

The sum of the widths of the gingival sulcus, junctional epithelium and connective tissue attachment to root cementum is referred to as the *dentogingival complex* and the sum of the width of the junctional epithelium and connective tissue attachment is known as the *biologic width* (Fig. 21.1).[1,3,6] The normal physiology of the dentogingival complex depends on the preservation of the biologic width. In humans, the sulcus tends to be about 0.7 mm deep, the junctional epithelium just under 1 mm and the connective tissue attachment just over 1 mm, for a total of about 2.75 mm from free gingival margin to alveolar margin.[6,18] In dogs and cats, the dimensions are much more variable, influenced by patient size and the specific tooth. At the canine tooth of a large-breed dog, the biologic width may be 5 mm or more, whereas around an incisor tooth of a cat, it may be less than 1 mm. Whatever the biologic width for a specific tooth, any periodontal surgery should have as a priority the preservation or recreation of this relationship. Therefore, if the free gingival margin is to be moved 3 mm apically, so must the alveolar margin.[6]

The gingiva's apical margin is the mucogingival junction, which is seen as a distinct line buccally on both the mandible and maxilla and on the lingual side of the mandible. On the maxilla, the palatal gingiva blends imperceptibly with the palatal mucosa (See Figs 18.2 and 18.3).

Healthy gingiva is very firm, dense and inelastic. The oral mucosa is much thinner, softer and more pliable/elastic. Therefore, any repositioning of the gingiva typically relies on extending the flap into the more mobile alveolar mucosa.

Topographical anatomy

When elevating the flaps for crown-lengthening of the maxillary canine tooth, it will be necessary to make an incision between the maxillary third incisor tooth and the canine tooth. There is a branch of the major palatine artery that passes through this space to anastomose with the lateral nasal artery.[19,20] This artery will be severed in creation of the flaps and though it bleeds significantly at first, hemorrhage can typically be controlled with direct pressure.

When elevating the buccal flap at the mandibular canine tooth, care should be taken to not damage the neurovascular structures emerging from the mental foramina, particularly the middle mental foramen, located ventrolateral to the apex of the canine tooth or ventral to the first or second premolar teeth.[19,20]

Crown-lengthening of the maxillary fourth premolar tooth calls for caution to avoid damaging neurovascular elements emerging from the infraorbital foramen, located dorsal to the apex of the distal root of the maxillary third premolar tooth.[19,20] Dorsal to the distal portion of the maxillary fourth premolar tooth is the parotid papilla and dorsal to the distal aspect of the maxillary first molar tooth is the main zygomatic papilla.[20,21] Care should be taken to avoid severing or ligating either of these salivary ducts.

SPECIAL INSTRUMENTS AND MATERIALS

In addition to the standard set of periodontal instruments (see Ch. 19), bone chisels such as Ochsenbein #1 (Hu-Friedy®, Chicago, IL) and Kramer-Nevins #1/2 (Hu-Friedy®, Chicago, IL) can be used for ostectomy and osteoplasty (Fig. 21.2).

THERAPEUTIC DECISION-MAKING

Staging

If the crown-lengthening surgery is done in preparation for prosthodontic restoration, the crown will need to be prepared and impressions obtained for the dental laboratory. Crown preparation involves shaping the natural tooth structure to accept the prosthetic covering. An important feature of crown preparation is the placement of the finish line or crown margin. This is the line that marks where the prosthetic crown should end. It is recommended to place the finish line approximately 1 mm supragingivally in order to reduce the

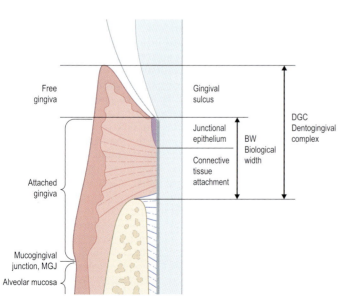

Fig. 21.1 The 'biologic width' is the sum of (a) sulcus depth + (b) junctional epithelium width + (c) connective tissue attachment.

Free gingiva

Attached gingiva

Mucogingival junction, MGJ

Alveolar mucosa

Gingival sulcus

Junctional epithelium

Connective tissue attachment

BW Biological width

DGC Dentogingival complex

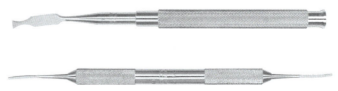

Fig. 21.2 Ochsenbein #1 (Hu-Friedy®, Chicago, IL) (*top*) and Kramer-Nevins #1/2 (Hu-Friedy®, Chicago, IL) (*bottom*) bone chisels. (*Courtesy of Hu-Friedy®, Chicago, IL.*)

impact of the prosthesis on the periodontium.[1,2,22,23] Another goal is to have the maximum surface area prepared for coverage by the prosthesis to improve retention. Though it might seem advantageous to do the crown preparation and impressions during the same anesthetic episode as the crown-lengthening procedure, this can lead to suboptimal results. Following the surgery, the soft tissues will often shrink and contract during healing, further lengthening the crown.[6] Waiting for 2–4 weeks after surgery can net another millimeter of clinical crown for prosthetic retention. Also, if impressions are obtained immediately following the surgery, the suture material may become trapped in the impression material, making it difficult to remove the impressions without tearing the sutures and damaging the flap margins. Therefore, it is best to do the crown-lengthening procedure at one visit and wait a few weeks for the tissues to heal. Then the crown can be prepared with a finish line placed 1 mm coronal to a stable gingival margin and impressions can be obtained without damage to tissues and sutures.

Prosthetic crown retention

The long-term success of a prosthetic crown largely depends on its retention and resistance, which must be sufficient to withstand the dislodging forces the prosthesis will meet during clinical use. Retention and resistance are influenced by a number of factors including the total surface area of clinical crown in contact with the luting agent and the shape of the crown preparation.[12] For full-crown coverage of the canine teeth in dogs, a minimum of 6 mm of clinical crown is suggested.[24] Less than that will provide insufficient surface area of tooth–cement–prosthesis interface for retention. Crown fractures may result in less than 6 mm of natural tooth structure remaining above the gingiva. In such cases, crown-lengthening can provide the necessary clinical crown length for restoration.

The shape of the crown preparation is important in that it will determine the angle at which dislodging forces meet the prosthesis and, by extension, the cement film. All luting agents are strongest in compression, intermediate in shear and weakest in tension. Developing a crown preparation that maximizes the mechanical retention of the prosthesis while minimizing tension forces on the cement film will increase the chances of success. An ideal preparation would have nearly parallel sides with each opposing axial wall tapering coronally at approximately 3 degrees, giving a total convergence angle of 6 degrees.[12] The conical shape of an undamaged canine in a dog typically imposes a far greater degree of taper and some fractures result in even greater taper.[25] Crown build-up with bonded restoratives can reduce this effect, though these represent another interface at which failure under load can occur. If the fracture to the crown is such that a type-II crown-lengthening procedure will not result in sufficient clinical crown length and acceptable clinical crown shape for adequate retention and resistance then a prosthetic crown is likely to fail.

SURGICAL TECHNIQUES

Type-II crown-lengthening involves raising full-thickness flaps buccally and lingually, ostectomy to move the alveolar margin apically, and apical repositioning of the flaps. When a fracture or caries extends below the preoperative free gingival margin, the new alveolar margin should be placed 2 mm or more apical to the most apical extent of the lesion.[6,10] As gingiva and periodontal ligament will not attach firmly to restorative materials, it is essential to expose some root cementum apical to the restoration for gingival attachment and reestablishment of biologic width. The lesion can then be restored to reestablish the desirable cervical anatomy and emergence profile.[26]

When increasing crown length in preparation for prosthodontic work, the alveolar margin should be a minimum of 3 mm apical to the planned new free gingival margin location, to allow for the reestablishment of biologic width and a gingival sulcus.[6]

Techniques for maxillary and mandibular canine teeth, and for the maxillary fourth premolar tooth in the dog, will be described. The principles discussed can be applied to other teeth as well.

Maxillary Canine Tooth[5]

If the crown needs only be lengthened by a few millimeters and there is abundant healthy gingiva, a simple gingivectomy (type-I crown-lengthening) may suffice. In considering this approach it is important to maintain the biologic width.

Type-II crown-lengthening starts with the creation of extended envelope flaps buccal and palatal to the tooth (Fig. 21.3). The gingiva is incised from the distal aspect of the third incisor tooth up to the mesial aspect of the second premolar tooth, including sulcular incisions of the canine and first premolar teeth. A full-thickness flap is raised. The buccal flap is reflected dorsally and the palatal flap is retracted toward the midline. If necessary, the envelope flap may be extended mesially or distally or vertical releasing incisions may be added.

Bone chisels are used to remove alveolar margin bone. Power rotary instruments should preferably not be used, to avoid damaging the root cementum.[18] However, bulk bone removal far removed from the root surface may be more efficient with well-irrigated rotary instruments. A smooth transition should be created between the surrounding bone and the newly created alveolar margin.[10] With the level of the alveolar bone established, the alveolar margin should be shaped to recreate the thin profile of normal marginal bone. This can be achieved by paring the bone with a well-sharpened periodontal curette. The curette can also be used to root-plane the exposed root surface in preparation for gingival attachment.

Debris from under the flap should be carefully removed. The flaps are then apposed around the tooth and the amount of crown-lengthening achieved is evaluated. If necessary, the flaps are elevated again and more bone is removed until the goal of the procedure has been met. The buccal and palatal flaps are then sutured where they meet interdentally. As it is not possible to suture the margin of a flap to the adjacent tooth wall, sling sutures may be used to draw the gingiva into close apposition with the buccal and palatal tooth walls.[27] For the palatal flap, the needle passes through the flap near the mesiopalatal line angle, around the tooth on the buccal side to the distopalatal line angle, through the flap and then back around the buccal aspect to meet itself where it started. As the knot is pulled snug, the palatal flap is drawn tight against the tooth surface. A similar suture can be used to draw the buccal flap against the tooth if needed.

Mandibular canine tooth[5]

A buccal flap is elevated starting with an intrasulcular incision buccally to the third incisor tooth, continuing interproximally, buccally around the canine tooth, through the gingiva along the dorsal margin of the mandible distal to the canine tooth and buccally around the first premolar tooth (Fig. 21.4). The gingiva between the mandibular canine and first premolar teeth is a fairly narrow band that runs along the dorsal margin of the mandible. Since the gingiva holds a suture well, it is recommended to keep the incision within this narrow strip of gingiva. Once the incision has been made, the flap is reflected ventrally, taking care to identify and protect the

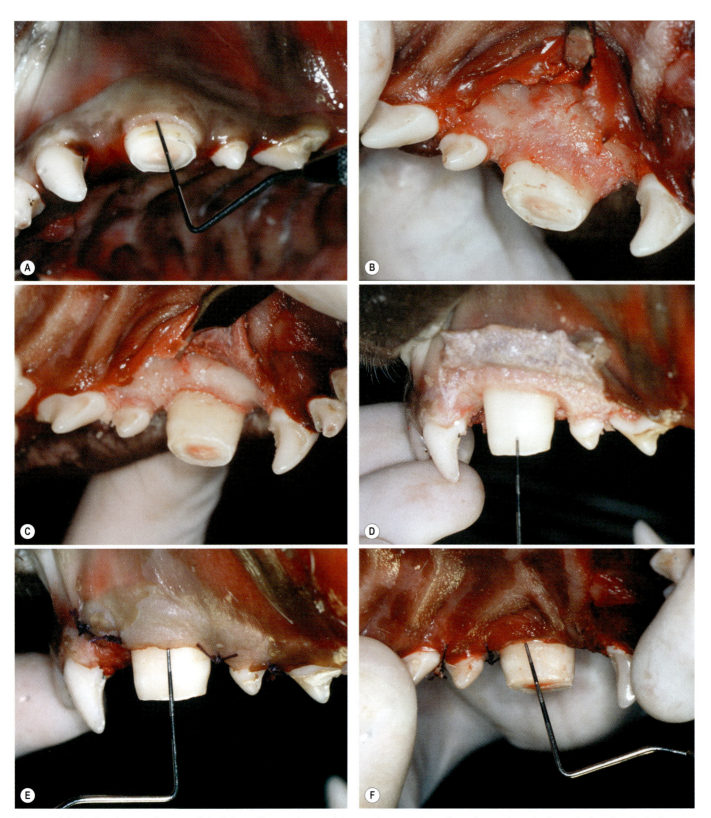

Fig. 21.3 (**A**) Simulated crown fracture of the left maxillary canine tooth in a cadaver specimen (lateral recumbency); the periodontal probe indicates a clinical crown length of 3 mm. (**B**) Palatal envelope flap raised, showing the height and shape of the alveolar margin. (**C**) The palatal aspect of the tooth following ostectomy and osteoplasty. (**D**) The buccal aspect of the tooth following ostectomy and osteoplasty, with the periodontal probe indicating the preoperative level of the clinical crown length. (**E**) The buccal and palatal flaps have been repositioned and sutured; the clinical crown length is now 7 mm on the buccal aspect. (**F**) Palatal view showing 6 mm of clinical crown length. *(Reproduced with permission from: Hale FA. Crown lengthening for mandibular and maxillary canine teeth in the dog. J Vet Dent 2001;18:219–221.)*

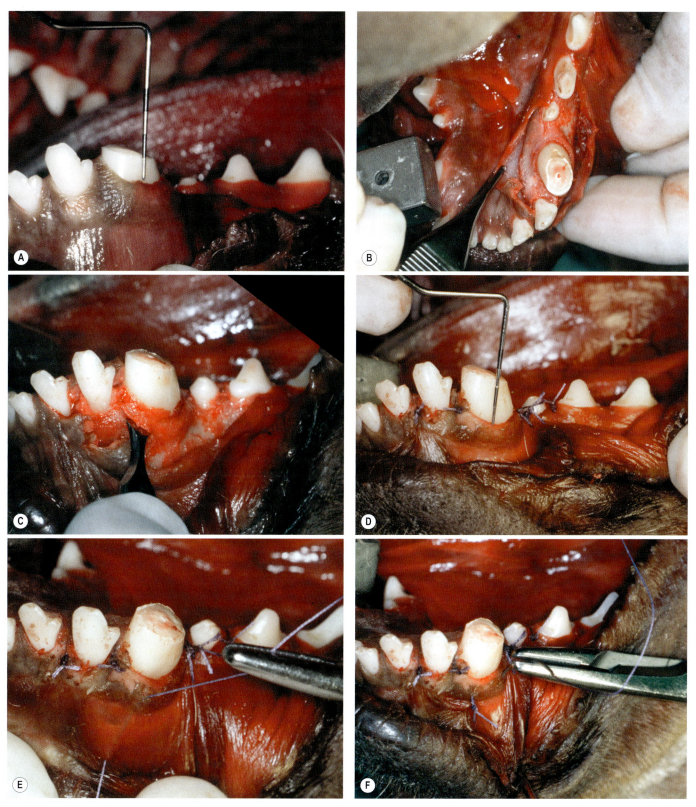

Fig. 21.4 (**A**) Simulated crown fracture of the left mandibular canine tooth in a cadaver specimen (lateral recumbency); the periodontal probe indicates a clinical crown length of 3 mm. (**B**) Buccal and lingual flaps have been raised following interproximal and intrasulcular incisions. (**C**) Ostectomy is performed with an Ochsenbein chisel. (**D**) The flaps have been repositioned and sutured; the clinical crown length is now 7 mm on the buccal aspect. (**E**) To prevent the buccal flap from sliding coronally, a tacking suture is placed on the mesial aspect to anchor the gingiva to the ventral mandibular periosteum. (**F**) The mesiobuccal tacking suture has been placed and the distobuccal tacking suture is now placed. *(Reproduced with permission from: Hale FA. Crown lengthening for mandibular and maxillary canine teeth in the dog. J Vet Dent 2001;18:219–221.)*

neurovascular structures emerging from the mental foramina. A lingual flap is elevated in a similar fashion. If necessary for adequate exposure, the flaps may be extended mesially or distally.

With the flaps reflected, hand chisels and rotary instruments are used for ostectomy to create a new alveolar margin approximately 3 mm apical to the planned position of the free gingival margin. The bone and tooth surfaces are finished as described above.

The proximity of the third incisor tooth on the mesial aspect of the mandibular canine tooth can pose a challenge. At times, achieving the operative goals for salvage of the canine tooth may lead to severe compromise of the periodontal support of the incisor tooth, and extraction of the incisor tooth may be indicated.

Closure is similar to the procedure for the maxillary canine tooth. Some gingivoplasty or gingivectomy may be necessary to allow proper adaptation of the flaps. Since the roots of the third incisor and the canine teeth converge apically, the interdental gingiva may be too wide to fit into the tighter interdental space. The lingual flap may lie against the tooth in its original location despite removal of the underlying bone. In both cases, trimming of the gingiva to improve tissue apposition is indicated.

The buccal flap has a tendency to slide up the crown of the canine tooth toward its original location. To hold the flap in a more apical position during healing, a tuck suture can be employed. The needle is passed through the gingiva of the flap near the distobuccal line angle of the canine tooth, passes below the flap ventrally, engages the periosteum near the ventral border of the mandible and emerges through the oral mucosa at the base of the buccal vestibule. The suture is then brought back up to the entry point and tied. As the knot is snugged down, the mobile flap will be pulled ventrally toward the immobile ventral periosteum. A second tuck suture can be placed in a similar fashion at the mesiobuccal line angle of the canine tooth. The sutures should be pulled tight enough to place the free gingival margin of the flap at the desired location to achieve sufficient crown-lengthening without compromising biologic width.

Maxillary fourth premolar tooth

Crown-lengthening of the maxillary fourth premolar tooth typically involves an apically repositioned flap on the buccal side only, as the injury is almost always a subgingival slab fracture of the buccal wall. The main limiting factor in crown-lengthening for the maxillary fourth premolar tooth, or any multirooted tooth, is furcation involvement. Careful evaluation of the animal's overall periodontal health and the level of home care anticipated are essential in deciding if salvage or extraction is more appropriate.

In a periodontally sound patient who will receive daily dental home care, some crown-lengthening may be possible, though the buccal flap cannot be apically repositioned such that the furcation would be left exposed.

Given the tight interdental contacts between the maxillary fourth premolar and the adjacent third premolar and first molar teeth, an envelope flap may not provide sufficient exposure or allow sufficient apical repositioning without compromising the adjacent teeth. Therefore, vertical releasing incisions may be made at the distobuccal line angle of the third premolar or the mesiobuccal line angle of the first molar teeth. An intrasulcular incision severs the gingival attachment and the flap is elevated dorsally.

With the flap reflected, the extent of the subgingival damage can be assessed; hairline cracks and fracture fragments must be identified. As previously described, the alveolar margin is reduced with hand instruments to a level 2 mm apical to the extent of the damage. If this cannot be done without going more than a few millimeters apical to the furcation, then extraction is indicated.

With the lesion exposed, any lost root tissue is replaced with restorative materials to reestablish a desirable emergence profile. The flap is then apically repositioned and sutured in place interdentally.

The free gingival margin should be 2 mm coronal to the furcation to allow gingival reattachment; however, it should not be more than 3 mm coronal to the apical extent of the restoration to which gingiva cannot attach or a deep periodontal pocket will be the result. If a releasing incision was made, there will be a step from the unmoved free gingival margin down to the apically repositioned free gingival margin. It is important to ensure that the repositioned gingiva has some contact with the adjacent gingiva such that there can be a contiguous band of gingiva around the teeth. This is another factor that can limit the degree of crown-lengthening that can be achieved.

POSTOPERATIVE CARE AND ASSESSMENT

Following surgical crown-lengthening, clients should be instructed to feed only soft food. The patient should be denied access to hard or abrasive chew toys. These measures are intended to protect the flaps from mechanical forces that might disrupt or delay healing.

Toothbrushing should be suspended for 2 weeks, or the operative side of the mouth should be avoided. Rinsing the surgical site with a chlorhexidine oral solution or a zinc ascorbate gel twice daily is indicated in a cooperative patient, provided that this can be achieved without any tension or pressure being applied to the surgical site. However, if the patient is likely to struggle in a way that would put tension on the sutures and possibly disrupt healing, it would be best to instruct the client to leave the mouth alone for 2 weeks. An Elizabethan collar should be sent home with the patient to prevent the animal from pawing at the mouth and disrupting healing.

After healing but prior to crown preparation, the periodontal health status of the tooth (and adjacent teeth) should be assessed. The tissues should be examined to evaluate the healing and the circumference of the tooth gently probed to evaluate the level and quality of attachment. Any periodontal concerns must be addressed prior to proceeding with the prosthodontic treatment.

COMPLICATIONS

The most significant complication of type-II crown-lengthening is dehiscence of the gingival flaps. This can happen if the flaps are under tension or if the animal engages in behavior (chewing, pawing) that stresses the suture line. Should this occur, there will usually be retraction of the flaps away from the surgical site, exposing bone and the periodontal space to contamination. There will also be some loss of gingival tissue.

Treatment of dehiscence begins with reflecting the flaps to expose the underlying tissues for debridement of gross debris and contaminated tissue. The flaps may need to be undermined further to allow tension-free apposition. The flap margins may be covered with epithelium, which will need to be removed to allow apposition of fresh connective tissue margins. Since the initial surgery will have decreased the blood supply to the flaps, delayed healing and dehiscence may occur with subsequent surgery.

Other complications include compromise of the periodontal status of treated or adjacent teeth. Excessive bone removal leading to a poor crown-length : root-length ratio and tooth mobility may necessitate extraction of adjacent teeth.

Gouging of the alveolar bone at the treated tooth can cause the free gingiva to invert instead of properly adapting to the tooth surface. This results in entrapment of food and debris.

REFERENCES

1. Wolf HF, Rateitschak EM, Rateitschak KH, et al. Perio-prosthetics 2, supplemental measures, esthetics. In: Rateitschak KH, Wolf HF, editors. Color atlas of dental medicine: periodontology. 3rd ed. Stuttgart, Germany: Thieme; 2004. p. 489–509.

2. Spear FM, Cooney JP. Restorative interrelationships. In: Newman MG, Takei HH, Klokkevold PR, et al, editors. Carranza's clinical periodontology. 10th ed. Philadelphia, PA: WB Saunders; 2006. p. 1050–69.

3. Wiggs RB, Lobprise HB. Operative dentistry: crowns and prosthodontics. In: Wiggs RB, Lobprise HB, editors. Veterinary dentistry – principles and practice. Philadelphia, PA: Lippincott-Raven; 1997. p. 395–434.

4. Sozio RB. Prosthodontics. In: Sonis ST, editor. Dental secrets. Philadelphia, PA: Hanley & Belfus; 1994. p. 131–48.

5. Hale FA. Crown lengthening for mandibular and maxillary canine teeth in the dog. J Vet Dent 2001;18:219–21.

6. Melnick PR. Preparation of the periodontium for restorative dentistry. In: Newman MG, Takei HH, Klokkevold PR, et al, editors. Carranza's clinical periodontology. 10th ed. Philadelphia, PA: WB Saunders; 2006. p. 1039–49.

7. Marucha PT. Treatment of acute gingival disease. In: Newman MG, Takei HH, Klokkevold PR, et al, editors. Carranza's clinical periodontology. 10th ed. Philadelphia, PA: WB Saunders; 2006. p. 706–13.

8. Marucha PT. Acute gingival infections. In: Newman MG, Takei HH, Klokkevold PR, et al, editors. Carranza's clinical periodontology. 10th ed. Philadelphia, PA: WB Saunders; 2006. p. 391–403.

9. Schroeder HE. Development and structure of the dental attachment apparatus. In: Schroeder HE, editor. Oral structural biology. New York: Thieme Medical Publishers; 1991. p. 187–293.

10. Lindhe J. Esthetics and periodontal therapy. In: Lindhe J, editor. Textbook of clinical periodontology. 2nd ed. Copenhagen: Munksgaard; 1989. p. 477–514.

11. Harvey CE. Management of periodontal disease: understanding the options. Vet Clin North Am Small Anim Pract 2005; 35:819–36.

12. Shillingburg HT, Jacobi R, Brackett SE. Biomechanical principles of preparation. In: Shillingburg HT, Jacobi R, Brackett SE, editors. Fundamentals of tooth preparations. Chicago, IL: Quintessence Publishing; 1987. p. 13–44.

13. Wiggs RB, Lobprise HB. Operative and restorative dentistry. In: Wiggs RB, Lobprise HB, editors. Veterinary dentistry – principles and practice. Philadelphia, PA: Lippincott-Raven; 1997. p. 351–94.

14. Fiorellini JP, Kim DM, Ishikawa SO. The gingiva. In: Newman MG, Takei HH, Klokkevold PR, et al, editors. Carranza's clinical periodontology. 10th ed. Philadelphia, PA: WB Saunders; 2006. p. 46–67.

15. Wolf HF, Rateitschak EM, Rateitschak KH, et al. Structural biology. In: Rateitschak KH, Wolf HF, editors. Color atlas of dental medicine: periodontology. 3rd ed. Stuttgart, Germany: Thieme; 2004. p. 7–20.

16. Wiggs RB, Lobprise HB. Oral anatomy and physiology. In: Wiggs RB, Lobprise HB, editors. Veterinary dentistry – principles and practice. Philadelphia, PA: Lippincott-Raven; 1997. p. 55–86.

17. Schroeder HE. Marginal periodontium. In: Oral structural biology. New York: Thieme Medical Publishing; 1991. p. 230–64.

18. Cohen ES. Resective osseous surgery. In: Cohen ES, editor. Atlas of cosmetic and reconstructive periodontal surgery. 2nd ed. Philadelphia, PA: Lea & Febiger; 1994. p. 259–83.

19. Evans HE. The heart and arteries. In: Evans H, editor. Miller's anatomy of the dog. 3rd ed. Philadelphia, PA: WB Saunders; 1993. p. 586–681.

20. Gioso MA, Carvalho VGG. Oral anatomy of the dog and cat in veterinary dental practice. Vet Clin North Am Small Anim Pract 2005;35:763–80.

21. Evans HE. The digestive apparatus and abdomen. In: Evans HE, editor. Miller's anatomy of the dog. 3rd ed. Philadelphia, PA: WB Saunders; 1993. p. 385–462.

22. Visser CJ. Restorative dentistry. Vet Clin North Am Small Anim Pract 1998;28:1273–84.

23. Shillingburg HT, Jacobi R, Brackett SE. Finish lines and the periodontium. In: Shillingburg HT, Jacobi R, Brackett SE, editors. Fundamentals of tooth preparations. Chicago, IL: Quintessence Publishing; 1987. p. 45–59.

24. Harvey CE, Emily PP. Restorative dentistry. In: Harvey CE, Emily PP, editors. Small animal dentistry. St. Louis, MO: Mosby; 1993. p. 213–65.

25. Holmstrom SE, Frost P, Eisner ER. Restorative dentistry. In: Holmstrom SE, Frost P, Eisner ER, editors. Veterinary dental techniques for the small animal practitioner. 2nd ed. Philadelphia, PA: WB Saunders; 1998. p. 319–34.

26. Summit JB. Fundamentals of operative dentistry: a contemporary approach. 2nd ed. Chicago, IL: Quintessence Publishing; 2000.

27. Takei HH, Carranza FA. The periodontal flap. In: Newman MG, Takei HH, Klokkevold PR, et al, editors. Carranza's clinical periodontology. 10th ed. Philadelphia, PA: WB Saunders; 2006. p. 926–36.

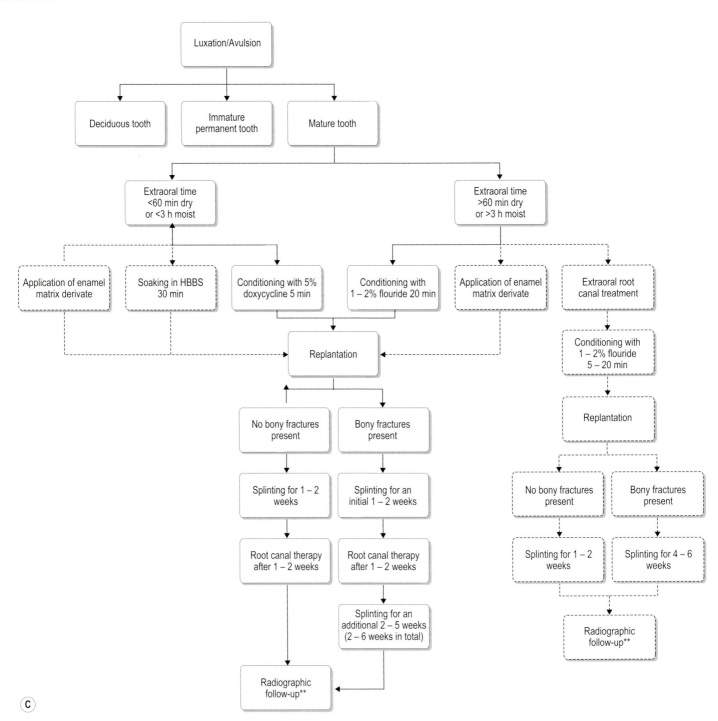

Fig. 22.4, cont'd.

Differences are mainly due to the need for general anesthesia for dental procedures in animals. Treatment includes replantation, management of bony and soft tissues injuries, and endodontic treatment, as in the majority of cases the blood supply to the pulp is disrupted as a consequence of the trauma.

Storage media for avulsed teeth

Successful replantation of avulsed teeth depends on the existence of viable periodontal fibroblasts that are capable of proliferating over the damaged root areas.[31] Teeth can be replanted without complications if reinserted into the alveolus within 60 minutes, even if stored dry.[29,32,33] Unfortunately, this is rarely possible in veterinary patients. After 60 minutes of extraoral time, the periodontal ligament begins to necrotize, which leads to extensive replacement resorption and ankylosis. If the tooth is placed in a suitable transport medium, however, it can be stored for up to 3 hours before successful replantation.[32] The optimal storage medium should be able to preserve the viability of the injured periodontal fibers, and should have correct osmolality and pH.[34] Tap water has been demonstrated to be almost as harmful to monkeys' periodontal fibers as long-term dry storage because it is hypotonic and results in rapid cell lysis.[31]

Several commercial tissue culture media (e.g., Hank's balanced salt solution – HBSS (Save-a-Tooth, SmartPractice.com, Phoenix, AZ, USA)) have been shown to be effective for storing and transporting avulsed teeth, because of their ability to reconstitute periodontal ligament cells and therefore prevent root resorption.[31,32,35-40] These media, however, may not be readily available. Low-fat milk has also been shown by studies on human and canine periodontal ligament fibers to be an excellent storage medium.[31,32,35,37,41,42] Milk is able to effectively maintain the viability of periodontal cells for up to 6 hours, particularly if used at cool temperature (4°C).[33,37,41,42] It contains important nutritional substances, such as amino acids, carbohydrates and vitamins, it has physiological osmolality and low bacterial content. Milk products such as sour milk and yoghurt provide poor conditions for cell survival because of their low pH.[42] Milk, however, has no restorative effect when periodontal ligament has already become dehydrated.[41] It has been recommended to soak in HBSS for 30 minutes teeth that have been kept extraorally for more than 15 minutes or that have previously been stored in milk, before replantation.[39] If a tooth cannot be immediately replanted or stored in a physiologic medium it should be wrapped in plastic foil to prevent air drying.[43] The IADT recommend not to replant immature teeth (teeth with an open apex) that have been dry for 60 minutes or longer, as they have a very poor prognosis and may potentially develop severe complications.[23,29] The same may be true for dogs and cats.

Prereplantation treatment of the tooth and alveolus

The tooth should be minimally manipulated, and curettage of either the root or the alveolus should be avoided to preserve healthy periodontal ligament from being removed.[26,44] The alveolus should not be air dried, and surgical flaps should be avoided unless bony fragments prevent replantation. Medicaments, disinfectants, or chemicals should never be applied to the root surface.[18] Very gentle irrigation with saline or the careful use of cotton pliers are recommended to remove blood clots and gross debris.[2,26,45] The removal of the blood clot prior to replantation of experimentally avulsed dog teeth resulted in less ankylosis and resorption.[45] A chemotactic stimulus may be released from the fibrin clot if left in place, attracting neutrophils and monocytes that have detrimental effects upon the tissues through the release of lysosomal enzymes.[45]

When used topically at the time of replantation, doxycycline was shown to decrease the frequency of ankylosis and inflammatory root resorption, and increase the frequency of complete pulp revascularization of replanted immature monkeys' teeth.[46] Tetracyclines have also been shown to have antiresorptive properties in addition to antibacterial properties.[47] It may therefore be useful to soak avulsed teeth in a 5% doxycycline solution for 5 minutes to kill the bacteria on the root surface and in the pulp before replantation.[39] This treatment has also been shown to enhance revascularization of immature replanted teeth in dogs.[48] On the other hand, the application of the tetracycline derivative antibiotic minocycline (Arestin™, OraPharma Inc., Warminster, PA, USA) to replanted dog teeth after extended dry times did not show any benefit in the attenuation or prevention of external root resorption,[49] but it may be beneficial for pulp revascularization of immature teeth.[50]

Coating the crowns of the teeth with an unfilled resin in an attempt to decrease the chances of bacterial invasion of pulp tissues was shown to be ineffective in dogs.[48]

After 60 minutes of dry storage, the periodontal cells can be assumed to be necrotic. In this case, or even if the tooth is stored in one of the recommended mediums longer than the advised time, the periodontal ligament may be mechanically or chemically removed before replantation. Soaking these teeth in a citric acid solution for 3 minutes, followed by a 1% stannous fluoride solution for 5–15 minutes, and finally a 5% doxycycline solution for 5 minutes may prevent or minimize root resorption.[39,51-55] However, other studies have questioned the efficacy of such treatments.[56] In humans, it is currently recommended to immerse avulsed permanent teeth in a 2% sodium fluoride solution for 20 minutes before replantation.[30]

Oral administration of nonsteroidal antiinflammatory drugs in dogs has proven ineffective in preventing resorption.[57] However, the topical use of dexamethasone supplemented to HBSS was shown to be of some use to enhance healing and decrease resorption complications in replanted dogs' teeth.[58]

To arrest any hemorrhage and to avoid contamination of the surgical field with dental materials, lacerated soft tissues should be sutured and bony fractures should be stabilized at the time of replantation before splinting the displaced teeth. Bone fragments with adequate soft tissue attachment should not be discarded if possible, and the facial and lingual plates should be manually compressed to adhere to the tooth surface.[2,18]

Splinting

A dental splint is defined as 'a rigid or flexible device or compound used to support, protect or immobilize teeth that have been loosened, replanted, fractured or subjected to certain endodontic procedures.'[59] The purpose of splinting is to stabilize the tooth for as long as is required to ensure that there is no further injury and to protect the attachment apparatus in order to allow the periodontal fibers to regenerate.[59]

As rigid fixation has been associated with a high degree of ankylosis and root replacement resorption, flexible splints are preferred for the treatment of displaced teeth.[60] It has been shown that the normal masticatory stimulus can prevent and eliminate small external resorption areas on the root surface of replanted teeth, promotes pulpal healing and is necessary for normal bone remodeling.[59,60] However, a recent evidence-based review of splinting luxated, avulsed and root-fractured teeth has questioned the hypothesis that prognosis for these teeth is determined by factors associated with splinting.[61] Despite the fact that the type of splint and the fixation period seem to be generally not significant variables when related to healing outcomes, the authors still concluded that 'current recommended splinting treatment protocols should still be considered "best practice"'.[61]

Teeth of dogs used experimentally in periodontal trauma models are often either not splinted or secured only with a sling suture after reimplantation.[40,49,50,62,63] However, these teeth may exfoliate and get lost,[40,62] which may be acceptable in an experimental study evaluating a large number of animals and roots, but obviously undesirable in clinical cases. Therefore, splinting is always recommended following replantation.

Animal studies have proven that acid-etched splints (with or without wire) produce adequate lateral support for replanted teeth while allowing slight mobility, which improves periodontal healing.[59,60] These splints are very reliable, easy to apply and remove, well tolerated by dogs, easy to clean for the client, and relatively inexpensive.

The splinting technique involves:

- Scaling and polishing the teeth to be included in the splint. Nonfluoride pumice is used for polishing, as fluoride interferes with the setting of the composite and resin materials.
- Splinting the displaced teeth to the adjacent teeth utilizing orthodontic or stainless steel wire (Fig. 22.5 A-C). The splint should extend 1 to 3 teeth mesially and distally from the displaced ones. The size of the wire depends on the size of the dog and the teeth. The wire is shaped with the aid of orthodontic pliers to passively conform to the dental surface, and is positioned a few millimeters coronal to the gingival

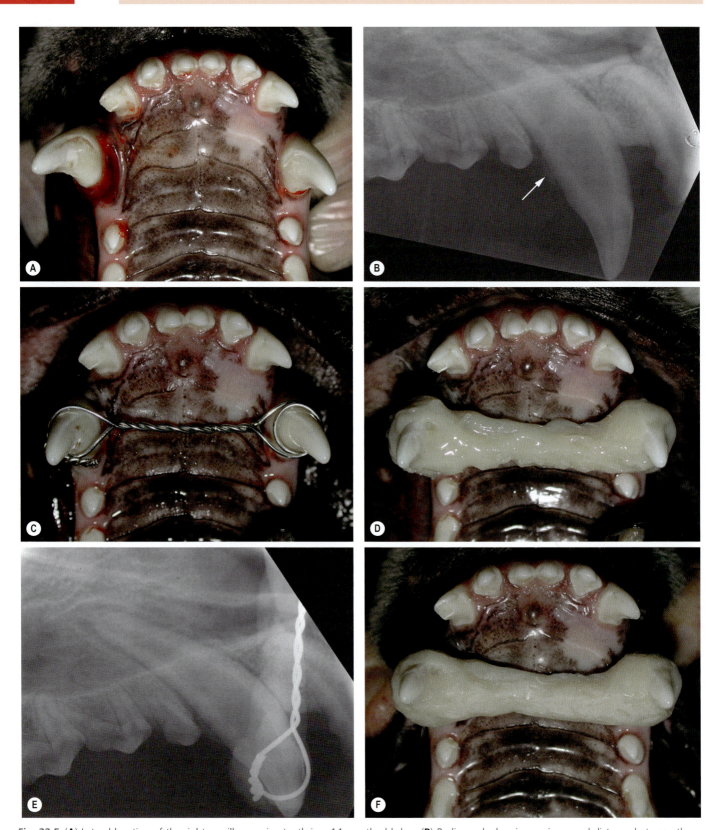

Fig. 22.5 (**A**) Lateral luxation of the right maxillary canine tooth in a 14-month-old dog. (**B**) Radiograph showing an increased distance between the tooth root and the alveolar walls, and a small bony fragment attached to the distal surface of the tooth (*arrow*). (**C**) Wire-splinting of the displaced tooth. (**D**) Composite resin was added to cover the wire to avoid tongue laceration. (**E**) Radiograph following replantation showing correct tooth repositioning. (**F**) The composite resin was smoothed.

margin to avoid contact with the soft tissue. To prevent occlusal interference, the wire and the bulk of the resin should be placed on the buccal side of the maxillary teeth and on the lingual aspect of the mandibular teeth. In brachycephalic breeds, positioning may be necessarily different.

- Acid-etching of the surface of the teeth to be included in the device with phosphoric acid etching gel or liquid for 15 seconds. Acid-etching can be avoided if the shape of the teeth included in the splint assures good mechanical retention for the splinting material.
- Applying a bonding material on the teeth and the wires. Bonding can be avoided if the shape of the teeth included in the splint assures good mechanical retention for the splinting material.
- Applying composite material or acrylic resin to secure the wire (Fig. 22.5D). Polymerization of light-cured composite is started from the noninjured teeth and finished with the displaced teeth, that can be held in position by digital pressure. After polymerization, the distal ends of the wire may be smoothed with burs. To avoid inflammation, the acrylic or composite material should not be in contact with the soft tissues.

- Obtaining a radiograph to verify the repositioning (Fig. 22.5E).
- Trimming and smoothing the splint (Fig. 22.5F).
- Inspecting the occlusion before allowing the patient to recover.

It is almost impossible to stop dogs from using the splinted teeth, but biting may be kept to a minimum by feeding a soft diet and limiting access to chew toys. Proper oral hygiene should be instituted with daily brushing using a soft toothbrush and a 0.1% chlorhexidine gel. A clinical reexamination of all replanted teeth should be scheduled 1–2 weeks after treatment to check stability and integrity of the splint, extent of gingival inflammation or any undesired orthodontic movements.

Duration and retention of the splint depends on the age of the animal and the extent of the dental and bony lesions. In human patients, the splint is removed in 7–10 days, as prolonged splinting may induce replacement resorption and increase the frequency of pulp necrosis and inflammatory resorption.[1,18,64] If no bony fractures are present, this time is sufficient to secure adequate periodontal healing. The splint should be left in place longer, up to 4–6 weeks in case of extensive bony fractures.[1] After radiographically confirming bone and periodontal healing (Fig. 22.6A), the splint is removed by

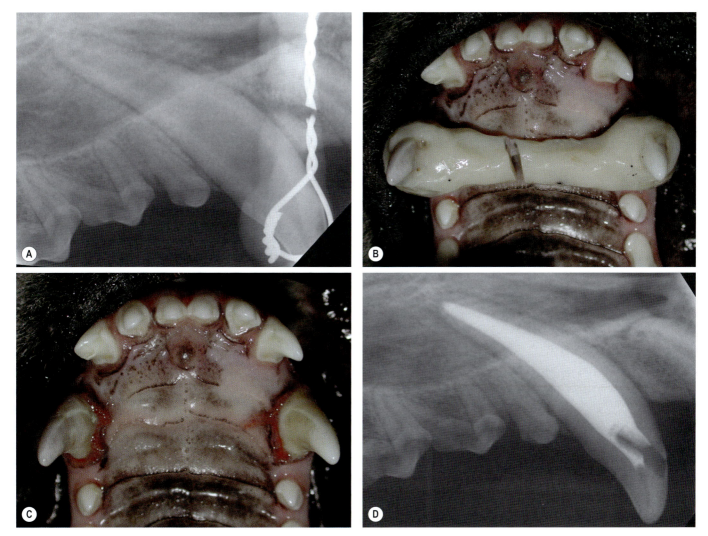

Fig. 22.6 Four-week follow-up of the patient in Fig. 22.5. (**A**) Radiograph (after dividing the splint) showing periodontal healing. (**B**) Before removal, the splint was divided and tooth mobility was evaluated manually. Note the pink discoloration of the right canine tooth, indicating pulp damage. (**C**) As the tooth was stable, the splint was removed. Mild gingivitis developed underneath the splint, but resolved within a few days. (**D**) Radiograph showing root canal treatment before placement of the final restoration.

gouging the splinting material with the appropriate burs on a high-speed handpiece and abundant water cooling. Particular care should be taken not to damage the tooth surface. To easily distinguish the resin from the dental structure, a shade distinctly different from the color of the teeth should be used. If possible, the splint should be initially divided in such a way that tooth mobility can be manually assessed (Fig. 22.6B). If significant mobility is still present, the splint should be repaired and left in place for a longer period. Otherwise, orthodontic bracket removal pliers (Bracket removal pliers, Ormco, Orange, CA, USA) are used to gently break off the material. After splint removal, the teeth should be polished.

Systemic antibiotic treatment

If started preoperatively or immediately postreplantation, systemic antibiotic therapy prevents bacterial invasion of the pulp and inflammatory resorption. If, however, antibiotic therapy is instituted some time after replantation, there is no reduction of the incidence of inflammatory root resorption.[34,47] Both postreplantation tetracycline hydrochloride (20 mg/kg PO TID for 7 days) and amoxicillin (22 mg/kg PO BID for 7 days) treatments have been shown to be effective in limiting inflammatory root resorption secondary to pulpal infection in dogs,[65] and should therefore always be administered in all cases of replantation. In humans, penicillin V is also recommended.[4,30]

Endodontic treatment

As a result of dental displacement, the vascular supply to the pulp is often partially or totally severed, leading to degenerative changes in the pulp tissues. Therefore, standard root canal treatment is generally necessary following replantation.[1] Endodontic treatment should be performed when the tooth is in its alveolus.[1] Extraoral filing before replantation always results in ankylosis, due to the fact that root canal treatment prolongs the extraoral period. Furthermore, pressure and damage to the periodontal ligament caused by incorrect handling of the teeth may induce further replacement resorption.[64] Only if more than 1 hour has elapsed before replantation and the avulsed tooth has been stored dry during this time, endodontic therapy may be accomplished extraorally.[11,39] The tooth should be washed thoroughly and held by the crown in moist, sterile gauze.

Generally, endodontic treatment should be performed 7–14 days after replantation, at the time of splint removal.[1] To minimize trauma to the newly formed periodontal fibers, endodontic treatment may be performed before physically removing the dental splint by creating an access hole through the splinting material. Initially, calcium hydroxide is used as filling material.[1] Calcium hydroxide is bactericidal and is apparently able to inhibit root resorption, probably by creating an alkaline environment which stimulates tissue repair while reducing the resorptive process.[66] This treatment, repeated every 3–6 months as the calcium hydroxide dissipates, is followed by permanent filling with gutta-percha approximately 1 year after replantation. In dogs and cats, because of the need for anesthesia for each procedure, short-term treatment with calcium hydroxide or single-stage root canal therapy with gutta-percha at the time of splint removal may be an acceptable treatment option (Fig. 22.6D).

Promising results on the use of a corticosteroid (1% triamcinolone) and antibiotic (3% demeclocycline) containing paste (Ledermix™, Lederle Pharmaceuticals, Wolfrantshausen, Germany) as a filling material have been shown in a recent study using a canine dental trauma model.[67] It was demonstrated that intracanal placement of the tested paste immediately following an avulsion injury and before replantation decreases tooth resorption and favors healing.[67] Also, the use of a 1% triamcinolone cream as filling material was shown to be as effective at inhibiting external root resorption as the triamcinolone–demeclocycline paste.[68] These researchers suggested that intracanal placement of corticosteroids should be used as standard treatment protocol at emergency visit for traumatic injuries in which root resorption is predicted.[68]

Endodontically treated teeth should be restored using zinc oxide-eugenol or glass ionomer cements (temporary restoration following temporary endodontic treatment), or acid-etch composite resins (permanent restoration).[29] In both instances, a >4 mm deep restoration is recommended to minimize the risk of coronal leakage and bacterial contamination.[29]

If the trauma is minimal, such as in case of concussion or subluxation, the pulp may survive and the tooth should be monitored radiographically at 1, 3, 6 and 12 months before endodontic treatment is performed.[1,2]

Finally, in case of immature teeth with an open apex, revascularization of the pulp tissues within 3–4 weeks is possible after immediate replantation.[48,50,69,70] Revascularization is accomplished by in-growth of new cell-rich and well-vascularized connective tissue.[63,71] In these patients, endodontic treatment is delayed and radiographic reexaminations are recommended every 2–4 weeks until continued root development is evident. In case of pulp necrosis or root resorption, temporary endodontic treatment with calcium hydroxide can be performed to achieve apexification before permanent obturation of the canal.

COMPLICATIONS FOLLOWING TRAUMA AND REPLANTATION

Animal studies have shown that healing of the periodontal ligament starts soon after clot formation within the periodontal space. After replantation, new junctional epithelium is reestablished within 7 days.[72,73] At 2 weeks, new collagen fibers extend from the cementum to the alveolar bone, and periodontal healing is complete in 2–4 weeks.[74] However, complications following dental displacement are common, more so in mature than immature teeth.[24]

Pulpal healing complications

Coronal discoloration

Discoloration of the crown soon after injury may be a sign of damage to the pulp (Fig. 22.6B). The discoloration is often transient.[25]

Pulp necrosis

The most common complication of severe dental displacement is pulp necrosis.[1,24,64] The necrotic pulp is also often infected as a result of contact with saliva, plaque or extraoral material. Whether pulp necrosis will occur following trauma depends on the type of injury and stage of root development (Fig. 22.7).[25] Risk of pulp necrosis is least after concussion and subluxation, and greatest in extrusion, lateral luxation and intrusion, in that order.[25] Pulp necrosis is more common in teeth with completed rather than uncompleted root development.[25] In immature teeth with an open apex, revascularization following luxation or avulsion may occur.[69,72,73]

Pulp necrosis following dental displacement is diagnosed in humans based on the presence of loss of pulpal sensitivity, gray crown discoloration or periapical radiolucency, and confirmed by pulp vitality testing.[25] As vitality tests are unreliable in dogs and cats, the diagnosis of pulp necrosis in these patients should be based mainly on radiographic and clinical signs (i.e., coronal discoloration).[75]

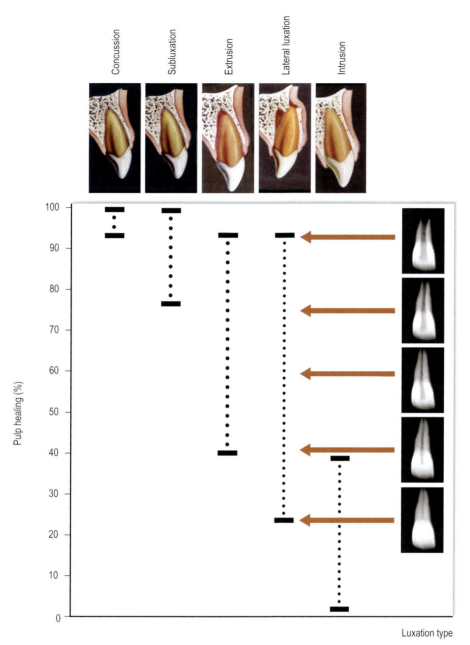

Fig. 22.7 Relationship between luxation diagnosis, stage of root development and pulpal healing after trauma in human beings. Each bar represents the level of pulp survival 1 year after injury. The upper set of bars represents pulp survival for teeth with incomplete root formation, and the lower set pulp survival for teeth with complete root formation. *(From Andreasen JO, Andreasen FM, Andersson L, eds.* Textbook and color atlas of traumatic injuries to the teeth. *4th ed. Oxford: Blackwell Munksgaard, 2007, with permission.)*

In humans, a small but significant proportion of extruded and laterally luxated mature teeth may develop transient apical breakdown (TAB), visible radiographically as a periapical radiolucency appearing spontaneously some time after injury and disappearing without treatment.[76] In some cases the radiographic abnormalities persist over an extended period of time, and may either spontaneously return to normal or be accompanied by surface resorption and pulp canal obliteration.[1,76] Strict monitoring of these teeth for at least a year is mandatory to confirm pulp and periapical healing. If there is any doubt about the client's compliance with long-term radiographic examinations, endodontic treatment should be performed as soon as a periapical lesion is diagnosed.

Root canal obliteration

Root canal obliteration should be considered a normal reaction of vital pulp to a moderate trauma. In humans, it is more common following displacement of teeth with incomplete rather than complete root formation, in particular after luxation injuries.[59,64] It is rarely seen after concussion and subluxation, when little damage to the pulp occurs.[25]

Root canal obliteration can usually be diagnosed within the first year after injury.[25] In approximately 1–16% of human traumatized teeth it is followed by pulpal necrosis.[1]

Root resorption

Root resorption is a serious complication associated with replantation, and represents the major cause of failure following treatment of displaced teeth. In humans, it occurs more frequently in avulsed than in luxated teeth.[1] Root resorption progresses more rapidly in younger than older replanted teeth, and is negatively influenced by the presence of concomitant fractures of the alveolar bone or by an extended period of splinting.

Root resorption is directly related to an injury to the periodontal tissues. The presence of a vital periodontal ligament has been shown to inhibit invasion of bone cells. In particular, the intermediate cementum is thought to resist root resorption and bone invasion, and its loss as a result of trauma may predispose to resorption.[77] The intermediate cementum cannot be regenerated once it has been damaged; therefore successful replantation is directly related to the preservation of the periodontal ligament and superficial layer of the root.[34] Root resorption is classified into three types: (1) surface resorption, (2) inflammatory resorption, and (3) replacement resorption.[1] The same tooth may develop a combination of surface resorption, followed by cemental healing, and osseous replacement.[49] Internal resorption only occurs in 4% of displaced teeth, mainly after luxation injuries.[24]

Surface resorption

Surface resorption is characterized by small, localized resorption cavities affecting the cementum and the superficial layer of dentin.[1] It is apparently caused by drying of the periodontal membrane and cementum during the extra-alveolar time and by pressure directed onto the root surfaces.[59] Surface resorption can be recognized within 1 week after replantation, becomes more prominent at 2 weeks and may heal spontaneously with reparative cementum within a few weeks.[34] It is usually asymptomatic and cannot be visualized on routine radiographs.[2] When dentin is resorbed, healing may occur with an altered root outline that may become radiographically visible.[78,79]

Inflammatory resorption

The development of inflammatory root resorption is directly related to damage of the root surface and periodontium at the time of the traumatic insult and the presence of bacteria within the root canal and dentinal tubules.[1] Under normal circumstances, if the pulp becomes infected, the cemental layer does not allow the toxins from the pulp to reach the periodontal space. After an avulsion, the cemental covering may be damaged and the toxins from the necrotic and infected pulp may pass through the dentinal tubules and stimulate an inflammatory response in the corresponding periodontal ligament space. Root substance and bone are then destroyed.

This process is accelerated in the young patient and following an extended extra-alveolar period due to increased chances of infection.[1] If inflammatory resorption is not resolved, rapid destruction of the root, progressive tooth mobility and eventually tooth loss may occur.[72]

Consequently, control of root canal infection with adequate root canal therapy after replantation is critical for the prevention and/or treatment of inflammatory root resorption. If endodontic treatment is delayed, it is difficult to eliminate resorption once it begins.[2] If the inflammation subsides, ankylosis often results.

Inflammatory resorption consists radiographically of bowl-shaped resorption cavities of the root and radiolucent areas of the adjacent bone.[3] These progressive changes can be seen as early as 2–3 weeks after avulsion (Fig. 22.8).[59,72]

Dentoalveolar ankylosis and replacement resorption

In replacement resorption, a large amount of root hard tissue is resorbed and filled with alveolar bone, causing the tooth to be anchored tightly in its alveolus. The clinical signs include reduced

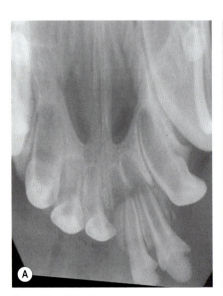 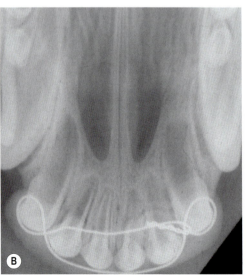 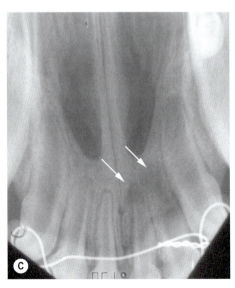

Fig. 22.8 (**A**) Radiograph of a 5-month-old beagle with lateral luxation of the left maxillary first and second incisor teeth. (**B**) Radiograph showing correct positioning after replantation and splinting. (**C**) Three-week follow-up radiograph showing lack of root development, apical root resorption and periapical radiolucency of the replanted teeth (*arrows*).

motility and a metallic, high percussion sound. Human teeth with less than 10% of ankylosed root surface, though, exhibit normal percussion sound and mobility, and a high-pitched percussion tone has been shown to develop only when at least 20% of the root surface is ankylosed.[33] Radiographically, the distinction between the root and surrounding bone is lost, the periodontal ligament space is absent and a moth-eaten appearance results.[2,3]

However, visualization is not always possible because of overlapping structures and bone marrow spaces.[33,59] Radiographic signs usually appear after a few weeks from replantation, when the resorption cavities have increased to more than 1–2 mm in diameter.[59]

As long as the protective covering of cementum is intact and periodontal cells are healthy, resorption will not occur.[44] Factors such as extraoral time, use of a suitable storage medium, and the type and duration of splinting are critical for the prevention of replacement resorption.[37] When the periodontal membrane and cementoblasts are damaged, the root is exposed to colonization by osteoclasts, cells of the same hematological origin as osteoclasts that from the adjacent bone marrow migrate into the damaged areas.[1,2]

The ultimate outcome of replacement resorption is destruction of the root, which leads to either infection via the gingival sulcus, crown fracture due to loss of support, or exfoliation of the tooth.[2,33]

The use of agents inhibiting osteoclastic activity has been studied in dogs to evaluate the possibility to decrease root resorption following displacement and replacement.[80] An enamel matrix derivative (Emdogain®, Biora, Malmö, Sweden) has been shown to exhibit a positive effect in regenerating cemental and periodontal ligament fibers in dogs' exarticulated teeth.[81] However, a subsequent study showed inability of the same product to protect the root of reimplanted canine teeth from replacement resorption.[82]

The topical use of recombinant human bone morphogenetic protein-12 (rhBMP-12), a member of the transforming growth factor-b/BMP gene family, failed to reestablish normal periodontal ligament fibers and to prevent ankylosis and root resorption of dogs' reimplanted teeth.[62]

Fluoride is considered to promote osteoblastic activity or to inhibit osteoclastic activity by reducing the susceptibility of bone and dental hard tissues to resorptive processes.[34]

Loss of marginal bone

Loss of marginal bone support following dental displacement may develop because of mechanical irritation of the splint, plaque accumulation or directly because of the trauma.[59,64] It increases with the severity of the injury, being very common in case of intrusion and extrusion.[1,2]

PROGNOSIS

The prognosis of traumatized teeth is generally better in younger patients and in those having intact soft tissues, no root fractures, and maximal bone support.[11] The presence of an intact, viable periodontal ligament is the most important factor in assuring healing without resorption, the critical extra-alveolar time being 60 minutes.[1,30] Healing is also dependent upon the extent of the injury: severely displaced teeth show a higher incidence of healing complications than subluxated teeth.[24] Intrusive displacement is second only to avulsion in severity, as root resorption, ankylosis and pulp necrosis will frequently occur.[1] Duration of immobilization has also been shown to influence the prognosis of luxation injuries: the longer the splinting time, the higher the incidence of complications.[64]

It is important to consider that teeth affected by resorption and ankylosis may be exfoliated or may fracture months or years after the initial injury. Because of the possible development of late complications, radiographic follow-up examinations are recommended in humans for 2–5 years post replantation.[1,8,29] Further studies are needed to evaluate the incidence and rate of development of late complications in veterinary patients.

REFERENCES

1. Andreasen JO, Andreasen FM, Andersson L. Textbook and color atlas of traumatic injuries to the teeth. 4th ed. Oxford, UK: Blackwell Munksgaard; 2007.
2. Trope M, Blanco L, Chivian N, et al. The role of endodontics after traumatic injuries. In: Cohen S, Hargreaves KM, editors. Pathways of the pulp. 9th ed. St. Louis, MO: Elsevier Mosby; 2006. p. 610–49.
3. White SC, Pharoah MJ. Trauma to teeth and facial structures. In: White SC, Pharoah MJ, editors. Oral radiology. principles and interpretation. 4th ed. St Louis, MO: Mosby; 2004. p. 615–38.
4. Flores MT, Andersson L, Andreasen JO, et al. Guidelines for the management of traumatic dental injuries. I. Fractures and luxations of permanent teeth. Dent Traumatol 2007;23:66–71.
5. Nakane S, Kameyama Y. Root resorption caused by mechanical injury of the periodontal soft tissue in rats. J Period Res 1987;22:390–5.
6. Tziafas D. Pulpal reactions following experimental acute trauma of concussion type on immature dog teeth. Endod Dent Traumatol 1988;4:27–31.
7. Mulligan TW, Aller MS, Williams CA. Atlas of canine and feline dental radiography. Trenton, NJ: Veterinary Learning System; 1998.
8. Gracis M, Orsini P. Treatment of traumatic dental luxation in six dogs. J Vet Dent 1998;15:65–72.
9. Kraaijenhagen P. Luxatie van een hoektand met fractuur van de alveolaire wand van het os maxillare bij een hond [Displacement of a canine tooth associated with fracture of the alveolar wall of the maxilla in a dog]. Tijdschr Diergeneeskd 1986;111:1260–1.
10. Ulbricht RD, Manfra Marretta S, Klippert LS. Mandibular canine tooth luxation injury in a dog. J Vet Dent 2004;21:77–83.
11. Powers MP, Quereshy FA, Ramsey CA. Diagnosis and management of dentoalveolar injuries. In: Fonseca RJ, Walker RV, Betts NJ, et al, editors. Oral and maxillofacial trauma. 3rd ed. St. Louis, MO: Elsevier Saunders; 2005. p. 427–77.
12. Ebeleseder KA, Santler G, Glockner K, et al. An analysis of 58 traumatically intruded and surgically extruded permanent teeth. Endod Dent Traumatol 2000;16:34–9.
13. Turley PK, Joiner MW, Hellstrom S. The effect of orthodontic extrusion on traumatically intruded teeth. Am J Orthod 1984;85:47–56.
14. Turley PK, Crawford LB, Carrington KW. Traumatically intruded teeth. Angle Orthod 1987;57:234–44.
15. Cunha RF, Pavarini A, Percinoto C, et al. Pulpal and periodontal reactions of immature permanent teeth in the dog to intrusive trauma. Endod Dent Traumatol 1995;11:100–4.
16. Cunha RF, Pavarini A, Percinoto C, et al. Influence of surgical repositioning of mature permanent dog teeth following experimental intrusion: a histologic assessment. Dent Traumatol 2002;18:304–8.
17. Rubin LD. Ectopic implantation of a canine tooth displaced by trauma.

Vet Med Small Anim Clin 1979; 74:68.

18. Grossman LI, Oliet S, Del Rio CE. Replantation, transplantation, and endodontic implants. In: Grossman LI, Oliet S, Del Rio CE, editors. Endodontic practice. 11th ed. Philadelphia, PA: Lea & Febiger; 1988. p. 329–48.

19. Sherman Jr P. Intentional replantation of teeth in dogs and monkeys. J Dent Res 1968;47:1066–71.

20. Runyon CL, Rigg DL, Grier RL. Allogeneic tooth transplantation in the dog. J Am Vet Med Assoc 1986;188:713–17.

21. Spodnick GJ. Replantation of a maxillary canine tooth after traumatic avulsion in a dog. J Vet Dent 1992;9:4–7.

22. Briggs RA. Treatment of tooth luxations in dogs. Proceedings, Veterinary Dentistry Congress, New Orleans, USA, 1989.

23. Flores MT, Malmgren B, Andersson L, et al. Guidelines for the management of traumatic dental injuries. III. Primary teeth. Dent Traumatol 2007;23:196–202.

24. Crona-Larsson G, Bjarnason S, et al. Effect of luxation injuries on permanent teeth. Endod Dent Traumatol 1991;7:199–206.

25. Andreasen FM. Pulpal healing after luxation injuries and root fracture in the permanent dentition. Endod Dent Traumatol 1989;5:111–31.

26. Trope M. Clinical management of the avulsed tooth. Dent Clin North Am 1995;39:93–112.

27. Flores MT, Andreasen JO, Bakland LK. International Association of Dental Traumatology. Guidelines for the evaluation and management of traumatic dental injuries. Dental Traumatol 2001; 17:97–102.

28. American Association of Endodontists. Treatment of the avulsed permanent tooth. Recommended Guidelines of the American Association of Endodontists. Dent Clin North Am 1995;39:221–5.

29. Trope M: Clinical management of the avulsed tooth: present strategies and future directions. Dent Traumatol 2002; 18:1–11.

30. Flores MT, Andersson L, Andreasen JO, et al. Guidelines for the management of traumatic dental injuries. II. Avulsion of permanent teeth. Dent Traumatol 2007;23: 130–5.

31. Ashkenazi M, Sarnat H, Keila S. In vitro viability, mitogenicity, and clonogenic capacity of periodontal ligament cells after storage in six different media. Endod Dent Traumatol 1999;15:149–56.

32. Pettiette M, Hupp J, Mesaros S, et al. Periodontal healing of extracted dogs' teeth air-dried for extended periods and soaked in various media. Endod Dent Traumatol 1997;13:113–18.

33. Barrett EJ, Kenny DJ. Avulsed permanent teeth: a review of the literature and treatment guidelines. Endod Dent Traumatol 1997;13:153–63.

34. Hammarström L, Pierce A, Blomlöf L, et al. Tooth avulsion and replantation. A review. Endod Dent Traumatol 1986;2:1–8.

35. Hupp JG, Trope M, Mesaros SV, et al. Tritiated thymidine uptake in periodontal ligament cells of dogs' teeth stored in various media for extended time periods. Endod Dent Traumatol 1997;13:223–7.

36. Hupp JG, Mesaros SV, Aukhil I, et al. Periodontal ligament vitality and histologic healing of teeth stored for extended periods before transplantation. Endod Dent Traumatol 1998;14:79–83.

37. Trope M, Friedman S. Periodontal healing of replanted dog teeth stored in ViaSpan, milk and Hank's balanced salt solution. Endod Dent Traumatol 1992;8:183–8.

38. Trope M, Hupp JG, Mesaros SV. The role of the socket in the periodontal healing of replanted dogs' teeth stored in ViaSpan for extended periods. Endod Dent Traumatol 1997;13:171–5.

39. Krasner P, Rankow HJ. New philosophy for the treatment of avulsed teeth. Oral Surg Oral Med Oral Pathol Oral Radiol Endod 1995;79:616–23.

40. Buttke TM, Trope M. Effect of catalase supplementation in storage media for avulsed teeth. Dent Traumatol 2003;19: 103–8.

41. Blomlöf L, Lindskog S, Andersson L, et al. Storage of experimentally avulsed teeth in milk prior to replantation. J Dent Res 1983;62:912–16.

42. Blomlöf L, Lindskog S, Hammarström L. Periodontal healing of exarticulated monkey teeth stored in milk or saliva. Scan J Dent Res 1981;89:251–9.

43. Blomlöf L, Lindskog S, Andersson L, et al. Periodontal healing of replanted monkey teeth prevented from drying. Acta Odontol Scand 1983;41:117–23.

44. Löe H, Waerhaug J. Experimental replantation of teeth in dogs and monkeys. Arch Oral Biol 1961;3:176–84.

45. Matsson L, Klinge B, Hallström H. Effect on periodontal healing of saline irrigation of the tooth socket before replantation. Endod Dent Traumatol 1987;3:64–7.

46. Cvez M, Cleaton-Jones P, Austin J, et al. Effect of topical application of doxycycline on pulp revascularization and periodontal healing in reimplanted monkey incisors. Endod Dent Traumatol 1990;6:170–6.

47. Sae-Lim V, Wang CY, Choi GW, et al. The effect of systemic tetracycline on resorption of dried replanted dogs' teeth. Endod Dent Traumatol 1998;14: 127–32.

48. Yanpiset K, Trope M. Pulp revascularization of replanted immature dog teeth after different treatment methods. Endod Dent Traumatol 2000; 16:211–17.

49. Bryson EC, Levin L, Banchs F, et al. Effect of minocycline on healing of replanted dog teeth after extended dry times. Dent Traumatol 2003;19:90–5.

50. Ritter ALS, Ritter AV, Murrah V, et al. Pulp revascularization of replanted immature dog teeth after treatment with minocycline and doxycycline assessed by laser Doppler flowmetry, radiography, and histology. Dent Traumatol 2004;20:75–84.

51. Klinge B, Nilvéus R, Selvig KA. The effect of citric acid on repair after delayed tooth replantation in dogs. Acta Odontol Scand 1984;42:351–9.

52. Bjorvatn K, Selvig KA, Klinge B. Effect of tetracycline and SnF2 on root resorption in replanted incisors in dogs. Scand J Dent Res 1989;97:477–82.

53. Selvig KA, Bjorvatn K, Claffey N. Effect of stannous fluoride and tetracycline on repair after delayed replantation of root-planed teeth in dogs. Acta Odont Scand 1990;48:107–12.

54. Selvig KA, Bjovartn K, Bogle GC, et al. Effect of stannous fluoride and tetracycline on periodontal repair after delayed tooth replantation in dogs. Scand J Dent Res 1992;100:200–3.

55. Lin S, Zuckerman O, Fuss Z, et al. New emphasis in the treatment of dental trauma: avulsion and luxation. Dent Traumatol 2007;23:297–303.

56. Skoglund A. A study on citric acid as a proposed replacement resorption inhibitor. Swed Dent J 1991;15: 161–9.

57. Walsh JS, Fey MR, Omnell LM. The effects of indomethacin on resorption and ankylosis in replanted teeth. ASDC J Dent Child 1987;54:261–6.

58. Sae-Lim V, Metzger Z, Trope M. Local dexamethasone improves periodontal healing of replanted dogs' teeth. Endod Dent Traumatol 1998;14:232–6.

59. Oikarinen K. Tooth splinting: a review of the literature and consideration of the versatility of a wire-composite splint. Endod Dent Traumatol 1990;6:237–50.

60. Oikarinen K, Andreasen JO, Andreasen FM. Rigidity of various fixation methods used as dental splints. Endod Dent Traumatol 1992;8:113–19.

61. Kahler B, Heithersay GS. An evidence-based appraisal of splinting luxated, avulsed and root-fractured teeth. Dent Traumatol 2007; doi: 10.1111/j.1600-9657.2006.00480.x

62. Sorensen RG, Polimeni G, Kinoshita A, et al. Effect of recombinant human bone morphogenetic protein-12 (rhBMP-12) on regeneration of periodontal attachment following tooth replantation in dogs. A pilot study. J Clin Periodontol 2004;31:654–61.

63. Claus I, Laureys W, Cornelissen R, et al. Histologic analysis of pulpal revascularization of autotransplanted immature teeth after removal of the original pulp tissue. Am J Orthod Dentofacial Orthop 2004;125:93–9.

64. Oikarinen K, Gundlach KKH, Pfeifer G. Late complications of luxation injuries to

teeth. Endod Dent Traumatol 1987;3: 296–303.

65. Sae-Lim V, Wang CY, Trope M. Effect of systemic tetracycline and amoxicillin on inflammatory root resorption of replanted dogs' teeth. Endod Dent Traumatol 1998; 14:216–20.

66. Trope M, Moshonov J, Nissan R, et al. Short vs. long-term calcium hydroxide treatment of established inflammatory root resorption in replanted dog teeth. Endod Dent Traumatol 1995;11:124–8.

67. Bryson EC, Levin L, Banchs F, et al. Effect of immediate intracanal placement of Ledermix Paste® on healing of replanted dog teeth after extended dry times. Dent Traumatol 2002;18:316–21.

68. Chen H, Teixeira FB, Ritter AL, et al. The effect of intracanal anti-inflammatory medicaments on external root resorption of replanted dog teeth after extended extra-oral dry time. Dent Traumatol 2007; doi: 10.1111/j.1600-9657.2006. 00483.x

69. Skoglund A, Tronstad L. Pulpal changes in replanted and autotransplanted immature teeth of dogs. J Endod 1981;7:309–16.

70. Yanpiset K, Vongsavan N, Sigurdsson A, et al. Efficacy of laser Doppler flowmetry for the diagnosis of revascularization of reimplanted immature dog teeth. Dent Traumatology 2001;17:63–70.

71. Skoglund A, Tronstad L, Wallenius K. A micro-angiography study of vascular changes in replanted and autotransplanted teeth of young dogs. Oral Surg Oral Med Oral Pathol 1978;45:17–28.

72. Andreasen JO. A time related study of periodontal healing and root resorption activity after replantation of mature permanent incisors in monkeys. Swed Dent J 1980;4:101–7.

73. Nasjleti CE, Caffesse RG, Castelli WA, et al. Healing after tooth replacement in monkeys. A radioautographic study. Oral Surg Oral Med Oral Pathol 1975;39: 361–75.

74. Yamada H, Maeda T, Hanada K, et al. Re-innervation in the canine periodontal ligament of replanted teeth using an antibody to protein gene product 9.5: an immunohistochemical study. Endod Dent Traumatol 1999;15:221–34.

75. Hale FA. Localized intrinsic staining of teeth due to pulpitis and pulp necrosis in dogs. J Vet Dent 2001;18:14–20.

76. Andreasen, FM. Transient apical breakdown and its relation to color and sensibility changes after luxation injuries to teeth. Endod Dent Traumatol 1986;2: 9–19.

77. Andreasen JO. The effect of pulp extirpation or root canal treatment upon periodontal healing after replantation of permanent incisors in monkeys. J Endod 1981;7:245–53.

78. Andreasen JO. Analysis of topography of surface and inflammatory root resorption after replantation of mature permanent incisors in monkeys. Swed Dent J 1980;4: 135–44.

79. Andreasen JO. Luxation of permanent teeth due to trauma. A clinical and radiographic follow-up study of 189 injured teeth. Scand J Dent Res 1970;78: 273–86.

80. Levin L, Bryson EC, Caplan D, et al. Effect of topical alendronate on root resorption of dried replanted dog teeth. Dent Traumatol 2001;17:120–6.

81. Iqbal MK, Bamaas NS. Effect of enamel matrix derivative (Emdogain) upon periodontal healing after replantation of permanent incisors in Beagle dogs. Dent Traumatol 2001;17:36–45.

82. Araujo M, Hayacibara R, Sonohara M, et al. Effect of enamel matrix proteins (Emdogain) on healing after re-implantation of 'periodontally compromised' roots. An experimental study in the dog. J Clin Periodontol 2003;30:855–63.

Chapter | **23** |

Principles of endodontic surgery

Edward R. Eisner

DEFINITIONS[1–3]

Apicoectomy: see Root canal therapy, surgical

Dilaceration: a developmental problem resulting in a crown or root structure that is bent or curved

Direct pulp capping: the procedure that includes exposing the pulp and treating it medically to stimulate repair of the injured tissue followed by covering it with a surface restoration

Endodontic surgery: endodontic therapy to prevent or treat periapical pathosis by surgical means, which generally includes apicoectomy and also may include abscess drainage, hemisection/root amputation, replantation (see Ch. 22), and other corrective procedures

Hemisection: removing one root and half of the crown of a two-rooted tooth, combined with appropriate endodontic treatment of the remaining tooth fragment

Lateral (accessory) canal: a small canal communicating from the root canal to the periodontal space, usually in the apical one-third of the tooth root

Root amputation: removal of one root of a multirooted tooth, leaving most of the crown intact, and combined with appropriate endodontic treatment of the remaining dental structure

Root canal therapy, standard (nonsurgical, conventional): a pulpectomy and obturation performed via a normograde fashion through the crown of the tooth

Root canal therapy, surgical: the surgical removal of the apex of the tooth root (apicoectomy) combined with the sealing of the opening of the remaining pulp cavity in a retrograde fashion

INTRODUCTION

In most cases of endodontic disease, standard root canal treatment, in which the approach to the dental pulp is made through a coronal access site, is successful, with a reported failure rate in dogs of 5.5%.[4] In certain specific cases, however, only surgical endodontic treatment can salvage the affected teeth.[5–7] In most cases where surgical root canal therapy is employed, it is preceded by standard root canal therapy.[6–11]

Surgical root canal therapy is a retrograde procedure that involves elevating a mucoperiosteal flap, removing bone to expose the affected root tip(s) and sealing the apical end of the root canal in a retrograde fashion.[8] Surgical and standard root canal therapy are complementary and should not be performed by a clinician with inadequate equipment or limited experience in endodontic treatment.[6–8,12]

Surgical endodontic treatment is indicated only occasionally in dogs and rarely in cats, but can salvage cases of aberrant intracanal anatomy, roots fractured in the apical third, inflammatory root end resorption, and selected cases of failed standard root canal procedure. Surgical endodontic treatment can almost always salvage a tooth that can no longer be treated by other endodontic means and that might otherwise require extraction.[10,13] The teeth most often requiring surgical root canal therapy are the maxillary and mandibular canine teeth, the maxillary fourth premolar and the mandibular first molar teeth in the dog, and the maxillary and mandibular canine teeth in the cat.[8–12,14,15] Although the results of surgical endodontic treatment in animals have not been documented, the procedure may have a high success rate in treating difficult cases.[12,14]

THERAPEUTIC DECISION-MAKING

Surgical endodontics versus other treatment options

Surgical endodontics versus re-treatment

The success rate of nonsurgical root canal treatment is very high and, in most instances, it is indicated to repeat a standard root canal procedure if the apical root structures are intact, rather than to treat the case surgically.[6,8,9,16] In a retrospective study of 253 root canal treatments on dogs, only 4 (1.5%) required surgical procedures and 3 of those were identified prior to initial therapy, because of the peracute nature of the infection, where a two-stage root canal treatment might have been indicated.[13,17] Failure to resolve an abscess when performing standard root canal therapy is typically due to an inadequate apical seal.[6,15] If the apex is intact, re-treating the canal to establish a solid fill of the apical one-third of the canal usually resolves the problem.[9,14,18] Coronal leakage at the restoration margin is another indication for re-treatment, rather than surgical root canal therapy.

In some cases it may be advantageous to repeat the root canal treatment in two stages. During the first stage, the pulp cavity is cleaned, shaped and dried. It is subsequently filled with calcium hydroxide paste and a temporary restoration is placed. Two or three weeks later the restoration and calcium hydroxide are removed and the pulp cavity is filled with gutta-percha. The intracanal medication with calcium hydroxide aids in the disinfection of the canal and the healing of the periapical tissues. Re-treatment in two stages may be indicated in the following instances: (1) iatrogenic perforation of the apex or pulp cavity occurs during the procedure; (2) early inflammatory resorption is present; (3) the pulp cavity is found to be filled with exudate; or (4) a large periapical lesion is present.[19]

Repeating the nonsurgical root canal treatment may be impractical or impossible, for example, if a prosthetic crown is present, especially when a post was used.[16] Removing a prosthetic crown is difficult and can often not be achieved without destroying the prosthesis. Therefore, if a periapical lesion develops on a tooth that was successfully restored using a prosthetic crown, it is justifiable to resort to surgical endodontic treatment rather than to repeat the root canal procedure.

Root amputation/hemisection versus surgical endodontics

Occasionally, hemisection is an appropriate treatment in a multi-rooted tooth in which advanced periodontal vertical bone loss involves only one root, but threatens the tooth with impending ascending endodontic infection. Another situation lending itself to hemisection therapy is an inaccessible furcational abscess. A viable endodontic therapeutic option may be to hemisect the tooth and remove the affected root and overlying crown, so that effective periodontal treatment may be performed.[18] This may be recommended if the affected tooth is in a breed that requires full dentition, or the tooth is functionally important. At the time of sectioning, if the pulp in the chamber appears healthy, direct pulp capping may be performed over the exposed pulp. On the other hand, if the pulp in the chamber appears infected, standard root canal therapy is indicated for the remaining root(s). Standard root canal therapy may also precede hemisection or root amputation if there is evidence of endodontic disease prior to the procedure.

Root amputation is the treatment of choice on a root where surgical root canal treatment is theoretically indicated but technically impossible to perform, for anatomical reasons. The most common example of this is the mesiopalatal root of the maxillary fourth premolar tooth in the dog, the apex of which is almost impossible to approach. It is generally accepted that amputating this root is a more practical alternative, although it has been documented that this weakens the tooth considerably.[13]

Indications

Indications for surgical root canal therapy include anatomical barriers or irretrievable material preventing complete debridement and obturation, intraoperative complications of standard root canal therapy, transverse fracture of the apical third of the root with pulp necrosis, inflammatory root resorption, and failure of well-performed standard root canal therapy to resolve an apical lesion.[8,11,12,20] The goal is to remove persistent infection and the potential causes for chronic or recurrent periapical or periradicular inflammatory disease.[9,16]

Anatomical problems preventing standard normograde root canal treatment

Preoperative intraoral radiographs may reveal anatomical aberrations such as dilaceration that may make standard root canal therapy difficult. A pulp stone obstructing the passage of an endodontic file, a calcified or constricted canal preventing the smallest endodontic file from reaching the apex, and lateral canals preventing the formation of a complete seal of the canal may also act as a barrier to successful standard root canal therapy. Standard root canal treatment should be attempted first, but apicoectomy is indicated if debridement and obturation cannot be achieved in order to prevent future complications.

Transverse fracture of the apical third of the root with pulp necrosis

It is possible for transverse fractures of the apical third of the root to heal and remain asymptomatic. However, if the pulp undergoes necrosis, a periapical lesion may form, associated with the root fragment. In this case, the fragment is surgically removed and a standard root canal treatment performed on the remaining root.[16] Retrograde sealing of the root canal may also be indicated at this time.[20]

Advanced apical root resorption

Occasionally, a unilateral serous or purulent nasal discharge is present in patients with a periapical abscess or there is a draining tract at the mucogingival junction. When the maxillary canine tooth is involved, the draining tract is seen above the maxillary first or second premolar tooth. For the maxillary fourth premolar tooth, drainage is seen near the mucogingival junction or suborbitally directly dorsal to the maxillary fourth premolar tooth. A draining tract in the skin on the ventral aspect of the mandible indicates an abscess of the canine or the first molar tooth. This is most commonly seen ventral to the first or second premolar or first molar teeth. Radiographic evaluation is indicated in patients with any of the above signs. It is common in these cases to see evidence of extensive apical root resorption. Severe abscessation and advanced root resorption increase the chances that standard treatment will fail.[4] Some of these cases may be treated by means of two-stage nonsurgical root canal treatment, but if adequate debridement and obturation is impossible, surgical root canal treatment is indicated.[16]

Endodontic instrument separation and procedural errors

Surgical root canal therapy is effective in salvaging intraoperative complications of standard root canal therapy that prevent re-treatment or the creation of a successful apical seal. These complications include: (1) a separated file tip that cannot be bypassed; (2) iatrogenic perforation of the apex (overinstrumentation); or (3) apical root resorption with severe overfilling ('apical blowout').[14] During standard root canal therapy, it is important to obtain intraoperative radiographs so that the therapeutic plan can be adjusted in a timely fashion.

During attempted re-treatment of a failed root canal treatment, the canal may be obstructed by debris and materials from the initial procedure. If this cannot be removed completely it may interfere with debridement and obturation, in which case surgical root canal treatment is indicated.

Large unresolved periapical lesion or pain following root canal treatment

Surgical endodontic therapy is most commonly needed in patients with recurrent swelling over the apex of the tooth root.[14] Typically, purulent swellings recur at two- to three-month intervals following repeated courses of oral antibiotics. A periapical cyst may form as a result of the proliferation of epithelial rests from within the periodontal ligament, surrounding a longstanding, disintegrating periapical granuloma.[12] Pain may be exhibited following standard root canal therapy if the canal has been incompletely debrided. Such pain is an indication to consider either re-treating or performing surgical root canal therapy.

Contraindications for surgical root canal therapy

Unidentifiable cause of root canal treatment failure

It is inappropriate to attempt to correct all standard root canal therapy failures by performing surgical root canal therapy. It should be considered reckless to perform this procedure if the cause of failure cannot be identified.[6,16] When re-treatment is an option, it should be strongly considered.

Re-treatment is possible

In the majority of standard root canal therapy failures, for example in cases where failure was due to incomplete debridement and obturation, or restorative leakage, re-treating the canal in normograde fashion will likely remedy the problem. Periapical lesions will resolve if this is done correctly.

Medical concerns

If possible, surgical treatment should be avoided in patients with hemorrhagic disorders, history of previous radiation therapy, or patients in poor health that pose a significantly increased anesthetic risk that will be associated with the stress of an invasive procedure.[8,10,18]

There are no specific contraindications for endodontic surgery that would not be similar to other types of oral surgical procedures.[16]

Anatomical limitations

Treatment should be avoided if there is high risk of destruction or serious compromise to the mandibular canal, maxillary recess, mental foramen or the major palatine blood vessels, as indicated by the location or extent of disease.[8,12,18] Treatment of short-rooted teeth has a higher likelihood of failure because an unfavorable crown:root ratio is more likely to result in compromised stability. Cases with extensive root damage that would result postoperatively in too short a root may result in subsequent exfoliation due to trauma or inflammatory disease.[8,11,18] In cases in which there is a fair chance of failure, the treatment of choice may be extraction.

Other dental considerations

Surgical root canal therapy is contraindicated if restorability and periodontal prognosis is poor.[9] Teeth with advanced periodontal disease, teeth with vertically fractured roots, and small nonessential teeth are not good candidates for surgical root canal therapy. Idiopathic resorption in dogs and odontoclastic resorption lesions in cats are also contraindications for surgical root canal treatment.

When periodontitis is the primary cause of endodontic disease, both the periodontal and the endodontic disease will need to be treated in order to regain oral health. Cases like this have a higher likelihood of failure, especially in short-rooted teeth, where amputation of a portion of the root will significantly compromise the effectiveness of the root as an anchor for the tooth. In cases where periodontal disease is extensive, adequate debridement may also further weaken the mandible and significantly reduce the chances for successful treatment.[8]

REFERENCES

1. Shafer WG, Hine MK, Levy BM. Developmental disturbances of oral and paraoral structures. In: A textbook of oral pathology. 4th ed. Philadelphia, PA: W.B. Saunders; 1983. p. 2–85.

2. Holmstrom, SE, Frost P, Eisner ER. Dental records. In: Veterinary dental techniques. 3rd ed. Philadelphia, PA: WB Saunders Co; 2004. p. 1–38.

3. Boucher CO, Zwemer TJ. Boucher's clinical dental terminology – a glossary of accepted terms in all disciplines of dentistry. 4th ed. St. Louis, MO: Mosby – Year Book; 1993.

4. Kuntsi-Vaattovaara H, Verstraete FJM, Kass PH. Success rate of root canal treatment in dogs: 127 cases (1995–2000). J Am Vet Med Assoc 2002;220: 775–80.

5. Markowitz K. Tooth sensitivity: mechanisms and management. Compend Contin Educ Dent 1993; 14:1032–45.

6. Harvey CE, Emily PP. Endodontics. In: Small animal dentistry. St. Louis, MO: Mosby – Year Book; 1993. p. 157–212.

7. Eisner ER. Endodontics in small animal practice: an alternative to extraction. Vet Med 1992;87:418–34.

8. Holmstrom SE, Frost P, Eisner ER. Endodontics. In: Veterinary dental techniques. 3rd ed. Philadelphia, PA: WB Saunders Co; 2004. p. 339–414.

9. Matthew IR, Frame JW. Surgical endodontics. In: Pedlar J, Frame JW, editors. Oral and maxillofacial surgery. Philadelphia, PA: Churchill Harcourt International; 2001. p. 71–87.

10. Carr GB. Surgical endodontics. In: Cohen S, Burns RC, editors. Pathways to the pulp. 6th ed. St. Louis, MO: Mosby – Year Book; 1994. p. 531–67.

11. Wiggs RB, Lobprise HB. Advanced endodontic therapies. In: Veterinary dentistry: principles & practice. Philadelphia, PA: Lippincott-Raven; 1997. p. 325–50.

12. Kim S. Endodontic microsurgery. In: Cohen S, Burns RC, editors. Pathways of the pulp. 8th ed. St. Louis, MO: Mosby – Year Book; 2002. p. 683–725.

13. Eisner ER. 353 sequential canine and feline endodontic cases: a retrospective study in an urban veterinary practice. J An Anim Hosp Assoc 1992;28(6):533–8.

14. Eisner ER. Performing surgical root canal therapy in dogs and cats. Vet Med 1995; 90:648–61.

15. Lyon KF. Endodontic therapy in the veterinary patient. Vet Clin North Am Small Anim Pract 1998;28: 1203–36.

16. Walton RE. Principles of endodontic surgery. In: Peterson LJ, Ellis III E, Hupp JR, et al, editors. Contemporary oral and maxillofacial surgery. 3rd ed. St. Louis, MO: Mosby – Year Book; 1998. p. 433–55.

17. Eisner ER. Standard and surgical root canal therapy performed as a one-stage procedure in a dog. Vet Med 1995;90: 680–6.

18. Grossman LI, Oliet S, Del Rio CE. Endodontic surgery. In: Endodontic practice. 11th ed. Philadelphia, PA: Lea & Febiger; 1988. p. 289–312.

19. Dorn SO, Gartner AH. Case selection and treatment planning. In: Cohen S, Burns RC, editors. Pathways of the pulp. 6th ed. St. Louis, MO: Mosby – Year Book; 1994. p. 60–76.

20. Eisner ER. Dentistry: Endodontic and restorative treatment planning. In: Ettinger SJ, Feldman EC, editors. Textbook of veterinary internal medicine. 5th ed. Philadelphia, PA: WB Saunders Co; 2000. p. 1135–42.

Chapter 24

Apicoectomy techniques

Edward R. Eisner

DEFINITIONS[1-4]

Alveolar jugum: the palpable convexity of the buccal alveolar bone overlying a large tooth root

Apical delta: the diverging branches of the root canal at the apical end of the tooth root typically seen in carnivores

Apicoectomy: see Root canal therapy, surgical

Draining tract: a tract originating from a focus of suppuration, such as a periapical abscess, and discharging pus. Most tracts are lined by chronic inflammatory cells. In longstanding cases the lining may epithelialize, in which case the term 'fistula' may be used

Lateral (accessory) canal: a small canal communicating from the root canal to the periodontal space, usually in the apical one-third of the tooth root

Line angle: an imaginary vertical line forming the intersection of two adjacent vertical dental surfaces; they denote specific positions on a tooth and are important surgical landmarks

Parulis: a sessile, hyperplastic nodule on the gingiva or at the mucogingival junction at the site where a draining tract, usually from a periapical abscess, reaches the surface

Root amputation: removal of one root of a multirooted tooth, leaving most of the crown intact, and combined with appropriate endodontic treatment of the remaining dental structure

Root canal therapy, surgical: the surgical removal of the apex of the tooth (apicoectomy) combined with the sealing of the opening of the remaining pulp cavity in a retrograde fashion

PREOPERATIVE CONCERNS

Standard root canal therapy first

Surgical and standard root canal therapy are complementary procedures. Standard root canal therapy is performed as a first step, unless technically impossible.[1-3,5] Cases requiring surgical root canal therapy are more complex and the crucial preoperative consideration is to identify the indications or contraindications for surgical endodontic treatment (see Ch. 23). The cause for failure of root canal therapy is generally detectable by clinical or radiographic examination, but, in the cases where it is not, the etiology will almost always be apparent when surgical therapy is performed.[5]

SURGICAL ANATOMY

To perform this procedure, a clinician must be familiar with the anatomy of the tooth to be treated and the adjacent structures.[6] In most instances swelling or a draining tract will help to identify the location of the involved root apex and the site of the persistent infection (Fig. 24.1).[7] Evaluation of dental radiographs will also help identify and locate the root apex and lesion. When it is difficult to locate the apex surgically, it is often helpful to superimpose a radiopaque pointer, such as a gutta-percha point or a hypodermic needle, over the affected area and again evaluate radiographically. The teeth most frequently in need of surgical root canal therapy in the dog are the maxillary canine, mandibular canine, maxillary fourth premolar and mandibular first molar teeth, and the canine teeth in the cat. The apices of these teeth lie in close proximity to important structures, such as the infraorbital canal, nasal cavity and mandibular canal.

Dog

Maxillary canine tooth in the dog

Abscessation may be identified by a localized erythematous, painful swelling over the area of the apex, on the dorsolateral aspect of the muzzle dorsal to the second premolar, or by a parulis at, or dorsal to, the mucogingival junction at the first or second premolar tooth (Fig. 24.1A). The proximity of the root can be identified and palpated as the alveolar jugum arching dorsocaudally from the base of the tooth's crown. The alveolar bone on the palatal aspect, separating the alveolus from the nasal cavity, is very thin (Fig. 24.2A).[6]

DOI: 10.1016/B978-0-7020-4618-6.00024-5

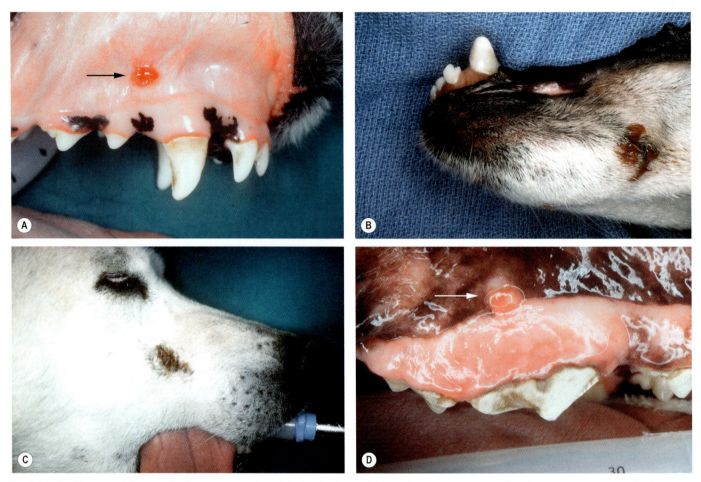

Fig. 24.1 Swelling or draining tract indicates the location of the involved root: (**A**) Parulis (*arrow*) at the exit of a draining tract from a periapical abscess of the maxillary canine tooth. (**B**) Cutaneous draining tract originating from the mandibular canine tooth. (**C**) Cutaneous draining tract originating from the distal root of the maxillary fourth premolar tooth. (**D**) Parulis (*arrow*) and draining tract originating from the mesiobuccal root of the maxillary fourth premolar tooth. *(Fig. 24.1C from Verstraete FJM. Self-assessment color review of veterinary dentistry. 1st ed. Ames: Iowa State University Press, 1999.)*

Mandibular canine tooth in the dog

Abscessation may be identified by localized swelling of the area of the mandibular canine apex, parasagittal to the caudal aspect of the mandibular symphysis (Fig. 24.1B). Alternatively, a parulis may be seen, typically near the mucogingival junction, at the level of the second premolar tooth. The apex of the mandibular canine tooth lies just ventral to the second premolar tooth. It is medial, caudal and ventral to the middle mental foramen (Fig. 24.2B).[6]

Maxillary fourth premolar tooth in the dog

This tooth has three roots: mesiobuccal, mesiopalatal, and distal. The root canals of all normal multirooted teeth communicate via the pulp chamber within the crown of the tooth. The palatal root of the maxillary fourth premolar tooth cannot be easily accessed surgically and, if affected, will require amputation. The distance from the gingival margin to the apices of the maxillary fourth premolar tooth is approximately equal to the distance between the buccomesial and buccodistal line angles. Abscessation of this tooth is seen as a localized swelling, with or without a draining tract, either at the caudodorsal aspect of the muzzle or suborbitally (Fig. 24.1C). Alternatively, a draining tract may be seen at the mucogingival junction (Fig. 24.1D) or, if the palatal root is affected, as a unilateral serous or mucopurulent nasal discharge. The alveolar juga of the mesiobuccal root and, to a lesser

extent, the distal root, are usually palpable. The infraorbital canal lies immediately dorsal to the apices of the two buccal roots and is separated from the apices by a thin layer of bone (Fig. 24.2B, Fig. 24.3A).[6] The rostral superior alveolar branches, which course through the infraorbital canal on the ventral aspect of the infraorbital nerve, enter the incisivomaxillary canal just dorsomedial to the apex of the mesiobuccal root of the maxillary fourth premolar tooth in most dogs. The infraorbital canal lies relatively more ventral, between the mesiobuccal and palatal roots, in small breeds. The nerve and vessels exit through the infraorbital foramen dorsomedial to the apex of the distal root of the third premolar tooth.[8] The parotid and zygomatic papillae lie in close proximity to the apices of the tooth roots and should be identified prior to creating a flap for apicoectomy.

Mandibular first molar tooth in the dog

Most commonly, a periapical abscess of this tooth is observed as a localized swelling or drainage on the ventral border of the mandible ventral to the affected tooth. The apices lie in close proximity to the mandibular canal (Fig. 24.2C).[6] It is possible to avoid exposing the mandibular canal when operating on the mandibular first molar teeth in large-breed dogs. The apices of the roots of the first molar tooth often lie just medial to the mandibular canal, especially in small breeds, and exposing the canal is unavoidable (Fig. 24.3B, C). The

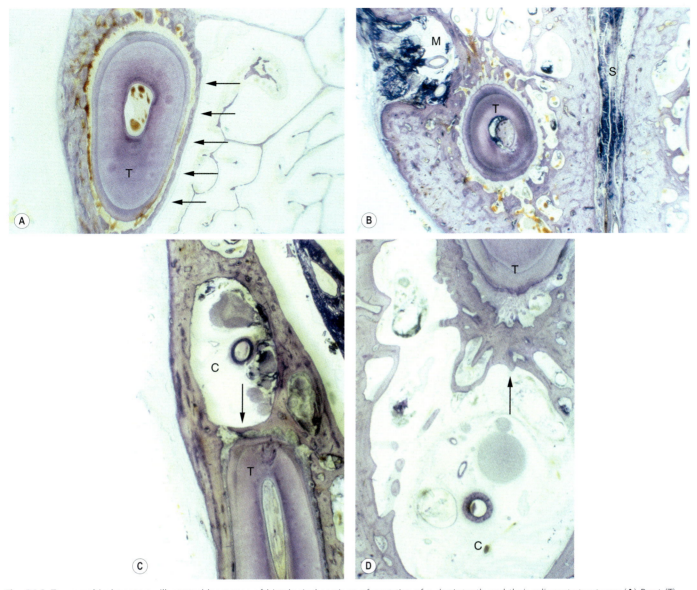

Fig. 24.2 Topographical anatomy illustrated by means of histological sections of root tips of a dog's teeth and their adjacent structures: (**A**) Root (T) of the maxillary canine tooth – note the thin layer of bone separating the alveolus from the nasal cavity (*arrows*). (**B**) Root (T) of the mandibular canine tooth in close proximity to the middle mental foramen (M) and mandibular symphysis (S). (**C**) Mesiobuccal root (T) of the maxillary fourth premolar tooth – note the thin layer of bone separating the alveolus from the infraorbital canal (C) (*arrow*). (**D**) Mesial root (T) of the mandibular first molar tooth – note the thin layer of bone separating the alveolus from the mandibular canal (C) (*arrow*). *(From Manfra Marretta S, Eurell JA, Klippert L. Development of a teaching model for surgical endodontic access sites in the dog. J Vet Dent 1994;11:89–93.)*

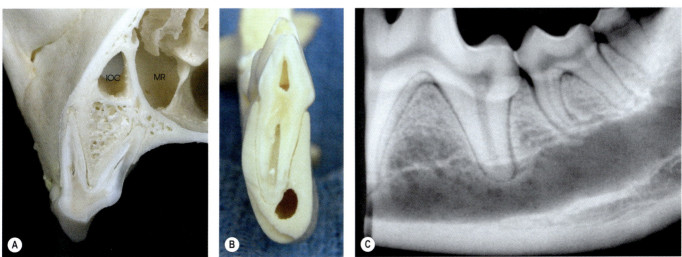

Fig. 24.3 Topographical anatomy illustrated by means of osteological specimens and radiograph: (**A**) Transverse section through the mesiobuccal and mesiopalatal roots of the maxillary fourth premolar tooth – note the proximity of the infraorbital canal (IOC) and maxillary recess (MR). (**B**) Transverse section through the mesial root of the left mandibular first molar tooth of a small dog – note that the apex of the tooth is located medial to and partly invaginated into the mandibular canal. (**C**) Radiograph of the specimen shown in (**B**) showing the radiographic illusion of the roots of the first molar tooth seemingly being located within the mandibular canal.

apex of the mesial root typically is located on a vertical line drawn through the developmental groove in the crown.[6]

Cat

Because of the small size of the teeth of domestic cats, apicoectomy is almost always performed only on the canine teeth, and even then seldomly, because of the shortness of the canine tooth roots.

Maxillary canine tooth in the cat

Periapical abscess of the maxillary canine tooth of the cat is most often seen as a suborbital swelling or drainage opening. Dacryocystitis and ocular discharge may be present if infection has invaded the lacrimal duct. The proximity of the root can be identified and palpated, in a similar way as with the dog, as the alveolar jugum arching dorsocaudally from the base of the tooth's crown. The root is not as caudally curved as in the dog, but the shortness of the face results in the apex of the tooth being relatively closer to the eye than in most dogs. The alveolar bone on the palatal aspect which separates the alveolus from the nasal cavity is, similarly, very thin.

Mandibular canine tooth in the cat

Periapical abscess in the mandibular canine tooth of the cat is most often clinically evident either by a localized ventral swelling and drainage tract on one side of the chin or a dorsal drainage tract midway between the canine and the third premolar teeth. The apex of the root of the mandibular canine tooth lies just rostral to the mesial root of the third premolar tooth. It is medial and ventral to the middle mental foramen, but occasionally the apex may be rostral or caudal to the middle mental foramen. Preoperative radiographs will aid in its surgical location, and a ventral incision over the apex will better assure that the mental nerve will not be injured as the apex is approached.

SPECIAL INSTRUMENTS AND MATERIALS

The practitioner who is already equipped to perform standard root canal therapy will require relatively few additional instruments. The practice of endodontic microsurgery with ultrasonic or sonic root end preparation, however, does require special instruments (Fig. 24.4). A selection of specific instruments for endodontic surgery suitable for use in dogs and cats is listed in Table 24.1.

SURGICAL TECHNIQUE – APICOECTOMY AND RETROGRADE FILLING

Before performing the procedure on a dog or cat, familiarization with technique can be gained by assisting and by performing the procedure on a laboratory specimen.[6] Aseptic technique is employed.[3] As in standard root canal therapy, it is important to take intraoperative radiographs to evaluate progress so the therapeutic plan can be appropriately adjusted in a timely fashion.

Flap design

Dogs and cats often have a limited amount of attached gingiva. The apicoectomy exposure does not necessarily need to include the attached gingiva, but priority should be given to visualization of the surgical field. The flap must be tension free, full thickness,

Table 24.1 Instruments for apicoectomy and root-end preparation in dogs and cats

Description	Details
General	
Surgical loupe	
Small suction tip	Frazier #6[a]
Instruments for approach and apical exposure	
Scalpel handle	#3[a] or #5 (round)[a]
Scalpel blade	#11; #15C[b]
Periosteal elevator	#24G[a]
Surgical curette (used as periosteal elevator)	Molt #2; Molt #4[a]
Tissue forceps	Adson 1X2[a], Adson-Brown 7X7[a]
Tissue scissors	Goldman–Fox #16[a]
Tissue retractors	Senn #5[a]
Surgical curette	Lucas #85[a]
Excavator (used as a surgical curette)	#33L[a]
Bone curette	Molt #5L[a]
Carbide burs	#2, 701L, and 1558L[c]
Instruments for apicoectomy and root-end preparation	
Micro-handpiece	Intralux miniature head; Intralux micro head[d]
Sonic or ultrasonic root-end preparation instruments	Sonicflex Retro[d]
Carbide burs	# ½ round; #33 ½ inverted cone; #3 rose[c]
Retrograde carriers	Retro-filling amalgam carrier 1.2 mm (3/64') or 2 mm (5/64')[e]
Retrograde filling plugger	#1; #2; #9/10[a]
Endodontic micromirrors	3-mm round and rectangular[a]
Instruments for closure	
Small needle holder (tungsten carbide inserts)	Hegar–Baumgartner[a]; Halsey (NH-5036)[a]

[a]Hu-Friedy, Chicago, IL
[b]BD Bard Parker, Franklin Lakes, NJ
[c]Brasseler USA, Savannah, GA
[d]KaVo America, Lake Zurich, IL
[e]Moyco Union Broach, York, PA

mucogingival or mucosal, have an adequate blood supply and expose the apex and periapical tissues. One notable exception is the mandibular canine tooth, in which case the incision is through the skin just rostral and lateral to the caudal aspect of the mandibular symphysis.[9]

Triangular (three-cornered) flap

A three-cornered flap is triangular in shape and particularly useful for procedures involving incisor teeth in large dogs, or teeth in smaller dog breeds and cats. A full-thickness flap is raised by making

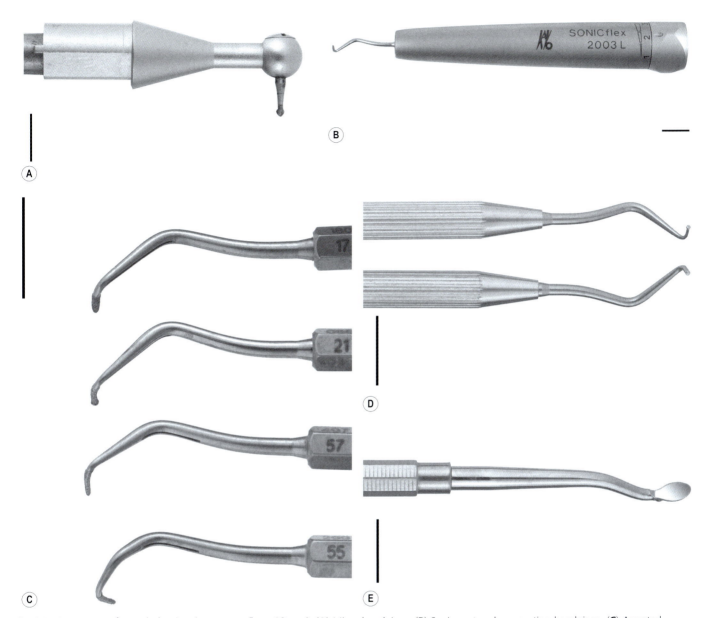

Fig. 24.4 Instruments for endodontic microsurgery (bar = 10 mm): (**A**) Micro-handpiece. (**B**) Sonic root end preparation handpiece. (**C**) Assorted diamond-coated tips for the sonic handpiece. (**D**) Retrograde filling pluggers. (**E**) Endodontic micromirror.

a releasing incision with a #15C or #11 scalpel blade, perpendicular to the gingival margin of the mesiobuccal line angle of the tooth to be treated, the mesiobuccal or distobuccal line angle of the tooth mesial to it, or interproximal if this space is wide enough. The vertical releasing incision extends past the mucogingival junction and into the alveolar mucosa beyond the level of the apex. The releasing incision is preferably perpendicular to the alveolar margin, although a slightly divergent incision to obtain a wider flap base has been recommended until recently.[10,11] The second incision is made, entering through the epithelial attachment of the gingival sulcus and extending from the first incision to a point one-half to one tooth farther than the affected tooth (Fig. 24.5A). Alternatively, the sulcular incision is made first and the vertical releasing incision second. Instead of a sulcular incision, a submarginal incision can be made into the attached gingiva (Fig. 24.5B, D).[10,11] The latter approach offers the advantage that the gingival contour is not disrupted. Surgical closure is also easier, compared to the sulcular incision technique, as there is tissue available for closure of the horizontal incision of the triangular flap. Using a triangular flap with a sulcular incision in the presence of periodontitis is contraindicated.[1] The full-thickness flap is raised, beginning in the releasing incision and progressing toward the attached gingiva. One or both incisions may be extended as necessary to permit adequate access and visualization of the apex.

Surgical wound retractors or periosteal elevators used as retractors are important to facilitate good exposure. Most difficulties encountered during flap management result from inadvertent crushing, tearing, or ischemic damage that occurs during incision, elevation, retraction or suturing.[1,11] Appropriate flap design is essential for the overall success of the procedure.[11]

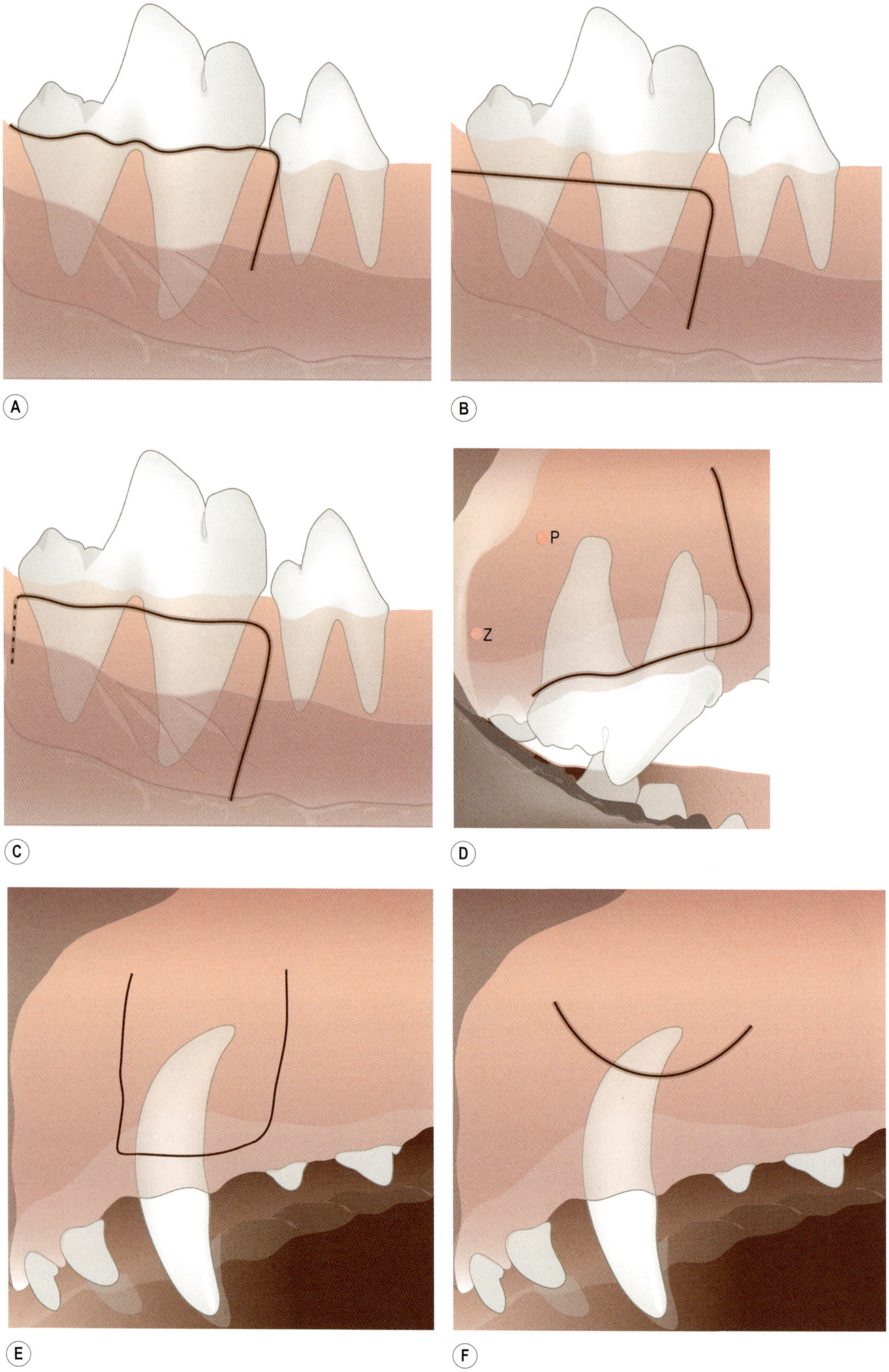

Fig. 24.5 Flap design for surgical endodontics: (**A**) Triangular flap with sulcular incision for approaching the roots of the mandibular first molar tooth. (**B**) Triangular flap with submarginal incision for approaching the roots of the mandibular first molar tooth. (**C**) Pedicle flap with submarginal incision for approaching the roots of the mandibular first molar tooth. (**D**) Triangular flap with submarginal incision for approaching the roots of the maxillary fourth premolar tooth – note the proximity of the parotid (p) and zygomatic papillae (z). (**E**) Pedicle flap with submarginal incision for approaching the root of the maxillary canine tooth. (**F**) Semilunar incision into the alveolar mucosa for approaching the root of the maxillary canine tooth.

Pedicle (four-cornered) flap

A pedicle flap design is required when a larger flap is necessary, as is the case with multirooted teeth and canine teeth in dogs. It is essentially a three-cornered flap that has had an additional vertical releasing incision originating at the attached gingiva on the distobuccal line angle of the tooth involved, the mesiobuccal or distobuccal line angle of the tooth distal to it, or interproximal if this space is wide enough. Similar to a triangular flap, the horizontal incision can be made in either the gingival sulcus or in the attached gingiva (Fig. 24.5C, E).[10,11] For teeth with long roots and/or little attached gingiva, the horizontal incision can be made in the alveolar mucosa. It is currently recommended to make the two vertical releasing incisions parallel, although divergent incisions have been recommended until recently.[10,11] Slightly rounded corners are preferred in the design of the mucoperiosteal flap.[8,10,11]

Semilunar flap

Though other flap designs are currently more frequently employed in human endodontic surgery,[1,10,11] in veterinary dentistry the semilunar flap is the flap still commonly used for most teeth (Figs. 24.5F). The exception to this is the mandibular canine tooth, for which a straight rostrocaudal skin incision is made (Fig. 24.6A). The semilunar incision is in the shape of $\frac{3}{8}$ of a circle and is made entirely in the alveolar mucosa and penetrates to the bone. The apex of the flap is approximately at the coronal one-third of the root(s) and ends apically just dorsal to, and half a tooth mesial and distal from, the apex or apices of the affected maxillary tooth or ventral to the apices of mandibular teeth. The semilunar flap offers relatively limited exposure.[10,11]

Approach and exposure

Maxillary canine tooth in the dog

To expose the maxillary canine tooth apex, a pedicle flap (Fig. 24.5E) or semilunar incision can be made through the alveolar mucosa at the swelling or drainage site (Fig. 24.5F). The pedicle or semilunar flap should be wide enough to allow adequate exposure. Both flaps are full thickness and their base is located dorsally.

Mandibular canine tooth in the dog

To expose the mandibular canine tooth apex, an extraoral incision is made through the aseptically prepared skin. The incision is directed rostrocaudally on the ventral border of the mandible over the affected site. The apex of the mandibular canine tooth lies just lateral to and slightly rostral to the caudal border of the mandibular symphysis. The incision is extended beyond the swollen area, rostrally and caudally to permit visualization and access to the periapical tissues (Fig. 24.6).[3] A draining tract may guide the surgeon to the apex, but generally it will be necessary to remove a bony window to expose the apex.[9–12]

Maxillary fourth premolar tooth in the dog

To expose the maxillary fourth premolar tooth, a triangular flap with the vertical releasing incision on the mesial aspect of the tooth can be used (Fig. 24.5D). Care should be taken to avoid damage to the parotid and zygomatic papillae and ducts. A semilunar incision can also be made through the alveolar mucosa coronal to the root apices. To aid in locating the apices of the buccal roots of the maxillary fourth premolar tooth, one can visualize that they are located at the dorsal end of an imaginary square, the ventral base of which is the

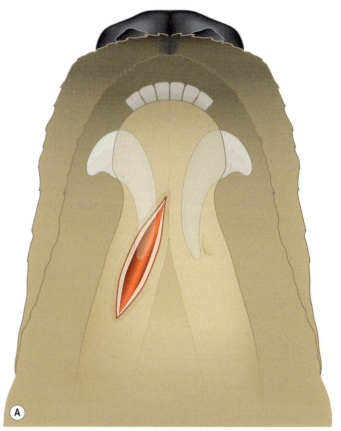

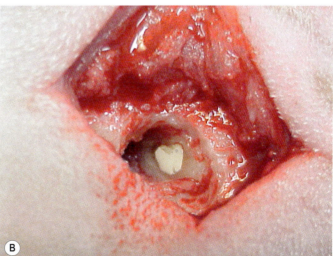

Fig. 24.6 Transcutaneous approach to the mandibular canine tooth: (**A**) Line drawing illustrating the landmarks for the soft tissue incision. (After Eisner ER. Performing surgical root canal therapy in dogs and cats. *Vet Med* 1995;90:648–661.) (**B**) Intraoperative view of a completed apicoectomy and retrofilling using this approach – note that the apicoectomy was correctly performed near-perpendicular to the long axis of the root. *(Courtesy of Dr. T.M. Woodward.)*

mesiodistal length of the fourth premolar tooth at the gingival margin. The incision should be long enough to adequately visualize the root to be treated. The semilunar mucoperiosteal flap is raised, with its base located dorsally. The palatal root of the maxillary fourth premolar tooth cannot be easily accessed surgically and will require amputation if affected.

Mandibular first molar tooth in the dog

The apices of the mandibular first molar tooth can be exposed by making a ⅜-circle, semilunar rostrocaudal incision in the alveolar mucosa, at the level of the apical two-thirds of the two roots. A full-thickness flap, based dorsally to permit enlargement as necessary for increased exposure, is elevated. Adequate exposure with this approach can be difficult to obtain, especially in small brachycephalic breeds. Two alternatives are available to obtain better visualization. A triangular flap with the vertical releasing incision on the mesial aspect of the first molar tooth or the distal aspect of the fourth premolar tooth can be made (Fig. 24.5A, B). Alternatively, a pedicle flap can be used (Fig. 24.5C). An extraoral approach through the skin overlying the ventral border of the mandible has been described but this approach may have a higher likelihood of trauma to the neurovascular structures in the mandibular canal.[6]

Bone removal and debridement

Bone removal is accomplished by removing superficial bone with an irrigated cutting bur such as a #331L pear-shaped, #2 round, #701L tapered crosscut, or #1558L domed crosscut bur. Ideally a surgical handpiece or a high-speed handpiece without air outflow should be used to prevent tissue emphysema (see Ch. 6).[10] A repeated delicate brush-stroke motion is used, with alveolar bone being removed with the side of the bur. This procedure is continued until the unique texture of the tooth root is recognized. A trench is carved around the apex with the bur while exposing at least 5–6 mm of root end, being careful that exposure includes peripherally healthy-appearing tissue. It is imperative that the trench penetrates to the medial wall of the alveolus and that the resultant channel created consists visually of healthy-appearing bone. It is important to irrigate during cutting to prevent bone necrosis. The periradicular tissues are debrided, including the removal of any extruded root canal sealant material, with a small cutting bur and curets (see Table 24.1). Granulomatous soft tissue is removed as completely as possible before performing the apicoectomy.[10]

Apicoectomy

Complete amputation of the apex is very important in surgical root canal procedures because most endodontic failures occur secondary to apical seal leakage.[8,11] Current technique dictates resecting the affected apex at a slightly oblique angle, approximately 80° to the long axis of the root (Fig. 24.7).[11] The purpose of the amputation of the apex is to remove the apical delta, along with any potential lateral canals and any necrotic root that could be a source for residual infection.[9] The goal is to amputate at least 4 mm of apex and make a nearly transverse cut that will still provide visualization of the root canal. This will reduce the chance of leaving residual apical delta or lateral canals on the palatal/lingual wall of the apical end of the remaining root.[1,11] The amount of apex to be amputated is determined by the visual health of the root, the length of root, and the amount of bone support remaining to maintain a stable tooth subsequent to the procedure. Until recently, a 45° angle was thought to be optimal, but this does increase the risk of unidentified persistent residual infection.[1,3,5,9,11] The 45° angle was based on convenience (ease of retrograde filling, and convenience of inspection), rather than on a scientific basis.

Once the apicoectomy has been performed, the newly exposed periradicular tissue should be curetted and irrigated with saline to remove granulomatous tissue and debris. The standard of care in human oral surgery is to submit the periapical tissue that is removed for histopathological examination.[13] The diagnostic yield of this

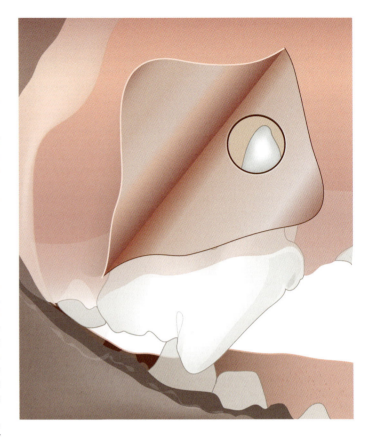

(A)

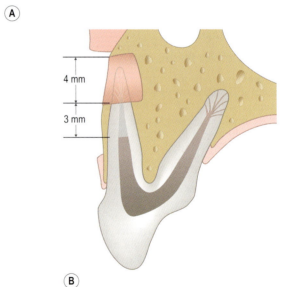

4 mm

3 mm

(B)

Fig. 24.7 Apicoectomy and retrograde filling of the mesiobuccal root of the maxillary fourth premolar tooth: (**A**) Lateral view illustrating the bony window created. (**B**) Transverse view illustrating the near-perpendicular angle of the apicoectomy and the 3-mm retrofilling without undercut.

practice, however, is low, and may not be economically justifiable.[14] An acceptable compromise in veterinary dentistry may be to submit lesions that are suspicious in nature, based on the history, preoperative evaluation, and intraoperative findings.

Visualization is enhanced by using suction equipment. Hemorrhage is controlled by using an appropriate local hemostatic agent (see Ch. 7). Cotton pellets should preferably not be used, as cotton strands left in the surgical site delay healing and result in an inflammatory reaction.[9,11] Bone wax can also be used in apicoectomy procedures to aid in hemostasis, but care should be taken to remove it completely before surgical closure.

Once the root is isolated and hemostasis in the surgical field is achieved, the retrograde filling can be placed.

Retrograde preparation, filling and restoration

As stated above, most root canal therapy failures are due to apical leakage. Therefore the retrograde sealing of the canal is very important for therapeutic success. The restorative preparation at the apicoectomy site is made so that its outline is parallel to the shape of the root canal, with minimal or no undercut (Fig. 24.8).[1,11] Microhead or miniature handpieces are recommended and small round or inverted-cone burs are used to prepare retention of a 3-mm root end filling. Ultrasonic or sonic root end preparation should be performed under magnification, either with an operating microscope or with a high-quality loupe. The apical root canal is prepared with a suitable sonic or ultrasonic tip to a depth of 3 mm and is more conservative, removing less tooth structure, than when a bur is used.[11] Following preparation, the interior canal walls are inspected using a micromirror.

The periapical tissues are air dried, then packed appropriately, to trap any excess filling material and to contain any moisture from bleeding before the placement of the restorative material. The sealant is packed into the prepared site in small increments with a 1.2- or 2.0-mm diameter retro-carrier and the material condensed with appropriately sized and shaped condensers, pluggers, or packers. The material is allowed to set according to manufacturer's directions and the restoration smoothed. Marginal integrity of the restoration is verified with an explorer because a marginal defect will be an avenue for leakage and failure.

Choice of materials for retrofilling

Newer non-zinc amalgams (Dispersalloy, Dentsply Caulk, Milford, DE) have a higher copper content that results in less marginal deterioration than those with a lower copper content. Products available as comminuted particles (lathe-cut and pulverized particles) are available as both zinc (those containing more than 0.01% Zn) and non-zinc (less than 0.01% Zn) alloys. Even so, studies have shown that amalgam is only 75% effective in preventing microleakage due to corrosion.[5] In comparison, intermediate restorative material (IRM) (IRM Intermediate Restorative Material, Dentsply Caulk, Milford, DE) has been used with better results (94%), because it seals well and expands little after setting. Zinc-free amalgam should be chosen because of concerns of precipitation of zinc carbonate into the tissues.[15] Zinc-containing amalgam, if placed in a moist environment, will expand by 4% and may result in procedural failure due to creep, restorative expansion or root fracture, or loss of apical seal.[9] Amalgam and SuperEBA have historically been the two most commonly used materials in human apicoectomies.[16,17] The use of amalgam does require that an undercut be made.

Intermediate Restorative Material (IRM) is a zinc oxide-eugenol cement reinforced by adding 20% polymethacrylate to the powder.[17] This material has a milder tissue reaction than zinc oxide-eugenol and it compares favorably with other currently used retrofilling materials; it is easily delivered using a dental syringe delivery system (Centrix, Shelton, CT).[3]

Ethoxybenzoic acid cement (SuperEBA) (SuperEBA, Harry J. Bosworth Co., Skokie, IL), is also a reinforced zinc oxide (60%) – eugenol cement, with 34% aluminum oxide (alumina) added – making it a

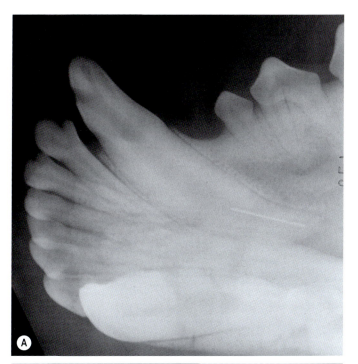

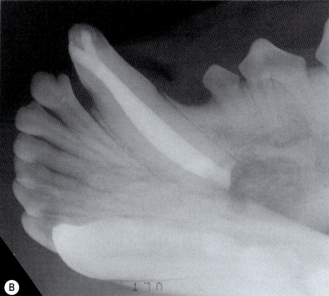

Fig. 24.8 (A) File separation occurred during standard root canal treatment on a mandibular canine tooth in a dog, and the file fragment could not be retrieved through the coronal access openings. **(B)** Postoperative radiograph following apicoectomy, removal of the file fragment, normograde root canal treatment and retrograde filling using glass-ionomer; note that there is only a minimal undercut present.

stronger cement.[11] It is 95% effective against microleakage, is inexpensive, is the strongest and least soluble of the zinc oxide-eugenol formulations, and is user-friendly.[11] It also has excellent antibacterial properties.[18] SuperEBA is readily delivered using a dental syringe delivery system (Centrix, Shelton, CT).

Composites may also be used, but must be delivered in an absolutely dry field. They can provide as good a seal as the other filling materials mentioned here, but are not chosen by most endodontists because they are so technique-sensitive.[11]

Glass-ionomer restoratives have been used, but reports of their efficacy as retrograde restoratives are inconsistent.[19] Ketac Silver (Ketac Silver Applicap, 3M ESPE Dental Products, St. Paul, MN) was compared to zinc oxide-eugenol and amalgam and was found to be superior in both in vitro and in vivo applications.[20,21]

Mineral trioxide aggregate (MTA) (ProRoot MTA, Dentsply Tulsa Dental, Tulsa, OK) has a high pH, like $Ca(OH)_2$, but is a hard-setting nonabsorbable compound with cavity adaptation and sealing ability superior to SuperEBA and other materials.[20,22,23] Its other advantages are that it is the least toxic of all the filling materials, has excellent biocompatibility, is hydrophilic, and is reasonably opaque. Its disadvantage is that it is also technique-sensitive and has a long setting time.

All of the above materials have been used with good results for retrofilling and it is possible to find data in the literature to support their use.[15,17,19]

Wound closure

After the apicoectomy, debridement and restoration have been completed, the surgical site should be irrigated with physiological saline solution to remove debris. Alternatively, a solution of 0.05% chlorhexidine gluconate or 1% povidone-iodine solution may be used. The mucoperiosteal flap is replaced and sutured with a single row of 5–0 or 4–0 absorbable suture in a simple continuous or interrupted pattern. In procedures involving the extraoral approach, the periosteum and subcutaneous tissues are closed using absorbable suture and nonabsorbable sutures are used in the skin (see Ch. 7).

SURGICAL TECHNIQUE – AMPUTATION OF THE PALATAL ROOT OF THE MAXILLARY FOURTH PREMOLAR TOOTH

A surgical crosscut bur (e.g., # 1558L or # 701L) or a tapered diamond bur is used to sever the palatal root from the tooth with an oblique, sagittal cut between the palatal cusp and the palatal wall of the major cusp of the tooth (Fig. 24.9A). After its epithelial attachment is severed, the root is removed by elevation or luxation (see Ch. 11) (Fig. 24.9B). The bone periapical to the palatal root will often be weakened by the inflammatory process and dorsal pressure may cause intrusive luxation of the root into the maxillary recess.[7] The resultant pulp chamber exposure in the remaining portion of tooth is prepared and a surface restoration installed.

POSTOPERATIVE CARE AND ASSESSMENT

Postoperatively, a radiograph is obtained to verify the root end filling (Fig. 24.8B). The radiograph is used when comparing follow-up radiographs.

If a cutaneous draining tract or abscess was present, gentle debridement and lavage with 0.05% chlorhexidine gluconate are indicated. In general, a draining tract or a drained abscess rapidly resolves following apicoectomy.

A 10-day postoperative course of oral broad-spectrum antibiotics is indicated (see Ch. 3). If there are clinical indications of persistent infection, such as osteomyelitis, a longer course with a narrow-spectrum antibiotic based on a bacterial culture and antibiogram is occasionally necessary.[3] The client is instructed to feed only soft food, withhold all hard biscuits and chew toys, and deny oral play for 2

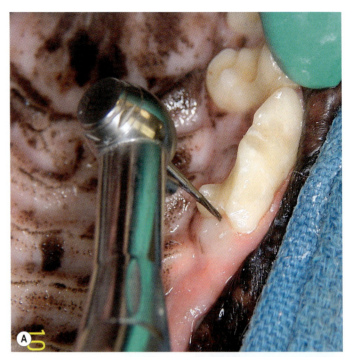
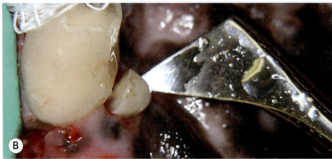

Fig. 24.9 (A) The proper angle for resection of the mesiopalatal root of the maxillary fourth premolar tooth, with a # 701L tapered crosscut bur on a high-speed handpiece. (B) Use of a Cryer elevator for elevation of the palatal root.

weeks until the incision has healed. The incision is rechecked in 2 weeks and any remaining sutures are removed at that stage. A 3-month recheck under general anesthesia and with radiographs is recommended, especially if any swelling persists or drainage is evident. Further radiographic examination should be performed at the time of subsequent routine annual dental care and continued annually, as endodontic failure may occur years later.[24]

COMPLICATIONS

Complications related to the surgical approach

Too small an exposure, or an incomplete exposure, may predispose to retention of unnoticed necrotic or infected material that might lead to recurrent infection.

Hemorrhage may be encountered if a major vessel is invaded. Pressure, for a few minutes, will usually provide hemostasis. If hemorrhage is persistent, a local hemostatic agent or bone wax will control the bleeding. Bone wax must be removed to reduce the risk of delayed healing or a foreign body reaction.[5]

When using high-speed air-powered drills, subcutaneous emphysema will occur occasionally. Use of the equipment should be stopped and the emphysema 'milked' manually toward the incision. There is risk of infection when subcutaneous emphysema occurs and antibiotics should be administered and dispensed, if not otherwise indicated. Rarely, when using high-speed handpieces or when using the air syringe extensively, air embolism occurs and is occasionally fatal in humans.[25] High-speed handpieces (Impact-Air 45 Handpiece, Palisades Dental, Englewood, NJ) are now available devoid of air at their working end. These newly devised handpieces reduce the risk of tissue emphysema as well as air embolism.[1] The possibility of air embolism with fatal outcome has been reported in an experimental study in the dog.[25]

Swelling and pain are common postoperative concerns. Clients should be advised preoperatively of these possibilities and that the degree of swelling is not proportional to the success of the procedure. Retractor-related bruising is most often the cause for postsurgical swelling. The clinician, being focused on the root end procedure, is often unaware of this complication until it is too late.[1]

Damage to adjacent anatomical structures

Drilling into the nasal cavity medial to the apex of the maxillary canine tooth can result in epistaxis or rhinitis. The insult will generally heal with the closure of the surgical site.

Perforation into the maxillary recess may occur during amputation of the palatal root of the maxillary fourth premolar tooth. Exudate present in the recess should be drained and the palatal root, if it has been displaced into the recess, should be removed.

The rostral superior alveolar nerve courses through the infraorbital canal and exits just rostral to the mesiobuccal root of the maxillary fourth premolar tooth in the dog. It may be damaged during instrumentation where it passes between the mesiobuccal and palatal roots in small dogs. The roots of the mandibular premolar and molar teeth, particularly in small breeds, are invaginated into the mandibular canal and apicoectomy puts the inferior alveolar nerve at risk (see Fig. 24.6). It innervates the mandible, teeth, gingiva and rostral aspect of the lower lip. Paresthesia may occur if either of the above-mentioned nerves is traumatized and infection may spread along the nerve.[10]

Hemorrhage from the cut surface of the alveolar bone may obscure visualization, increasing the risk for iatrogenic damage to an adjacent root or apex, especially in patients where crowded and rotated teeth are present.

Incomplete apicoectomy

Employing a bevel angle greater than 10°, in a transverse amputation of the necrotic apex, may predispose to leaving a portion of the infected or necrotic apical delta or one or more lateral canals that may happen to be present.[11] Hemorrhage may interfere with complete amputation of the apex.

Failure of the retrograde filling

The retrograde filling may be dislodged following inadequate site preparation or materials placement. Persistent or recurrent infection might occur secondary to inadequate debridement, insufficient apical amputation, or iatrogenic contamination. An incomplete sealing of the apical canal leaves to chance a reinoculation of periapical tissues with bacteria from an incompletely debrided apical canal.[26]

Filling material inadvertently deposited periapically is a mistake that may be made by inexperienced clinicians, in which case, retreatment is necessary. A postoperative radiograph should be taken immediately after restoration, prior to closure, so that an inadequate root end filling can be remedied at the time.

If amalgam is used and amalgam particles are present they sometimes will be seen later as black 'pigmentation' in the mucosa. This phenomenon is referred to as an 'amalgam tattoo' and, though unaesthetic, does not pose a problem.

PROGNOSIS

The treatment plan may change intraoperatively; therefore, no guarantee for a successful outcome should be given prior to procedure. However, as long as attention is paid to detail, the tissues are adequately instrumented and the materials used in accordance with the manufacturer's instructions, the success rate of surgical root canal therapy can be expected to be very high when preceded by standard root canal therapy.

REFERENCES

1. Carr GB. Surgical endodontics. In: Cohen S, Burns RC, editors. Pathways of the pulp. 6th ed. St. Louis, MO: Mosby – Year Book; 1994. p. 531–67.

2. Eisner ER. Dentistry: endodontic and restorative treatment planning. In: Ettinger SJ, Feldman EC, editors. Textbook of veterinary internal medicine. 5th ed. Philadelphia, PA: WB Saunders Co; 2000. p. 1135–42.

3. Holmstrom SE, Frost P, Eisner ER. Endodontics. In: Veterinary dental techniques. 3rd ed. Philadelphia, PA: WB Saunders Co; 2004. p. 339–414.

4. Simon JHS. Periapical pathology. In: Cohen S, Burns RC, editors. Pathways of the pulp. 6th ed. St. Louis, MO: Mosby – Year Book; 1994. p. 337–62.

5. Matthew IR, Frame JW. Surgical endodontics. In: Pedlar J, Frame JW, editors. Oral and maxillofacial surgery. Philadelphia, PA: Churchill Harcourt International; 2001. p. 71–87.

6. Manfra Marretta S, Eurell JA, Klippert L. Development of a teaching model for surgical endodontic access sites in the dog. J Vet Dent 1994;11:89–93.

7. Eisner ER. Performing surgical root canal therapy in dogs and cats. Vet Med 1995; 90(7):648–61.

8. Harvey CE, Emily PP. Endodontics. In: Small animal dentistry. St. Louis, MO: Mosby – Year Book; 1993. p. 157–212.

9. Wiggs RB, Lobprise HB. Advanced endodontic therapies. In: Veterinary dentistry: principles & practice.

Philadelphia, PA: Lippincott-Raven; 1997. p. 325–50.

10. Walton RE. Principles of endodontic surgery. In: Peterson LJ, Ellis III E, Hupp JR, et al, editors. Contemporary oral and maxillofacial surgery. 4th ed. St. Louis, MO: Mosby – Year Book; 2003. p. 380–404.

11. Kim S. Endodontic microsurgery. In: Cohen S, Burns RC, editors. Pathways of the pulp. 8th ed. St. Louis, MO: Mosby – Year Book; 2002. p. 683–725.

12. Grossman LI, Oliet S, Del Rio CE. Endodontic surgery. In: Endodontic practice. 11th ed. Philadelphia, PA: Lea & Febiger; 1988. p. 289–312.

13. Ellis GL. To biopsy or not. Oral Surg Oral Med Oral Pathol Oral Radiol Endod 1999;87:642–3.

14. Walton RE. Routine histopathologic examination of endodontic periradicular surgical specimens – is it warranted? Oral Surg Oral Med Oral PatholOral Radiol Endod 1998;86:505.

15. Spanberg L. Instruments, materials, and devices. In: Cohen S, Burns RC, editors. Pathways of the Pulp. 8th ed. Philadelphia, PA: Mosby; 2002. p. 521–72.

16. Trope M, Lost C, Schmitz HJ, et al. Healing of apical periodontitis in dogs after apicoectomy and retrofilling with various filling materials. Oral Surg Oral Med Oral Pathol Oral Radiol Endod 1996;81:221–8.

17. Jou Y, Pertl C. Is there a best retrograde filling material? Dent Clin North Am 1997;41:555–61.

18. Torabinejad M, Hong CU, Pitt Ford TR, et al. Antibacterial effects of some root end filling materials. J Endod 1995;21:403–6.

19. Torabinejad M, Pitt Ford TR. Root end filling materials: a review. Endod Dent Traumatol 1996;12:161–78.

20. Blackman R, Gross M, Seltzer S. An evaluation of the biocompatibility of a glass ionomer-silver cement in rat connective tissue. J Endod 1989;15:76–9.

21. Pissiotis E, Sapounas G, Spangberg LSW. Silver glass ionomer cement as a retrograde filling material: a study in vitro. J Endod 1991;17:225–9.

22. Torabinejad M, Smith PW, Kettering JD, et al. Comparative investigation of marginal adaptation of mineral trioxide aggregate and other commonly used root-end filling materials. J Endod 1995; 21:295–9.

23. Torabinejad M, Watson TF, Pitt Ford TR. Sealing ability of a mineral trioxide aggregate when used as a root end filling material. J Endod 1993;19:591–5.

24. Eisner ER. 353 sequential canine and feline endodontic cases: a retrospective study in an urban veterinary practice. J Am Anim Hosp Assoc 1992;28(6):533–8.

25. Rickles NH, Joshi BA. A possible case in a human and an investigation in dogs of death from air embolism during root canal therapy. J Am Dent Assoc 1963; 67:397–404.

26. Lyon KF. Endodontic therapy in the veterinary patient. Vet Clin North Am Small Anim Pract 1998;28:1203–36.

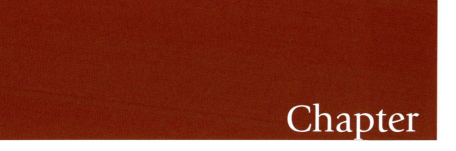
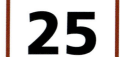

| 25 |

Chapter

Principles of maxillofacial trauma repair

Randy J. Boudrieau & Frank J.M. Verstraete

Most maxillofacial fractures are of traumatic origin and there usually is a history of significant blunt trauma, most often due to motor vehicle trauma. Pathologic fractures associated with severe periodontitis, with its associated bone loss, occur most commonly in small-breed dogs, where the teeth occupy a relatively larger portion of the mandible and periodontal disease is more frequent. In these breeds, fractures may occur iatrogenically during routine dental treatment and extractions. Pathologic fractures also may be associated with neoplasia.

dorsal aspect, the condylar process caudally, and the angular process caudoventrally.

The maxillary teeth are located in the maxillary and incisive bones. The term maxillary fractures in veterinary surgery often refers to fractures involving the incisive, palatine, zygomatic, lacrimal, frontal and nasal bones, in addition to the maxillary bone proper. The close proximity of the nasal cavity, maxillary recess, orbit, infraorbital canal and cranial nerves and associated blood vessels are of great importance in the management of fractures in this area.

ANATOMY[1,2]

The mandibles, incisive bones and maxillas have several unique features complicating fracture management. These bones differ from the rest of the skeleton in that they contain teeth. Most of the dorsal two-thirds of the body of the mandible is occupied by dental roots (Fig. 25.1). The ventral third includes the mandibular canal, containing the inferior alveolar nerve and associated blood vessels. The inferior alveolar nerve provides sensory innervation for the teeth and leaves the bone through three mental foramina as the mental nerves. These nerves are sensory to the soft tissues of the rostral part of the lower jaw. The blood vessels in the mandibular canal are most important, as they supply all of the teeth. Ventral to the mandibular canal there is only a single layer of dense cortical bone.

The lower jaw consists of two mandibles, joined at the symphysis, which consists of a synchondrosis between the slightly irregular bony surfaces. The symphysis remains a true joint throughout life in the dog and cat. The term symphyseal separation is therefore more accurate than symphyseal fracture. The mandible consists of a body (often incorrectly referred to as the horizontal ramus), which is the tooth-bearing part, and a ramus, which is the caudal, nontooth-bearing part. The body of the mandible can further be divided into an incisive part and a premolar/molar part. Fractures involving the incisive part are typically discussed together with symphyseal separations, while discussions of fractures of the body of the mandible focus on the premolar/molar part of the mandible. The ramus of the mandible contains three prominent processes: the coronoid process on the

GENERAL CONSIDERATIONS

Initial management

A mandibular fracture usually is an obvious lesion; a potential pitfall exists in that other less obvious but equally serious problems may go unnoticed. The diagnosis of a fracture of the mandible usually can be made by inspection and/or palpation. The ventral margins of both

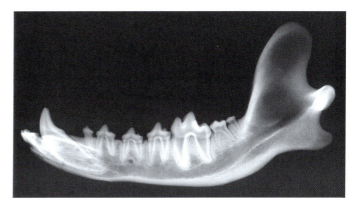

Fig. 25.1 Lateral radiographic view of the mandible. The volume that the teeth occupy can readily be appreciated, encompassing approximately two-thirds of the dorsoventral height of the mandible.

DOI: 10.1016/B978-0-7020-4618-6.00025-7

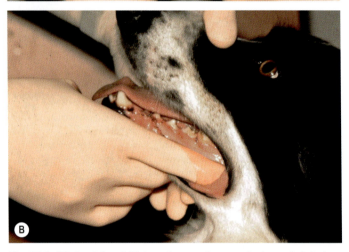

Fig. 25.2 (A) Cranial and **(B)** lateral gross photograph views of digital palpation of the mandible. **(A)** The index fingers are positioned along the gingival alveolar margin under the lips. **(B)** The mouth may also be gently opened during this palpation to allow a visual evaluation.

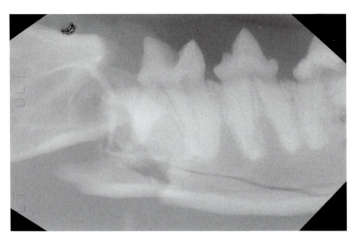

Fig. 25.3 Dental radiograph of a mandibular fracture in a cat showing fine trabecular detail and tooth involvement.

mandibles should be gently palpated for asymmetry and discontinuity by placing the fingers in the patient's mouth adjacent to the alveolar margin (Fig. 25.2). Some patients will permit gentle opening of the mouth, which will allow a visual assessment. As most fractures are open to the oral cavity, any discontinuity in the dental row, or gingival laceration or bony discontinuity usually are easily palpable or visible. Fractures caudal to the teeth, however, are much more difficult to assess on physical examination. The nature and extent of the fracture is best assessed under general anesthesia by gentle palpation and diagnostic imaging.

Diagnostic imaging is necessary to visualize the fracture site(s) and to diagnose any concomitant dental trauma. Conventional radiography may be difficult to interpret due to the many overlying structures of the skull and the bilateral nature of the regional anatomy. Standard radiographic views include ventrodorsal and lateral projections, and both right and left lateral oblique views. Oral radiography using dental film is preferred to conventional skull radiography, but also is limited to the areas of the dental arches. Dental radiographs provide fine detail of the trabecular structure of the bone and document the involvement of teeth in maxillofacial fractures (Fig. 25.3). Fractures

involving the ramus or condylar process of the mandible, and maxillary fractures may be observed with standard radiographs, but are best visualized using computed tomography (Fig. 25.4).

Fractures in the nasal area may be difficult to diagnose as the bone fragments usually are stable (commonly occurring as impaction fractures), and radiographic evidence may be difficult to interpret due to superimposition of the bones and the complex ethmoid and turbinate patterns (Fig. 25.5).[3] Fractures that involve the nasal turbinates may interfere with breathing. Longitudinal fractures along the center of the nose also are commonly observed with very stable position of the fragments (occurring more frequently in cats than in dogs). Swelling, pain on palpation, and nasal bleeding may be clues that maxillary fractures are present. Computed tomography is the most useful diagnostic tool utilized if any fractures are suspected (Fig. 25.6). When evaluating maxillary fractures it is important to recognize upward or lateral deviation of the nose so that proper nasal passage alignment and dental occlusion can be attained with fragment reduction and subsequent fixation. Recognition of mild nasal malalignment can be difficult when coexisting fractures of the mandibular rami are present since dental occlusion cannot be used to evaluate the accuracy of reduction. Similarly, fractures of or near the orbit may involve supporting structures of the eye. Due to the absence of circumferential bone, these injuries require special attention to reconstruct the supporting soft-tissue structures.

Large bone fragments involving the maxilla or incisive bones also may involve the attached dental structures. Open reduction and fixation of these large fragments are recommended not only to attain appropriate repositioning of the nasal cavity, but also of the dental arches so as to ensure appropriate occlusion.[4] Fractures through the dental arches elevate and/or tear the gingival mucosa, which also must be addressed after fracture reduction and fixation. It may be necessary to mobilize the labial mucosa to ensure soft tissue closure.

Maxillofacial trauma is most successfully managed by early definitive fracture fixation and often is performed as the initial emergency treatment once the patient has been stabilized. Such immediate fracture treatment facilitates the associated soft-tissue management and most quickly restores function.[4-6] Most patients will resume eating very quickly if so treated, provided the reduction restores occlusion and the fixation applied provides rigid stability. The patient's cosmetic appearance also is quickly restored. Nutritional support must still be considered, as in instances of severe trauma, where the animal

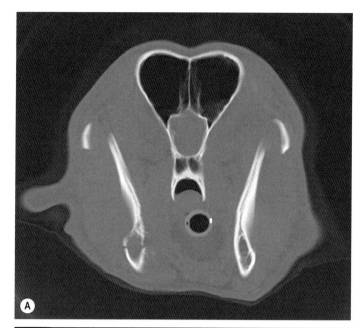

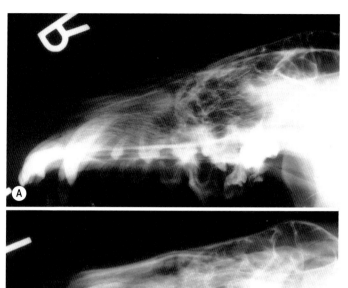

Fig. 25.5 (**A**) Lateral and (**B**) lateral oblique radiographic views of the maxilla in a dog with comminuted maxillary fractures. The location and the extent of the fractures are difficult to evaluate due to the superimposition of the bones in this area and the overlying complex ethmoid and turbinate patterns.

Assessment of teeth

Trauma to the teeth frequently occurs with maxillofacial fractures. Fracture of a tooth may expose the pulp cavity, or compromise the blood supply as a result of a fracture adjacent to the tooth root. Significant patient morbidity will result if such lesions are not appropriately addressed. Continuous tongue licking, reluctance to chew resulting in a diminished appetite, and sensitivity to heat or cold are all clinical signs consistent with ongoing dental issues.

An increased frequency of complications with fracture healing has been observed when teeth are removed due to their involvement with fractures of the dental alveoli.[7] Previously, it has been recommended to extract teeth located within a fracture line.[8,9] The rationale suggested that as a consequence of the fracture, tooth blood supply was disrupted and the pulpal tissue underwent an inflammatory response that subsequently resulted in a periapical abscess, which in turn delayed or prevented fracture healing. However, despite this possibility, it is not often observed. Furthermore, removal of teeth may increase complications due to disruption of the blood supply and iatrogenic trauma to the adjacent tissues, including the following: further displacement of the fractured bone fragments; elimination of occlusal landmarks useful in realigning bone segments to allow functional occlusion; elimination of available structures for use in the fixation of bone fragments; and creation of a large bony defect adding to the difficulty of the reduction and stabilization. These latter factors are much more significant and common, resulting in complications of prolonged healing and infection. Several studies in humans have long established that teeth remaining in a fracture line did not increase the complication rate or morbidity associated with mandibular fractures.[10,11] Preservation of teeth involved within a fracture line in mandibular fractures also has been reported to have a favorable

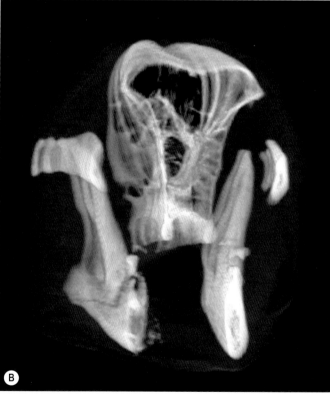

Fig. 25.4 (**A**) Transverse computed tomography (CT) single slice and (**B**) tridimensional reconstruction in the same area demonstrating a fracture at the base of the ramus; this is a pathologic fracture through an acanthomatous ameloblastoma. The CT also allows the extent of the tumor invasion to be evaluated.

may remain inappetent. Those patients in which a definitive procedure is delayed must be managed with temporary bony support (muzzle) and adjunct nutritional supplementation (bypassing the oral cavity). Delay of definitive repair should be avoided, however, as pain control and soft-tissue management are very difficult to administer successfully.

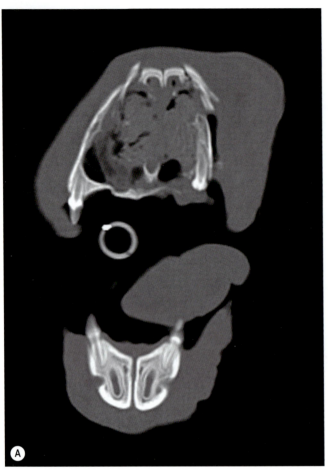
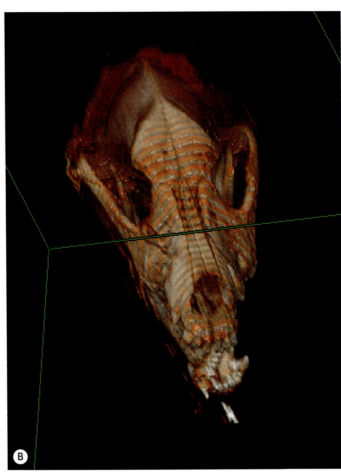

Fig. 25.6 (**A**) Transverse computed tomography (CT) single slice and (**B**) tridimensional reconstruction in the same area demonstrating multiple fractures of the maxilla – including a bilateral depression of the nasal bones and bilateral maxillary fractures.

prognosis if optimal reduction and stabilization of the jaw has been achieved.[12] Therefore, removal of teeth is not advised unless involved teeth are fractured (even here, universal removal is not recommended if the tooth contributes to the stabilization, i.e., the fracture of the tooth does not involve the root) or loose and cannot be stabilized (Fig. 25.7). It is preferable to allow long-term observation to assess the final outcome of possible pulpal damage in situations in which the vitality of a tooth is in question. Current recommendations by human oral surgeons are to preserve teeth whenever possible in the presence of a fracture.[12–14] Preservation of teeth in small animals is similarly recommended – especially considering the much greater relative area of bone that the teeth occupy in small animals, and their greater importance in maintaining bony continuity/stability.

Fracture of the alveolar bone or fracture of a tooth root will usually result in a loose tooth. If only the alveolar bone is fractured and the tooth structure is intact, the preferred treatment is to leave the tooth in place and to stabilize the fracture.[15] Teeth that are avulsed may be reimplanted provided the alveolus remains intact[9,14,16] or can be reestablished with stable fixation.[12,14] A pulpectomy is required in these cases once the tooth is stable, but need not be performed at the time of the initial fracture repair.[14,17] If the fracture involves the tooth, treatment approaches vary. Teeth that are not salvageable and not essential to the stability of the fracture repair should be removed. These extractions most commonly involve the incisors or smaller premolars. Fractured teeth with small mobile coronal fragments are preserved; these fragments are removed and enamel bonding of the defect performed

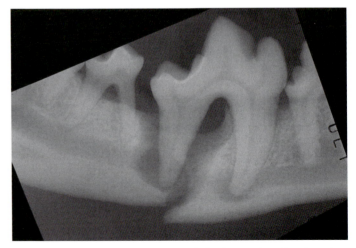

Fig. 25.7 Dental radiograph of a mandibular fracture in a dog through the alveolus of the distal root of the first molar tooth with severe periodontal disease and a large periapical lesion.

if the pulp cavity is not invaded. In the case of a fractured tooth with exposure of the pulp cavity, an endodontic procedure should be performed at the time of the initial fracture repair. Endodontic treatment consists of either pulp capping, pulpotomy or pulpectomy. The indications for these techniques vary with the severity of the damage to the pulp.[17,18] Pulp capping and pulpotomy are procedures designed to treat and preserve vital pulp. If the vitality of the tooth in the fracture area is uncertain, the fracture is treated and the tooth is reevaluated both during and after fracture healing. If the tooth loses vitality, endodontics are performed. If a periapical abscess develops, extractions must be performed, but this usually is delayed until fracture healing has occurred.

Sequential clinical and radiographic examination of the teeth in the fracture line is performed to evaluate suspected dental injury. Loss of alveolar bone, periapical abscess formation, or tooth root resorption may be observed radiographically. Endodontics and/or restorations, or extractions may need to be performed if any problems with the teeth are identified.

Fractures in the presence of periodontal disease further complicate fracture management (see Fig. 25.7). In simple fractures, the recommended therapy involves periodontal treatment and appropriate extractions. Loose teeth must be removed due to the presence of underlying bone disease as alveolar bone resorption already is present, which inhibits healing. Periodontal treatment includes supragingival scaling, and periodontal debridement or root planing. Scaling may be followed by selective polishing of the crown and exposed root. As noted, extraction is indicated if the tooth is mobile, implying that a majority of the supporting alveolar bone has been destroyed. Periodontal disease produces significant loss of alveolar bony support, and removal/debridement of the alveolar socket further weakens this diseased bone; subsequent fractures are not uncommon. Fracture management usually is very difficult in cases with complex fractures and severe osteolysis due to the presence of pre-existent periodontal disease, and nonunion and fixation failures are common. Fracture healing is inhibited in the presence of the existing bony destruction as a result of the ongoing osteitis. This poor bone quality does not hold metal implants well, as they frequently pull through the soft, diseased bone. The goal in these patients simply is to retain a functional mandible, and successful outcomes include fibrous as opposed to bony unions. A fibrous union is more likely to occur in the presence of a unilateral mandibular fracture, where some stability is maintained by the intact, opposite side. However, in the presence of bilateral mandibular fractures, there is no inherent stability, and these cases are much more difficult to manage. Therefore, any attempt of a bony repair in the face of severe periodontal disease must be performed judiciously. A rostral mandibulectomy may be the only recourse in these patients. Regardless, a goal of a fibrous union or mandibulectomy needs the appropriate client education regarding outcome and/or potential complications.

Anesthetic and surgical positioning

Treatment of maxillofacial trauma poses unique problems of appropriate surgical access. Special attention must be given to maintaining an adequate airway, including appropriate tracheal access, and proper patient positioning so as to secure the head and simultaneously permit unimpeded approach to the bones of the skull and mandible. Routine induction and endotracheal intubation per os for anesthetic maintenance and surgery is performed in the management of simple fractures (large fracture fragments without comminution). Anatomic realignment and reduction of the fracture fragments, rather than dental occlusion, is used to determine the accuracy of surgical reduction in these instances. Alternatively, dental occlusion must be used to access the accuracy of the surgical reduction in cases of severely

comminuted fractures or those with bone loss (e.g., gunshot). In these instances, the endotracheal tube must be re-placed so as to bypass the mouth (endotracheal intubation via pharyngotomy) so that the mouth can be fully closed to assess occlusion (see Ch. 4).

Patient positioning must include consideration for both unimpeded surgical access to the head and anesthetic management that does not interfere with the surgical procedure. Most often, this includes positioning the patient such that the head is reversed and at the opposite end of the surgical table from the anesthetic machine (Fig. 25.8A). Additionally, the head must be securely fixed to the table so as to remain stable during surgical manipulation; this is accomplished by taping the maxilla/mandible to the table with waterproof tape that traverses across the upper or lower canine teeth, dorsal versus ventral recumbency, respectively (the tape and oral cavity is additionally surgically prepped – Fig. 25.8B). Finally, the tongue must be reflected caudally (into the pharynx) to allow an unobstructed intraoperative assessment of occlusion (Fig. 25.9). Such surgical access and patient positioning complicates anesthetic monitoring, as the routine evaluation of eye position and reflexes and assessment of jaw tone is not possible. Therefore, greater reliance is placed on monitoring the heart rate and rhythm, respiratory depth and rate, pulse character, and blood pressure (see Ch. 6).

Aseptic preparation of the surgical field, including the mouth, is accomplished by routine methods. The eyes must be protected with an ophthalmic ointment. In simple fractures, where endotracheal intubation per os is performed, the oral cavity is not included in the draping. In those cases where occlusion is to be used to assess the reduction, and the endotracheal tube bypasses the mouth, draping is performed to include full access to the oral cavity. As previously noted, the tongue is reflected back on itself into the pharynx to avoid its interference with intraoperative assessment of dental occlusion (Fig. 25.8B).

Surgical goals

Proper dental occlusion is the primary objective, which ensures appropriate fracture reduction; however, rigid skeletal fixation is also a necessary adjunct. Both of these goals are interrelated objectives that cannot be compromised. Malocclusion after fracture reduction and fixation, in addition to adversely affecting function, will result in abnormal leverage against the fixation devices. These abnormal forces likely will result in disruption of the fixation, leading to motion at the fracture site and subsequent loosening of these implants. The bone fragment motion and loose implants will interfere with revascularization and healing, and also contributes to the development of infection. Mandibular fracture stability may be even more important than in other fracture locations because bone fragment motion also will inhibit healing of the oral mucosa. Any gaps in the oral mucosa allow saliva and food particles access to the fracture site, further compromising the healing process and predisposing the area to infection.

The goal of any internal skeletal fixation procedure is rigid/stable fixation and an early/rapid return to function. These goals are magnified in maxillofacial fracture repair where any failure to attain these goals results in early complications and a great deal of difficulty with patient management (pain, inappetence, infection). Many different techniques and devices are described for this purpose. Uncomplicated healing without infection is obtained only with a full knowledge of the unique biomechanical requirements of this location, and knowledge of both the advantages and limitations of the different methods of fixation. Appropriate reapposition and rigid fixation of bone fragments without further compromise of the blood supply, and appropriate management of skin and mucosal lacerations, i.e., judicious soft-tissue debridement, create optimal conditions for uncomplicated healing without infection.[19-21] Antibiotic administration is

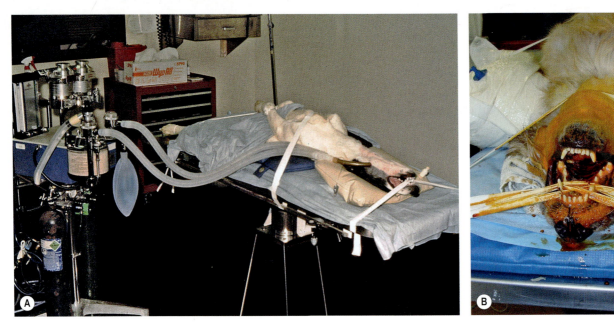

Fig. 25.8 (**A**) Positioning of the dog with a mandibular fracture. The dog is in dorsal recumbency with both forelegs pulled caudally (the forelimbs also are crossed, which helps to stabilize the positioning). The upper jaw is secured near the end of the table with waterproof tape placed over the maxillary canine teeth. The endotracheal tube has bypassed the oral cavity by being placed through a left pharyngotomy. The anesthetic machine is placed at the other (caudal) side of the dog. Sufficient access is obtained by a surgical field that surrounds the entire end of the table. Notice that the tilting mechanism for the table also is under this end of the table so that additional height may be gained by elevating this end of the table. Similar positioning, but in ventral recumbency, is performed for access to the upper jaw. (**B**) Rostral view of a dog with bilateral comminuted mandibular fractures at the junctions of the bodies of the mandibles with the rami. The maxilla has been secured to the table as described in (**A**) with waterproof tape. In addition to the ventral surface of the mandible, the oral cavity (and the tape) has been prepped for the surgical procedure. Notice that the tongue is not visible (reflected into the pharynx – see Fig. 25.9).

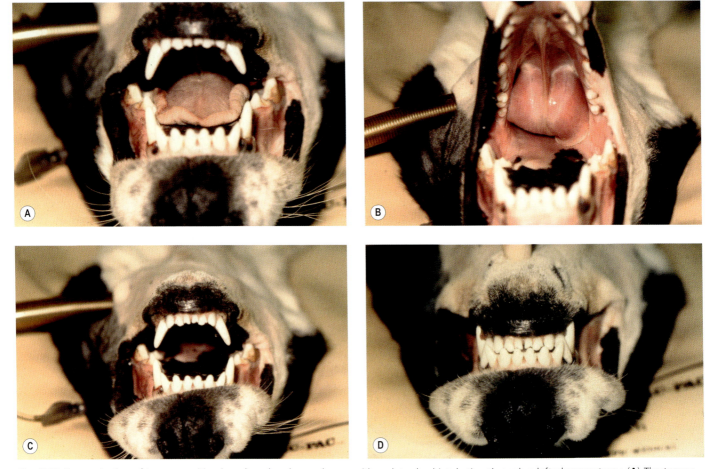

Fig. 25.9 Demonstration of tongue position in a dog, dorsal recumbency, with endotracheal intubation through a left pharyngotomy. (**A**) The tongue can be seen resting normally. (**B**) The mouth is opened and the tip of the tongue reflected caudally into the pharynx. (**C**) The tongue can no longer be seen. (**D**) Full closure of the mouth can be obtained in order to assess occlusion; the tongue no longer interferes with this assessment.

recommended in all cases, as open fractures occur in a majority of these cases (which are open to the oral cavity) and inevitably are contaminated.[22-24] Despite the agreement in antibiotic use perioperatively, continued postoperative use has been questioned.[25]

BIOMECHANICS

The biomechanics of the masticatory system and, in particular, the muscular forces acting on the mandible, are of utmost importance in the management of fractures of the body of the mandible. The temporal, masseter and medial pterygoid muscles are responsible for closing the mouth, and in so doing can generate tremendous occlusal forces. The static force exerted by these muscles also tends to lift the mandible. As the muscular insertions are located on the caudal part of the mandible, this part in particular will be lifted when a fracture of the body of the mandible has occurred; the resultant force exerted by these muscles is in a rostrodorsal direction. The relatively small digastricus muscle, with its relatively small area of insertion at the angle of the jaw, is responsible for opening the mouth. The rostral fragment of a fractured mandible thus displaces in a caudoventral direction. Alternatively, the maxilla is broadly attached to the skull and supports the dental arch with areas of thickened bone (or buttresses) that disperse the forces over a wide area. Application of the fixation devices used for the repair of maxillofacial fractures must include a complete understanding of this functional anatomy. These biomechanical aspects dictate the ideal placement of the various internal fixation devices; furthermore, these factors also play a role in the selection of the most appropriate fixation devices.

Mandible

Bending forces are the primary forces acting on the mandible during functional stress (mastication).[26,27] A continuum of tensile to compressive stresses exists from one side of the bone to the other during bending stress.[28] Maximal tensile stresses exist at the oral (alveolar) surface and maximal compressive stresses exist at the aboral surface.[29] At the ramus, shear forces are maximal, whereas rostrally (symphysis) rotational forces are maximal.[26,27] Distraction of the oral margin therefore will occur after a mandibular fracture, and is magnified with any mandibular muscular contraction (Fig. 25.10). The anatomic configuration of a long lever arm with an absence of any further supplemental support is unique to the mandible and must be considered with any fixation method. Therefore, application of the fixation must consider both the tension and compression surfaces of the bone. Because all fixation devices are strongest in tension (all stresses acting parallel to the longitudinal axis of the implant), they are ideally placed on the tension surface of the bone, or in cases of mandibular fractures, along the alveolar border. The basic biomechanical principle to be considered is tension-band fixation.[30] Depending upon the type of fixation to be used, the fixation may not be suitable for application to this location due to interference with tooth roots and neurovascular structures adjacent to the tooth roots. In the dog and cat, the tooth roots encompass approximately two-thirds of the bone adjacent to the alveolar margin, severely limiting the type of implant that can be applied.

Maxilla

The term 'maxilla' is used here to refer to the incisive, palatine, zygomatic, lacrimal, frontal and nasal bones, in addition to the maxillary bone proper. By definition, the forces exerted on the mandible also

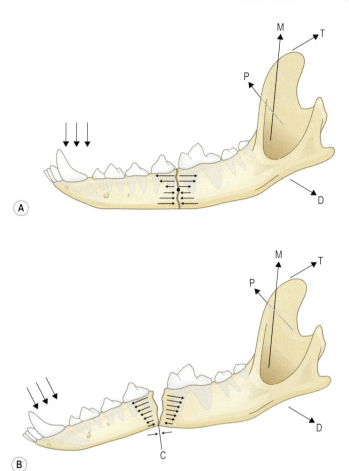

Fig. 25.10 (**A**) Line drawing of the intact mandible demonstrating the normal lines of stress (*small arrows*) through the body of the mandible with muscular contraction and any external force applied to the rostral portion of the jaw (biting, chewing – *medium arrows*). (**B**) Bending forces are the primary forces acting on the mandible during functional stress; with a fracture at this level there is distraction along the alveolar surface of the bone; the point C shows that the ventral portion of the bone is the only area where compressive stresses exist – if there is contact. (P, M. pterygoideus; M, M. masseter; T, M. temporalis; D,M. digastricus.) (*From Boudrieau RJ, Mandibular and Maxillofacial Fractures. In: Tobias KM and Johnston SA (eds). Veterinary Surgery Small Animals, Elsevier 2012, with permission.*)

are exerted on the maxilla. However, the distribution of these forces is much different, and it is generally accepted that the maxilla is subject to much less strain. The maxillofacial area can most easily be thought of as an 'outer facial frame,' which acts as a link between the base of the skull and the occlusal surfaces.[31] The support of the facial region is provided by a series of anatomic buttresses that distribute the masticatory forces to the head. These buttresses exist in the horizontal, vertical and coronal planes.[31-34] There are three primary buttresses: rostral (medial), lateral, and caudal (Fig. 25.11).[31-34] These buttresses also can be defined anatomically: the rostral (medial) as the nasomaxillary buttress, the lateral as the zygomaticomaxillary buttress, and the caudal as the pterygomaxillary buttress. The anatomic definitions mirror the bones of the skull that compose these buttresses. The caudal buttress (which is not readily accessible) is composed of the lacrimal, palatine and pterygoid bones. In the presence of a fracture, the facial frame can be adequately reconstructed with two of the three buttresses: medial and lateral (see below). Therefore, the palatine and lacrimal bones are more likely to be dealt with

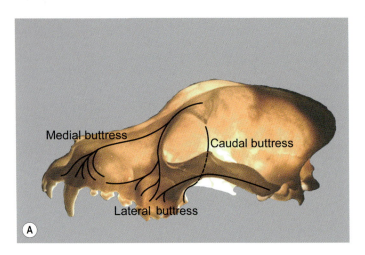

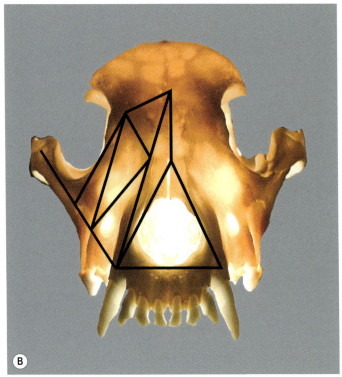

Fig. 25.11 (**A**) Right lateral and (**B**) cranial view of the skull, which is transilluminated to reveal the buttressing. The lines drawn indicate a pyramidal arrangement: The nasomaxillary (medial) buttress is seen rostrally, and the zygomaticomaxillary (lateral) buttress is seen caudally; the pterygomaxillary (caudal) buttress is shown with the dashed line.
(Modified from: Boudrieau RJ. Fractures of the maxilla. In: Johnson AL, Houlton JEF, Vannini R, eds. AO principles of fracture management in the dog and cat,. *Stuttgart: Georg Thieme Verlag, 2005;116–129.)*

secondarily, i.e., with primary stabilization of other fractures of the skull. The incisive bones are not part of the buttresses, and therefore may not need to be stabilized as this area generally does not provide essential support to the skull, or can effectively be treated by other means (see Ch. 28). The nasal bones also may be fractured without disturbing the medial buttress. Fixation of these areas still may be useful in these areas in either providing the support for the incisors or reestablishing the cosmetic appearance of the nasal area when depressed fractures occur.[5] Similarly, maxillary fractures often may not require stabilization unless the buttresses are compromised.[4] In the

latter case, occlusion or support of the orbit is compromised, and fixation (most often plate) is ideally suited to stabilize these fractures and reestablish the medial buttress. Likewise, if the lateral buttress is compromised, which often will affect the orbit, plate fixation again is ideally suited for stabilization and to reestablish this buttress (Ch. 31).[4,5]

An evaluation of the facial support of these buttresses reveals that they are designed as a basic 'truss' or 'frame,' which is a triangle; in three dimensions the basic truss is a tetrahedron (three-sided pyramid) – simply four triangles that can resist distortion in any direction three-dimensionally.[31] In humans, the vertical buttresses of the midface are the clinically most important with regards to the management of midface fractures.[32,33] These buttresses are divided into three principal areas, as previously noted: nasomaxillary (anterior or medial) buttress, zygomaticomaxillary (lateral) buttress, and pterygomaxillary (posterior) buttress.[31–34] These areas all represent thicker bone designed to support the maxilla in humans in the vertical dimension. These buttresses are quite strong in resisting vertically directed stresses; however, they cannot withstand forces of similar magnitudes in the transverse plane. There is no similar detailed description of the maxillary buttresses in the dog or cat; however, a similar anatomic arrangement to the human skull has been suggested (see Fig. 25.11).[4] These trusses can be visualized in the skull as pillars of reinforced bone. In the dog, the medial and caudal buttresses provide similar vertical support as in humans; although, due to the configuration of the skull, these buttresses are better designed to also withstand transverse forces as compared to humans. The lateral buttress also appears to primarily function to withstand forces in the vertical plane. It also further supports the other two buttresses so as to better withstand the increased shearing forces in the premolar/molar region in these species. The lateral buttress in the dog also appears to more effectively neutralize forces in the transverse plane, despite lacking the secondary lateral support adjacent to the orbit (orbital ligament in the dog and cat as compared to bony support in humans, the latter of which also contributes to the lateral buttress). The attachment of the maxilla to the base of the skull, therefore, appears to have greater bony support as compared to humans.

SURGICAL APPROACHES

Treatment planning

Occlusion is used to determine the accuracy of the fracture reduction when comminution or gaps in the bone are present. Simpler fractures may be reconstructed anatomically. Performing anatomic reconstruction, without relying on occlusal evaluation, should be performed with caution, especially in comminuted fractures, as it is not unusual to have a malocclusion despite what appears to be a 'perfect' reconstruction on the accessible outer (nonalveolar) bony surface. Usually, one side of the head/face is more severely injured (since the inciting trauma is rarely directed along the midline); therefore, a common-sense approach is to repair the side with the simplest fractures first. In most instances the mandible is repaired first, which serves as the 'base' for subsequent facial repairs. The mandible should be repaired from caudal to rostral, with symphyseal separations secured as the last step. After mandibular reconstruction has been completed, the maxilla is then addressed, concentrating first on the lateral, and then medial, maxillary buttresses (in humans the medial buttress is addressed first in order to preserve midface height). Performing temporary maxillomandibular fixation provides for appropriate occlusal realignment, which serves as a further template for the reconstruction, and also provides some degree of stabilization during application of the definitive fixation. Securing the medial and lateral buttresses in this manner permits exact rostrocaudal positioning of the maxilla, and also corrects height and projection. Direct reconstruction of the caudal buttress is unnecessary as the reconstructed medial and lateral buttresses are sufficient to maintain appropriate alignment. Direct exposure of all fractures in order to ensure accurate anatomic realignment of all bone fragments, and the ensuring application of the implants for appropriate reconstruction of the entire face cannot be overemphasized.

Mandibular fractures

Although the fractured bone fragments often may be visualized within the mouth, due to the extensive lacerations of the gingiva that usually accompany these fractures, separate ventral mandibular approaches are the preferred surgical access (see Ch. 27). The ventral approach to each mandible facilitates exposure and bone fragment manipulation, including the ability to perform an accurate reduction and stabilization; furthermore, a route for ventral drainage can easily be established should it be required.

A separate lateral approach is required to expose the temporomandibular joint (see Chs 27 and 33). The mandibular ramus dorsal to this joint need not be repaired.

Maxillary fractures

Skin incisions generally are made directly over the fracture in nasal, maxillary, or frontal areas (see Ch. 27). Dorsal midline incisions may be best to avoid neurovascular structures along the nose and most easily expose the maxillary buttresses (Fig. 25.12).[4,5]

SUMMARY

Maxillofacial trauma sufficient to result in fractures generally results in gross and usually severe patient disfigurement, and often results in the inability to function appropriately, e.g., an inability to eat and/or drink, and may even cause respiratory issues due to possible upper airway obstruction. These fractures are exceptionally rewarding cases to treat as simple techniques usually can be performed, resulting in a successful functional outcome most often within 24 hours after fracture stabilization. Once post-traumatic inflammation and edema resolve, a markedly improved cosmetic appearance rapidly follows.

The primary principles of fracture treatment, i.e., restoring occlusion and providing stable fixation to the bone fragments, may be successfully used only through an appreciation and proper application of the most appropriate implants (and techniques), dependent upon an understanding of the biomechanical principles. Knowledge that bending forces (divided into their tensile and compressive components) are the primary forces to be neutralized in mandibular fractures dictates the use of the fixation devices. Similarly, an understanding of the importance of the maxillary buttresses is also of paramount importance for the fixation methods applied to these areas.

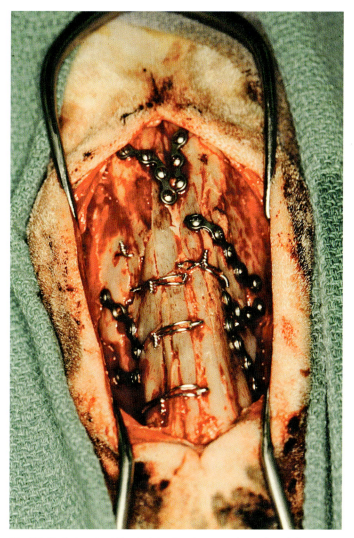

Fig. 25.12 A dorsal midline incision has been made to allow full access to the maxillary buttresses in order to apply internal fixation in this dog with multiple comminuted fractures of the nasal and maxillary bones. This approach also can be combined with a direct gingival approach next to the alveolar bone to provide additional exposure to the lateral buttress.

Successful treatment is predicated on obtaining a cosmetically acceptable and functional result. Anatomic reduction and rigid fixation of fractures that can be reconstructed piece-by-piece creates optimal conditions for uncomplicated healing. Fractures in which bone loss or severe comminution exists, and which cannot be anatomically reconstructed, must be reduced using dental occlusion as the template for fracture fixation, thereby avoiding malocclusion.

REFERENCES

1. Evans HE, Christensen GC. The skeleton: The skull. In: Evans HE, Christensen GC, editors. Miller's anatomy of the dog. 2nd ed. Philadelphia, PA: WB Saunders; 1979. p. 113–59.

2. Evans HE, Christensen GC. Muscles: Muscles of the head. In: Evans HE, Christensen GC, editors. Miller's anatomy of the dog. 2nd ed. Philadelphia, PA: WB Saunders; 1979. p. 273–303.

3. Buchet M, Boudrieau RJ. Correction of malocclusion secondary to maxillary impaction fractures using a mandibular symphyseal realignment in 8 cats. J Am Anim Hosp Assoc 1999;35:68–76.

4. Boudrieau RJ. Miniplate reconstruction of severely comminuted maxillary fractures in two dogs. Vet Surg 2004;33:154–63.

5. Boudrieau RJ, Kudisch M. Miniplate fixation for repair of mandibular and maxillary fractures in 15 dogs and 3 cats. Vet Surg 1996;25:277–91.

6. Rudy RL, Boudrieau RJ. Maxillofacial and mandibular fractures. Semin Vet Med Surg (Small Anim) 1992;7:3–20.

7. Henney LHS, Galburt RB, Boudrieau RJ. Treatment of dental injuries following craniofacial trauma. Semin Vet Med Surg (Small Anim) 1992;7:21–35.

8. Manfra-Maretta S, Tholen MA. Extraction techniques and management of associated complications. In: Bojrab MJ, Tholen M, editors. Small animal oral medicine and surgery. Philadelphia, PA: Lea and Febiger; 1990. p. 75–95.

9. Rossman LE, Garber DA, Harvey CE. Disorders of teeth. In: Harvey CE, editor. Veterinary dentistry. Philadelphia, PA: Saunders; 1985. p. 79–105.

10. Kahnberg K-E, Ridell A. Prognosis of teeth removed in the line of mandibular fractures. Int J Oral Surg 1979;8:163–72.

11. Neal DC, Wagner WF, Alpert B. Morbidity associated with teeth in the line of mandibular fractures. J Oral Surg 1978;36:859–62.

12. Gerbino G, Tarello F, Fasolis M, et al. Rigid fixation with teeth in the line of mandibular fractures. Int J Oral Maxillofac Surg 1997;26:182–6.

13. Flores MT, Andersson L, Andreasen JO, et al. Guidelines for the management of traumatic dental injuries. I. Fractures and luxations of permanent teeth. Dent Traumatol 2007;23:66–71.

14. Flores MT, Andersson L, Andreasen JO, et al. Guidelines for the management of traumatic dental injuries. II. Avulsion of permanent teeth. Dent Traumatol 2007; 23:130–6.

15. Eisenmenger E, Zetner K. Tooth fracture and alveolar fractures. In: Eisenmenger E, Zetner K, editors. Veterinary dentistry. Philadelphia, PA: Saunders; 1985. p. 83–112.

16. Tholen MA. Periodontal surgery. In: Tholen MA, editor. Concepts in veterinary dentistry. Edwardsville, IL: Veterinary Medicine Publishing; 1983. p. 99–113.

17. Williams CA. Endodontics. Vet Clin North Am Sm Anim Pract 1986;16:875–93.

18. Goldstein GS, Anthony J. Basic veterinary endodontics. Compend Contin Educ Pract Vet. 1990;12:207–17.

19. Burri C. Post-traumatic osteomyelitis. Bern, Switzerland: Hans Huber Publications; 1975.

20. Rittman W-W, Pusteria C, Matter P. Frulund Spatinfektionen bei offenen Frakturen. Helv Chir Acta 1969;36:537–40.

21. Rittman W-W, Perren SM. Cortical bone healing after internal fixation and infection: Biomechanics and biology (Corticale Knockenheilung nach Osteosynthese und Infektion). New York: Springer-Verlag; 1974.

22. Umphlet RC, Johnson AL. Mandibular fractures in the dog. A retrospective study of 157 cases. Vet Surg 1990;19:272–5.

23. Umphlet RC, Johnson AL. Mandibular fractures in the cat. A retrospective study. Vet Surg 1988;17:333–7.

24. Chole RA, Yee J. Antibiotic prophylaxis for facial fractures. A prospective, randomized clinical trial. Arch Otolaryngol Head Neck Surg 1987;113:1055–7.

25. Lovanto C, Wagner JD. Infection rates following perioperative prophylactic antibiotics versus postoperative extended regimen prophylactic antibiotics in surgical management of mandibular fractures. J Oral Maxillofac Surg 2009;67:827–32.

26. Spiessl B. Principles of rigid internal fixation in fractures of the lower jaw. In Spiessl B, editor. New concepts in maxillofacial bone surgery. Berlin: Springer-Verlag; 1976. p. 21–34.

27. Coletti DP, Caccamese Jr JF. Diagnosis and management of mandible fractures. In: Fonseca RJ, Turvey TA, Marciani RD, editors. Oral and maxillofacial surgery, Volume II, 2nd ed. St. Louis, MO: Saunders; 2009. p. 139–61.

28. Özkaya N, Nordin N. Biomechanics of bone. In: Fundamentals of biomechanics: equilibrium, motion, and deformation, 2nd ed. New York: Springer Science+ Business Media; 1999. p. 206–10.

29. Küppers K. Analyse der funktionellen Struktur des menschlichen Unterkiefers. Adv Anat 1971;44:3–90.

30. Pauwels F. The significance of a tension band for the stressing of the tubular bone with application to compression osteosynthesis. In: Biomechanics of the locomotor apparatus: Anatomy of the locomotor apparatus (Gesammelte Abhandlunger zur funktionellen Anatomie des Bewegungsapparates). New York: Springer-Verlag; 1980. p. 430–49.

31. DuBrul EL: Architectural analysis of the skull. In: Sicher's oral anatomy. 7th ed. St. Louis, MO: Mosby; 1980. p. 85–93.

32. Forrest CR, Phillips JH, Prein J. Le Fort I–III Fractures. In: Prein J, editor. Manual of internal fixation in the cranio-facial skeleton: Techniques recommended by the AO/ASIF maxillofacial group. Berlin: Springer-Verlag; 1998. p. 108–26.

33. Reddy LV, Pagnatto M. Midface fractures. In: Fonseca RJ, Turvey TA, Marciani RD, editors. Oral and maxillofacial surgery, Volume II, 2nd ed. St. Louis, MO: Saunders; 2009. p. 239–55.

34. Champy M, Blez P. Anatomical aspects and biomechanical considerations. In: Härle F, Champy M, Terry BC, editors. Atlas of craniomaxillofacial osteosynthesis: Miniplates, microplates, and screws. Stuttgart, Germany: Thieme; 1999. p. 3–7.

Chapter 26

Facial soft tissue injuries

Steven F. Swaim

DEFINITIONS[1]

Axial-pattern flap: a pedicle flap of skin and subcutaneous tissue that incorporates a direct cutaneous artery and vein into its base

Debridement: excision of devitalized tissue and foreign material from a wound

Rotation flap: a semicircular flap of skin and subcutaneous tissue that moves about a pivot point by a combination of rotation, transposition and stretching into a defect; it is particularly useful for triangular-shaped wounds

Single-pedicle advancement flap: a flap of skin and subcutaneous tissue that is mobilized by undermining and advanced into a defect without altering the plane of the pedicle; they are particularly useful for square and rectangular-shaped wounds

Transposition flap: a flap of skin and subcutaneous tissue that is generally rectangular in shape; it turns on a pivot point to reach an adjacent defect to be covered, which is usually at a right angle to the axis of the flap; it is particularly useful for square and rectangular-shaped wounds

PREOPERATIVE CONCERNS

Perioperative wound management

Facial soft tissue wounds are often caused by blunt or sharp trauma resulting in devitalized, contaminated or infected tissue in the wound. Management entails administration of systemic antibiotics, preferably within the first 3 hours after trauma. The antibiotic selected should be effective against the bacteria expected in the wound (see Ch. 3).

Wound debridement and lavage are performed. Debridement should be done using color and attachment as guides. Tissues that are very dark, very white or that are separating from underlying tissue should be debrided. Questionable tissue is left for reevaluation the next day as part of the staged debridement technique. Wound lavage should be done with tap water, sterile isotonic saline or balanced electrolyte solution, or a 0.05% solution of chlorhexidine gluconate liquid delivered under moderate pressure.[1–3]

SURGICAL ANATOMY

The surgical anatomy of the lips is described in Chapters 44 and 48.

SURGICAL TECHNIQUES

When repairing facial soft tissue injuries, three principles should be kept in mind. First, due to the scarcity of soft tissue on the rostral area of the face, reconstruction requires moving soft tissue from caudal to rostral (Fig. 26.1). Second, soft tissue can be effectively affixed back to the skull and mandibles by transosseous placement of wires and sutures. Third, mucosal grafts from the sublingual area and inside of the upper lips can be used to reconstruct the nasal plane, nares and vestibule.

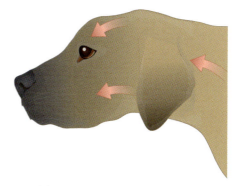

Fig. 26.1 Repair of facial wounds requires moving soft tissue (*arrows*) from caudal where skin is more abundant (*light area*) to rostral where skin is less abundant (*progressively darker shading*).

DOI: 10.1016/B978-0-7020-4618-6.00026-9

Lip lacerations and defects

Minor lip lacerations

Lip lacerations and defects with a minimal amount of tissue missing should be sutured in layers, with the number of layers being dependent upon the lip thickness. For lacerations caudal to the fourth premolar, a thin wire loop should be inserted into the parotid papilla to identify the parotid duct during suturing. A 'figure-of-eight', vertical mattress, or near–far suture should first be placed at the lip margin for perfect alignment. Four layers (submucosa or mucosa, muscle fascia, subcutis and skin) may be necessary for closure on a thick lip.[1] Small animals with thin lips may require fewer layers. A submucosal suture pattern may be used, excluding sutures in the mucosa. Thus, mucosal inversion is avoided.[4–6] Additional suture layers can be placed in the fascial/muscle layer if needed to help align the skin edge or minimize tension on the skin closure.[4,6] If a simple continuous suture is used in the mucosa, care should be taken to avoid mucosal inversion, which can interfere with healing.[5] The appropriate types and sizes of suture material are used (see Ch. 7). Interrupted fine monofilament stainless steel sutures in the skin may discourage licking at a surgical site around the lips (Fig. 26.2).[1] An alternative technique for closure of an upper lip defect is to close the deeper layers from dorsal to ventral first, followed by skin closure. However, skin closure begins at the lip edge and progresses dorsally; this assures a smooth lip edge.

Wedge closure

Lip trauma may result in defects necessitating conversion into a wedge shape or the creation of various flaps for closure. Closure of labial defects in cats and breeds of dogs with tight lips may cause problems. However, one-third to one-half of the lip may be resected on dogs with large pendulous lips with direct apposition of the wound edges, and no deformity or malfunction will result.[5] Wedge-shaped debridement should avoid creating narrow flaps with compromised vasculature at the lip edge, which could result in dehiscence. Debriding incisions should be perpendicular to the lip edges. Significant disparity of the wound edges may be corrected by removing a triangle of tissue (known as a Bürow's triangle) from the longer edge near the wedge apex. Closure of the defect is as stated above (Fig. 26.3).[1,6]

Square and rectangular defects

A rectangular lip defect may be closed in a similar manner as a laceration or wedge defect, except that after the initial lip edge-approximating suture is placed, closure in the deeper layers of the lip begins in the upper corners of the defect, progressing ventrally with a resulting 'Y-shaped' closure of the deep tissues and skin (see Fig. 44.5).[4,6]

Flap closure

Because of the size, location, and/or scar tissue around a lip defect, it may be necessary to incise the lip tissue to create various types of flaps for lip reconstruction. In general, all of these flaps entail moving tissue from caudal to rostral for reconstruction.

Rotation flap

A full-thickness rotation flap is semicircular in shape. It is made dorsally to the level of the junction of labial and gingival mucosa. As the incision progresses caudally, the parotid papilla should be watched for and the parotid duct cannulated with a lacrimal needle, an

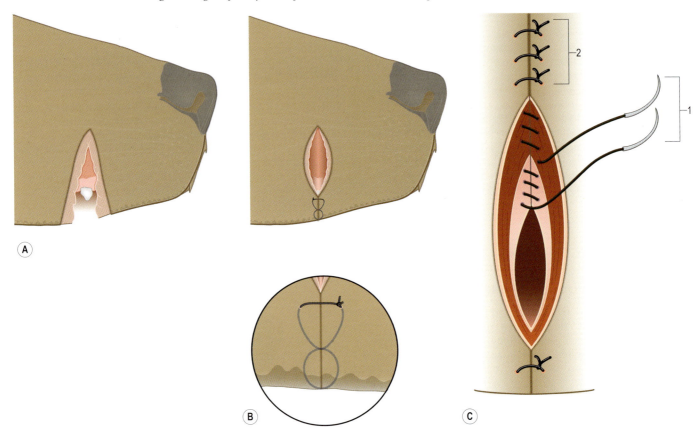

Fig. 26.2 Suturing lip laceration. (**A**) Lip laceration. (**B**) Placement of 'figure-of-eight' suture at lip margin, detail of suture (inset). (**C**) Layer closure of lip. (1) continuous suture layers in deeper layers (2) interrupted stainless steel sutures in skin. (*After Swaim SF, Henderson RA. Small animal wound management. 2nd ed. Baltimore: Williams and Wilkins, 1997; page 192, with permission. http://lww.com.*)

over-the-needle catheter or a folded-over segment of stainless steel wire to identify the duct for preservation, if possible. If it cannot be preserved, it should be ligated proximal to the lesion.[5] The flap is then rotated rostrally to close a defect. When placing buried sutures, the flap is advanced using 'walking'-type sutures. The first bite of the first suture is placed near the base of the flap. The second bite is taken a short distance rostrally in the dorsal edge of the defect. When tied, the suture advances the flap rostrally a small amount. Subsequent sutures are placed in like fashion to advance the flap into position (Fig. 26.4).

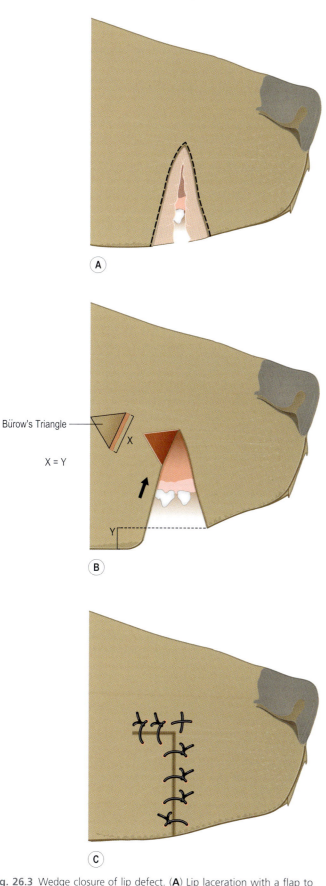

Fig. 26.3 Wedge closure of lip defect. (**A**) Lip laceration with a flap to be debrided (*broken line*) to create a wedge-shaped defect. (**B**) Disparity of wound edges corrected by removing Bürow's triangle from longer lip edge and shifting tissue (*arrow*) for closure. (**C**) Wound closed. *(After Swaim SF, Henderson RA. Small animal wound management. 2nd ed. Baltimore: Williams and Wilkins, 1997; page 194, with permission. http://lww.com.)*

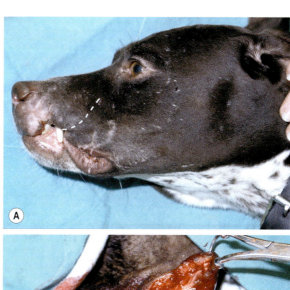

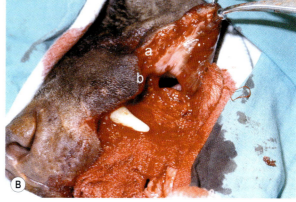

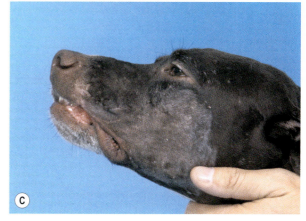

Fig. 26.4 Rotation flap to close a lip defect. (**A**) Lip defect with incision line for flap (*broken line*). (**B**) Flap incised and reflected; (a) where first bite of the first 'walking' suture will be placed (b) where second bite of the first 'walking' suture will be placed – rostral to first bite. (**C**) Defect closed by advancing tissues with 'walking' sutures.

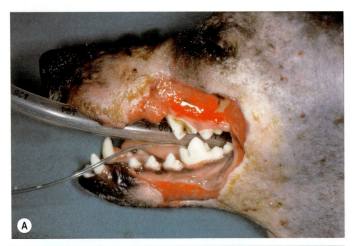

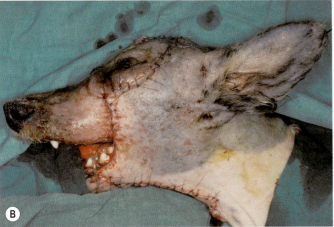

Fig. 26.5 A full-thickness single-pedicle advancement labial flap to close a traumatic defect of the lips. (**A**) A large rectangular upper labial defect with a similar smaller lower labial defect. (**B**) A full-thickness single-pedicle advancement flap as explained in Fig. 44.6 has been used to correct both upper and lower labial defects.

Single-pedicle advancement flap

A full-thickness single-pedicle advancement labial flap can be used to reconstruct large rostral square or rectangular defects in the upper lips (Fig. 26.5).[1,4-6] These are defects involving one-third to one-half of the lip, and incising the flap may require transecting the infraorbital vessels and nerve.[4] When incising upper lip mucosa, a 5-mm strip of mucosa is left along the gingival border for better suture-holding strength. A 25–50-mm length of mucosa is incised first to see if enough relaxation is gained to close the defect without a flap. If not, the mucosal incision is continued, and the skin is incised parallel to the lip edge from the dorsal defect edge to a point caudal to the oral commissure. Identification of the parotid duct should be done as previously described. Tension bands that can be palpated as the flap is advanced are carefully divided at the flap base, avoiding damage to the flap vasculature. The rostrodorsal corner of the flap can be trimmed for better apposition of this area into the rostral aspect of the labial defect. The lip margin apposition suture, submucosal and labial muscle sutures are placed. A continuous subcuticular suture and an intradermal suture are placed followed by interrupted skin sutures (see Fig. 44.6).[1,4,5]

A similar flap can be used for a lower labial defect, incising the mucosa first in a staged fashion, then the skin, to create the necessary flap length. 'Walking' sutures can also be used to advance the flap into position when placing the mucosal sutures. Mucosal sutures are

placed interproximally at the mandibular canine and first premolar teeth to help prevent lip sag. A 6-mm diameter Penrose drain may be placed under the flap before skin closure. The drain is removed by day 3 (see Fig. 44.11).[6]

Buccal or commissure rotation flap

For very large upper lip defects, a buccal or commissure rotation flap (lower labial pedicle rotation flap) can be used for correction.[1,4,8] With this technique, the abundant cheek pouch present in many dogs is taken advantage of in creating the flap. The principles of a full-thickness single-pedicle advancement labial flap are followed. However, the base of the flap is more ventral and the labial edge of the flap directly includes the oral commissure (see Fig. 44.8).[1,4,5]

Intermandibular wounds

Single-pedicle advancement flap

Some skin defects resulting from injury in the rostral intermandibular area can be repaired using a single-pedicle advancement flap from the caudal intermandibular area. With the animal in dorsal recumbency and the head and neck extended, skin incisions are made from the caudal aspect of each side of the defect caudally following the ventral aspect of the bodies of the mandibles (Fig. 26.6A). The incisions are made incrementally with undermining of the skin and subcutaneous tissue until a flap of sufficient length has been created to advance to cover the lesion with minimum tension. 'Walking' sutures of fine synthetic absorbable suture material are used to advance the flap into position (Fig. 26.6B). The same suture material is used to place continuous subcuticular sutures along each edge of the flap, and nonabsorbable monofilament simple interrupted sutures are used for skin closure (Fig. 26.6C).[1,5]

Axial-pattern flaps

Axial-pattern flaps based on the caudal auricular vessels have been described to repair head wounds, including intermandibular wounds.[5,6,9-11] Skin defects in the intermandibular area may be so large that intermandibular skin is not available for closure, especially on cats and brachycephalic dogs. In such cases, a caudal auricular axial-pattern flap may be considered for repair (see Ch. 48).[5,11]

A measurement is obtained from the lateral aspect of the atlas wing to the rostral aspect of the wound. A second measurement is taken from the atlas wing along the lateral cervical area to note how far along the neck a flap will have to be designed to transpose cranially to close the defect. Keeping this flap as short as possible reduces the chance of partial flap necrosis, which is occasionally noted if a flap has to be extended to the cranial or midscapular area to be long enough to reach the cranial aspect of the wound.[4,6] Thus, these flaps are more indicated for the caudal intermandibular area or on cats and brachycephalic dogs.

The flap is created by palpating the lateral aspect of the wing of the atlas. Two full-thickness skin incisions are made parallel to the cervical spine. The dorsal incision is close to the dorsal midline, while the ventrolateral incision extends caudally from the palpable depression between the base of the ear and the lateral wing of the atlas. It is parallel to the dorsal incision. The width of the flap will be to some extent determined by the width of the intermandibular lesion to be corrected. The two parallel incisions are connected to create the distal end of the flap. The flap is then elevated from caudal to cranial to include the sphincter colli superficialis muscle, cutaneous vessels, and the caudal auricular vessels. The free end of the flap is transposed cranially to the intermandibular lesion. It is trimmed to fit the defect and sutured in place. The flap's edges, which extend from the base of the ear to the tip sutured into the defect, can be sutured into a tube

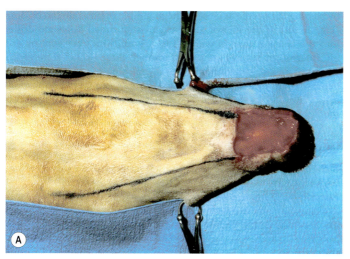

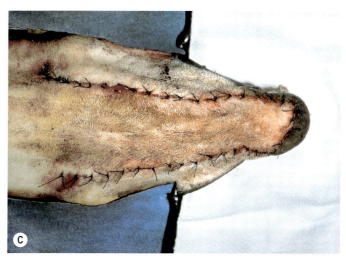

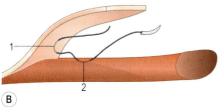

Fig. 26.6 Single-pedicle advancement flap for intermandibular wound. (**A**) Skin defect in the cranial intermandibular area with single-pedicle advancement flap drawn following ventral aspects of mandibular bodies. (**B**) Placement of 'walking' sutures to advance flap rostrally, second bite (2) is rostral to the first bite (1). (**C**) Flap sutured in place. *(A and C from Swaim SF, Henderson RA. Small animal wound management. 2nd ed. Baltimore: Williams and Wilkins, 1997; page 250, with permission. http:// lww.com.)*

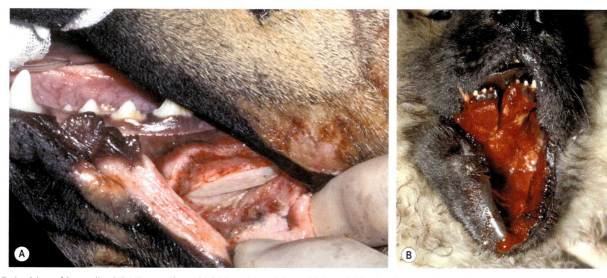

Fig. 26.7 Avulsion of lower lip. (**A**) Minor unilateral labial avulsion. (**B**) Total bilateral labial avulsion with mandibular symphyseal separation. *((B) from Miller WM, Swaim SF, Pope ER. Labial avulsion repair in the dog and cat. J Am Anim Hosp Assoc 1985;21:435–438, with permission.)*

or they can be sutured to the edges of a bridging incision made in the lateral cervical skin. The subcutaneous tissue and skin of the donor site are closed in routine fashion.[5,11]

Aftercare consists of a light bandage over the area, and an Elizabethan collar to protect the flap. If the flap has been tubed, 2–3 weeks after the flap has been placed and the distal end has developed a blood supply from the recipient site, the tube can be excised.[5,11]

Avulsion of the lower lip

Avulsion of the lower lip from the mandible caused by caudally directed forces on labial and gingival mucosa as well as subcutaneous tissue can result in separations of varying severity. Such injuries range from minor unilateral tissue separation to major bilateral avulsion back to the oral commissures (Fig. 26.7).[5] Usually, the avulsion occurs along the mucogingival junction, leaving only the mucosa and gingiva in the interdental space to reattach the lip, and this can present complications.[5] The degree of tissue separation governs the technique for repair.

Suturing techniques

With minor lower labial avulsion, the soft tissue flap can be replaced after cleaning and debridement. The soft tissues can be kept in contact with the bone using a single large horizontal mattress monofilament suture which is passed through the chin and around the canine teeth.

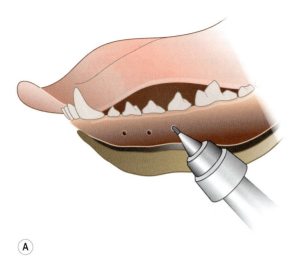
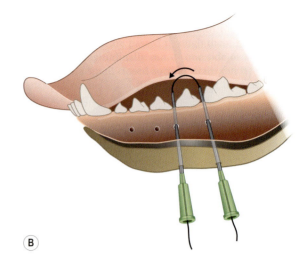
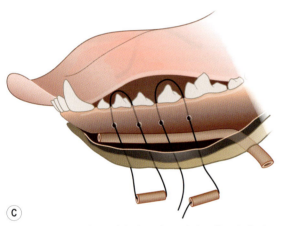
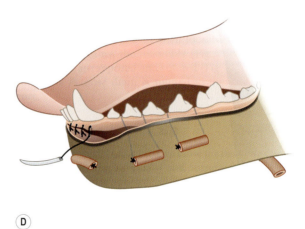

Fig. 26.10 Extensive lower labial avulsion. (**A**) Drilling holes between teeth for transosseous tension sutures/wires. (**B**) A 20-gauge hypodermic needle passed through the skin and mandible for placing sutures/wire. (**C**) Two transosseous suture/wires placed and Penrose drain in place. (**D**) Transosseous sutures/wires tied through rubber tube stents and interrupted gingivolabial sutures are being placed. *(After Swaim SF, Henderson RA. Small animal wound management. 2nd ed. Baltimore: Williams and Wilkins, 1997; page 199, with permission. http://lww.com.)*

loose skin in the cervical area. If the flap's base cannot be incorporated into the edge of the defect, a bridging incision can be made between the edge of the wound and base of the flap. Thus, the flap base can be completely sutured in place. This avoids tubing the flap base over intact skin. For cosmetics, a strip of skin can be excised along the bridging incision so the flap base lies flat. A drain may be necessary in the donor area because seromas are common due to movement in the cervical area.[5]

Axial-pattern flaps

Axial-pattern flaps based on the caudal auricular vessels can be used for repair of dorsal cranial wounds.[4–6,9,10] The flap is reflected dorsally to repair wounds on the dorsal aspect of the head and facial area (see Ch. 48).

Large frontal and lateral facial wounds

Random-pattern flap-closure

A random-pattern transposition flap taken from the ventrolateral cervical area has been described for repair of a large lateral facial defect on a brachycephalic dog.[14] For such a flap, a dorsally based rectangular flap is designed on the ventrolateral cervical area of such a length that the diagonal across the flap from its pivot point is equal to the diagonal from the pivot point to the far corner of the defect (Fig. 26.14A). This compensates for the loss of effective length of the flap as it is rotated into position.[1] The flap is transposed into position and sutured as described above. A drain can be placed under the flap to prevent seroma formation (Fig. 26.14B).

A semicircular rotation flap of skin and subcutaneous tissue can be used to repair wounds on the head and face, to include the lateral

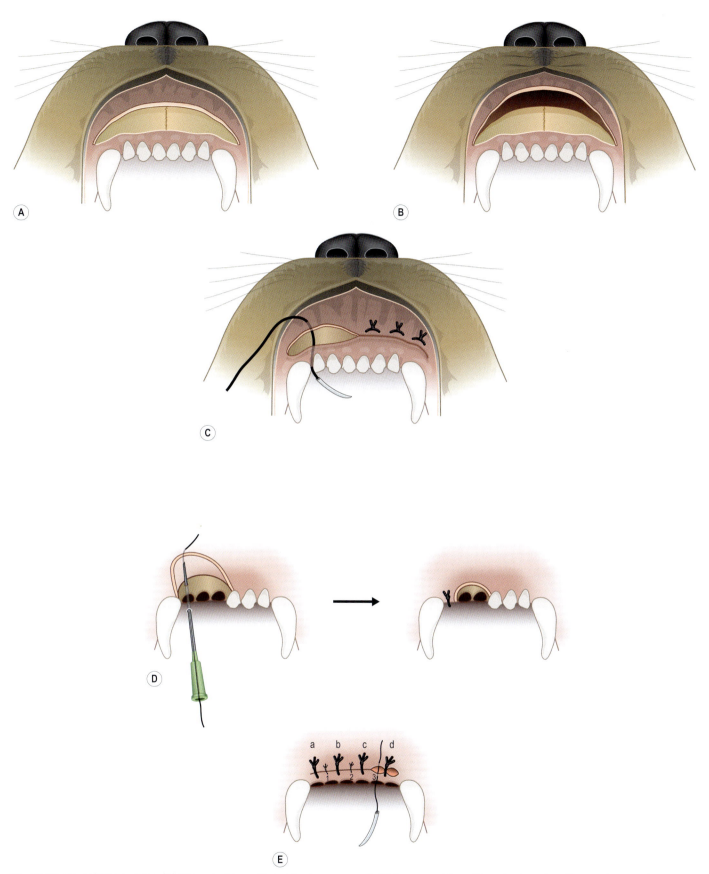

Fig. 26.11 Upper labial avulsion. (**A**) Minor avulsion with incisive bone exposed. (**B**) Severe avulsion with avulsed nasal cartilage and oronasal communication. (**C**) Minor avulsion correction with incisor teeth present – interrupted horizontal mattress suture through labial–gingival mucosa and looped around incisor teeth. (**D**) Minor avulsion with incisor teeth missing. Left: hole drilled in incisive bone with 20-gauge hypodermic needle through hole, suture through mucosal edge and through needle; right: needle removed, and suture tied. (**E**) Severe upper labial avulsion with all incisor teeth missing – four transosseous sutures (a–d) with intervening interrupted mucosal sutures (1–3). ((**A**), (**B**), (**C**), (**E**) *After Swaim SF, Henderson RA. Small animal wound management. 2nd ed. Baltimore: Williams and Wilkins, 1997; page 200–201, with permission. http://lww.com. (**D**) after Pavletic MM. Atlas of small animal wound management and reconstructive surgery. 3rd ed. Ames, Iowa: Wiley-Blackwell, 2010;447, with permission.)*

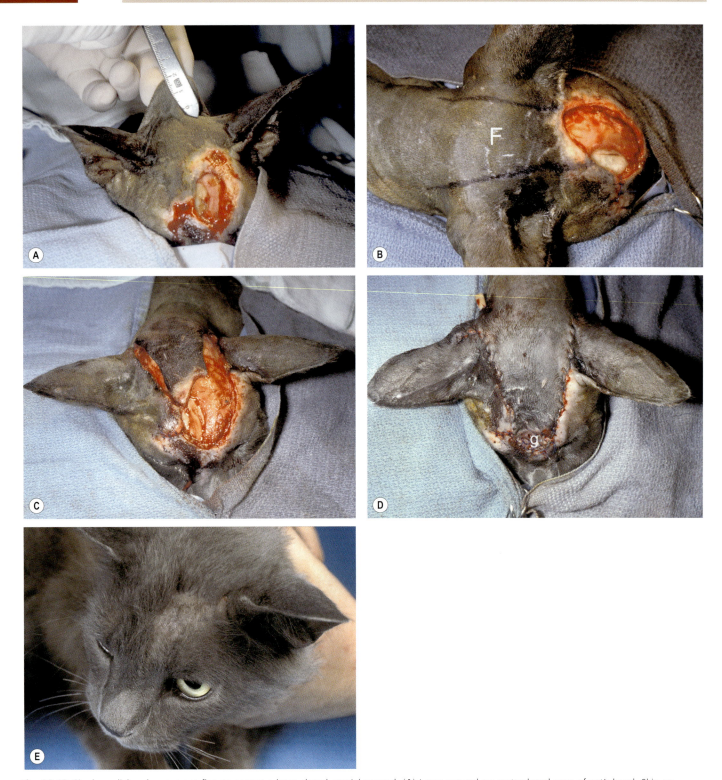

Fig. 26.12 Single-pedicle advancement flap to correct a large dorsal cranial wound. (**A**) Large wound on rostrodorsal area of cat's head. Skin on cranial cervical and caudal cranial area measured for flap creation. (**B**) Flap (F) drawn on caudal cranial and cranial cervical skin. (**C**) Flap incised. (**D**) Flap advanced into place. A small mesh graft (g) was placed at the rostral-most end of defect. (**E**) Flap and graft healed. *(From Swaim SF, Henderson RA. Small animal wound management. 2nd ed. Baltimore: Williams and Wilkins, 1997; page 250–251, with permission. http://lww.com.)*

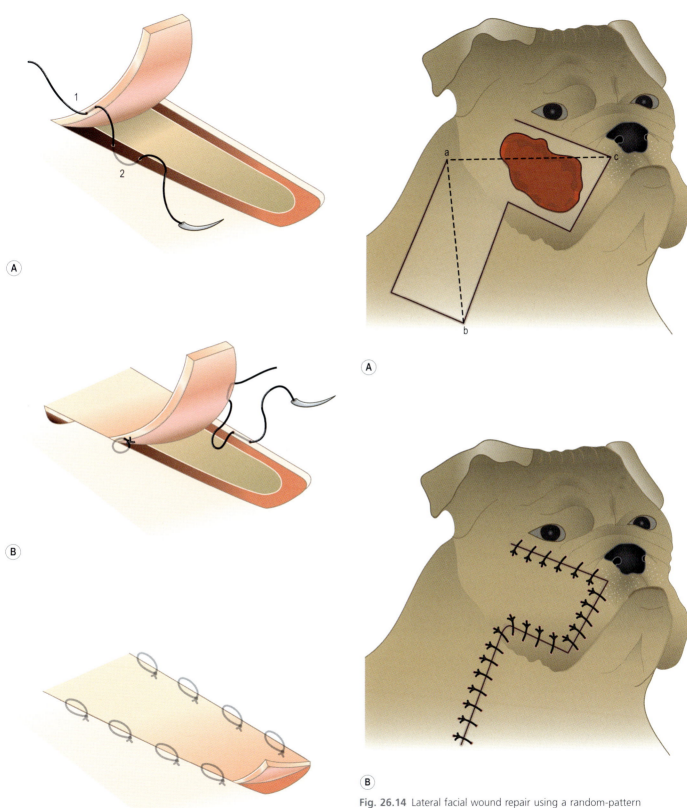

A

B

C

Fig. 26.13 'Walking' sutures at the edge of the flap when bone is exposed. (**A**) First bite (1) is in edge of the flap, and the second bite (2) is advanced in the edge of the adjacent skin. (**B**) Second 'walking' suture being placed on the opposite side of the wound. (**C**) 'Walking' sutures have advanced the flap into position. *(After Swaim SF, Henderson RA. Small animal wound management. 2nd ed. Baltimore: Williams and Wilkins, 1997; page 255, with permission. http://lww.com.)*

A

B

Fig. 26.14 Lateral facial wound repair using a random-pattern transposition flap. (**A**) A dorsally based rectangular transposition flap designed on the ventrolateral cervical area. Diagonal across the flap from its pivot point is equal to the diagonal from the pivot point to the far corner of the defect (a–b=a–c). (**B**) Flap in position with donor site closed.

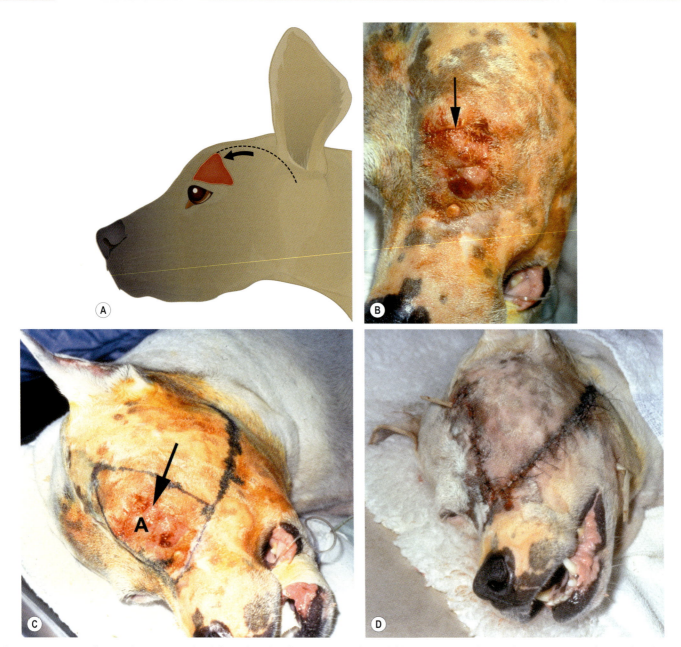

Fig. 26.15 Rotation flap to close a triangular defect when skin for closure is only available on one side of the defect. (**A**) Rotation flap to close lesion over an eye. (**B**) Fibrosarcoma in area of previous eye enucleation (*arrow*). (**C**) Area to be excised (A). Direction of flap movement (*arrow*) for reconstruction. (**D**) Flap sutured in place. *(Courtesy of Dr. WW Miller.)*

facial area, caudal bridge of the nose, and especially around the eyes to minimize tension on the eyelids.[1–4] The flap is moved by a combination of rotation, transposition, and stretching to close triangular wounds that only have skin available for closure on one side of the wound (Fig. 26.15).[1,6] A semicircular flap is drawn on the skin, with the leading edge of the flap being one edge of the wound. It should be large enough so there is no tension across it when it is sutured in place. The flap and associated subcutaneous tissue are then raised incrementally with sharp undermining until it can be rotated across the wound without excess tension. Making a small back cut at the end of the incision opposite the wound allows the flap to rotate and transpose into position easier (Fig. 26.16). However, the larger the back cut, the greater are the chances of cutting into vasculature supplying the flap. Back cuts should be made judiciously. 'Walking'

sutures can be used to help move the flap into position. The flap edge is sutured in place with a synthetic absorbable continuous subcuticular suture and simple interrupted sutures in the skin. If a line of tension develops across the flap as it is sutured in place, a small stab incision perpendicular to the line of greatest tension will help relieve the tension. The 'dog ear' of skin that forms adjacent to the base of the flap as it is sutured in place is removed and the defect is closed.[1]

Axial-pattern flaps

The caudal auricular axial-pattern flap can be considered to repair frontal and lateral facial wounds (see Ch. 48).[4–6,9,10]

An axial-pattern flap based on the cutaneous branch of the superficial temporal artery has been described experimentally in cats,[4,15] and

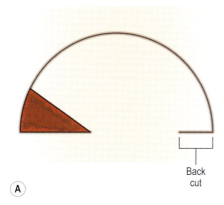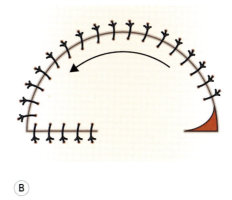

Back-
cut

Ⓐ   Ⓑ

Fig. 26.16 Back-cut in a rotation flap. (**A**) A small back-cut along the diameter line of a rotation flap's base. (**B**) Flap rotates into place easier. *(After Swaim SF, Henderson RA. Small animal wound management. 2nd ed. Baltimore: Williams and Wilkins, 1997; page 245, with permission. http://lww.com.)*

experimentally on mesaticephalic dogs, as well as a clinical case in a dog.[4,16] To perform the procedure, the animal is placed in ventral recumbency. The landmarks for the base of the flap are the caudal aspect of the zygomatic arch caudally and the lateral orbital rim rostrally, i.e., the base is the width of the zygomatic arch. Parallel lines are drawn from these points across the top of the head to the level of the middle of the dorsal orbital rim of the contralateral eye, where the lines are connected, forming the distal flap-end. The flap and underlying frontalis muscle are incised and the flap is undermined and reflected back to its base. To enhance flap rotation, a small superficial branch of the rostral auricular nerve plexus at the rostral border of the flap over the eye and adjacent to the flap base is divided. The flap can be rotated rostrally as far as the nasal plane.[13,14]

The omocervical cutaneous flap can be used to repair frontal and facial wounds.[4,6] It tends to be more successful in cats. The flap is based on the superficial cervical vessels that exit the musculature cranial to the shoulder at the level of the prescapular lymph node and the cranial shoulder depression. The vessels course craniodorsally. Flap boundaries are: ventrally, the acromion of the scapula; caudally, the scapular spine; cranially, a line parallel to the caudal border, i.e., twice the distance from the scapular spine to the prescapular lymph node. The dorsal midline is a safe distal border. However, it may extend to the contralateral shoulder area, especially in cats.[4]

Mucosal grafts to reconstruct nasal plane, nares or vestibule

Occasionally it is necessary to reconstruct large intraoral or eyelid defects, the nasal plane, nares or vestibule. Mucosal grafts can be harvested from under the tongue or from the upper lips for this purpose.[4,17] For reconstruction of the nares it is necessary to have some wound tissue in the area where the nares will be reconstructed. This can be in the form of edges of labial flaps that have been used to reconstruct the area or by cutting holes in such a flap that will serve as the 'nares' openings. Silicone tubes are placed between the edges of the flaps and back into the nasal passages as the edges are sutured together, or into the holes cut in a flap. The tubes are sutured in place by interrupted sutures through the tube and adjacent skin (Fig. 26.17A). The tubes are left in place for approximately 2 weeks to allow granulation tissue to form around them. At this time, rectangular mucosal grafts of sufficient width to go around the silicone tube and of sufficient length to traverse the length of the granulation tube that has formed are harvested bilaterally from under the tongue.

The grafts may be harvested by hydrodissection. This requires injecting 5–10 mL of dilute solution of lidocaine with epinephrine (25 mL of 1% lidocaine/epinephrine per liter of lactated Ringer's solution) submucosally on the ventral tongue surface. This allows easy collection of the graft because of separation of the mucosa from the underlying tissue.[4]

The grafts are sutured submucosal-side out around the silicone tubes that had been in the nasal cavity. Two double-traction sutures of synthetic monofilament suture are placed in each end of the graft 180° apart. The two sutures in the end of the graft to be placed in the nasal cavity are threaded back through the end of the tube they are closest to and out the other end of the tube (Fig. 26.17B, C). With traction on all four sutures to keep the graft smooth, each tube with its graft is reinserted in the nasal cavity. The rostral edge of the graft and tube are affixed to the skin at the edge of the 'nares' opening with simple interrupted sutures after all traction sutures are pulled out (Fig. 26.17D). Seven days later, the sutures are removed, and the tubes are easily removed, leaving cylindrical 'nares' openings with healed mucosal grafts lining the area (Fig. 26.17E). Because there is no cartilaginous support of the openings, they usually collapse with time. Thus, they are not effective for breathing, but due to their mucosal graft linings, they do not heal closed. They remain open to allow drainage of nasal secretions.

POSTOPERATIVE CARE AND ASSESSMENT

Elizabethan collars are indicated to prevent animals from molesting lip and facial reconstruction areas. If wounds were infected prior to debridement, systemic antibiotics are indicated. For more extensive flaps, intermittent moist cool compresses for 72 hours after surgery may help keep the wound clean and reduce edema.[1] Nonabsorbable skin sutures are removed 7–10 days postoperatively.

If a drain was used in the repair of a minor lip avulsion, it is usually removed in 3 days. For major avulsions, the drain is removed after 4–5 days and the transosseous sutures or wires are removed after 10–14 days.[1]

Following upper lip avulsion no attempts should be made to examine the surgical site during the first 7 days unless problems are suspected. If the area is examined, sedation or anesthesia should be used to prevent the animal from resisting examination and damaging the surgical site.[1] Nonabsorbable sutures used for transosseous fixation can be removed at 10–14 days.

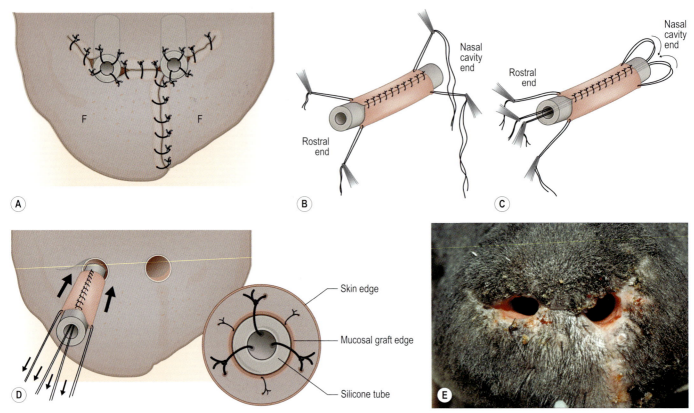

Fig. 26.17 (**A**) Silicone tubes placed between labial flaps (F) and back into the nasal passages. Tubes are sutured to the skin edges to hold them in place. Mucosal graft preparation for placement. (**B**) Graft sutured, submucosal side out, around silicone tube with two double-traction sutures 180° apart at each end. (**C**) Sutures at end of graft to go into nasal cavity are passed back through tube. (**D**) Placement of mucosal grafts into granulation tissue-lined 'nares.' Tube with graft is inserted into 'nares' (*large arrows*) with traction on traction sutures (*small arrows*) to hold graft smooth. (*Inset*) Graft and tubes sutured to the skin. (**E**) Mucosal grafts healed in place, lining the 'nares.' ((**A–E**) *after Welch JA, Swaim SF. Nasal salvage/reconstruction in a dog following severe trauma. J Am Anim Hosp Assoc 2003;39:407–415.*)

COMPLICATIONS

Lip lacerations and defects

If the mucosa and submucosa are sutured together, the mucosa may invert, which can impair healing. Thus, submucosa only should be sutured and, if mucosa is sutured, it should be sutured separately from within the oral cavity.[1] When it is necessary to create a new mucocutaneous junction on the upper lip, haired skin can be pulled into the area normally occupied by the labial mucosa, which can result in an unaesthetic appearance with hair growing in the mouth and becoming matted with saliva. To prevent this, the skin should be trimmed back so that suturing skin to mucosa either results in edge-to-edge apposition at the lip edge or pulls labial mucosa to the outside.

Simple closure of labial defects in cats and dogs with relatively tight lips may result in excessive tension or interference with function.[5] For instance, labial advancement flaps are more difficult in cats because there is less free lip margin and a smaller commissure from which to construct a flap.[1] With large defects, the flap procedures pull the oral commissure rostrally.[1,6] In addition, contraction of a full-thickness single-pedicle advancement labial flap may result in distortion of the nasal plane, but this usually subsides in 2–3 weeks.[6]

Intermandibular wounds

If a single-pedicle advancement flap is designed too short and not anchored sufficiently to underlying intermandibular musculature, tension on the flap could cause caudal displacement of the lower lip to expose the mandibular canine and incisor teeth. However, when an animal recovers from anesthesia and resumes a normal head and neck flexion posture, it helps take tension off of the flap.

If a caudal auricular axial-pattern flap is designed too long, the tip of the flap may necrose from lack of perfusion.[4,6] If initial measurements indicate that the flap will have to be long, another form of reconstruction may be needed, such as a skin graft. A disadvantage of these flaps is the difference in type, direction, and length of hair growth in the reconstruction area since skin from the caudal cervical area will be placed in the intermandibular area.[11] On long-haired dogs and cats, periodic trimming of their 'beard' may be necessary.

Lower lip avulsion

In both minor and major labial avulsions, if tissues are properly debrided, lavaged, drained and sutured, they heal uneventfully. However, if not properly handled, wound infection, abscessation, and tissue slough could possibly result. It is difficult to suture the gingiva on the buccal surface of the teeth because the gingiva is tightly attached to the underlying bone, resulting in sutures tearing out. Suturing through just the interdental space mucosa may not provide sufficient support to hold the tissues apposed until adequate healing has occurred. Use of swaged taper-cut needles may help prevent sutures from tearing out. However, if major avulsions are not stabilized with transosseous tension sutures, tension on the simple gingival–labial sutures may arise as tissues swell and weight of the lip tissues increases.[1,5,6,12]

Upper lip avulsion

When properly debrided, lavaged, and sutured, minor and major upper labial avulsions usually heal uneventfully. However, due to their location, sutures can be easily molested by the animal's tongue, resulting in wound disruption. If wire is used for the transosseous fixation, the sharp ends of the tags help discourage such suture molestation. Absorbable mucosal sutures placed between transosseous sutures may tear through the mucosa.[1]

Large wounds on the dorsum of the cranium

Because single-pedicle advancement flaps tend to have more tension on them, there is the potential for causing distortion of the upper eyelids if they are used to close large dorsal cranial wounds and have tension associated with them. Movement of the cervical area may result in seroma formation at the donor site of a transposition flap used to repair a dorsal cranial defect.[5] If a caudal auricular axial-pattern flap is designed too long, the distal end may undergo avascular necrosis when used over a dorsal cranial defect.[4,6]

Large frontal and lateral facial wounds

The caudal auricular axial-pattern flap has the same complications when used for frontal and lateral facial wound repair as when used for repair of intermandibular and dorsal–cranial wounds. Likewise, transposition flaps from the ventrolateral cervical area may have similar complications.

An axial-pattern flap based on the cutaneous branch of the superficial temporal artery is not indicated for rostrally located lesions on dolichocephalic breeds due to discrepancy in flap length and skull length. The procedure is reserved for cats and mesaticephalic dogs.[15,16] Other reconstructive techniques have to be considered for dolichocephalic dogs. The direction and length of hair growth on the flap is less cosmetic, with skin being taken from the top of the head and rotated 90° onto an area with shorter hair. Other complications of this flap are facial nerve paralysis, transection of the axial-pattern blood supply with partial flap necrosis, difficulty closing the eyelids if the flap is designed too wide, and dehiscence of the donor site.[4]

Rotation flaps have the disadvantage of causing tension on eyelids when used on the face. It is important to design these flaps large enough to relieve tension.

REFERENCES

1. Swaim SF, Henderson RA. Small animal wound management. 2nd ed. Baltimore, MD: Williams and Wilkins; 1997. p. 191–274.
2. Pope ER. Lavage of open wounds: Chlorhexidine solution recommended. Vet Med Rep 1990;2:185.
3. Fossum TW, Hedlund CS, Hulse DA, et al. Small animal surgery. 3rd ed. St. Louis, MO: Mosby; 2007. p. 159–259.
4. Degner DA. Facial reconstructive surgery. Clin Tech Small Anim Pract 2007;22:82–8.
5. Pope ER. Head and facial wounds in dogs and cats. Vet Clin North Am Small Anim Pract 2006;36:793–817.
6. Pavletic MM. Atlas of small animal reconstructive surgery. 3rd ed. Philadelphia, PA: WB Saunders; 2010.
7. Pavletic MM. Nasal and rostral labial reconstruction in the dog. J Am Anim Hosp Assoc 1983;19:595–600.

8. Smeak DD. Lower labial pedicle rotation flap for reconstruction of large upper lip defects in two dogs. J Am Anim Hosp Assoc 1992;28:565–9.
9. Smith MM, Payne JT, Moon ML, et al. Axial pattern flap based on the caudal auricular artery in dogs. Am J Vet Res 1991;52:922–5.
10. Spodnick GJ, Hudson LC, Clark G, et al. Use of a caudal auricular axial pattern flap in cats. J Am Vet Med Assoc 1996;208:1679–82.
11. Aber SL, Amalsadvala T, Brown JE, et al. Using a caudal auricular axial pattern flap to close a mandibular skin defect in a cat. Vet Med 2002;97:666–71.
12. Miller WM, Swaim SF, Pope ER. Labial avulsion repair in the dog and cat. J Am Anim Hosp Assoc 1985;21:435–8.
13. Olmstead ML, Stoloff DR, O'Keefe CM. Avulsion of the upper lip in two dogs.

Vet Med Small Anim Clin 1976;71:1228–9.
14. Gibson KL, Dean PW. Using a transposition flap in the resection of a large facial tumor. Vet Med 1991;86:1100–3.
15. Fahie MA, Smith MM. Axial pattern flap based on the superficial temporal artery in cats: An experimental study. Vet Surg 1997;26:86–9.
16. Fahie MA, Smith MM. Axial pattern flap based on the cutaneous branch of the superficial temporal artery in dogs: An experimental study and case report. Vet Surg 1999;28:141–7.
17. Welch JA, Swaim SF. Nasal salvage/reconstruction in a dog following severe trauma. J Am Anim Hosp Assoc 2003;39:407–15.

Chapter 27

Surgical approaches for mandibular and maxillofacial trauma repair

Frank J.M. Verstraete, Boaz Arzi & Abraham J. Bezuidenhout

PRINCIPLES AND CLASSIFICATION

Principles

An acceptable surgical approach to a bone or joint is the least traumatic yet effective method of exposing the bone or joint, as determined by the topographical anatomy of the region. Major blood vessels, nerves, and salivary glands and ducts must be avoided or retracted.[1] It is therefore essential to be familiar with the normal anatomy. Muscles should be separated by blunt dissection of the intermuscular septa rather than incised or transected. To expose an area of bone that serves as an origin or insertion of a muscle, or where muscle loosely attaches to the bone, one of several techniques may be applicable, depending on the nature of the attachment. In most cases, muscle that adheres to the underlying bone must be elevated subperiosteally. The periosteum is exposed by blunt dissection between two muscle bellies, incised, and elevated using a periosteal elevator. A periosteal elevator designed for oral surgery (see Ch. 6) can be used for this purpose; alternatively a small orthopedic periosteal elevator is suitable.[1]

The surgeon is encouraged to regain the maximum function of injured skin or mucosa with the least possible deformity and scarring. This may be achieved by evaluating the static and dynamic skin tensions on the surrounding skin.[2] Static tension lines exist within the skin and are oriented in specific but variable directions.

Extraoral approaches

The extraoral or transfacial approaches are most commonly used in veterinary surgery.[1] In order to obtain an optimally healing wound, the extraoral surgical incision should follow the relaxed skin tension line direction within these areas. Skin tension lines are usually oriented perpendicularly to the underlying muscles.[2] Utilization of an extraoral approach is usually performed for open reduction of fractures followed by plating (e.g., mini-plating, locking reconstruction plates), screw applications, and certain wiring techniques. When such an approach is used, the facial neurovascular structures are potentially at risk and therefore the surgeon must be aware of and consider the relevant topographic anatomy.

Intraoral approaches

Intraoral or transoral approaches are most commonly used in humans, in order to avoid cutaneous scars.[2,3] They are infrequently used in veterinary surgery and mainly for fractures of the maxilla and incisive bone (see Chs 30 & 31). The typical intraoral incision lines for exposure of either the maxilla or the mandible are made within the unattached mucosa 3–4 mm away from the mucogingival junction. To expose the caudal part of the mandible the incision line is placed directly over the ramus of the mandible.

Approach through a traumatic wound

The approach through a traumatic wound should, as a general rule, be avoided.[1] It is occasionally indicated for avulsion of the lip or other oral soft tissues, usually due to car accidents.

In general, the approach should not add unnecessary trauma to that which the injured area has already sustained. The incision may be extended beyond the traumatic wound to allow adequate exposure to better analyze the destruction of anatomic and physiologic functions of the area invaded. In certain instances, a small exposure will force the surgeon to exert excessive pressure when manipulating the wound which will further injure the muscles and impairs circulation to the area.

ANESTHETIC CONSIDERATIONS[4]

A cuffed endotracheal tube and secured pharyngeal pack should be used to prevent aspiration during surgery. Restoring occlusion is the mainstay of proper repair of maxillary and mandibular fractures. When performing the fixation procedure in many patients, particularly in the more complicated cases, a pharyngotomy intubation is done to maintain anesthesia. This technique ensures an open airway while the animal's mouth is closed and the teeth can be occluded during the procedure, ensuring adequate reduction during application of fixation. After the surgery is completed, the endotracheal tube is removed and the pharyngotomy opening is allowed to heal by second intention.

© 2012 Elsevier Ltd
DOI: 10.1016/B978-0-7020-4618-6.00027-0

SURGICAL ANATOMY

Regional anatomy

In the upper jaw the incisive and maxillary bones carry teeth and form most of the dorsolateral surface of the face. Alveolar juga of the canine and shearing teeth are features of this surface. The infraorbital foramen, through which the infraorbital nerve and blood vessels emerge, lies dorsal to the septum between the third and fourth premolar teeth. Nasal bones complete the face dorsally, and the lacrimal and zygomatic bones complete the caudal aspect of the face rostral and ventral to the orbit. The temporal process of the zygomatic bone and the zygomatic process of the squamous temporal bone are the only contributors to the zygomatic arch. The orbital ligament connecting the zygomatic process of the frontal bone and the frontal process of the zygomatic bone completes the rim of the orbit caudally.

The body of the mandible has alveolar and ventral margins, and lingual and buccal/labial surfaces. The alveolar border is indented by conical alveoli for the roots of the incisor, canine, premolar and molar teeth. In mesaticephalic skulls the ventral border is slightly curved (convex), in brachycephalic skulls this convexity is more pronounced, while in dolichocephalic skulls the ventral border is almost straight. Rostrally the buccal surface carries two or three mental foramina through which the mental nerves and blood vessels emerge. The middle mental foramen is the largest, and lies ventral to the septum between the first two premolar teeth. The position of the caudal foramen is variable; it is generally located at the level of the distal root of the third premolar tooth, but may be rostral or caudal to it. Caudally, at the angle of the mandible, the body meets the ramus, the non-tooth-bearing portion of the mandible. Dorsally the ramus bears two processes, the coronoid process for the attachment of the temporal muscle, and a transversely elongated condylar process that articulates with the zygomatic process of the temporal bone to form the temporomandibular joint. The two processes are separated from each other by the mandibular incisure. The masticatory branch of the mandibular nerve to the masseter muscle passes from medial to lateral over the incisure. The lateral and medial surfaces of the coronoid process are concave, forming a masseteric fossa laterally and a pterygoid fossa medially. Ventrally, at the angle of the mandible, the ramus bears an angular process for the attachment of the masseter and medial pterygoid muscles. The mandibular foramen for the inferior alveolar nerve and blood vessels lies medially between the base of the coronoid process and the angular process, caudal to the last molar tooth. Left and right mandibles are rostrally united to each other by a slightly flexible, rough-surfaced fibrous joint, the symphysis of the mandible.

A thin articular cartilage (disk) lies between the condylar process of the mandible and the mandibular fossa of the temporal bone, completely dividing the joint space into dorsal and ventral compartments. The joint capsule attaches to the cartilage and is strengthened by the lateral ligament.

The extensive but thin platysma muscle extends from the dorsum of the neck to the angle of the mouth and ventrally as far as the midline. The mentalis muscle radiates from the alveolar border of the mandible near the third incisors into the lower lip. More caudally, the orbicularis oris muscle extends from the commissural region into the lips near their free borders.

The masseter muscle is attached to the zygomatic arch and the lateral surface of the ramus of the mandible. It projects slightly beyond the ventral and caudal borders of the mandible, some fibers attaching on the ventromedial surface. The temporal muscle has a broad attachment to the temporal fossa of the cranium and extends to the medial and lateral surfaces of the coronoid process, medially as far distally as the mandibular foramen and laterally as far distally as the ventral ridge of the masseteric fossa. The robust medial pterygoid muscle extends from the lateral surface of the pterygoid, palatine and sphenoid bones to the medial and caudal surfaces of the angular process of the mandible. The lateral pterygoid muscle extends from the sphenoid bone to the medial surface of the condylar process, just distal to the articular condyle. Other muscles associated with the mandible are the digastric, mylohyoid, geniohyoid and genioglossus muscles. The mylohyoid muscle is the most superficial, extending from the mylohyoid line of the mandible (along the lingual surface just ventral to the alveoli) to the basihyoid bone, forming a transverse sling for the tongue. The geniohyoid muscle extends along the midline from the caudal edge of the mandibular symphysis to the basihyoid bone; the genioglossus extends from the same area of the symphysis and radiates dorsally into the tongue. The digastric muscle originates from the paracondylar process and is attached along the ventromedial border of the mandible up to the level of the canine tooth. An indistinct myotendinous intersection separates the caudal and rostral bellies of the muscle.

The parotid, mandibular and monostomatic sublingual salivary glands lie caudal to the ramus of the mandible. The parotid duct crosses the lateral surface of the masseter muscle, ventral to the dorsal branch of the facial nerve, to open in the vestibule on the parotid papilla located opposite the caudal margin of the upper fourth premolar tooth. The ducts from the mandibular and sublingual salivary glands are closely related to each other throughout their course. The two ducts pass between the masseter and mandible laterally and the digastric muscle medially, then arches rostrally in the intermuscular septum between the genioglossus and mylohyoid muscles. Both ducts open on the sublingual caruncula.

SURGICAL APPROACHES

Approach to the incisive part and mandibular symphysis

The patient is positioned in dorsal recumbency with the neck extended and supported with a padded area. Forceps may be used to retract the skin of the ventral mandible to better visualize the oral mucosa. The buccal mucosa is incised a minimum of 3–5 mm from the mucogingival junction; the incision extends through the submucosa, muscles and periosteum (Fig. 27.1).[2,5] Sharp dissection is performed using scalpel or periosteal elevator to incise soft tissues, including the oral mucosa, and mentalis and orbicularis oris muscles. Closure may be done in two layers. The periosteum and elevated muscles constitute the first layer, and the submucosa and mucosa are closed in a second layer. In certain instances, a single mucosal and submucosal layer is elected.

Ventral approach to the body of the mandible

The patient is positioned in dorsal recumbency with the neck extended. The skin incision is made medial to the palpable ventral border of the mandible (Fig. 27.2A). If both rostral mandibles have to be exposed, a single midline incision can be made. However, if the entire body of both mandibles needs to be visualized, two separate incisions are recommended. The incised skin is then moved over the prominent ventral border. The subcutaneous fascia, the thin platysma muscle and periosteum are then incised with a single

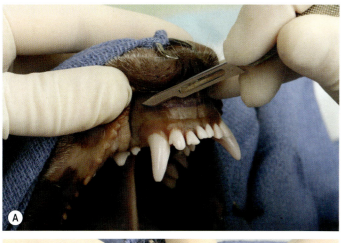

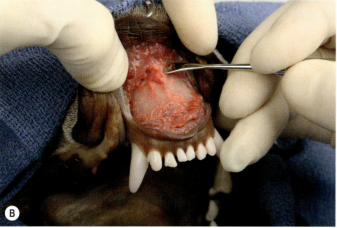

Fig. 27.1 Intraoral approach to the incisive part of the body of the mandible and the mandibular symphysis shown in a cadaver head. (**A**) The first incision is made 3–5 mm from the mucogingival junction. (**B**) The incision is then extended through the submucosa, muscles and periosteum.

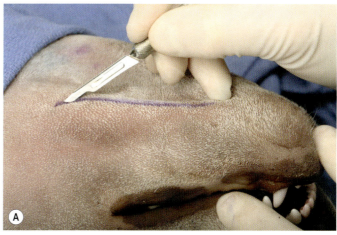

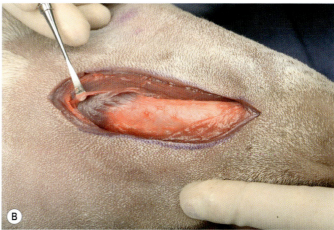

Fig. 27.2 Ventral approach to the body of the mandible shown in a cadaver head. (**A**) The skin incision is made medial to the ventral border of the mandible. (**B**) The ventral body of the mandible is exposed, avoiding the sublingual branch of the facial artery and vein.

full-thickness incision, which ends caudally at the insertion of the rostral belly of the digastricus muscle, thereby avoiding the sublingual branches of the facial artery and vein that cross it (Fig. 27.2B). All soft tissues can then be elevated subperiosteally and retracted medially and laterally, respectively. This includes the mylohyoideus muscle on the medial aspect and the insertion of the genioglossus and geniohyoideus muscles caudal to the symphysis. Care should be taken as one approaches the mucogingival junction during the elevation and retraction of soft tissues, as perforation can easily occur. It is usually not necessary to elevate the attached gingiva. When exposing the middle and caudal mental foramina, located at the level of the mesial root of the second and third premolar teeth, respectively, care should be taken to retract the associated neurovascular structures.

If the most caudal aspect of the body and the ramus of the mandible need to be exposed, the approach can be extended more caudally.[1]

Closure is usually achieved in three layers. The periosteum and elevated muscles constitute the first layer. The platysma and subcutaneous tissue are closed in a second layer, followed by the skin. The skin suture line is located medial to the ventral border thereby minimizing the risk of a visible scar. With comminuted fractures, the lacerated oral mucous membrane may require surgical debridement and additional sutures.

Ventral approach to the caudal part of the body and to the ramus of the mandible

The patient is positioned in dorsal recumbency with the neck extended. The skin incision is made medial to the palpable ventral border and angular process of the mandible (Fig. 27.3A). The incised skin is then moved over the prominent ventral border. The subcutaneous fascia and the thin platysma muscle are then incised. The rostral belly of the digastricus muscle on the ventromedial aspect of the mandible and the masseter muscle on the lateral aspect are identified. The intermuscular septum is divided by blunt dissection until the periosteum and insertion of the masseteric fascia are reached. The periosteum is subsequently incised and the two muscles subperiosteally elevated and retracted (Fig. 27.3B).[1] In order to expose the very caudal aspect of the mandible, the insertion of the medial pterygoid muscle has to be elevated. The sublingual artery, a branch of the facial artery and one of the facial veins cross the rostral belly of the digastricus muscle in a rostromedial direction, which may have to be ligated if they cannot be sufficiently retracted. Care is taken not to damage the facial artery and vein, which are located lateral to the incision.

The masseter and temporal muscles can be elevated from the masseteric fossa as far dorsally as the rostrodorsal margin of the coronoid process (often referred to as coronoid crest), to allow mini-plate

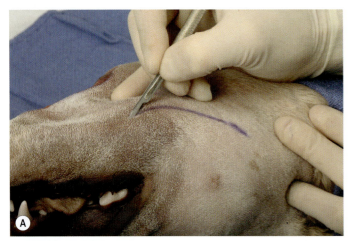

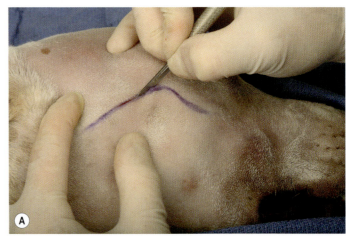

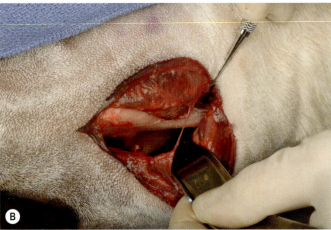

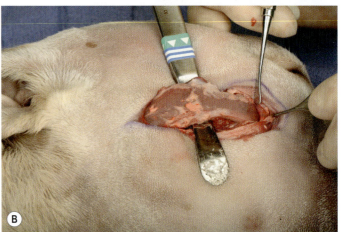

Fig. 27.3 Ventral approach to the caudal part of the body and to the ramus of the mandible shown in a cadaver head. (**A**) The skin incision is made medial to the palpable ventral border and angular process of the mandible. (**B**) After incising the subcutaneous fascia and platysma muscles, the intramuscular septum of the masseter muscle and digastricus is separated and retracted. Note the sublingual artery, a branch of the facial artery and one of the facial veins cross the rostral belly of the digastricus muscle in a rostromedial direction.

Fig. 27.4 Lateral approach to the zygomatic arch shown in a cadaver head. (**A**) The skin incision follows the ventral or dorsal border of the zygomatic arch. (**B**) Following periosteal incision, the masseter and temporal muscles are elevated and retracted.

placement in this biomechanically favorable position (see Ch. 31).[6] The exposure on the medial aspect is more limited due to the presence of the mandibular foramen and the neurovascular bundle associated with it.

Closure is usually achieved in three layers. The periosteum and elevated muscles constitute the first layer. The platysma and subcutaneous tissue are closed in a second layer, followed by the skin.

A combination of a ventrolateral approach to the caudal part of the body and to the ramus of the mandible, and the lateral approach to the temporomandibular joint, has been described.[4] This requires the subperiosteal elevation of the masseteric muscle from its insertion on the ventral border of the mandible in a dorsal direction, as well as freeing its origin on the zygomatic arch. This can potentially compromise the blood and nerve supply to this muscle. In addition, the two incisions create a relatively narrow strip of skin.

Lateral approach to the zygomatic arch

The patient is positioned in lateral recumbency with the neck extended and supported with a padded area. Once the zygomatic arch has been identified by digital palpation, the skin incision follows the ventral or dorsal border of the zygomatic arch and is extended as needed caudally or rostrally (Fig. 27.4A). The periosteum is subsequently incised, and the masseter and temporal muscles subperiosteally elevated and retracted using scalpel blade and periosteal elevator (Fig. 27.4B). The medial aspect of the zygomatic arch is separated from its muscular attachment using a periosteal elevator. The entire lateral and medial aspects of the zygomatic arch can be easily exposed.[3] Closure is usually achieved in three layers. The periosteum and elevated muscles constitute the first layer. The platysma and subcutaneous tissue are closed in a second layer, followed by the skin.

Lateral approach to the temporomandibular joint (TMJ)[4]

The patient is positioned in lateral recumbency with the neck extended and supported with a padded area. Once the zygomatic arch has been identified by digital palpation, the skin incision follows the ventral border of the zygomatic arch and crosses the TMJ caudally (Fig. 27.5A). The platysma muscle, directly under the skin, is incised on the same line. The origin of the masseter muscle is incised on the ventral border of the zygomatic arch and elevated using a periosteal elevator. The masseter muscle is retracted in rostroventral direction, avoiding nearby neurovascular structures. The TMJ is identified on the caudal

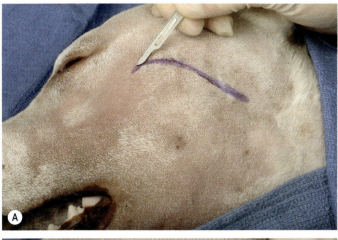

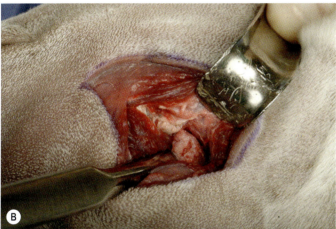

Fig. 27.5 Lateral approach to the TMJ shown in a cadaver head. (**A**) The skin incision follows the ventral border of the zygomatic arch and crosses the TMJ caudally. (**B**) Following elevation and retraction of the origin of the masseter muscle and incising the fibrous capsule, the TMJ is identified.

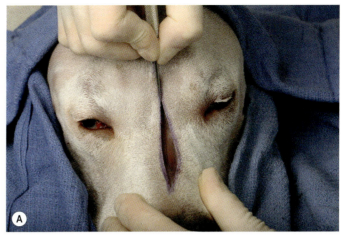

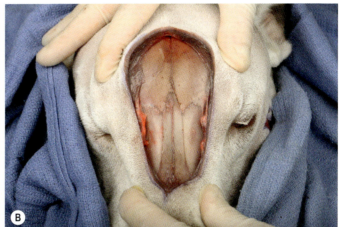

Fig. 27.6 Extraoral approach to the maxillae, nasal bones and frontal sinuses shown in a cadaver head. (**A**) A dorsal midline incision is made depending on the location of the fracture. (**B**) Following periosteal incision, the tissues are retracted to expose the bones.

aspect of the zygomatic arch (Fig. 27.5B). If possible (e.g., the jaw is not locked) opening and closing the jaw may help to identify the joint. The joint capsule is incised rostrolaterally and the condylar process partially visualized by manipulating the mandible. Closure is usually achieved in three layers. The periosteum and elevated muscles constitute the first layer. The platysma and subcutaneous tissue are closed in a second layer, followed by the skin.

Extraoral approach to the maxillae, nasal bones and frontal sinuses[7]

The patient is positioned in sternal recumbency with the head elevated on a padded area. A dorsal midline skin incision is made (Fig. 27.6A). If the fractures are at the maxillae or nasal bones, the incision is made beginning at the caudal end of the incisive bones and extends caudally to the area parallel to the zygomatic process of the frontal bones, midline between the orbits. If the frontal sinus must be exposed, the dorsal midline incision is centered on the location that parallels the zygomatic process of the frontal bone, beginning from midline between the orbits and extending caudally to the rostral end of the sagittal crest. The periosteum is incised on the midline and reflected using a periosteal elevator to expose the bones (Fig. 27.6B). Care

should be taken since the bone plates in these areas are very thin and can be perforated in the fractured area with excessive force. Closure is performed in two layers: the periosteum and connective tissue in one layer and the skin in the second layer. Often, a Stent bandage is used to prevent postoperative emphysema.

Intraoral approach to the maxilla[2,3,5]

The patient is positioned in dorsal or lateral recumbency with the neck extended and supported with a padded area. The incision is usually placed 3–5 mm away from the mucogingival junction, leaving the unattached mucosa on the alveolus to facilitate closure (Fig. 27.7A). This tissue is elastic and contracts following incision, although during closure the tissue can be grasped and holds sutures well. Alternatively, a sulcular incision using a scalpel blade and elevation of the attached gingiva and the mucosa with a periosteal elevator, as performed for surgical extractions, could be performed. The incision extends as far caudally and rostrally as needed, depending on the fractured area, to provide exposure.[2,3] Using a periosteal elevator, subperiosteal dissection and elevation proceeds to elevate the mucosa, submucosa and facial muscles, exposing the underlying tissue. The infraorbital neurovascular bundle is identified by dissecting medially and laterally to the location of the infraorbital canal, working toward the bundle

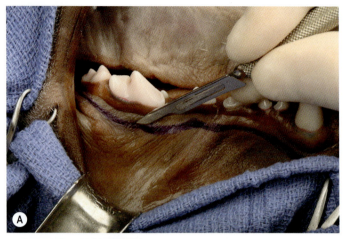

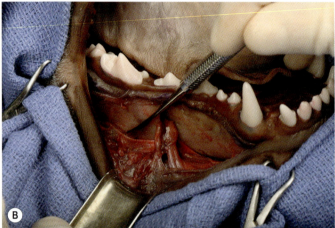

Fig. 27.7 Intraoral approach to the maxillae in a cadaver head. (**A**) The incision is placed 3–5 mm away from the mucogingival junction and extends caudally and rostrally as needed. (**B**) Subperiosteal dissection using a periosteal elevator exposes the underlying tissues. Note the location of the infraorbital foramen and its associated vasculature, as damage to these structures should be avoided.

(Fig. 27.7B). The bundle is encountered and the periosteum is dissected completely around the foramen if needed. In general, the infraorbital artery, vein and nerves should be avoided, as damaging them may cause impairment to blood supply to the fractured area and loss of sensation. If the incision should extend to the caudal maxilla, the facial vein will be encountered as it joins the deep facial vein near the levator nasolabialis muscle. The rostral aspect of the zygomatic bone will be exposed at the level of the maxillary molar teeth. If needed, the masseter muscle attachments can be elevated using a periosteal elevator. Closure is usually achieved in one layer for the submucosa and mucosa in a simple interrupted pattern.

POSTOPERATIVE CARE AND ASSESSMENT

Postoperative care is dependent on the fracture site and severity as well as on the general health of the patient. However, general guidelines apply to all mandibular and maxillofacial trauma repairs. During the immediate postoperative period, soft food and pain management are indicated, and mouth play or chewing activity should be avoided. Thereafter, the patient should be stimulated to use its jaws actively. Antibiotic therapy may be indicated, depending on the extent of the trauma. Postoperative nutritional support via feeding tube should be considered, especially in cats. If an extraoral approach was used, the skin sutures should be removed after 10–14 days. Absorbable sutures are typically used for an intraoral approach, so suture removal is not necessary in these cases. A 0.05% chlorhexidine gluconate solution can be used as an oral antiseptic rinse to keep the wound or incision area clean and to limit the negative effects of food accumulation. As a general rule, maxillofacial fracture repair typically is evaluated radiographically at 6 weeks postoperatively. Following confirmation of adequate healing, the pet may return to normal eating, playing and chewing activities.

REFERENCES

1. Piermattei DL, Johnson KA. The head. In: Piermattei DL, Johnson KA, editors. An atlas of surgical approaches to the bones and joints of the dog and cat. 4th ed. Philadelphia, PA: Elsevier – Saunders; 2004. p. 33–45.

2. Härle F. Surgical approaches. In: Härle F, Champy M, Terry BC, editors. Atlas of craniomaxillofacial osteosynthesis. Stuttgart & New York: Thieme; 1999. p. 15–26.

3. Ellis III E, Zide MF. Surgical approaches to the facial skeleton. Baltimore, MD: Williams & Wilkins; 1995.

4. Piermattei DL, Flo GL, DeCamp CE. Fractures and luxations of the mandible and maxilla. In: Piermattei DL, Flo GL, DeCamp CE, editors. Brinker, Piermattei, and Flo's handbook of small animal orthopedics and fracture repair. 4th ed. Philadelphia, PA: Elsevier – Saunders; 2006. p. 717–36.

5. Smith MM, Waldron DR. Oral and maxillofacial surgery. In: Smith MM, Waldron DR, editors. Atlas of approaches for general surgery of the dog and cat.

Philadelphia, PA: WB Saunders; 1993. p. 58–71.

6. von Werthern CJ, Bernasconi CE. Application of the maxillofacial mini-plate compact 1.0 in the fracture repair of 12 cats/2 dogs. Vet Comp Orthop Traumatol 2000;13:92–6.

7. Smith MM, Waldron DR. Ear, nose, and throat surgery. In: Smith MM, Waldron DR, editors. Atlas of approaches for general surgery of the dog and cat. Philadelphia, PA: WB Saunders; 1993. p. 16–21.

Chapter 28

Symphyseal separation and fractures involving the incisive region

Ulrike Matis & Roberto Köstlin

CLASSIFICATION AND INCIDENCE

Mandible

Injury to the incisive region of the mandible may involve the mandibular symphysis and the alveoli of the first incisor, second incisor and/or third incisor teeth, as well as the canine teeth. In dogs, alveolar fractures and separation of the mandibular symphysis occur with nearly equal frequency, whereas in cats, symphyseal separation is by far the most common injury. The second most frequent injury is fracture of the distal aspect of the alveolus of the canine tooth; in cats, the alveoli of the incisor teeth are seldom involved.

The percentage of mandibular injuries involving the rostral region ranges from 30% to 45% in dogs and from 56% to 78% in cats.[1–7] Symphyseal separations in dogs and cats have been classified based on the amount of tissue damage.[8] In type I lesions no soft tissue laceration is present. Type II lesions are characterized by soft tissue laceration, while in type III lesions major soft tissue trauma, comminution and exposure of bone, and fractured teeth are present. The proportion of open fractures among all fractures in the incisive region has been reported to be 90% in the dog.[2]

Maxilla and incisive bone

In dogs, injury to the rostral maxilla involves mainly alveolar fractures with luxation or subluxation of the incisors and/or canine teeth. In contrast, midline separation of the hard palate is the most common injury in cats, with about a third of all injuries involving the interincisive suture and the remainder the maxillary palatine process and the horizontal part of the palatine bone.[5] Overall, maxillary fractures occur less frequently than mandibular fractures. Of 171 canine and 428 feline jaw fractures, only 16% and 37% involved the maxilla, respectively.[3,5]

Concomitant injuries

Concomitant trauma to the skull and brain are common in animals with jaw injuries, particularly maxillary fractures. Ocular injuries may complicate the clinical presentation. Blunt trauma to the thorax as well as limb injuries may also occur. Multiple injuries are particularly common in cats that incur jaw fractures, which occur mainly after falling from a great height; according to one author, as many as 70% of these cats may be affected by multiple injuries.[5] In dogs, the most frequent causes of multiple injuries are being hit by a car and fighting with another dog. Thus, a thorough physical examination is imperative to recognize and treat life-threatening injuries promptly. Thoracic radiographs are of great importance in cats to assess anesthetic risks and should be obtained routinely in trauma patients.

DIAGNOSIS

Clinical findings

Characteristic signs of jaw injuries are malocclusion, abnormal movement and abnormal position of teeth. Non-specific signs include pain, epistaxis, ptyalism, often with blood-tinged saliva, and anorexia or reluctance to eat. A diagnosis can usually be made based on the clinical signs. However, radiography or other imaging modalities are necessary to determine precisely the course of the fracture.

Diagnostic imaging

Correct radiographic views are generally obtained by using the parallel technique; the X-ray beam is at a right angle to the film, which is parallel to the body part being radiographed. Because this is not possible within the oral cavity, the bisecting angle technique may be used to provide a reasonable radiographic image with linear accuracy, although the dimensional accuracy of the parallel technique may be lacking. Both techniques can be used for extraoral views. For images of the incisive region, intraoral projections with the X-ray beam at right angles to the film may also be adequate.

Complex fractures that involve not only the rostral jaw area but also the skull and temporomandibular joint, in particular, are best imaged using computed tomography. Magnetic resonance imaging is useful for the assessment of soft tissue lesions. Three-dimensional reconstruction using transverse computed tomographic images provides rapid topographical information, which is needed for establishing a

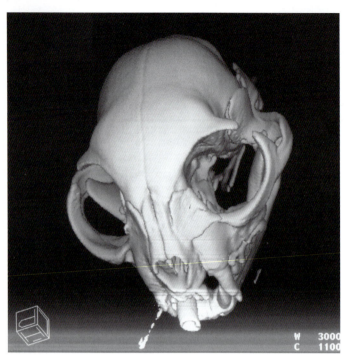

Fig. 28.1 Three-dimensional reconstruction of multiple skull fractures in a cat with a fracture of the left maxilla and an impression fracture further caudally in the parietal region. *(Reprinted with permission from: Beck W, Hecht S, Matis U. Dreidimensionale Rekonstruktion aus CT-Transversalbildern zur Darstellung komplexer Schädelfrakturen bei der Katze. Tierärztl Prax 2000;28:219–224.)*

prognosis and treatment plan for patients with multiple fractures (Fig. 28.1). However, fissures and small cracks that are easily seen on transverse images may be obscured and therefore missed in three-dimensional reconstructions.

ANESTHETIC CONSIDERATIONS

Life-threatening injuries must be ruled out and the patient stabilized before anesthesia is carried out (see Ch. 4). Pharyngotomy endotracheal intubation (see Chs 4 and 57) is typically not required for fractures of the rostral mandible or maxilla. When the jaws must be fixed in a closed position, drugs that are known to cause vomiting are contraindicated because of the risk of aspiration. As well, one must ensure that the patient can breathe adequately. This is particularly important in animals with complex fractures of the maxilla.

SURGICAL ANATOMY

Topographical anatomy

The mandibular symphysis joins the bodies of the right and left mandibles and is composed of fibrocartilage and connective tissue, which remain as such for life without being converted to bone (*synchondrosis et sutura intermandibularis*). The dorsal edge of the incisive region (*pars incisiva*) contains the alveoli of the incisor and canine teeth. The mandibular incisor and canine teeth are closer together than those of the maxilla. This enables the lingual surface of the maxillary incisor teeth to slide past the buccal or labial surface of the mandibular incisor teeth upon jaw closure. However, there are exceptions to the normally

secodont occlusion of carnivores; depending on the breed, maxillary brachygnathism can occur in brachycephalic dog and cat breeds and a relative mandibular prognathism in dolichocephalic dog breeds (e.g., dachshund, collie and some of the terrier breeds).

The maxillary incisor teeth are anchored in the alveoli (*alveoli dentales*) of the incisive bone (*os incisivum*). Its nasal process (*processus nasalis*) forms part of the rostral border of the nasal cavity, and its palatine process (*processus palatinus*), together with the palatine process of the maxillary bone (*processus palatinus*) and the palatine bone (*os palatinum*) caudally, form the hard palate. The interincisive suture, and the median palatine sutures (*sutura palatina mediana*) of the palatine processes of the maxillary bones and of the palatine bones are where these three structures unite in the midline to form a bony plate that serves as the roof of the oral cavity as well as the floor of the nasal cavity.

The roots of the incisor and canine teeth both in the upper and lower jaws are surrounded by only a thin layer of bone. Thus, it can be difficult to secure implants, particularly in the incisive region of the mandible. In the upper jaw, the roots of the incisor teeth are oval and laterally compressed in cross-section and are situated in separated alveoli, which converge medially. In contrast, the smaller incisor teeth of the lower jaw have roots that are straighter and sit in alveoli that may not be fully separated from each other. From mesial to distal, that is from the first to the third incisor teeth, the teeth increase in strength and size in both the mandible and maxilla. When the mouth is closed, the mandibular canine teeth occupy the interval between the maxillary third incisor and canine teeth, and the maxillary third incisor teeth occupy the interproximal space between the third incisor and canine teeth of the lower jaw.

The canine teeth sit between the third incisor and first premolar teeth. The conical and pointed crown is slightly curved caudally. In adult dogs, the large root of the canine tooth overlays the roots of the first and second premolar teeth. In cats, the incisor teeth are very small and thin, and their dagger-like canine teeth point slightly outwards. As in dogs, the mandibular canine teeth of cats sit between the maxillary third incisor and canine teeth when the mouth is closed and the occlusion is normal. The maxillary canine teeth, whose tips have a slightly buccal orientation, occlude between the mandibular canine and first premolar teeth.

In addition to establishing correct dental occlusion, care must be taken to preserve the vascular perfusion and innervation of the tissue. The infraorbital artery (*arteria infraorbitalis*), which is a branch of the maxillary artery (*arteria maxillaris*), supplies the rostral part of the maxilla. The inferior alveolar artery (*arteria alveolaris inferior*), also a branch of the maxillary artery, supplies the rostral part of the mandible. The infraorbital nerve (*nervus infraorbitalis*), which is the largest branch of the maxillary nerve (*nervus maxillaris*), innervates the maxillary incisor area including the canine teeth, and the mandibular incisive region is innervated by the inferior alveolar nerve (*nervus alveolaris inferior*), which is a branch of the mandibular nerve (*nervus mandibularis*). In the mandible, the majority of vessels and nerves exit the mandibular canal through three mental foramina, the most rostral of which is situated below the second incisor tooth. The middle and caudal foramina are located at the level of the second and third premolar teeth in dogs and interproximal between the canine and third premolar teeth and at the level of the third premolar tooth in cats. Provided that these structures are not already damaged by the initial trauma, care must be taken to preserve them during preparation, repositioning and fixation of the fracture.

Biomechanical considerations

As mentioned before, the roots of the canine and incisor teeth occupy almost the entire rostral region of the mandible and maxilla. Thus, the stabilization technique used must not depend on implants that are anchored in the bone. To obtain maximum stability with small implants, naturally occurring biomechanical forces must be taken advantage of. In human beings, the forces exerted on the mandible and maxilla during functional use have been investigated, and it appears that the biomechanical conditions are similar to those in dogs and cats. It is known that the greatest tractional forces occur along the alveolar process of the maxilla and mandible and that, in turn, the greatest compression forces occur along the ventral border of the body of the mandible. The bending moments on the mandible increase from cranial to caudal, whereby not only tractional and compression forces occur but also shearing and torsional forces. Torsional forces are particularly prominent rostral to the canine teeth and are greatest in the mandibular symphysis. Thus, by following the principles of tension band fixation, stabilization techniques in the rostral region of the jaw should be aimed at preventing the separation of bone fragments in the alveolar region.

THERAPEUTIC DECISION-MAKING

Conservative management versus surgical treatment

The goal of treatment is restoration of normal function and occlusion although anatomically perfect positioning of all the teeth may not always be possible. For practical purposes, this goal is achieved provided that unimpaired jaw closure is possible. The extraction of a tooth may be necessary to accomplish this. The decision between conservative and surgical treatment depends on the degree of malocclusion and the stability of the fracture. Non- or only mildly displaced fractures that are reasonably stable and allow normal occlusion, as judged by the position of the canine teeth, can be managed conservatively. For example, the majority of traumatic injuries to the hard palate can be left to heal on their own, and other, minimally displaced and fairly stable fractures of the maxilla do not require surgical

intervention. Details of conservative treatment are described in Chapter 29. Injuries of the rostral mandible usually require surgical repair, which is generally minimally invasive.

SURGICAL TECHNIQUES

Separation of the mandibular symphysis

These injuries are usually repaired using the circummandibular cerclage wiring technique. A transfixation pin is rarely indicated to secure the mandibles in position if there is loss of bone rostrally, and thus poor stability.

Cerclage wiring

Various modifications of this technique exist.[9] The authors prefer an intraoral approach. The lower lip is retracted, and a hypodermic needle is pushed through the junction of the attached gingiva and alveolar mucosa caudal to the canine tooth. It is advanced to the ventral surface of the mental region. A piece of orthopedic wire is inserted into the needle, which is then withdrawn, leaving the wire pointing in the desired direction. The needle is then inserted through the oral mucosa behind the canine tooth on the opposite side in an identical manner and the wire is located and inserted into the needle in a retrograde fashion. By advancing the wire and withdrawing the needle, the wire is advanced through the tissue without damaging it. The free ends of the cerclage wire are lightly twisted together caudolateral to one of the canine teeth at the interalveolar margin. After repositioning of the mandibles and confirming proper occlusion, the cerclage wire is tightened. The wire twist is shortened to two or three twists and, observing the direction of the twists, bent and positioned along the gingiva to prevent trauma to the tongue and lower lip (Fig. 28.2). In contrast to the ventral twist technique,[9] this method allows removal of the wire after consolidation of the mandibular symphysis

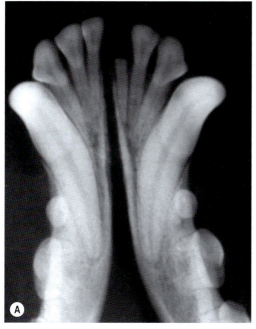 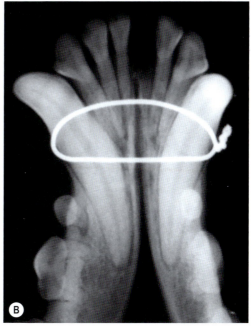

Fig. 28.2 Separation of the mandibular symphysis and fracture of the first incisor tooth in a 3-year-old dachshund: (**A**) before and (**B**) 3 months after extraction of the first incisor tooth and stabilization of the symphyseal separation using circummandibular cerclage wire. There is no ossification of the mandibular symphysis despite clinical consolidation of the fracture.

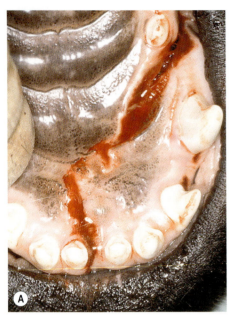
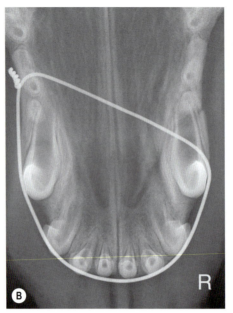
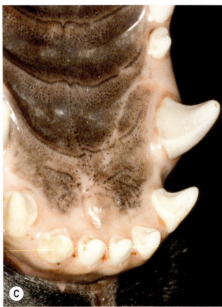

Fig. 28.3 (**A**) Fracture of the incisive bone and maxillary palatine process in a 1-year-old German shepherd dog; (**B, C**) the fractures were stabilized with cerclage wire placed over the facial surface of the incisor teeth and buccal surface of the canine teeth and between the roots of the contralateral second premolar tooth.

without making an incision. For removal, wire cutters are used to cut the cerclage wire on the side opposite the twist at the gingival margin. The twist is then grasped and the wire extracted. In this fashion, the contaminated intraoral section of wire is not pulled through the tissue during extraction. The cerclage wire is usually left in place for 6–12 weeks. In carnivores, the mandibular symphysis is usually not calcified so that consolidation should be assessed by clinical examination rather than by radiography.

Transfixation pin

In this technique, a Kirschner wire or Steinmann pin is placed through the mandibles caudal to the canine teeth without damaging the dental roots. To compress the symphysis, a cerclage wire can be placed in a figure-of-eight around the free ends of the pin, which are bent to cause small hooks at the ends. The wire twist should be situated such that it does not irritate the soft tissues. When a figure-of-eight cerclage wire is not used, a threaded K-wire or pin is recommended, the free ends of which are placed along the bone by bending. Because of the high risk of damage to the tooth roots and inferior alveolar nerve, this method should be limited to patients in which the mandibular symphysis cannot be adequately stabilized with circummandibular cerclage wire.

Palatine fractures

Suturing the gingiva is usually adequate for adaptation of bone fragments in relatively stable fractures. For unstable fragments that may result in malocclusion, osteosynthesis using cerclage wire and/or a transfixation pin or reconstruction of the dental arch using locking bone plate and screw systems is recommended.

Cerclage wiring

Oblique fractures, in which the isolated bone segment is displaced rostrolabially, can be stabilized by drawing the fragment in a contralateral direction with cerclage wire. After removing blood clots and devitalized tissue, the fragment is reduced with pointed reduction forceps. A cerclage wire is placed over the facial surface of the incisors and/or the buccal surface of the canine teeth and perpendicular to the palatine fracture line over the hard palate. Depending on the direction of the fracture line, the wire is placed caudal to the first premolar tooth on the opposite side or between the roots of the second premolar tooth. The two ends of the wire are then twisted together alongside the first premolar tooth (Fig. 28.3).

Transfixation pin

Fracture lines that run sagittally in the midline can be stabilized using a Kirschner wire, placed caudal to the canine teeth. After cleaning the fracture surfaces and compression of the fragments using pointed reduction forceps, the wire is pushed in a transverse direction through the thin palatine bony lamella until it appears on the contralateral side. The free end of the wire is bent to form a hook, and the wire is pulled back until the hook sits tightly against the maxilla. The other end of the wire end is also bent so that it lies tightly against the bone before it is shortened with side cutters (Fig. 28.4). Dislocation of the fragments does not normally occur when the pointed reduction forceps are removed. However, if it does occur, a figure-of-eight cerclage wire is placed around the bent ends of the wire and across the palate. The ends are twisted together laterally so that they do not injure the tongue or lips. Normal occlusion is achieved by closing the jaws during tightening of the cerclage wire.

Plate fixation

Plates are preferred for osteosynthesis of fractures that cannot be adequately stabilized using cerclage wire and/or transfixation pins.[10] In contrast to the mandible, plates can also be used in the incisive region of the upper jaw. Locking bone plate and screws systems are particularly well suited for this purpose because they allow a

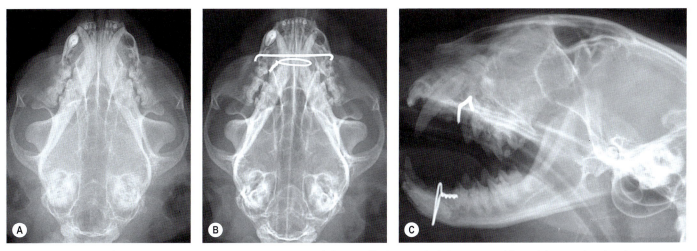

Fig. 28.4 (**A**) Fracture of the median palatine suture and separation of the mandibular symphysis in a 1-year-old cat; (**B**) ventrodorsal and (**C**) laterolateral radiographic views obtained after stabilization using a maxillary transfixation pin and circummandibular cerclage wire.

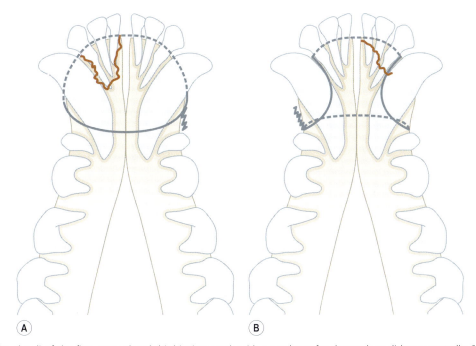

Fig. 28.5 Fracture of the alveoli of the first, second and third incisor teeth with a tendency for the teeth to dislocate rostrally. Stabilization can be achieved using cerclage wire over the facial aspect of the necks of the incisor teeth and (**A**) on the labial and (**B**) lingual surface of the necks of the canine teeth.

fixed-angle construct of the plate with screws placed between the tooth roots or proximal to the roots (see Ch. 31).

Intraoral acrylic or composite splints

Intraoral splints, which are made of self-hardening acrylic or composite, can be used to stabilize fractures of the hard palate and maxilla. The acrylic or composite can be held in position with transmaxillary wires, the free ends of which are bent to form hooks. More commonly, composite splints can also be attached to the teeth of the maxilla (see below).

Alveolar process fractures and (sub)luxation of mandibular and maxillary incisor teeth

Cerclage wiring

After removal of blood clots and devitalized tissue, the bone fragments and teeth are reduced and stabilized with a cerclage wire. One must be aware of the tendency for the teeth to dislocate. To prevent rostral displacement of teeth when the jaws are closed, the cerclage wire must be placed rostrally on the necks of the incisor teeth and caudally around the canine teeth (Figs 28.5–28.7). To prevent caudal

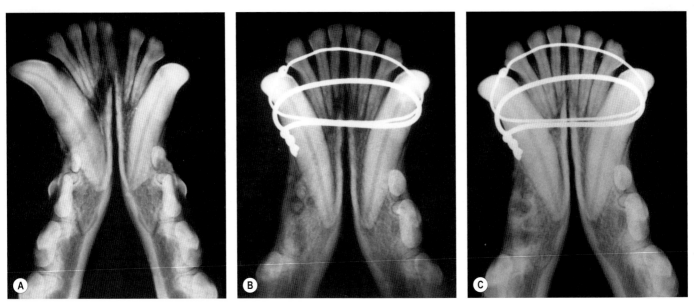

Fig. 28.6 (**A**) Fracture of the alveoli of the right mandibular canine tooth and incisor teeth and the contralateral first incisor tooth in a 3-year-old dachshund; (**B**) radiographs obtained immediately and (**C**) 6 weeks after placement of two cerclage wires on the facial surface of the incisor teeth and distal to the canine teeth.

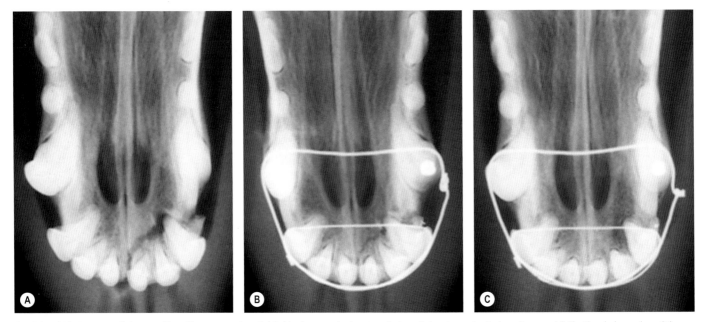

Fig. 28.7 (**A**) Fracture of the maxillary first, second and third incisor teeth that tended to dislocate rostrally in a 2-year-old Shetland sheepdog; (**B**) immediately and (**C**) 2 months after osteosynthesis using two cerclage wires on the facial surface of the necks of the incisor teeth and placed distal to the incisor and canine teeth, respectively.

displacement, the wire is placed on the caudal aspect of the neck of the reduced tooth and on the rostral surface of the necks of the normal teeth. The ends of the cerclage wire are twisted together on the labial aspect of the third incisor or the canine tooth. Rostral dislocation can also be prevented by placing an acrylic or composite splint on the incisor teeth (Fig. 28.8).

Intraoral acrylic or composite splints

Acrylic or composite splints using the acid-etch technique alone or in combination with interdental wiring or orthodontic brackets are available for the repair of alveolar process fractures and (sub)luxation of teeth (see Chs 22 and 29).[11] Intraoral splints are applied to the labial surface of the teeth in maxillary fractures and to the lingual surface of the teeth in mandibular fractures, if covering the entire crown would cause occlusal interference. An etching gel (~40% phosphoric acid gel) is applied to the enamel surface and, after cleaning and air-drying, a bonding agent is applied to the etched surface so that the composite material adheres securely. Depending on the material used, the composite splint either polymerizes on its own or is light-cured. During hardening, the fragments must be maintained in reduction with correct dental occlusion. The splint is then smoothed. The strength of the composite splint and the adhesive surface area can be increased

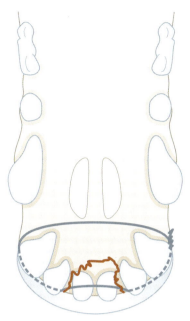

Fig. 28.8 Bilateral fracture of the alveoli of both first incisor teeth with a tendency to dislocate caudally and rostrally – these fractures can be stabilized with cerclage wire and a composite splint.

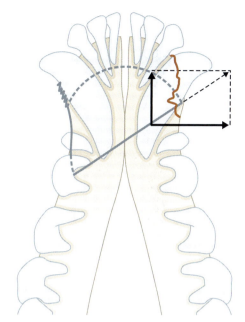

Fig. 28.9 Fracture of the alveolus of a canine tooth with a tendency to dislocate rostrally and laterally – stabilization can be achieved with cerclage wire placed around the necks of the canine and incisor teeth and between the roots of the contralateral second premolar tooth.

by integrating interdental wiring techniques. Brackets and buttons can be used with larger teeth.

After the fracture has healed, the splint is removed by sectioning the acrylic or composite material interdentally with a bur and removing the splint in segments using bond-removing forceps. The teeth are selectively polished after removal of the splint.

Alveolar process fractures and (sub)luxation of mandibular and maxillary canine teeth

Cerclage wiring

The techniques used are very similar to those used for stabilization of subluxation or luxation of the incisors. As with incisor teeth, the tendency for the canine teeth to dislocate must be considered before application of cerclage wire. When the affected tooth tends to move rostrally and labially upon jaw closure, the cerclage wire is placed rostrally around the necks of both canine teeth and around the first premolar tooth or between its roots on the side opposite the affected tooth. The ends of the wire are twisted together at the alveolar margin of the first premolar tooth (Figs 28.9 and 28.10). To prevent labial dislocation of a reduced canine tooth, the cerclage wire can be placed in a figure-of-eight around the necks of both canine teeth and the ends twisted together alongside the healthy canine tooth (Fig. 28.11). The different methods of cerclage wiring can be combined when needed. To prevent slippage, the cerclage wire can be secured to the teeth with composite.

Intraoral acrylic or composite splints

As described for alveolar process fractures, subluxation and luxation of the incisor teeth, intraoral splints, with or without brackets, buttons and interdental wiring, can be used to stabilize a canine tooth when wire alone is inadequate.

Labial reverse suture through buttons

This method is indicated for caudoversion of the canine teeth, which is sometimes seen in cats that have fallen from a great height. It can also be used to treat a jaw luxation that is unstable as well as concomitant fractures of the temporomandibular joint of cats. The mandible is stabilized with the mouth closed for 8–10 days, which allows consolidation of the injury with correct dental occlusion.

The caudally dislocated canine teeth are reduced to their normal position. Nonabsorbable suture material is then used to close the lips in a mattress pattern. The suture material is placed through buttons to distribute the pressure and tied loosely. The suture material is placed through the lips at their base at the mucogingival junction. The suture material is placed rostral to the canine teeth on both sides of the upper lip and through the midline of the lower lip (Fig. 28.12). Provided that the reduced canine teeth remain fairly stable, the suture can be tied loosely enough to allow the cat to lap up fluid with its tongue. However, if a tighter closure is required, a nasal, pharyngeal or esophageal feeding tube must be placed (see Ch. 5). A pharyngeal or esophageal feeding tube is preferred in patients with respiratory distress due to concurrent maxillary fractures. Cooperative cats can be fed fluid food with a syringe via the vestibulum of the lips. The advantage of labial reverse sutures for jaw stabilization is that, unlike the composite technique, the patient loses less saliva, thereby decreasing the risk of an acid–base imbalance.

POSTOPERATIVE CARE AND ASSESSMENT

Postoperative care consists of feeding wet food and the administration of antibiotics such as amoxicillin with clavulanic acid, clindamycin or a cephalosporin for 3–5 days, particularly in patients with open fractures (see Ch. 3). The client is encouraged to have the patient reassessed regularly. In uncomplicated injuries, such as separation of the mandibular symphysis, reevaluation is generally at 6–8 weeks

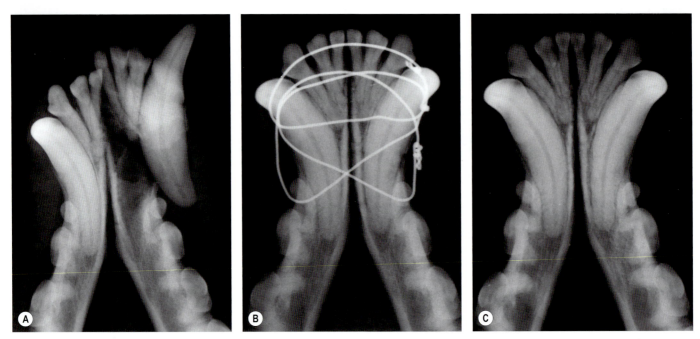

Fig. 28.10 Fracture of the alveoli of the canine tooth and the first, second and third incisor teeth with luxation of the teeth in a 4-year-old Münsterländer dog: (**A**) preoperative radiograph; radiographs obtained (**B**) immediately and (**C**) 4 months after fixation using three cerclage wires.

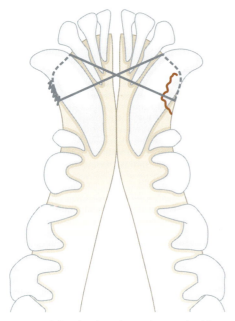

Fig. 28.11 Fracture of the alveolus of a canine tooth with a tendency to dislocate labially – the tooth can be stabilized with a figure-of-eight cerclage wire.

postoperatively, provided that the client can confirm normal food intake and occlusion. Alveolar process fractures that tend to be unstable should be reassessed at shorter intervals. Reexaminations should evaluate not only fracture healing but also whether the client is capable of performing the necessary oral hygiene in the patient. The latter includes routine removal of food particles without jeopardizing the stability of the fixation, particularly in animals with intraoral wires

and splints. In uncooperative patients, sedation or a brief anesthesia is recommended to carry out routine oral hygiene procedures. The authors advocate the use of a waterpick (Waterpik Dental Systems, Water Pik Technologies, Newport Beach, CA), set at low water pressure, for cleaning the oral cavity.

Fractures of the alveolar process are often associated with periodontal trauma and devitalization of teeth. Appropriate dental treatment is indicated if dental injuries and complications have occurred (see Ch. 22).[12]

COMPLICATIONS

Osteomyelitis is the most serious complication but rarely occurs after injuries of the incisive region of the mandible and maxilla (see Ch. 34). Osseous inflammation that is unresponsive to antibiotics is usually seen in fractures with inadequate fixation. It is important to remember that treating biomechanical deficits with antibiotics is futile. Thus, stabilization of jaw fractures is an absolute priority. For infections of the jaw bones, the choice of an appropriate antibiotic is discussed in Chapter 3. When the injury in the incisive region fails to heal, resection is possible without major functional impairment. However, incisivectomy and mandibulectomy of the incisive region due to injury are uncommon treatments.[13]

PROGNOSIS

There are numerous reports in the veterinary literature describing surgical methods and their indications, but not many that analyze the results of repair techniques in a representative group of patients. At the Ludwig Maximilians University in Munich, the authors carried out clinical and radiographic evaluations of 56 dogs with fractures of the incisive region and/or the alveolar process, which had been stabilized

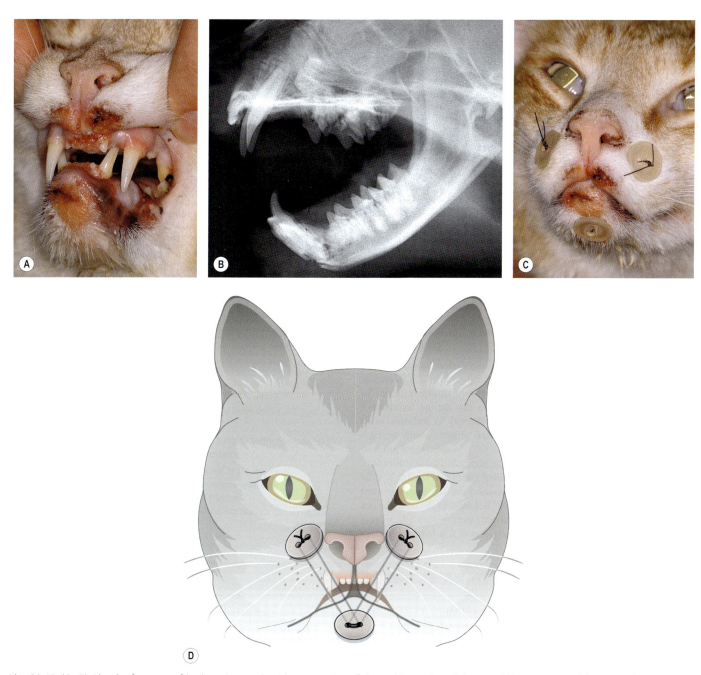

Fig. 28.12 (**A**, **B**) Alveolar fractures of both canine teeth with retroversion of the incisive region of the mandible in a 1-year-old cat; (**C**, **D**) the jaws were closed ensuring dental occlusion using a labial reverse suture through buttons.

with wire; 52 (93%) had normal jaw function after healing.[1] Of 45 dogs and 49 cats with injuries of the incisive region, 86% and 90%, respectively, had a good outcome.[2,4] We conclude therefore that the majority of rostral jaw fractures can be repaired successfully with a minimum of technical expenditure. For fractures that cannot be adequately stabilized with wire or additional intraoral splint techniques alone, alternative techniques such as maxillary/mandibular transfixation pins are available to restore normal jaw function. Partial jaw resection is a rarely used last resort. In the authors' experience, temporary lip closure using a labial reverse suture through buttons has a good prognosis in most feline cases requiring stability to the

mandible by the interdigitation of the canine teeth. With this relatively simple procedure, unimpaired jaw function was achieved in 67 of 72 (93%) cats that underwent clinical and radiographic reevaluation postoperatively.[14]

In human medicine, tooth luxation has a very guarded prognosis because of frequent tooth root resorption and crown fractures due to dental ankylosis. There is very little information about this subject in the veterinary literature (see Ch. 22). The authors have had only a few cases that were available for reevaluation over several months. However, it appears that the prognosis for tooth luxation in animals is better than that suggested in the human literature.

characteristics mandate that interdental methods be applied without interfering with occlusion. For example, since the premolar region is not occlusal, interdental acrylic or composite can be applied to both the buccal and lingual/palatal surfaces. However, the shearing occlusal characteristics in the caudal and rostral aspects of the oral cavity require unilateral acrylic or composite placement. Interdental material applied to the buccal aspect of the caudal mandibular teeth would be prone to failure following repeated biting forces emanating from the maxillary fourth premolar tooth.

When considering noninvasive techniques for mandibular fracture, tooth anatomy is also a factor. The majority of canine and feline teeth are conical or pyramidal in shape. The tooth neck is minimal, and located below the free gingival margin. These morphologic characteristics indicate that interdental wiring techniques must be applied to teeth in a subgingival location with subsequent gingivitis being a side effect of the procedure. Application of interdental wire coronal to the gingival margin is associated with fixation failure as the wire migrates or slips coronally.

Special instruments and materials

The equipment required for application of intraoral splints is not extensive or cost-prohibitive, and includes: acid-etchant, acrylic or composite, orthopedic wire, wire cutter, needle holder, and an acrylic bur.

Acid-etchants or conditioners are relatively strong acids (pH ≈ 1.0).[5] Phosphoric acid solutions and gels (37%, 35%, 10%) are considered to produce the most reliable etching patterns. These gels flow under slight pressure but, unlike liquids, do not flow under their own weight. The gel composition is preferred to avoid irritation to gingival tissues.

Enamel prisms are composed of hydroxyapatite crystals that form 89% of the enamel structure. Phosphoric acid etching of enamel dissolves enamel crystals in each prism. The etched enamel surface provides for micromechanical retention of restorative and acrylic materials.[5] Sufficient etching is obtained after application for the time specified by the manufacturer and is seen clinically by the appearance of a 'frosty' etching pattern on the enamel surface.

Polymethyl methacrylate polymers have been used as denture base materials since 1937.[5] Applications for acrylic polymers in prosthetic dentistry include denture repair materials, artificial teeth, facings in crown and bridge restorations, impression trays, record bases, temporary crowns, and obturation devices for cleft palate. The powder–liquid form of polymethyl methacrylate (Lang Jet acrylic, Henry Schein, Port Washington, NY) is chemically activated, or 'cold-curing,' which means no extrinsic heat is required for polymerization.[6] However, heat is produced during curing. This form of polymethyl methacrylate is inexpensive, but requires greater mixing times and produces a noxious odor compared with light-cured acrylics and composite materials. The heat generated during acrylic curing may cause thermal injury to the teeth, although a previous study indicated that there was no histopathologic evidence of thermal injury to the pulp 3 months following application of cold-curing polymethyl methacrylate splints in a canine bilateral mandibular fracture model.[7] Light-activated resins, supplied in premixed sheets, ropes or gel (Triad® VLC, Dentsply-Trubyte, York, PA) require no mixing and create no odor, but the incremental curing of large surfaces at 400–500 nm is time-consuming.[5]

Composite-based temporary crown and bridge materials (Maxi-Temp, Henry Schein, Port Washington, NY; Protemp 3 Garant, 3M-ESPE, Norristown, PA) are bisacrylate composites consisting of an organic matrix and inorganic fillers, similar to the composite restoratives. They have several advantages compared with conventional and light-cured acrylics (Fig. 29.1). The double-barreled, automix delivery system allows for quick, easy extrusion of the homogeneous material

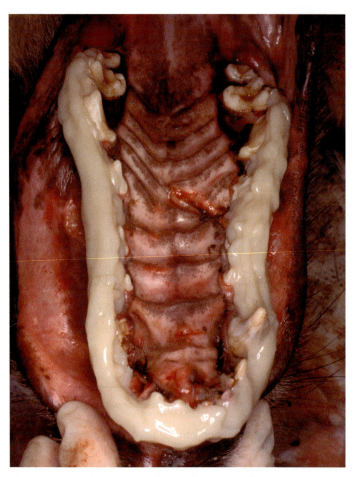

Fig. 29.1 Intraoral composite splint used for repair of a comminuted maxillary fracture in a dog. *(From Legendre L. Intraoral acrylic splints for maxillofacial fracture repair.* J Vet Dent *2003;20:70–78.)*

without voids. The self-curing polymerization process is not associated with noxious odors, and the composite material has similar mechanical properties to conventional acrylics. Although composite temporization materials are relatively expensive, each delivery system is multiuse, with a long shelf life.

Orthopedic wire measuring 24 gauge is recommended for application of interdental wire. A wire size of 26 gauge is considered too small, while 22 gauge is too large for most dogs. However, 22-gauge wire is an appropriate size for very large dogs, and for circumferential wiring of an acrylic or composite splint to the mandible.

THERAPEUTIC DECISION-MAKING AND TECHNIQUES

The operative goals for maxillofacial fracture repair include the application of stable fixation techniques that are minimally invasive and restore occlusion, providing for early return to function (see Ch. 25).[8–11]

Muzzle coaptation

Muzzle coaptation may be applied during the preoperative period to temporarily stabilize oral fractures. If used, the patient should be monitored to insure the muzzle does not interfere with breathing

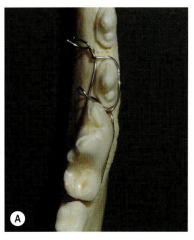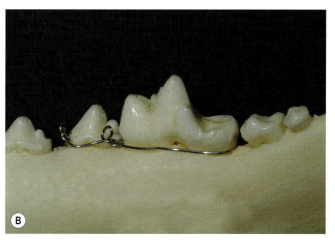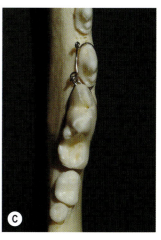

Fig. 29.2 Photographs of an osteological specimen of the right mandible showing application of the Ivy loop interdental wiring technique. (**A**) A length of wire is placed and twisted between two teeth with a resultant loop at the interdental space. (**B**) and (**C**) One free end is placed around the mesial aspect of the rostral tooth. The other free end is wrapped around the distal aspect of the caudal tooth and passed through the preformed interdental loop followed by the ends being twisted together and angled towards the coronal aspect.

status or cause unnecessary, potentially detrimental, excitement. In a 1990 study, muzzle coaptation was found to be the most common definitive stabilization technique for mandibular fractures in dogs at that time.[12] Its common use indicates that it is successful in providing bony union most of the time. However, complications and problems associated with muzzle application include malocclusion, aspiration of food secondary to vomiting, hyperthermia from impaired panting, and moist dermatitis. This fixation method is inexpensive and does not negatively affect fracture fragment vascular supply or tooth roots and neurovascular structures in the mandibular canal. Although often successful in providing fracture fragment stability sufficient to promote secondary bony healing, mandibular healing as a result of muzzle application may be associated with permanent malocclusion. Other potential complications which may occur during the treatment period include patient noncompliance, and delayed return to function related to restriction of normal mastication.[13,14] To create a custom-fitted tape muzzle, adhesive tape (2 inches in large dogs, 1 inch in smaller dogs) of appropriate length is folded on itself so that the nonsticky surface interfaces with the skin of the muzzle. The tape should limit the patient's ability to open its mouth while allowing the tongue to protrude between the incisor teeth. This degree of potential mobility allows the patient to drink water and eat food of gruel consistency. Side tapes are adhered to the muzzle tape, and then tied behind the patient's occipital area. The side tapes should be tied to a tightness level that barely allows the veterinarian's index finger between the tapes and the patient's skin. An optional third tape can be applied around the muzzle tape, coursing between the eyes, and attached to tied tapes at the occipital region. Prefabricated restraint muzzles can also be used for fracture stabilization, using the same tightness and fit guidelines mentioned previously. In general, interdental fixation methods are preferred since they restore and maintain occlusion with fewer potential complications.

Interdental wiring techniques

Interdental wire fixation methods for human maxillofacial fracture stabilization include Ivy loop, Stout loop, Risdon, and Essig wiring techniques.[15–17] The ability of these methods to provide mandibular fracture stabilization while avoiding iatrogenic complications inherent with other more conventional fixation methods makes them particularly desirable. The low cost of materials and relative ease

of application in dogs contribute to their potential uses in veterinary medicine. Their use is an economically viable alternative to muzzle coaptation since these techniques are more likely to restore occlusion while avoiding the potential complications associated with muzzles.

Ivy loop wiring technique

The objective of the Ivy loop wiring technique is to stabilize and align adjacent teeth.[17] A length of wire is placed and twisted between two teeth with a resultant loop at the interdental space. One free end is placed around the mesial aspect of the rostral tooth. The other free end is wrapped around the distal aspect of the caudal tooth and passed through the preformed interdental loop followed by the ends being twisted together (Fig. 29.2).[17]

Stout loop wiring technique

The Stout loop wiring technique supports a greater distance of the dental arch compared with the Ivy loop technique.[17] Therefore, it is more indicated as a stand-alone technique. This technique is a continuation of the Ivy loop technique whereby repetitive loops are placed around a minimum of two teeth on either side of the fracture. Loops are twisted tight as the wire is held taught in place along the teeth. The loops are twisted in a dorsal direction to lie flat against the coronal surface. Loops may be placed on the buccal or palatal/lingual surface with a preference for the side least likely to cause occlusal interference.

Risdon wiring technique

The Risdon wiring technique uses a base wire and individual interdental wires twisted around the base wire. This technique is particularly indicated for rostral fractures of the mandible and maxilla.[17] A wire is placed bilaterally around caudal anchoring teeth (mandibular first molars or maxillary fourth premolars), twisted to itself, followed by each base wire being twisted together in the first incisor region. Individual wires are placed interdentally around multiple teeth bilaterally and twisted to include the base wire (Fig. 29.3). For the aforementioned techniques, wire anchorage is best when placed in a subgingival location based on anatomic considerations mentioned previously.

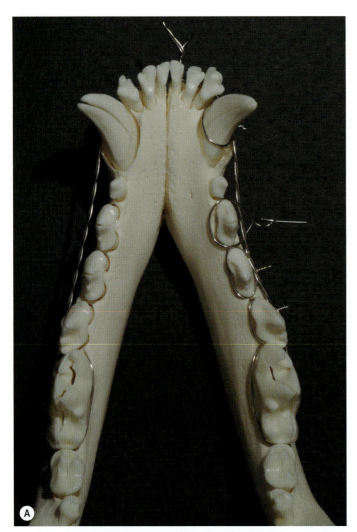

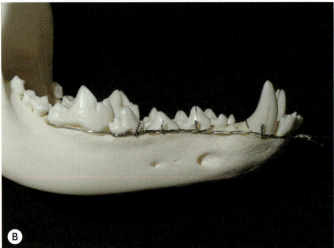

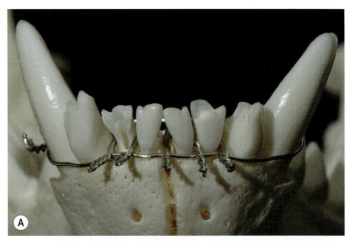

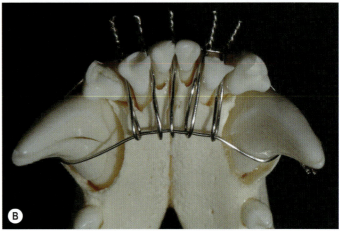

Fig. 29.4 Photographs of an osteological specimen showing application of the Essig interdental wiring technique. (**A**) The base wire is placed around canine teeth and along the rostral aspect of the incisor teeth. (**B**) Individual secondary wires are placed through the interproximal space and around the caudal and rostral aspects of the base wire. The interproximal wires are tightened to place tension on the base wire.

Essig wiring technique

Similar to the Risdon technique, the Essig wiring technique utilizes a base wire and individual wires for increased stability. The technique is particularly indicated for luxation or fracture/avulsion of canine teeth.[17] The base wire is placed around canine teeth and along the labial aspect of the incisor teeth. Individual secondary wires are placed through the interproximal space and around the caudal and rostral aspects of the base wire. The interproximal wires are tightened to place tension on the base wire. Twists are placed in a location least likely to cause occlusal interference (Fig. 29.4).

Intraoral splints combined with interdental wiring techniques

Strength in bending was determined for interdental apparati applied to canine cadaver mandibles osteotomized between the mandibular third and fourth premolar teeth. The bending strength of stainless steel wire applied using a Stout loop interdental wire technique and Erich arch bar anchored to teeth using individual interdental wires was increased by acrylic reinforcement.[18] Although acrylic does not adhere well to metal, it conforms to crown shape and interdigitates with the wire twists.[1]

Fig. 29.3 Photographs of an osteological specimen showing application of the Risdon interdental wiring technique. (**A**) A wire is placed bilaterally around the caudal anchoring teeth (mandibular first molars), twisted to itself, followed by each base wire being twisted together in the first incisor region. Individual wires are placed interdentally around multiple teeth bilaterally and twisted to include the base wire. (**B**) Wires are cut and turned coronally following tightening.

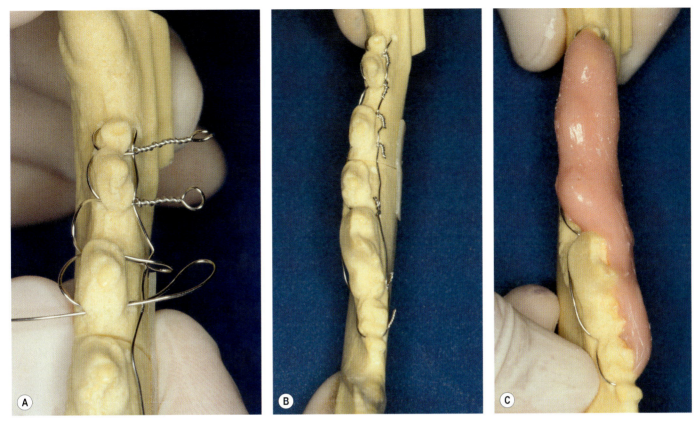

Fig. 29.5 Photographs showing application of interdental wire and acrylic in a canine mandible model. (**A**) In this example, the wire is placed using a modified Stout loop pattern. (**B**) Wire twists are located on the lingual aspect. (**C**) The acrylic is applied bilaterally in the premolar area and on the lingual aspect caudal to the mandibular first molar tooth in order to avoid occlusal interference.

Intraoral acrylic splints reinforced with interdental wiring techniques have been shown to provide for similar bony healing 16 weeks postoperatively compared with internal and external skeletal fixation.[7] Although interdental acrylic alone has superior strength in bending compared with interdental wiring techniques alone, breakage of the acrylic splint results in catastrophic failure and the necessity to restabilize the fracture. Wire-reinforced acrylic has superior strength in bending compared with either wire alone or acrylic alone.[19] Although it remains unknown how rigidly canine oral fractures must be fixed to support primary healing of bone, the combination of wire and acrylic or composite is recommended (Fig. 29.5).

Application of intraoral acrylic and composite splints

Endotracheal intubation via pharyngotomy is recommended in order to provide an unobstructed oral cavity to facilitate application of the intraoral acrylic or composite and to readily assess occlusion during the curing phase. Mandibular fracture repair using intraoral splints can be performed with the patient in sternal recumbency, contrary to the positioning for techniques requiring a ventral approach for open reduction (see Chs 6 and 25). Sternal recumbency is advantageous, as gravity facilitates the application of the acrylic or composite in this position. Maxillary fracture repair using intraoral splints is performed with the patient in dorsal recumbency.

Application of an intraoral acrylic or composite splint for fracture of the mandibular body does not specifically address the reduction of the fracture fragments. Rather, the technique emphasizes restoration of occlusion which secondarily results in bone apposition and secondary bone healing. Therefore, fracture fragment exposure and manipulation are avoided, while dental occlusion is relied upon to maintain acceptable bony alignment.

Sequentially, any exposed bone surfaces are debrided of necrotic or suspected devitalized tissue. Oral wounds and exposed bone fragments are lavaged with 0.12% chlorhexidine gluconate solution. The teeth to be incorporated into the splint are cleaned and polished using a nonfluoridated pumice wash. Polishing paste is not used because the glycerin present in polishing paste interferes with the etching and bonding processes and fluoride makes enamel more acid-resistant.[20,21] The teeth are placed in normal occlusion for the breed with bony alignment assessed by palpation of the ventral mandibles. The teeth that will receive the intraoral splint are acid-etched according to the manufacturer's directions, rinsed and dried. The acrylic or composite splinting material is applied to the acid-etched teeth. When applying the material to mandibular teeth, it is important to consider the normal occlusion of the maxillary arch in reference to the mandibular arch. Generally, it is recommended to apply the splinting material to both the lingual and buccal aspects of the premolar teeth since the maxillary and mandibular premolar teeth do not contact each other during occlusion. However, the bilateral splint application should be transitioned to lingual application only at the interdental space between the mandibular fourth premolar and first molar teeth. This spatial application of the splint avoids interference and potential implant failure during occlusion since the maxillary fourth premolar tooth and first molar tooth partially occlude on the buccal surface of the mandibular first and second molars. Additionally, application to the coronal surface of the distal aspect of the mandibular first molar and the mandibular second and third molar teeth are avoided for similar reasons. The advantage of placing an endotracheal tube via pharyngotomy is the ability to assess and maintain occlusion during the curing and hardening of the acrylic or composite. Extubation and reintubation per os during the curing phase contributes to the incidence of malocclusion postoperatively since minor discrepancies in tooth alignment may occur. Minimal discrepancies in normal tooth alignment may result in substantial malocclusion.[22] If the splinting material is applied to the occlusal surfaces of caudal mandibular teeth, occlusal assessment intraoperatively is mandatory, using a maneuver similar to taking an impression in order to minimize the amount of splinting material on the occlusal surface. If this latter technique is performed, a separating agent (such as petroleum jelly) should be applied to the teeth of the occluding quadrant. Once the splint is cured, any sharp or overhanging edges are removed using an acrylic bur. The intraoral acrylic or composite splint is unobtrusive and supports the mandible to allow early return to function with prehension of a softened, regular diet.

Intraoral splints combined with cerclage wires

Coronal application of acrylic and composite splints can be augmented using orthopedic wires to cerclage or compress the splint to the mandible (Fig. 29.6). A minimum of one wire is used to engage each fracture fragment. In order to pass each wire, a small skin incision is made ventral to the mandible. A wire is introduced ventral to the body of the mandible and slid along the buccal surface of the bone. The wire penetrates the buccal mucosa just ventral to the mucogingival junction, is looped over the dental quadrant and introduced

through a similar location on the lingual aspect of the mandible. The wire is then passed through the same ventral skin incision. The teeth are positioned in anatomic occlusion and the acrylic or composite is applied to the etched surfaces of the teeth as described previously. After the splinting material has cured to the doughy stage of polymerization, the wire ends are twisted to tighten the wire into the splint against the tooth surfaces. A final layer of acrylic or composite is added to cover the wires intraorally. A skin suture is usually not required for the ventral skin incisions.

Intraoral splints for treatment of maxillary fractures

Nondisplaced maxillary fractures may not require specific treatment. Unstable fractures causing malocclusion, facial deformity, oronasal communication or obstruction of nasal passages may also be repaired using intraoral acrylic or composite splints. The splint is applied using principles as described previously for mandibular fracture repair. However, unlike mandibular fracture repair, the splinting material is applied to the buccal surface of the maxillary teeth to avoid interference and disruption of the splint during occlusion.

Intraoral splints for salvage treatment of fractures of edentulous mandibles

Spontaneous pathologic or iatrogenic fracture of the mandible in the edentulous patient may be particularly challenging to repair. Fractures usually occur in the area of the mandibular first molar

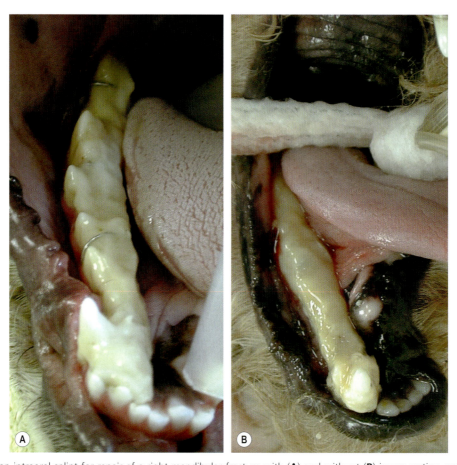

Fig. 29.6 Application of an intraoral splint for repair of a right mandibular fracture with (**A**) and without (**B**) incorporating cerclage wires placed around the mandible. *(From Legendre L. Intraoral acrylic splints for maxillofacial fracture repair. J Vet Dent 2003;20:70–7.)*

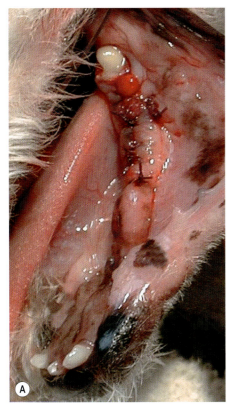 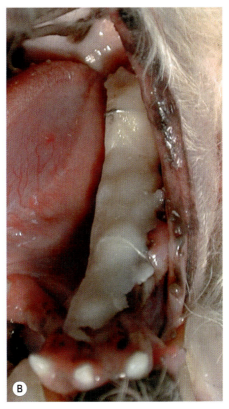 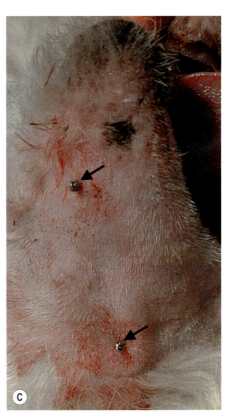

Fig. 29.7 Application of a composite splint to an edentulous left mandible: (**A**) Soft tissues are sutured, followed by (**B**) application of the splinting material directly to the mucosa, (**C**) including cerclage wires that are placed around the mandible and secured in a ventral location (*arrows*). *(From Legendre L. Intraoral acrylic splints for maxillofacial fracture repair. J Vet Dent 2003;20:70–78.)*

tooth. A typical signalment and history includes a geriatric toy-breed dog with chronic, advanced periodontal disease. Involved teeth, if still present, have to be removed. The poor bone quality makes the use of plates and screws difficult and intraosseous wiring contraindicated.

An intraoral acrylic or composite splint can also be used for mandibular fracture repair in the edentulous patient. The alveoli are debrided and lavaged with 0.12% chlorhexidine. Small mucogingival flaps may need to be raised and apposed with absorbable sutures to cover exposed alveoli (Fig. 29.7). An 18-gauge needle is inserted from the ventral edge of the mandible dorsally along the buccal surface of the mandible. A 22- or 24-gauge orthopedic wire is placed inside the needle and looped in the mouth. The needle is pulled back and redirected through the same hole but on the lingual surface of the mandible. The looped orthopedic wire is placed inside the needle and the needle is removed with both ends of the wire ventral to the mandible. Wires are placed on both the mesial and distal fragments of the mandible. Proper alignment of the mandible is confirmed, followed by application of a layer of acrylic or composite material along the length of the body of the mandible, incorporating both wire loops. The layer of splinting material should be 7–10 mm in diameter. After the material has cured to the doughy stage of polymerization, the wire ends are twisted to tighten the wire into the splint against the tooth surfaces. A final layer of splinting material is added to cover any intraoral exposure of the wires. Any rough edges or overhangs of the splinting material are removed as described previously. The intraoral splint conforms to the edentulous mandible and is secured in position by incorporation of the orthopedic wires that engage the mandibular fragments.

Maxillomandibular fixation – interdental bonding

Maxillomandibular fixation (also known as intermaxillary fixation) techniques are commonly used in humans.[23] They usually involve looping wire around teeth in both arches and subsequently joining these wires. Similar interdental wiring techniques are used rarely in the dog (see Ch. 32).[24] The use of intraoral screws and elastic bands for the more caudally located fractures in dogs has been described.[25] Screws are placed on the sides of both maxillas and mandibles. Elastic bands passed over the screw heads pull the mandible into occlusion. Placement of the screws is crucial. The bands can easily be removed should an emergency occur. Alternatively, a wire loop can be passed through holes drilled in the furcation bone of the maxillary fourth premolar and mandibular first molar teeth on both sides.[26] The same technique has been used in the cat, as well as a wire loop placed transversely through both maxillas and mandibles.[27,28]

The above techniques have largely been replaced by composite bonding of the canine teeth. Maxillofacial fractures in dogs and cats may be repaired by bonding the canine teeth together to promote secondary bony healing.[22] This technique is especially indicated for patients with multiple maxillofacial fractures not amendable to intraoral acrylic splints or other fixation techniques. It can also be used for immobilization of the temporomandibular joints following reduction of a luxation. Inclusion of the canine teeth into a composite pillar enables fixation of the mandibles and maxillas in a position that will result in restoration of occlusion following healing and removal of the bonding material.

The canine teeth are cleaned and acid-etched as described previously. The canine teeth are placed in occlusion, along with visual confirmation that the maxillary and mandibular dental arches are aligned correctly. The mouth is opened and the canine teeth are positioned to overlap by approximately one-third to one-half of the length of the crowns, allowing enough space for the patient to drink water and eat food with a liquid or gruel consistency (Fig. 29.8). A self-curing acrylic or composite is applied circumferentially around the teeth forming two posts or pillars of splinting material engaging the canine teeth (Fig. 29.9). Alternatively, the canine teeth may be placed into segments of syringe barrels or cases to serve as reinforcing molds during application and curing of the splinting material. The syringe barrel segments are left in place until removal of the splinting material.

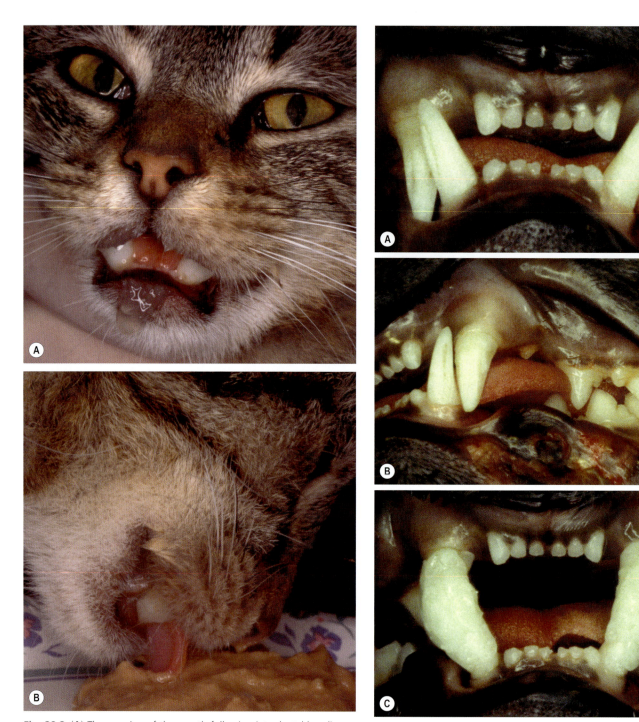

Fig. 29.8 (**A**) The opening of the mouth following interdental bonding. (**B**) The opening is sufficient for the cat to drink water and prehend food of gruel consistency. *(From Legendre L. Intraoral acrylic splints for maxillofacial fracture repair. J Vet Dent 2003;20:70–78.)*

Fig. 29.9 Occlusal assessment in a cat with maxillofacial fractures before (**A**, **B**) and after (**C**) interdental bonding. *(From Legendre L. Intraoral acrylic splints for maxillofacial fracture repair. J Vet Dent 2003;20:70–78.)*

POSTOPERATIVE CARE AND ASSESSMENT

Postoperative care

Nasoesophageal or esophageal feeding tube placement should be considered prior to anesthetic recovery, especially in patients receiving interdental bonding of canine teeth. It is not unusual for these patients to have a 24–48-hour adaptive period during which they are unwilling to eat or drink. It is easier to remove a feeding tube that is not needed than to reanesthetize the patient in order to provide oral bypass for alimentation.

The patient is usually discharged 24 hours following the procedure with instructions for the client to keep the patient supervised and provide soft food or a semiliquid diet until the examination at 5–7 days postoperatively. Chlorhexidine gluconate solution (0.12%) is provided for the client to irrigate the intraoral splint BID in order to decrease the accumulation of food and debris underneath and around the splint. A water flosser or dental water jet is also very effective for this purpose and is well-tolerated by animals.

The next examination is performed 6–8 weeks following surgery.[11] The patient is anesthetized and radiographs are obtained. Radiographic signs of bony union combined with palpable stability of the fracture indicates that the splint may be removed.

Appliance removal

The acrylic or composite splint may be scored with a cutting bur on a high-speed handpiece and removed in segments using bond removers (Direct bond remover with or without pad, Ormco, Orange, CA) or other suitable instruments (Fig. 29.10). The composite material is tooth-colored, making it imperative to remove the material very carefully in order to avoid damage to the underlying enamel. Acrylic and composite adhering to the tooth surface is removed in small increments using bond removers (Direct bond remover with or without pad, Ormco, Orange, CA) and scalers. The same method and instruments are used for removing the composite utilized for interdental bonding. Wire is cut with wire cutters or transected with the bur if embedded in acrylic or composites.

Following removal of the appliance, routine periodontal treatment including polishing is indicated to treat the gingivitis secondary to the intraoral splint and prevent long-term periodontal complications.

COMPLICATIONS

A common complication of intraoral acrylic and composite splints is inflammation of the gingiva due to trapping of food and debris between the appliance and gingiva. Sharp edges on the splint may also

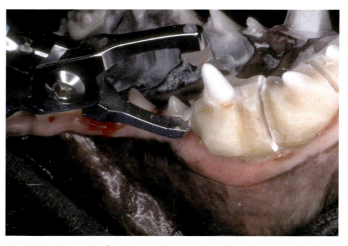

Fig. 29.10 Removal of an intraoral composite splint: the composite is scored interdentally with a cutting bur on a high-speed handpiece to facilitate composite removal with bond removing forceps.

contribute to the inflammation and should therefore be avoided. This complication may largely be prevented by meticulous oral care, as described above, and treated following removal of the appliance by routine periodontal treatment and continuation of home care.

Thermal damage to the pulp is possible when a large amount of cold-curing polymethyl methacrylate is used for making the splint.[7] This complication is rare and can be avoided altogether by using light-cured acrylics or composites.

Splint failure may be due to debonding at the composite– or acrylic–tooth interface or breakage of the material. This may be caused by material fatigue at weak spots, interference with occlusion, or self-inflicted trauma. Debonding may also be caused by technical problems, especially lack of moisture control during splint placement. Splint failure can largely be prevented by using correct technique. An Elizabethan collar may be indicated in cases of poor patient compliance.

Potential complications and problems associated with tape or nylon muzzle application include aspiration of food secondary to vomiting, hyperthermia from impaired panting, and moist dermatitis. Complications of maxillomandibular fixation using interdental bonding are also related to the inability to open the mouth while the fixation is in place.

REFERENCES

1. Weigel JP. Trauma to oral structures. In: Harvey CE, editor. Veterinary dentistry. Philadelphia, PA: WB Saunders Co; 1985. p. 140–55.

2. Strom D, Holm S, Clemensson E, et al. Gross anatomy of the craniomandibular joint and masticatory muscles of the dog. Arch Oral Biol 1987;33:597–604.

3. Cook WT, Smith MM, Markel MD, et al. Influence of an interdental full pin on stability of an acrylic external fixator for rostral mandibular fractures in dogs. Am J Vet Res 2001;62:576–80.

4. Renegar W, Leeds E, Olds R. The use of the Kirschner–Ehmer splint in clinical orthopedics: part I. long bone and mandibular fractures. Compend Contin Educ Pract Vet 1982;4:381–91.

5. Craig RG, Powers JM. Restorative dental materials. 11th ed. St. Louis, MO: Mosby; 2002.

6. Phoenix RD. Denture base resins. In: Anusavice KJ, editor. Phillips' science of dental materials. 11th ed.

Philadelphia, PA: WB Saunders Co; 2003. p. 721–57.

7. Kern D, Smith M, Stevenson S, et al. Evaluation of three fixation techniques for repair of mandibular fractures in dogs. J Am Vet Med Assoc 1995;12:1883–90.

8. Harvey CE, Emily P. Small animal dentistry. St. Louis, MO: Mosby–Year Book; 1993. p. 312–35.

9. Gorrel C, Penman S, Emily P. Small animal oral emergencies. New York: Pergamon Press; 1993. p. 37–45.

10. Wiggs RB, Lobprise HB. Veterinary dentistry: principles and practice. Philadelphia, PA: Lippincott-Raven; 1997. p. 259–79.

11. Smith MM, Kern DA. Skull trauma and mandibular fractures. Vet Clin North Am Small Anim Pract 1995;25:1127–48.

12. Umphlet RC, Johnson AL. Mandibular fractures in the dog. A retrospective study of 157 cases. Vet Surg 1990;19:272–5.

13. Withrow SJ. Taping of the mandible in treatment of mandibular fractures. J Am Anim Hosp Assoc 1981;17:27–31.

14. Dulisch M. Skull and mandibular fractures. In: Slatter DH, editor. Textbook of small animal surgery. 1st ed. Philadelphia, PA: WB Saunders Co; 1985. p. 2286–95.

15. Howard P, Wolfe SA. Fractures of the mandible. Ann Plast Surg 1986;17: 391–407.

16. Virolainen E, Aitasalo K. Surgical and conservative treatment of mandibular fractures. A follow-up study. Int J Oral Surg 1976;5:265–9.

17. Holmstrom SE, Frost P, Eisner ER. Dental orthopedics. In: Holmstrom SE, Frost P, Eisner ER, editors. Veterinary dental techniques. 2nd ed. Philadelphia, PA: WB Saunders Co; 1998. p. 470–7.

18. Black J. Orthopedic biomaterials in research and practice. New York: Churchill Livingstone; 1988.

19. Kern DA, Smith MM, Grant JW, et al. Evaluation of bending strength of five interdental fixation apparatuses applied to canine mandibles. Am J Vet Res 1993;54: 1177–82.

20. Baum L, Philips RW, Lund MR. Textbook of operative dentistry. 3rd ed. Philadelphia, PA: WB Saunders Co; 1995. p. 220–69.

21. van Amerongen JP, van Loveren C, Kidd EAM. Fundamentals of operative dentistry. A contemporary approach. 2nd ed. Quintessence Publishing Co; 2001. p. 70–90.

22. Bennett JW, Kapatkin AS, Manfra Marretta S. Dental composite for the fixation of mandibular fractures and luxations in 11 cats and 6 dogs. Vet Surg 1994;23:190–4.

23. Williams JL. Rowe and Williams' maxillofacial injuries. 2nd ed. Edinburgh: Churchill Livingstone; 1994.

24. Piermattei DL, Flo GL. Fractures and luxations of the mandible and maxilla. In: Piermattei DL, Flo GL, editors. Handbook of small animal orthopedics and fracture repair. 3rd ed. Philadelphia, PA: WB Saunders Co; 1997. p. 659–75.

25. Nibley W. Treatment of caudal mandibular fractures: a preliminary report. J Am Anim Hosp Assoc 1981;17:555–62.

26. Lantz GC. Interarcade wiring as a method of fixation for selected mandibular injuries. J Am Anim Hosp Assoc 1981; 17:599–603.

27. Lewis DD, Oakes MG, Kerwin SC, et al. Maxillary-mandibular wiring for the management of caudal mandibular fractures in two cats. J Small Anim Pract 1991;32:253–7.

28. Umphlet RC. Interarcade wiring: a method for stabilization of caudal mandibular fractures and temporomandibular joint luxations in the cat. Companion Anim Pract 1987;1(3):16–8.

Chapter | **30** |

Maxillofacial fracture repair using intraosseous wires

Randy J. Boudrieau

Intraosseous wire fixation has historically been the preferred method of maxillofacial fracture fixation in both veterinary and human medicine.[1-4] The rationale for its use was to place a small implant in a location where other modes of fixation were too large or too cumbersome to apply. The basic premise of wire fixation is to use the wire as a rigid suture to reappose and compress the fractured bone fragments together. A prerequisite for their use is that they must be placed along the lines of tension stress, which requires an understanding of the biomechanical stresses encountered. With this mode of fixation it is apparent that there is no stability imparted in compression, rotation or bending – the fixation is totally dependent upon tension and the compression provided between two perfectly apposed bone fragments. Intraosseous wire fixation therefore is limited to simple, relatively stable fractures, with well-interdigitating fracture fragments. Comminuted fractures and fractures with gaps cannot be addressed with this technique.

PREOPERATIVE CONCERNS

Objectives

Proper occlusion and rigid fixation are interrelated objectives; since fractures amenable to intraosseous wiring are relatively simple, they are treated by anatomic realignment and fixation of the bone fragments, which subsequently restores occlusion.[5-7] This anatomic reconstruction provides the necessary base for support of the soft tissues. In comminuted fractures and fractures with gaps, it is not possible to attain this degree of stability with intraosseous wire fixation; therefore, other methods need to be selected to provide the appropriate buttress support (see Chs. 29, 31 and 32).

BIOMECHANICAL, ANATOMICAL AND TECHNICAL CONSIDERATIONS

Lines of stress

The biomechanical principles of the fixation devices used for mandibular and maxillary fracture repair must include an understanding of the functional anatomy (see Ch. 25). Intraosseous wiring techniques rely on the static forces generated by the tension of the wire and by the frictional forces generated between the corresponding bone fragments.[2-4] Therefore, adequate stability for healing is provided only with accurate anatomic reduction and sufficient neutralization of two broad, opposing bone fragments.[2,3] Consequently, intraosseous wiring techniques are most successful if all bone fragments can be anatomically repositioned, thereby enabling the bone and implants to share any applied loads.[2-4] Significant comminution or bone loss precludes the ability to obtain precise anatomic apposition of the bone fragments, as it is not possible to achieve continuous interfragmentary compression across each/all bone fragments.[2-4] Intraosseous wires also only provide two-dimensional stability, as rotation continues to occur around the wires since they are passed through holes of slightly greater diameter than the wire.[2,4]

Because of the small implant size and their use as tight wires to compress two apposing fragments together, it is crucial that the biomechanical limitations of wire fixation be fully understood. These devices must be placed along the lines of tension stress in order that the distractive forces of mastication not overwhelm the implants, and yet still effectively neutralize these forces.[8] Application of the tension-band principle takes advantage of the fact that these fixation devices are strongest in tension (all stresses acting parallel to the long axis of the implant).[9]

© 2012 Elsevier Ltd
DOI: 10.1016/B978-0-7020-4618-6.00030-0

Man

In ap
surfac
prima
tralize
bendi
lel to
lar ar
mastie
using
the li
and s
the r:
bendi
fixatio
(see C

Max

The n
ble, w
facial
cated
not ir
methc
lapse
ments
and tl
on its
are qu

Ana

Bone

The th
to rec
Multij
recons
figura
stock

Avoi

The b
bone
appro
ously
availal
teeth 1
these

Bloo

Althot
progre
with \
healin
bones
is due
the lat
tissues

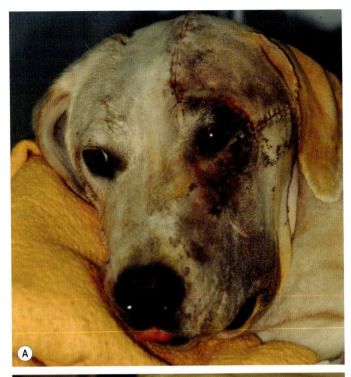

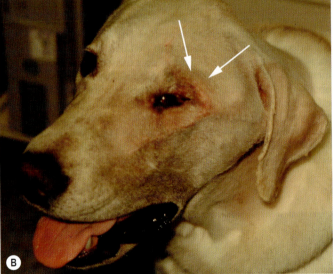

Fig. 31.2 (**A**) Dorsolateral view of left orbit: comminuted zygomatic and frontal bone fracture (zygomatic process) immediately postoperatively, and (**B**) months later, demonstrating contracture and scarring of the soft tissues around the lateral margin of the eye due to a lack of rigid (bony) support of the lateral canthal ligament (*arrows*).

compromised if malocclusion occurs; therefore, dental occlusion must be used to assess the accuracy of the surgical reduction.[1-4]

Other head trauma

Trauma to the eye/orbit is directly related to the support provided by the surrounding bone and soft tissues. Zygomatic arch fractures and fractures of the maxilla at the base of the orbit or zygomatic arch (medial and lateral buttresses) will directly affect both the cosmetic and functional result. Providing the necessary bony support, and thus

sufficient stabilization, in this area is difficult without the use of a buttress support. Miniplate fixation is best suited for these fractures.

ANESTHETIC CONSIDERATIONS

Patient positioning must allow unimpeded access to the head and face and simultaneously permit an avenue for anesthetic management (see Ch. 6). Dental occlusion must be used to guide the fracture reduction. Endotracheal intubation, therefore, is performed via a pharyngotomy access (see Ch. 57).[3,5]

When using occlusion to guide the subsequent orthopedic repair, standard practice in human maxillofacial trauma repair is to first secure maxillomandibular fixation (MMF), i.e., wiring the jaw shut so as to ensure appropriate occlusal apposition.[6-9] If MMF is not applied, as usually is the case in animals, it is essential that the draping include access to the oral cavity to assess occlusion intraoperatively (see Ch. 6).

BIOMECHANICS

The skull and mandible in the dog and cat may be arbitrarily divided into areas that are either more or less suited for miniplate fixation. These areas generally are the buttresses of the face (facial frame) and along lines of tensile stress of the mandible.

Miniplates may be used in most areas, but may be especially useful in the maxilla and in the mandible at the junction of the body and ramus. In the latter area, the rapidly changing bony contours and the thin bone of the masseteric fossa preclude the use of most other fixation devices.[10] Miniplates may either be used as the sole form of fixation, or combined with other techniques.

Lines of stress

The biomechanical principles of the fixation devices used for mandibular and maxillary fracture repair must include an understanding of the functional anatomy (see Ch. 25). Because of the small implant size, it is crucial that the biomechanical limitations of miniplates be fully understood. These devices must be placed along the lines of tension stress in order that the distractive forces of mastication not overwhelm the implants, and yet can effectively neutralize these forces.[11] Application of the tension-band principle takes advantage of the fact that all fixation devices are strongest in tension (all stresses acting parallel to the long axis of the implant).[12]

Maxilla

The maxillofacial area abuts the mandible directly, which might imply that the force distribution is identical to the mandible; however, the maxillofacial area is supported by a number of anatomical buttresses (an 'outer facial frame') that distributes the masticatory forces arising from the mandible (see Ch. 25). These buttresses are defined as present in the rostral/medial, lateral, and caudal planes, and are designed as a basic truss or frame that are considered as pillars of reinforced bone.[10,13,14] Reconstruction of such buttresses, or pillars, requires some form of inherent structural support, which is most readily provided with plate fixation. Because of the small size of these reinforced areas, and the thin bone adjacent to them, small plates that can be easily contoured to match the bone shape – and screws with a fine thread pitch (so as to purchase thin bone) – are required to effectively span these areas and simultaneously provide support.

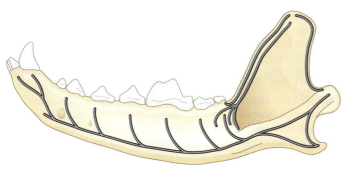

Fig. 31.3 Proposed trajectories of the mandible.

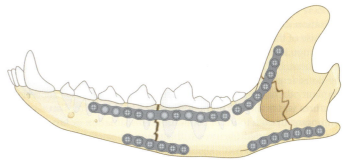

Fig. 31.4 Drawing of the mandible, which shows the relatively large size of the teeth in relationship to the bone. Miniplates can be contoured to match the alveolar bone and screws positioned without interfering with the tooth roots: both tension-band and stabilization plates demonstrating repair of fractures in the mandible and in the ramus. Single tension-band and stabilization plates could be used to span both fractures in cases of comminution. The ventral (stabilization) plate in the ramus could also be contoured such that it traverses along the condylar crest towards the condylar process. *(From Boudrieau RJ, Mandibular and Maxillofacial Fractures. In: Tobias KM and Johnston SA (eds). Veterinary Surgery Small Animals, Elsevier 2012, with permission.)*

Depressed fractures of the maxillofacial skeleton are uncommon in small animals; however, fractures that occur through these buttresses can disrupt the 'connection' with the base of the skull, and result in malocclusion or alter the anatomic support of the orbit. These fractures require reconstruction of this outer facial frame to rebuild this buttress support. It is along these lines of stress that the miniplate fixation needs to be applied in order to maximize their ability to stabilize the bone.

Mandible

Application of the fixation must consider the tension and compression surfaces of the bone, as bending forces are the primary distracting forces acting on the mandible that must be neutralized (see Ch. 25). The mandible acts as a long lever arm and resists bending forces with a strong compact layer of bone that lies parallel to the dental trajectory (Fig. 31.3).[14] This long lever arm extends from the temporomandibular joint, and also consists of the origins of the muscles of mastication on the ramus, which extend rostrally to the incisor teeth.[14] The dental trajectory also parallels the lines of tension stress of the mandible.[14] This bone is similar to a long bone, where the shape of the trabecular and compact bone is a result of the functional stress of mastication present.[14] Since, as already noted, all fixation devices are strongest in tension (stresses parallel to the longitudinal axis of the implant), these small implants (miniplates) must be placed along the lines of tensile stress, or on the tension surface of the bone. In cases of mandibular fractures, this location is along the alveolar margin, which most effectively neutralizes the bending forces.[11,12] Bending moments are the primary distractive forces that must be neutralized in the mandible, which are most easily addressed using the tension-band principle.[15–18] A sole tension-band device, however, will not effectively neutralize the additional shearing and torsional loads that also exist. Torsional and shear forces may be neutralized by applying two plates parallel to, and a few millimeters apart, from each other: a tension-band device placed on the traction side of the bone (alveolar margin) and a stabilization device placed on the pressure side of the bone (ventral margin) (Fig. 31.4).[15,19,20]

Anatomy

Bone shape and thickness

One of the issues with fixation of maxillary fractures, and also mandibular fractures in the ramus, is the lack of adequate bone purchase for most implant systems. This is evident in small animals when attempting to rebuild the maxillary buttresses, where limited space is available to place the implants, and where bone thickness usually is approximately 2 mm (although up to 4 mm may be present in the larger or giant breeds of dogs). Greater bone thickness is present in the mandible, although the masseteric fossa is generally less than 2 mm thick. If plate application is confined to the dental trajectory along the coronoid crest and the condylar crest of the ramus, this problem can be circumvented to some degree, as the masseteric fossa is avoided. However, implant placement in these locales is additionally complicated by the very rapid changes in bone contour.

The miniplates are quite adaptable to the rapid change in bone contour, as the plates can be shaped very easily in three dimensions with adequate room for their placement due to their small size. Securing these implants into the thin bone also is obtained without difficulty, again due to the small size of the implants. In addition, the screws have a fine (usually ≈1 mm) thread pitch, which enables at least two threads to be present within the available bone thickness, and thus is sufficient to attain adequate bone purchase.[12,17,20–22]

Avoiding dental trauma

The biomechanically ideal location of the implants, at the alveolar margin, may not always be obtained, as most fixation devices will interfere with the tooth roots and neurovascular structures adjacent to the tooth roots at this location. In the dog and cat, these structures comprise a majority of the bone volume in both the mandible and maxilla. Therefore, implants must be placed so as to avoid these structures, i.e., placed on the ventral aspect, or on the biomechanically disadvantageous side of the bone. Because of the ability to easily contour a miniplate, and the small size of the screws, it is easier to apply these implants without interfering with the tooth roots along the alveolar margin of the bone (Fig. 31.4), which is the biomechanically advantageous side.[23] The only limitation appears to be with rostral mandibular fractures, where the large size of the canine tooth roots fills almost the entire rostral mandible.[23]

Avoiding the tooth roots with any of the fixation devices is a time-honored principle with mandibular and maxillary fracture repair. The rationale is that any penetration of the tooth root at its apex likely will result in tooth death due to an interference with its vascular supply.[24,25] Furthermore, due to the alternative access created, e.g., screw placed into the root, there is a potential tract that can provide bacterial access to this location, resulting in an infection and subsequently a periapical lesion.[25]

2.0-mm outer thread diameter. A 2.3-mm screw is available as an emergency screw (with a 1.8-mm core diameter). The screw threads are of a self-tapping, standard thread design, with a 1-mm thread pitch. A bone tap is available for thicker bone (>3 mm) where self-tapping may prove to be difficult. The tip of the screw has a conical, rather than trocar, shape in order to provide more of a self-centering action in the drill hole for easier starting of the screw. Screws are available from 5 mm to 15 mm in length, with a straight, slotted head (Fig. 31.5). The screw head and plate design allows screw placement up to a 30° angle relative to the plate surface.

A specially designed plate bending pliers is used to contour the plate three-dimensionally (Fig. 31.6). An anvil and two circular prongs at the tip of the bending pliers provide the leverage necessary to bend the plate in any direction for a limited distance. Horizontal, or in-plane bending (parallel to the edge of the plate surface), is accomplished by inserting the two prongs into adjacent holes in the plate (the prongs are approximately the same diameter as the screw holes in the plate), and applying the anvil between these holes. The prongs prevent distortion of the plate holes during bending. Bending the plate perpendicular to its flat surface (out-of-plane bending), as is routinely performed with standard plates, also is performed with this instrument. The base of the prongs provides the support for bending against the anvil when applied in this fashion.

Synthes maxillofacial system (Synthes, Paoli, PA)[45,47]

The titanium miniplates are offered in various sizes: 1.0-mm, 1.3-mm, 1.5-mm, 2.0-mm, 2.4-mm, 3.0-mm and 4.0-mm systems (the 1.0–1.5-mm systems are considered microplate systems and the 2.4–4.0-mm systems, which are generally too big for use in the dog and cat, are not discussed). The 2.0-mm miniplates are 0.85 mm thick, and the straight plates are either 19.3 cm (30-hole) or 10 cm (20-hole); the former with a 6.5-mm spacing between the holes, and the latter with 5-mm spacing between the holes (Fig. 31.7). These plates are cut to the length desired. Specially designed plate cutters cut the plate without leaving a burr along the cut edge of the plate. A variety of pre-shaped plates also are available: curved, Y, T, X, H, right-angle, etc.

The screws have a 1.4-mm core diameter and a 2.0-mm thread diameter, with a 0.6-mm thread pitch. A 2.4-mm screw also is available as an emergency screw (with a 1.7-mm core diameter, and a 1-mm thread pitch). The screw threads and screw tip design are similar to the Martin system. A bone tap is available for thicker bone (>3 mm) where self-tapping may prove to be difficult. Screws are available from 4 mm to 18 mm in length, with a cruciate head or StarDrive recess. The screw head and plate design allows screw placement up to a 20° angle relative to the plate surface.

Specially designed plate bending pliers are used to contour the plate three-dimensionally (Fig. 31.7). Two pliers are used together in order to contour the plate. Each pair of pliers has a central pin that inserts into the hole in the plate, with two adjacent smaller pins that engage the outside of the plate on either side of the plate hole, thus ensuring preservation of the shape of the plate hole that prevents distortion of the plate during bending.

A 2.0-mm Locking Mandible System also is available. In this system, plates are available in 1.0 mm thickness and 4.8 mm width (mini), 1.3 mm thickness and 5.0 mm width (intermediate), 1.5 mm thickness and 6.5 mm width (large), and 2.0 mm thickness and 6.5 mm width (extra large). Only the mini is discussed here. Threaded plate holes are present within the plate, which accommodate either standard or locking screws. The locking screw has special double-lead threads beneath the screw head that engage and lock into the threaded plate holes. The screws are available in 5–18-mm lengths, with a thread pitch of 0.75 mm. The purpose of the locking screw design is to increase the construct stability and decrease the risk of screw

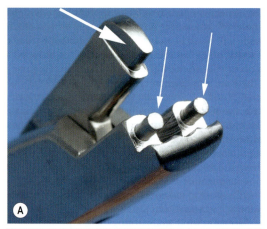

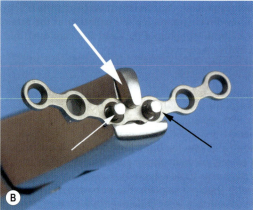

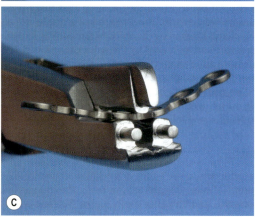

Fig. 31.6 (**A**) Martin bending pliers. The anvil (*large arrow*) and two circular prongs at the tip of the bending pliers (*small arrows*). (**B**) The plate is bent along its edge (in-plane bending) by inserting the circular prongs into two adjacent holes in the plate (*small arrows*) and depressing the anvil (*large arrow*) between the holes. The circular prongs prevent distortion of the holes within the plate. (**C**) The plate is bent perpendicular to its surface (out-of-plane bending) by using the base of the circular prongs as support while the anvil is depressed. (*From Boudrieau RJ, Mandibular and Maxillofacial Fractures. In: Tobias KM and Johnston SA (eds). Veterinary Surgery Small Animals, Elsevier 2012, with permission.*)

back-out with subsequent loss of reduction. The locking screws must be centered within the plate hole and inserted perpendicular to the plate surface; however, when using standard screws, they may be angled relative to the plate surface as noted previously. This system introduced the StarDrive recess in the head of the screw, and the corresponding screwdriver blade.

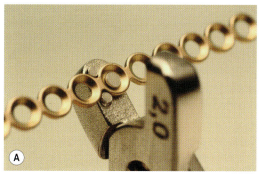

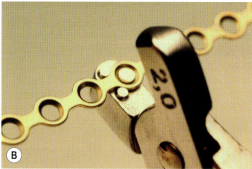

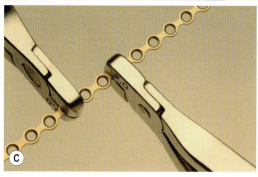

Fig. 31.7 Synthes bending pliers and plates. The pliers have a central pin that inserts into the hole in the plate, with two adjacent smaller pins that engage the outside of the plate on either side of the plate hole, thus ensuring preservation of the shape of the plate hole, which prevents distortion of the plate during bending. Bending pliers and plate: (**A**) 5-mm spacing between screw holes; (**B**) 6.5-mm spacing between screw holes. (**C**) Two pliers are required to bend the plate. *(From Boudrieau RJ, Mandibular and Maxillofacial Fractures. In: Tobias KM and Johnston SA (eds). Veterinary Surgery Small Animals, Elsevier 2012, with permission.)*

THERAPEUTIC DECISION-MAKING

Surgical approaches

The specific surgical approaches are discussed in Chapter 27. In general, a separate ventral approach to each mandible is used (a single midline incision may be used; however, access to the mandibular rami in bilateral fractures is obtained with considerable difficulty).[48,49] At the caudal extent of each individual incision, the digastricus m. is left attached to the bone whenever possible. This muscle may be retracted either medially or laterally; access to the ramus of the mandible generally is sufficient. If necessary, a lateral approach may be used to access the mandibular ramus;[50] however, this is rarely necessary as adequate access to the mandible can be obtained from the ventral approach. Furthermore, it is not necessary to repair fractures of the ramus above

the level of the condylar process. A lateral approach is necessary for fractures involving the condylar process.[51]

The maxillas and incisive bones usually can be adequately approached by an intraoral exposure – simply reflecting the gingiva and alveolar mucosa away from the alveolar bone adjacent to the base of the teeth. In cases of severe maxillary fractures with collapse of the nasal and maxillary bones (to rebuild the medial buttresses), or frontal bone, a dorsal midline approach also is utilized.

The zygomatic arch can be approached directly.[51] The lateral buttresses also can be accessed from the dorsal midline. The lateral aspect of the frontal bone and the adjacent orbit can be approached by combining an approach to the zygomatic arch and also reflecting the lateral soft tissue support to the eye and orbital ligament, attached to the zygomatic process of the frontal bone.

Sequence of repair

Simple fractures are reconstructed anatomically; however, comminuted fractures, or fractures with gaps, must be reconstructed using occlusion to determine the accuracy of the reduction. Plate fixation of the accessible bone surface with 'perfect' reduction, e.g., ventral mandibular surface, does not always result on the buccal surface of the bone. Reduction opposite the fracture repair will not always follow, since compression directly under the plate may cause distraction of the opposite cortex (this is a commonly acknowledged result of plate fixation, which requires pre-stressing or pre-bending of the plate directly over the fracture). When using occlusion to determine the accuracy of the reduction, temporary MMF should be strongly considered as a method to ensure that adequate reduction is obtained.

Reconstruction of any fracture should start with the more straightforward (simple) fracture first, and build toward the more difficult (comminuted) fractures (see Ch. 25). In cases of both maxillary and mandibular trauma, the mandible is usually repaired first, providing a base upon which to build the maxillary repair. For the maxilla, the lateral buttresses are repaired first, followed by the medial buttresses (the caudal buttress need not be addressed as reconstruction of two of the three buttresses ensures that the remaining buttress will be reduced). It is imperative that there is adequate surgical exposure in order to apply bridging plate fixation across all bone fragments.

Rigid fixation, buttress plate support, is placed while ensuring passive and accurate contouring of the miniplate(s). The plates must be accurately bent into the appropriate shape in order to passively fit the contours of the bone. If the plate is not accurately bent, the underlying bone will be pulled toward the plate, causing a corresponding shift at the occlusal level. A malocclusion, in addition to adversely affecting function, also may result in fixation failure as abnormal leverage is exerted against the fixation devices. The latter contributes to motion at the fracture site, and subsequent loosening of the fixation. Accurate contouring of plates to the anatomic irregularities of the mandibular and maxillary bone surface is difficult, especially with the standard plating systems, and is much more easily accomplished with miniplates.[33] All bone fragments are reconstructed with the plate(s). If the bone fragments are too small to reconstruct, they are removed, and any gaps are spanned with a plate(s). Further split-thickness bone grafting also needs to be considered to similarly span any defects.

The basic principles of fixation can be summarized as follows:

1. Mandibular reconstruction proceeds as the first step.
2. Reconstruction of the lateral maxillary buttresses is the key to maxillary repair.
3. Direct, and complete, exposure of the maxillary buttresses permits anatomic reconstruction.
4. Reinforcement of bone defects and unstable buttresses must be obtained with either bone grafts and/or miniplate fixation.

SURGICAL TECHNIQUES

Fractures involving the incisive and maxillary bones

Incisive and maxillary bone fractures may not occur as part of the structural support of the face, i.e., detachment of the occlusal surfaces from the skull; however, they can result in an alteration of the occlusal surface, which is interrupted by the fracture. This is best illustrated where a fracture line traverses the dental arch, and results in a step along the occlusal surface. Restoring the line of dentition may be easily accomplished via miniplate fixation using an intraoral approach – simply reflecting the alveolar mucosa away from its attachments to the alveolar bone adjacent to the base of the teeth. The incision should be made approximately 2 mm from the mucogingival junction, thereby preserving an area for suture placement with subsequent soft tissue closure. The entire dental arch, from the last molar tooth to the incisor teeth on both sides of the face, can be exposed with a single incision in the alveolar mucosa. Miniplate location is adjacent to the alveolar margin. Plate location is kept below the infraorbital foramen of the maxilla laterally; similarly, the plate is kept below the nasal cartilages and applied directly to the incisive bone rostrally (Fig. 31.8).

Screw placement is performed so as to avoid the tooth roots, angling the screws between the tooth roots of the same and adjacent teeth (Fig. 31.9). Closure of the alveolar mucosa is not impaired by the plate due to its low-profile design (Fig. 31.8).

Fractures involving the nasal and frontal bones

Fractures of the nasal and frontal bones are rarely involved with facial support; however, depressed areas will cause a cosmetic defect, and are easily repaired with miniplate fixation. A dorsal midline approach, sufficient to expose the entire fracture, is made and the soft tissue reflected laterally to identify intact adjacent maxilla or frontal bone. The miniplates are used as buttress devices to span across the fractured area(s) while secured in intact bone. Usually, these plates are oriented in the transverse plane. All small bone fragments also can be secured to these plates, effectively rebuilding the bony contour (Fig. 31.10).

One area of functional importance of the frontal bone is the zygomatic process. This area is the dorsal attachment of the orbital ligament. This ligament serves as the lateral attachment of the lateral palpebral ligament and orbicularis oculi muscle.[46] Loss of support of

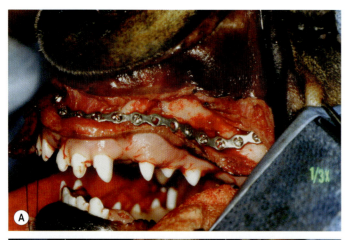

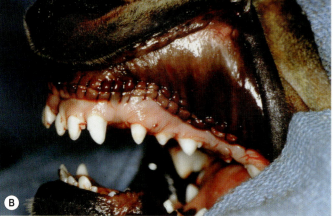

Fig. 31.8 (**A**) Intraoperative photograph of plate placement adjacent to the alveolar margin of the incisive and maxillary bones. Note that a single plate traverses from the level of the third incisor on the right to the fourth premolar on the left. (**B**) Intraoperative photograph of the mucosal closure over the miniplate fixation. *(From Boudrieau RJ. Fractures of the maxilla. In: Johnson AL, Houlton JEF, Vannini R (eds). AO Principles of fracture management in the dog and cat,. Georg Thieme Verlag, Stuttgart, 2005:116–129).*

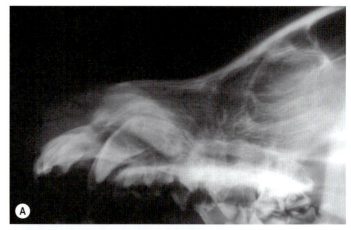

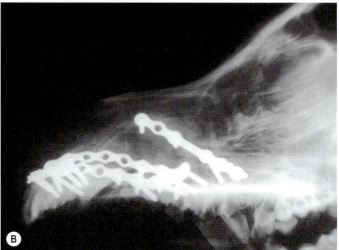

Fig. 31.9 (**A**) Preoperative lateral radiograph demonstrating comminuted maxillary fracture with dorsal displacement of the incisive and part of the maxillary bones. (**B**) Immediate postoperative lateral radiograph demonstrating multiple miniplate fixation to span the comminuted fracture fragments. The plates are placed adjacent to the alveolar border, and the screws are angled so as to avoid impingement with the tooth roots.

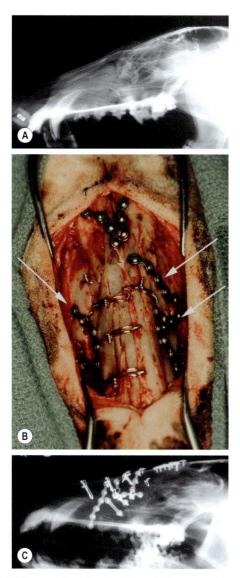

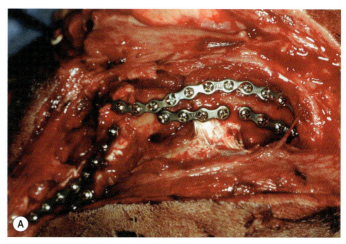

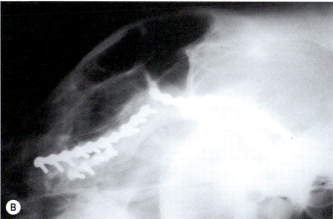

Fig. 31.11 (**A**) Intraoperative photograph demonstrating the multiple miniplate fixation that bridges the comminuted fracture of the left zygomatic bone. Short miniplates were used first to span the individual fractures, and then the zygomatic arch was spanned with two miniplates (dorsally) to finally stabilize the fractures. The dog is facing to the left. (**B**) Immediate postoperative lateral radiograph of the fracture repair. *(From Boudrieau RJ. Fractures of the maxilla. In: Johnson AL, Houlton JEF, Vannini R (eds). AO Principles of fracture management in the dog and cat. Georg Thieme Verlag, Stuttgart, 2005:116–129).*

Fig. 31.10 (**A**) Preoperative lateral radiograph demonstrating comminuted nasal and maxillary fractures with loss of the medial buttress. (**B**) Intraoperative photograph demonstrating the miniplate fixation that bridges the fracture lines and reestablishes the lateral buttress (*arrows*). Note that 'skewer-pins' and figure-of-eight wires also were used to support the nasal fractures, although miniplates also could have been used. (**C**) Immediate postoperative lateral radiograph demonstrating multiple miniplate fixation to span the comminuted fracture fragments.

the zygomatic process of the frontal bone will result in a lack of lateral support of the eye (Fig. 31.2).

Fractures involving the zygomatic arch

Fractures of the zygomatic bone are usually associated with trauma to the eye and orbit. This fracture may result in exophthalmos if the bone fragments have been displaced medially, or alternatively, either a caudal or ventral displacement of the eye if the lateral support provided by this bone is lost. A direct approach to the zygomatic arch is performed. The arch may be reconstructed either with a single plate that spans the arch or, in highly comminuted fractures, pieced together

with smaller plates across the individual fracture lines and then additionally spanned over the entire distance (Fig. 31.11). Caution must be exercised to protect the zygomatic branch of the facial nerve, which courses over the caudodorsal aspect of the zygomatic arch. Repair of fractures at the caudal aspect of the zygomatic arch must be approached with great caution due to the proximity of the facial nerve and maxillary artery. It may be more prudent to follow a conservative, noninterventional approach, for fractures at this location.

Fractures involving the maxillary (medial and lateral) buttresses

Fractures that cause a disconnect between the occlusal surfaces of the maxilla and the skull are a result of a loss of the support of the facial frame, i.e., the medial, lateral and caudal buttresses.[52] The caudal buttress need not be reconstructed directly since reconstruction of the medial and lateral buttresses will accurately reposition the caudal buttress, as was previously discussed. Approach to the medial and lateral buttresses can be obtained from a dorsal midline approach, and lateral soft tissue elevation in order to adequately expose the fractures. If necessary, the lateral buttress may be approached separately, either directly over the rostral aspect of the zygomatic bone or intraorally by elevating the alveolar mucosa apical to the fourth premolar tooth. Reconstruction should commence with the lateral buttress to reestablish continuity between the occlusal surfaces and the skull. Further reconstruction and fixation then proceeds rostrally (see Fig. 31.10).[52]

Fractures of the mandible

Body of the mandible

Separate ventral approaches to the mandible are used to access mandibular body fractures. Buccal exposure of the mandible is performed apical to the mucogingival junction. After fracture reduction, a miniplate is secured to the bone immediately adjacent to the alveolar margin. Screw placement is performed so as to avoid the tooth roots, angling the screws between the tooth roots of the same and adjacent teeth. This is the tension-band plate, which must be secured first in order to ensure that the occlusal surface is restored into anatomical alignment. A second miniplate then is secured parallel to the first miniplate, on the ventral mandibular margin (if possible below the level of the mandibular canal) (see Fig. 31.4). This plate functions as the stabilization plate. Rather than utilizing a miniplate as the second stabilization plate, a standard DCP or reconstruction plate may be used in large-breed dogs.[20] The argument in favor of the latter approach is that the masticatory forces of the mandible in animals may be sufficiently great to overwhelm the stability provided by the miniplate, despite the appropriate positioning of these plates along the lines of tensile stress. The importance of the more dorsally placed tension-band plate cannot be overemphasized, regardless of which size plate is used as the stabilization plate. Success has been documented with both approaches.[4,23,26,27] In the mandibular body there is sufficient space in all but the smallest dogs, or cats, to place a standard plate along the ventral mandibular border. The greater security provided by the addition of this larger plate may be a practical and sensible alternative to solely dual miniplate fixation in this area.

Large defects, due to either bone or tooth loss, can easily be spanned with buttress plate fixation; however, such large gaps may take a long time to heal, even if cancellous bone grafting is performed. There is a limited time where the fixation will remain stable as buttress fixation. Compression or neutralization fixation can be used if the fracture gap is spanned by a cortical bone graft (strut).[4] The advantage of the latter approach is less reliance on the implant as the only means of support. If continuity of bone across the fracture site can be reestablished, the applied shear and bending loads become shared between the bone and the implant, resulting in a more stable fixation than if only a buttress device is used.[53] In addition, when large mandibular gaps are present, the implant – regardless of the type of fixation – is of insufficient strength to counteract the considerable forces of mastication, and the fixation device tends to loosen before bony continuity is reestablished.[54] In the dog and cat, autogenous cortical bone can be obtained from the ulna or rib(s) with low morbidity.[4] Similar tension-band and stabilization plate fixation is applied to the mandible spanning the cortical autograft (see Fig. 31.12). The cortical bone graft is also supplemented with a cancellous bone graft. The length of a free (avascular) cortical bone autograft should not exceed 40 mm.[7,55]

Ramus of the mandible

Separate ventral approaches to the mandible again are used to access these fractures. A lateral approach generally is not necessary as adequate access to the ramus can be obtained from the ventral

approach. As in mandibular body fractures, the tension-band plate is the first fixation applied to the reduced fracture. This plate is secured along the coronoid crest, thus ensuring adequate screw purchase in the thicker bone of this region. The stabilization plate then is secured to the ventral mandibular margin, along the condylar crest (Fig. 31.13). In the larger breeds of dogs, a larger standard plate may be used, as was discussed for mandibular body fractures. Additional fixation, using miniplates, may be used to reconstruct defects within the masseteric fossa; this is limited to areas where the bone thickness is >1 mm. Fractures dorsal to a line connecting the occlusal surface with the temporomandibular joint need not be addressed.

Condylar process

Fractures of the condylar process must be approached directly from the lateral aspect. These fractures are difficult to repair due to the small size of the bone and, because of the necessity of a specific surgical approach, must be identified before surgery (Fig. 31.14). A fracture of the condylar process may be repaired using interfragmentary compression, using 2.0-mm or 1.5-mm screws (Fig. 31.14). Fractures just below this process, in the area of the mandibular notch, which isolates the condylar process, also may be repaired using interfragmentary compression by angling a screw along the coronoid crest (a trough is first created as a starting point for the screw) and into the condylar process. Alternatively, a miniplate may be used to span the fracture site along the coronoid process, and also possibly along the caudal and vertical border of the ramus. The small size of this area in most dogs and cats may, however, make such suggestions impractical.

POSTOPERATIVE CARE AND ASSESSMENT

Antibiotics

Postoperative antibiotic therapy is recommended in the dog[56] and cat,[57] much the same as in humans,[58] since open fractures occur in a majority of these cases.[3] Antibiotics generally are continued in the postoperative period; the choice of subsequent antibiotic therapy is determined by the results of bacterial cultures obtained intraoperatively, and subsequent susceptibility testing.[3]

Diet and activity restriction

With rigid skeletal fixation, there is no reason to avoid feeding per os. Animals so treated can, and will, eat and drink normally within 24 hours after surgery, only limited by the degree of postoperative swelling that is present. The ability for oral prehension is regained immediately postoperatively. The only limitation to the diet is to use soft food. Chewing on hard objects is not permitted for the first 4–6 weeks postoperatively. Playing with any toys, balls, sticks, etc., which the animal chews, is to be avoided.

COMPLICATIONS

Miniplate fixation has few complications if the principles of rigid skeletal fixation are followed and iatrogenic technical failures associated with implant application are avoided.

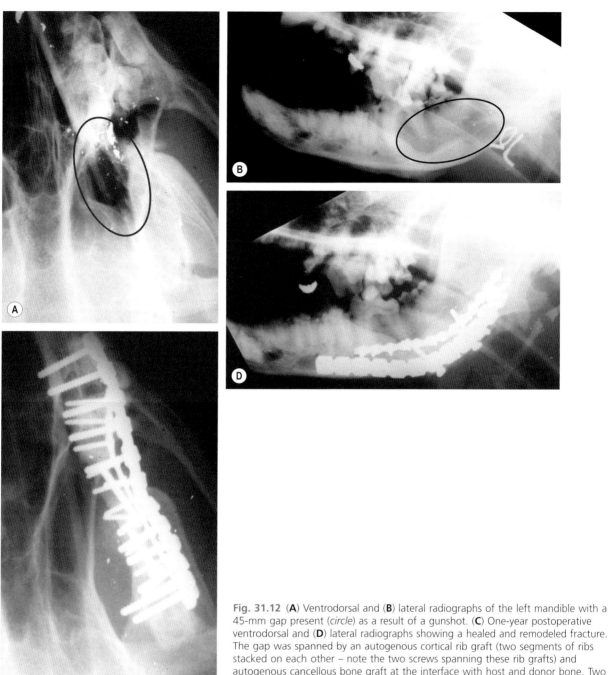

Fig. 31.12 (**A**) Ventrodorsal and (**B**) lateral radiographs of the left mandible with a 45-mm gap present (*circle*) as a result of a gunshot. (**C**) One-year postoperative ventrodorsal and (**D**) lateral radiographs showing a healed and remodeled fracture. The gap was spanned by an autogenous cortical rib graft (two segments of ribs stacked on each other – note the two screws spanning these rib grafts) and autogenous cancellous bone graft at the interface with host and donor bone. Two plates were used: a 13-hole miniplate as the tension band plate (placed first to restore occlusal alignment), and a 12-hole 2.7-mm reconstruction plate as the stabilization plate.

Technical failures

Incorrect plate/location (mandible)

Successful repair of mandibular fractures ultimately depends upon the strength of the fixation, and its ability to effectively withstand the masticatory forces. The simplest method to increase strength is with a stronger (larger) plate, a longer plate with additional screw fixation, compression across the fracture site, or use of multiple plates. In unstable fractures, i.e., those with comminution or segmentation, a plate of sufficient length is used in order to obtain a minimum of

three screws on either side of the fracture site; additionally, with severely comminuted fractures, or fractures with bone loss, a minimum of four screws is necessary (this recommendation dictates that this number of screws be secured in intact bone on both sides of the fracture).[15] The use of a plate that is too short, with screws placed too close to the fracture site, is one of the most common causes of failure of this method of internal fixation.[15,59]

Using the correct size of plate is particularly important once it is recognized that in most instances a standard plate is placed on the wrong side of the mandible, i.e., the pressure (ventral) surface. This plate must withstand far greater forces than it would if placed on the

303

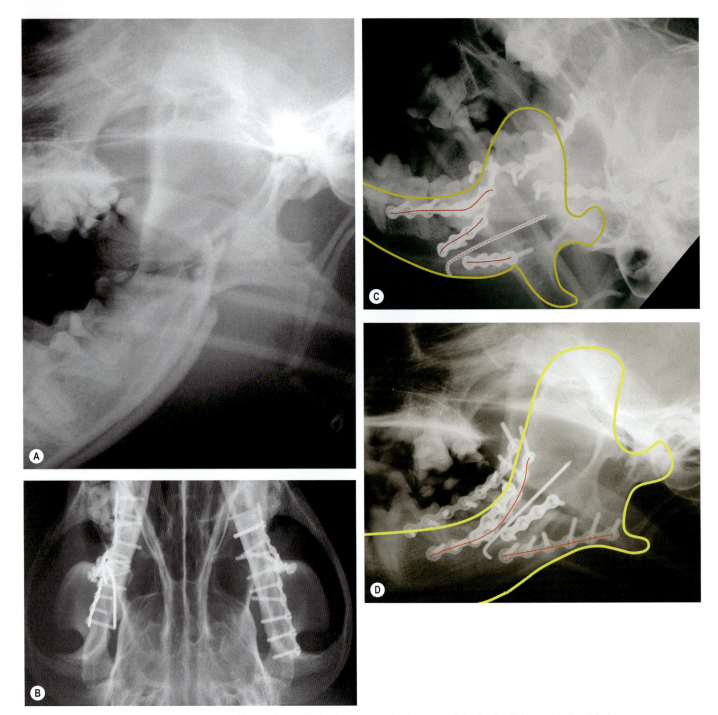

Fig. 31.13 (**A**) Preoperative lateral radiograph of bilateral mandibular fractures at the junction of the body of the mandible with the ramus. (**B**) Postoperative ventrodorsal, (**C**) right lateral oblique and (**D**) left lateral oblique radiographs (the yellow line outlines the right and left mandibles; the red lines parallel the fixation for the mandible outlined). The postoperative fixation demonstrates both the tension-band miniplates placed along the coronoid crest, and stabilization plates placed along the condylar crest.

tension-band (alveolar) surface; thus the emphasis on first spanning a fracture with a miniplate along the alveolar margin of the mandible. When using only miniplates, this principle becomes even more important, as multiple plates must be used in order to obtain adequate stability. Miniplates used in other than the alveolar margin, where they do not align along the lines of tension stress, are of insufficient strength to counteract the functional masticatory forces across the fracture site.

Incorrect plate/location (maxilla)

A poor result in this location usually is the result of not restoring the three-dimensional anatomy and not placing the plates along the maxillary buttresses, where the thicker bone enhances screw purchase. This generally is the result of an inadequate surgical exposure where all of the fracture fragments are not identified.[60] Similarly, maintenance of the fixation is compromised under similar conditions of poor surgical

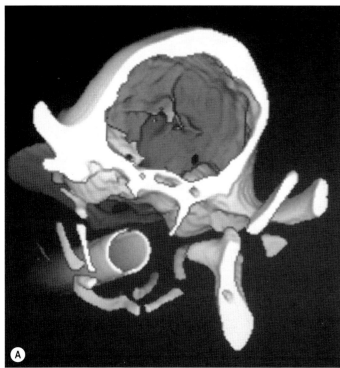

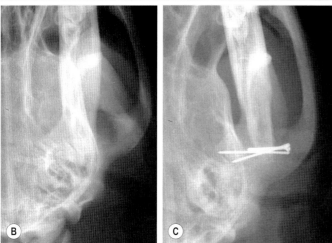

Fig. 31.14 (**A**) Three-dimensional reconstruction – spiral CT – of a dog with bilateral ramus fractures and a left-sided transverse fracture of the condylar process (and also a transverse fracture of the ramus dorsal to this level, which need not be repaired). (**B**) The fracture is not visible despite multiple radiographic views. (**C**) Immediate postoperative ventrodorsal radiograph of the fracture repair using a 2.0-mm screw placed in lag fashion and two 0.035″ K-wires. *(From Boudrieau RJ, Mandibular and Maxillofacial Fractures. In: Tobias KM and Johnston SA (eds). Veterinary Surgery Small Animals, Elsevier 2012, with permission.)*

exposure, as it leads to an inability to accurately place the fixation in the most appropriate location.[60]

Plate contour

The plates must be passively fitted to the contours of the mandible. If the plate is not accurately bent, the underlying bone will be pulled toward the plate, causing a corresponding shift at the occlusal level. Failure to take the time and trouble to bend the standard plates accurately is one of the most common causes of complications in rigid

fixation of the mandible.[59,60] By first placing a tension-band plate (miniplate), it is much easier to appropriately bend and place the second stabilization plate.[59,60]

The most difficult area for plate placement is at the angle of the jaw due to the rapidly changing contours of the mandible at this location.

Screw insertion

Accurate and atraumatic drill hole placement must be performed in order to prevent bone necrosis, which will result in premature screw loosening. In the thin bone of the maxilla, drilling should be accomplished at <1000 rpm, with sufficient cooling irrigation – both of which minimize bone necrosis. It also is essential that all drilling occur along a single axis. High-speed drilling and/or redirection during drilling will result in oval-shaped holes that fail to secure the screw adequately. Accurate measurement of drill hole depth ensures adequate screw fixation, which adds to the overall strength of the repair. If any doubt exists regarding screw purchase, an emergency screw should be used to replace the questionable screw.

Screw loosening leads to subsequent plate loosening and ultimate implant failure. Furthermore, the resulting motion inhibits bone healing and enhances the likelihood of infection and sequestration.[59]

Fracture gaps

Failure to bridge a fracture gap will lead to implant failure as the implant is of insufficient strength to counteract the considerable forces of mastication, and the fixation device will loosen before bony continuity can be reestablished.[54] Reestablishing bone continuity allows the applied shear and bending loads to be shared between the bone and the implant, resulting in a more stable fixation than if only a buttress device is used.[61] Therefore, cortical bone grafting should be strongly considered under these circumstances.

An alternative to cortical grafting is to utilize the locking screw/plate design, which increases the stability of the fixation. This must be combined with cancellous bone grafting to stimulate bone healing within the gap.

Malocclusion

Obtaining appropriate dental occlusion is absolutely essential. Even small errors will likely become problems, as function will be adversely affected. This is especially true with rigid internal (plate) fixation. Postoperative modification of the reduction/repair is not possible. Attempts to correct occlusion with such treatments as odontoplasty, or endodontic procedures, or both, and tooth extraction rarely are effective.[60]

Persistent malocclusion, in addition to adversely affecting function, also may result in fixation failure, as abnormal leverage is exerted against the fixation devices. The latter contributes to motion at the fracture site, and subsequent loosening of the fixation.

Soft tissue coverage/dehiscence

Adequate soft tissue coverage over the plates and screws is essential to ensure satisfactory healing and prevent infection. An exposed plate after fixation will not necessarily cause problems with wound healing, provided that it is rigidly fixed. Routine mouth and wound care generally will allow the wound to close over the plate.

Later wound dehiscence can occur, resulting in plate exposure, due to soft tissue necrosis (Fig. 31.15). If the bone has healed, the plate is simply removed. Because of the small size of the miniplates, a portion of the plate may be removed. This is performed using a high-speed bur at each extent of its exposure within the wound, while protecting the soft tissues from the metallic debris.

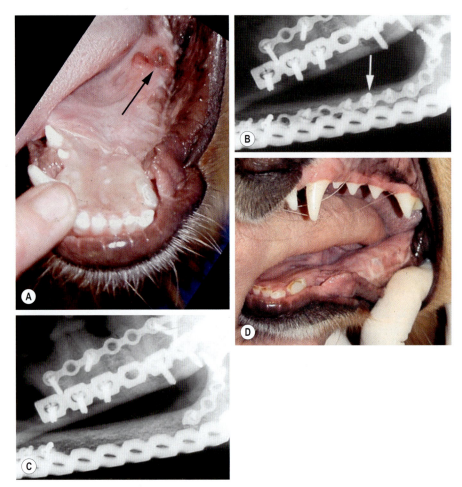

Fig. 31.15 (**A**) Mucosal dehiscence directly over a miniplate at the caudal mandible (*arrow*). The edge of the plate was no longer in contact with bone due to resorption from the remodeling process. (**B**) Left lateral oblique radiograph of the healed fracture; the arrow points to the portion of the plate that is exposed intraorally. (**C**) Left lateral oblique radiograph 4 months after partial plate removal and (**D**) photograph 4 months after partial plate removal (the plate was transected using a high-speed bur, and the bone covered with a single pedicle buccal mucosal advancement flap).

If bone healing is not complete, the plate is left in place, provided that it remains adequately fixed. Soft tissue covering can easily be accomplished using a single pedicle buccal mucosal advancement flap.

If the plates have loosened, dehiscence is the usual sequela, and plate exposure will occur, either externally or intraorally. These plates must be removed, since loose implants interfere with revascularization, and also act as a foreign body, both of which predispose to bone infection. Gaps that are present in the oral mucosa allow for additional bacterial contamination of the fracture site.

Perforation of the oral mucosa on the lingual aspect of the mandible may occur if screws that are too long are used. This may also lead to laceration of the tongue.

Infection

Infection generally is not a problem, despite the open nature of the original wounds. The excellent vascular supply of the head and the rigid stability imparted with plate fixation decrease this possibility. Antibiotic administration, based upon intraoperative bacterial cultures and sensitivity testing, helps to ensure appropriate treatment and the prevention of subsequent problems.

Infection will occur, despite appropriate antibiotic therapy, if any bone fragment instability is present. This is a result of implant loosening. Implant failure most commonly is the result of intraoperative technical failures, improper implant application or malocclusion.

Delayed/Nonunion

A delay or failure of bone healing is, once again, a result of instability. These are the same factors that predispose the bone (and soft tissues) to infection. Treatment is identical, and has been described previously.

Teeth

Interference with the teeth, or tooth roots, can result in pulp necrosis. There also exists the possibility that a periapical lesion will occur as a result of the compromised blood supply and alternative bacterial access (along the pathway of the implant). Treatment consists of either endodontic procedures or tooth removal. Tooth removal should await bone healing, as the creation of a large defect may adversely affect implant stability and subsequent fracture healing.

ACKNOWLEDGMENTS

The author would like to acknowledge Andrew Cunningham for the photos.

REFERENCES

1. Chambers JN. Principles of management of mandibular fractures in the dog and cat. J Vet Orthop 1981;2:26–36.

2. Marretta SM, Schraeder SC, Matthiesen DT. Problems associated with the management and treatment of jaw fractures. Probl Vet Med 1990;2:220–47.

3. Rudy RL, Boudrieau RJ. Maxillofacial and mandibular fractures. Semin Vet Med Surg (Small Anim) 1992;7:3–20.

4. Boudrieau RJ, Tidwell AS, Ullman SH, et al. Correction of mandibular nonunion and malocclusion by plate fixation and autogenous cortical bone grafts in two dogs. J Am Vet Med Assoc 1994;204: 744–50.

5. Hartsfield SM, Gendreau C, Smith CW, et al. Endotracheal intubation by pharyngotomy. J Am Anim Hosp Assoc 1977;13:71–4.

6. Yaremchuk MJ, Manson PN. Rigid internal fixation of mandibular fractures. In: Yaremchuk MJ, Gruss JS, Manson PN, editors. Rigid fixation of the craniomaxillofacial skeleton. Boston, MA: Butterworth-Heinemann; 1992. p. 170–86.

7. Gruss JS. Rigid fixation of complex mandibular fractures. In: Yaremchuk MJ, Gruss JS, Manson PN, editors. Rigid fixation of the craniomaxillofacial skeleton. Boston, MA: Butterworth-Heinemann; 1992. p. 195–208.

8. Gruss JS, Phillips JH. Rigid fixation of Le Fort maxillary fractures. In: Yaremchuk MJ, Gruss JS, Manson PN, editors. Rigid fixation of the craniomaxillofacial skeleton. Boston, MA: Butterworth-Heinemann; 1992. p. 245–62.

9. Klotch D: Use of rigid fixation in the repair of complex and comminuted mandible fractures. Otolaryngol Clin N Am 1987;20:495–518.

10. Forrest CR, Phillips JH, Prein J. Le Fort I–III Fractures. In: Prein J, editor. Manual of internal fixation in the cranio-facial skeleton: Techniques recommended by the AO/ASIF maxillofacial group. Berlin: Springer-Verlag; 1998. p. 108–26.

11. Champy M, Lodde JP. Étude des contraintes dans la mandibule fracturée chez l'homme. Mesures théoriques et vérification par jauges extensométriques in situ. Rev Stomatol Chir Maxillofac 1977;78:545–51.

12. Black J. Biomaterials for internal fixation. In: Heppenstall B, editor. Fracture treatment and healing. Philadelphia, PA: WB Saunders; 1980. p. 113–23.

13. Champy M, Blez P. Anatomical aspects and biomechanical considerations. In: Härle F, Champy M, Terry BC, editors. Atlas of craniomaxillofacial osteosynthesis: Miniplates, microplates, and screws. Stuttgart, Germany: Thieme; 1999. p. 3–7.

14. DuBrul EL: Architectural analysis of the skull. In: Sicher's oral anatomy. 7th ed. St. Louis, MO: Mosby; 1980. p. 85–93.

15. Spiessl B: Principles of the ASIF technique. In: Spiessl B, editor. Internal fixation of the mandible. A manual of AO/ASIF principles. New York: Springer-Verlag; 1989. p. 38–92.

16. Champy M, Lodde JP. Synthèses mandibulaires. Localisation des synthèses en fonction des contraintes mandibulaires. Rev Stomatol Chir Maxillofac 1976;77: 971–6.

17. Pauwels F. The significance of a tension band for the stressing of the tubular bone with application to compression osteosynthesis. In: Biomechanics of the locomotor apparatus: Anatomy of the locomotor apparatus. New York: Springer-Verlag; 1980. p. 430–49.

18. Küppers K: Analyse der funktionellen Struktur des menschlichen Unterkiefers. Adv Anat 1971;44:3–90.

19. Champy M, Pape H-D, Gerlach KL, et al. The Strasbourg miniplate osteosynthesis. In Krüger E, Schilli W, Worthington P, editors. Oral and maxillofacial traumatology. Chicago, IL: Quintessence Publishing; 1985. p. 19–43.

20. Prein J, Kellman RM: Rigid internal fixation of mandibular fractures – Basics of AO technique. Otolaryngol Clin N Am 1987;20:441–56.

21. Champy M, Lodde JP, Schmidt R, et al. Mandibular osteosynthesis by miniature screwed plates via a buccal approach. J Maxillofac Surg 1978;6:14–21.

22. Champy M, Lodde JP, Wilk A, et al. Probleme und Resultate bei der Verwendung von Dehnungsmeßstreifen am präparierten Unterkiefer und bei Patienten mit Unterkieferfrakturen. Dtsch Z Mund- Kiefer- Gesichts-Chir 1978; 2:41–3S.

23. Boudrieau RJ, Kudisch M. Miniplate fixation for repair of mandibular and maxillary fractures in 15 dogs and 3 cats. Vet Surg 1996;25:277–91.

24. Verstraete FJM, Ligthelm AJ. Dental trauma caused by screws in internal fixation of mandibular osteotomies in the dog. Vet Comp Orthop Traumatol 1992;5:104–8.

25. Tholen M, Hoyt RF: Oral pathology. In: Bojrab MJ, Tholen M, editors. Small animal oral medicine and surgery. Philadelphia, PA: Lea and Febiger; 1990. p. 25–55.

26. Boudrieau RJ, Mitchell S, Seeherman H. Mandibular reconstruction of a partial hemimandibulectomy in a dog with severe malocclusion. Vet Surg 2004;33:119–30.

27. Spector DI, Keating JH, Boudrieau RJ. Immediate mandibular reconstruction of a 5 cm defect using rhBMP-2 after partial mandibulectomy in a dog. Vet Surg 2007; 36:752–9.

28. Härle F. Bone repair and fracture healing. In: Härle F, Champy M, Terry BC, editors. Atlas of craniomaxillofacial osteosynthesis: Miniplates, microplates, and screws. Stuttgart, Germany: Thieme; 1999. p. 8–14.

29. Rahn BA: Direct and indirect bone healing after operative fracture management. Otolaryngol Clin N Am 1987;20:425–40.

30. Rever LJ, Manson PN, Randolph MA, et al. The healing of facial bone fractures by the process of secondary union. Plastic Reconstr Surg 1991;87:451–8.

31. Kellman RM, Schilli W: Plate fixation of fractures of the mid and upper face. Otolaryngol Clin N Am 1987;20:559–72.

32. Schilli W, Ewers R, Niederdellmann H: Bone fixation with screws and plates in the maxillofacial region. Int J Oral Maxillofac Surg 1981;10(Suppl. 1): 329–32.

33. Ewers R, Härle F. Experimental and clinical results of new advances in the treatment of facial trauma. Plastic Reconstr Surg 1985;75:25–31.

34. Schilli W, Niederdellmann H. Internal fixation of zygomatic and midface fractures by means of miniplates and lag screws. In: Krüger E, Schilli W, Worthington P, editors. Oral and maxillofacial traumatology. Chicago, IL: Quintessence Publishing; 1986. p. 177–96.

35. Ewers R, Schilli W. Metallplattenosteosynthese und Drahtosteosynthese zur Versorgung der periorbitalen Frakturen im experimentellen Versuch. Dtsch Zahnärztl Z 1977;32:820–3.

36. Champy M, Lodde JP, Jaeger JH, et al. Ostéosynthèses mandibulaires selon la technique de Michelet. I – Base biomécaniques. Rev Stomatol Chir Maxillofac 1976;77:569–76.

37. Champy M, Lodde JP, Jaeger JH, et al. Ostéosynthèses mandibulaires selon la technique de Michelet. II – Présentation d'un nouveau matériel. Resultats. Rev Stomatol Chir Maxillofac 1976;77: 577–83.

38. Luhr H-G: Vitallium Luhr systems for reconstruction of the facial skeleton. Otolaryngol Clin N Am 1987;20: 573–606.

39. Worthington P, Champy M: Monocortical miniplate osteosynthesis. Otolaryngol Clin N Am 1987;20:607–620.

40. de Zeeuw LM. Materials and instrumentation. In: Härle F, Champy M, Terry BC, editors. Atlas of craniomaxillofacial osteosynthesis: Miniplates, microplates, and screws. Stuttgart, Germany: Thieme; 1999. p. 27–30.

41. Altobelli DE. Implant materials in rigid fixation: Physical, mechanical, corrosion, and biocompatibility considerations. In:

Yaremchuk MJ, Gruss JS, Manson PN, editors. Rigid fixation of the craniomaxillofacial skeleton. Boston, MA: Butterworth-Heinemann; 1992. p. 28–56.

42. Reuther JF. The Würzburg titanium system for rigid fixation of the craniomaxillofacial skeleton. In: Yaremchuk MJ, Gruss JS, Manson PN, editors. Rigid fixation of the craniomaxillofacial skeleton. Boston, MA: Butterworth-Heinemann; 1992. p. 134–51.

43. Luhr HG. Specifications, indications, and clinical applications of the Luhr Vitallium maxillofacial systems. In: Yaremchuk MJ, Gruss JS, Manson PN, editors. Rigid fixation of the craniomaxillofacial skeleton. Boston, MA: Butterworth-Heinemann; 1992. p. 79–115.

44. Kahn J-L, Khouri M. Champy's system. In: Yaremchuk MJ, Gruss JS, Manson PN, editors. Rigid fixation of the craniomaxillofacial skeleton. Boston, MA: Butterworth-Heinemann; 1992. p. 116–23.

45. Yaremchuk MJ, Prein J. The AO/ASIF maxillofacial implant system. In: Yaremchuk MJ, Gruss JS, Manson PN, editors. Rigid fixation of the craniomaxillofacial skeleton. Boston, MA: Butterworth-Heinemann; 1992. p. 124–33.

46. Pollock RVH. The eye. In: Evans HE, Christensen GC, editors. Miller's anatomy of the dog. 2nd ed. Philadelphia, PA: WB Saunders; 1979. p. 1073–127.

47. Prein J, Rahn BA: Scientific background. In: Prein J, editor. Manual of internal fixation in the cranio-facial skeleton: Techniques recommended by the AO/ASIF maxillofacial group. Berlin: Springer-Verlag; 1998. p. 1–49.

48. Piermattei DL: Approach to the rostral shaft of the mandible. In: An atlas of surgical approaches to the bones and joints of the dog and cat. 3rd ed. Philadelphia, PA: Saunders, 1993. p. 32–3.

49. Piermattei DL: Approach to the caudal shaft and ramus of the mandible. In: An atlas of surgical approaches to the bones and joints of the dog and cat. 3rd ed. Philadelphia, PA: Saunders, 1993. p. 34–5.

50. Piermattei DL: Approach to the ramus of the mandible. In: An atlas of surgical approaches to the bones and joints of the dog and cat. 3rd ed. Philadelphia, PA: Saunders, 1993. p. 36–7.

51. Piermattei DL: Approach to the temporomandibular joint. In: An atlas of surgical approaches to the bones and joints of the dog and cat. 3rd ed. Philadelphia, PA: Saunders, 1993. p. 38–9.

52. Boudrieau RJ. Miniplate reconstruction of severely comminuted maxillary fractures in two dogs. Vet Surg 2004;33:154–63.

53. Pollock RA, Gruss JS. Craniofacial and panfacial fractures. In: Foster CA, Sherman JE, editors. Surgery of facial bone fractures. New York: Churchill Livingstone; 1987. p. 235–54.

54. Gruss JS, Phillips JH. Complex facial trauma: The evolving role of rigid fixation and immediate bone graft reconstruction. Clin Plastic Surg 1989;16:93–104.

55. Pape H-D, Gerlach KL: Mandibular reconstruction with free, non vascularized bone grafts. In: Härle F, Champy M, Terry BC, editors. Atlas of craniomaxillofacial osteosynthesis: Miniplates, microplates, and screws. Stuttgart, Germany: Thieme; 1999. p. 145–7.

56. Umphlet RC, Johnson AL. Mandibular fractures in the dog. A retrospective study of 157 cases. Vet Surg 1990;19:272–5.

57. Umphlet RC, Johnson AL. Mandibular fractures in the cat. A retrospective study. Vet Surg 1988;17:333–7.

58. Zallen RD, Curry JT. A study of antibiotic usage in compound mandibular fractures. J Oral Surg 1975;53: 431–4.

59. Gruss JS. Complications of rigid fixation of the mandible. In: Yaremchuk MJ, Gruss JS, Manson PN, editors. Rigid fixation of the craniomaxillofacial skeleton. Boston, MA: Butterworth-Heinemann; 1992. p. 217–32.

60. Assael LA. Complications in the rigid fixation of midface fractures. In: Yaremchuk MJ, Gruss JS, Manson PN, editors. Rigid fixation of the craniomaxillofacial skeleton. Boston, MA: Butterworth-Heinemann; 1992. p. 351–6.

61. Müller ME, Allgöwer M, Schneider R, et al, editors. Manual of internal fixation. 2nd ed. New York: Springer-Verlag; 1979.

Chapter | 32 |

Maxillofacial fracture repair using external skeletal fixation

Anson J. Tsugawa & Frank J.M. Verstraete

DEFINITIONS

Biplanar: external frame configuration that occupies two planes

External skeletal fixation: method of stabilizing bone segments with percutaneously placed fixation pins that are externally connected

Free-form fixators: fixator design that consists of full- or half-pins and acrylic columns for connecting bars

Full-pin: through-and-through fixation pin that penetrates both skin surfaces and cortices of the bone

Gunning splint: indirectly fabricated acrylic or composite intraoral splint secured to the mandible (or maxilla) with circumferential wires

Half-pin: fixation pin that penetrates the near skin surface and both cortices of the bone

Intraoral interdental full-pin: single intraoral pin anchored to the mandibular canine teeth using a figure-of-eight wire and a bridge of acrylic or composite between the canine and incisor teeth

Linear fixators: fixator design that consists of full- or half-pins, connecting bars and clamps

Type I: unilateral half-pin frame in a uniplanar or biplanar configuration

Type II: bilateral full-pin frame in a uniplanar configuration

Type III: bilateral combination half- and full-pin frame in a biplanar configuration

Uniplanar: external frame configuration that occupies a single plane

PREOPERATIVE CONCERNS

Pharyngotomy is the recommended route of intubation to provide uninhibited intraoperative assessment of occlusion and permit maxillomandibular fixation (MMF) if indicated. Temporary MMF is a method of establishing the proper occlusal relationship of teeth before reducing fractures of tooth-bearing bones (Fig. 32.1A–C).[1]

Teeth maintain a constant relationship to the bones of the maxilla and mandible, and aligning mandibular or maxillary fracture fragments without establishing pre-injury occlusion will predispose the patient to a suboptimal postoperative occlusion.[2] To obtain the normal occlusion in a dog, the mandibular canine teeth are positioned in the space between the maxillary third incisor and canine teeth, and the crowns of the mandibular fourth premolar teeth are aligned between the maxillary third and fourth premolar teeth.[3] External skeletal fixation provides rigid stability and patients rarely have to be maintained in postoperative MMF.

SURGICAL ANATOMY

The fixation pins of an external pin fixator are introduced percutaneously through small stab incisions in the skin and inevitably impale muscle tissue as they traverse a path into the bone. Pin placement, however, should not unnecessarily violate tooth roots and neurovascular structures, and an applied knowledge of the regional cross-sectional anatomy in combination with radiographs will facilitate achievement of this goal (see Fig. 25.1). This is especially challenging in pediatric patients with unerupted teeth; careful attention must be paid to avoid injuring the tooth buds during surgical reduction. If possible, the neurovascular bundle should be avoided when placing pins in the mandible. In humans, the canal can usually be avoided by placing pins within the inferior border of the mandible. In dogs and cats, the ventral margin of the mandible is usually not of substantial thickness to support pin placement, and as a compromise, pins are usually placed dorsal to the mandibular canal between tooth roots. This may be difficult as the bone that is available for pin insertion is extremely limited in certain areas (see Fig. 25.1).[4] Pins for mandibular fixators are placed in a bicortical fashion with only the pin tip protruding from the opposite cortex. Pin placement in a transmandibular fashion is not recommended because tongue function may be impaired.[5]

In comparison to the bones of the mandible, the maxillary bones are thin, and transmaxillary pin placement is necessary to achieve functional stability with maxillary external fixators. Damage to the nasal conchae and associated hemorrhage are inevitable with this

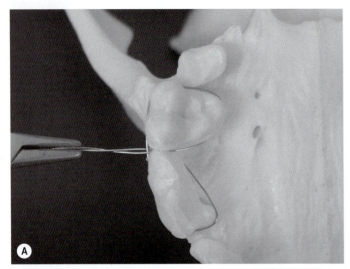

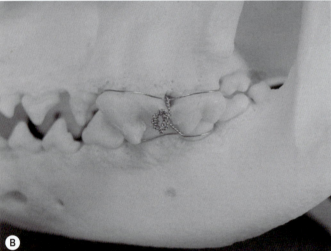

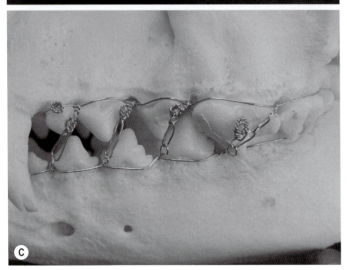

Fig. 32.1 Wire techniques for MMF demonstrated on the skull of a dog. Placement of the maxillary wire for an Ernst-type ligature around the fourth premolar and first molar teeth. (**A**) By convention, the wire ends are twisted in a clockwise direction to form a twist knot. (**B**) Completed Ernst-type ligature. (**C**) Stout continuous loop technique. Notice that the wire tails of the completed ligatures are cut short and finished in a 'rosette' configuration to minimize trauma to the oral soft tissues.

technique. Terminal branches of the facial nerve should be excluded from the skin incisions to avoid paralysis of the upper lip. The infraorbital neurovascular bundle can be readily palpated as it exits its foramen in the maxilla and is easily avoided.

SPECIAL INSTRUMENTS AND MATERIALS

Historical background

External skeletal fixation (ESF) of craniofacial fractures was first reported in 1939.[6] Veterinary application of ESF also dates back to the 1930s, and a veterinarian by the name of Stader was the first to introduce a half-pin splint that was widely used on human patients during World War II.[7] Treatment of a comminuted fracture of the mandibular ramus in a dog with a Stader splint was reported in 1947.[8] In the same year, Ehmer developed a veterinary modification of the Anderson splint.[9] As with many techniques currently used in veterinary oral and maxillofacial surgery, clinical experience with similar medical devices in human medicine usually preceded their use in veterinary medicine. An example of such a device is the biphasic external fixation splint (Joe Hall Morris appliance) for treatment of mandibular fractures that was first introduced in human oral and maxillofacial surgery in 1949, and was later adapted for use in veterinary medicine in the early 1980s.[10–12] Conversely, Becker in the 1950s developed a whole system consisting of threaded pins, bolts, acrylic, and special instruments that was first used in a variety of domestic animals and shortly thereafter in humans.[13,14] The acrylic connecting bar was secured in place over each pin by means of two nuts.

In the 1970s, the traditional tenets for external fixation were challenged with the introduction of miniplates and screws by Michelet and Champy.[15,16] Many of the comminuted fractures that could previously only be treated by external skeletal fixation are currently treated by rigid internal fixation (see Ch. 31). Despite a decline in popularity as a technique for maxillofacial fracture repair, external fixation devices have recently experienced a resurgence of interest with the development of distraction osteogenesis techniques.

Components

The basic components of an ESF system include fixation pins, clamps and connecting bars. The pins are inserted percutaneously on both sides of the fracture and are attached via clamps to an external connecting bar that provides immobilization of the fracture.

Fixation pins

Fixation pins used for ESF are constructed of implant-grade, hardened stainless steel. Pin shaft diameters vary with the type of ESF system selected. The pin shaft may be threaded or smooth. Threaded pins may be threaded at the end of the shaft (end-threaded) or centrally threaded. Fully threaded or regular Steinmann pins are weak, have a tendency to break, and are not recommended for ESF.[17] The thread pitch can be fine or coarse, fine-pitched for use in cortical bone and coarse-pitched for use in cancellous bone. The profile of a threaded fixation pin refers to whether the threads are machined into the core diameter of the shaft (negative profile) or raised above the core diameter of the pin (positive profile). Due to their reduced core diameter, negative-profile pins are of reduced strength and less resistant to bending forces than positive-profile pins and should not be used with unstable fractures.[18] The stress focal point of a negative-profile pin is at the threaded–non-threaded junction of the shaft.[19] Threaded pins have a biomechanical advantage over smooth pins because they are more resistant to axial extraction from the bone.[20,21] Smooth pins must rely upon the circumferential forces exerted by the surrounding bone on the pin (radial preload) for retention.[22] The axial extraction resistance of a smooth pin can be improved by increasing the porosity of the pin surface with a coating that encourages fibrous tissue and bone ingrowth.[23] Porous implants may be more prone to infection following contamination, which is a concern when pins are driven through the skin and oral cavity.[23] Pins are also supplied in variety of tip designs. Both fluted and nonfluted tips are available. T-tip pins are a type of nonfluted tip and are the most common tip used in veterinary medicine.[22] T-tip pins produce smaller holes in the bone compared to fluted-tip pins but incur greater tip temperatures during placement because they do not clear bone debris while cutting.[22] Fluted tip designs such as the hollow-ground tip also eliminate the need for predrilling of a pilot hole.[22]

Connecting bars and clamps

Metal (stainless steel or aluminum) clamps and stainless steel, aluminum, titanium or composite connecting bars are utilized in the currently available linear ESF systems. Free-form ESF systems use hand-molded acrylic around the external pin ends or acrylic-filled plastic/silicone tubing as substitutes for straight metal bars. The plastic tubing serves as a mold for the acrylic while it is curing. Because of the potential environmental safety hazard associated with the use of acrylics, other materials such as epoxy putty and nontoxic rigid polymers have been investigated as suitable alternatives.[24,25] Although realistically any flexible tubing of appropriate diameter can be used, it has been recommended that the diameter of the free-form connecting bar be 2 to 2.5 times the diameter of the bone being repaired.[26] In studies comparing the mechanical properties of stainless steel and acrylic connecting bars, 19-mm diameter acrylic columns were found to be stronger than 4.8-mm diameter metal connecting bars.[27,28]

External fixator systems

Linear and free-form ESF frames are used for maxillofacial fracture repair. Linear maxillofacial ESF frames are typically configured in a uniplanar type I or in a modified type II fashion with half-pins. Free-form frames may also be applied in uniplanar, unilateral or bilateral configurations, but are not classified into types. Half-pins are routinely used in the mandible. Fixation pins for maxillary fractures are placed transmaxillary (through two skin surfaces and four cortices), and are not used as half- or full-pins.

Linear

The Kirschner-Ehmer (KE) apparatus consists of clamps, connecting bars and fixation pins, and is the most well-known linear ESF system in veterinary surgery. Kirschner-Ehmer clamps and connecting bars are available in three sizes (small, medium and large), but generally only the small and medium sizes are used in veterinary orthopedics.[3] The large-size clamps and connecting bars are made of aluminum, but the small- and medium-size KE parts are stainless steel.[29] KE fixators are simple to use and affordable, but their stiffness is inferior to that of newer systems.[30] Stiffer ESF devices enhance the speed and quality of fracture healing.[31]

The Securos (Securos ESF System, Securos Veterinary Orthopedics, East Brookfield, MA) and SK (SK ESF System, IMEX Veterinary, Inc., Longview, TX) systems are recent additions to the veterinary ESF market that incorporate the use of modern materials and improved modularity over the traditional KE fixator. In comparison to the KE fixator, both the Securos and SK systems are more secure at the fixation pin/connecting bar junction, and include larger and stiffer connecting rods for increased biomechanical strength.[32] The Securos system uses fixation pins and connecting rods made of 316L stainless steel, and the SK system utilizes connecting rods composed of titanium, aluminum or carbon-fiber composite. The stiffness of the former can be increased by up to 450% with the use of augmentation plates.[33] SK fixators require a change in the type of connecting rod to adjust fixator stiffness. The clamps for each system are unique and cannot be readily interchanged. Both systems include drill guides that simplify the process of pin placement. The biggest difference between the two systems is that the Securos system gives the operator the option of progressively disassembling the frame (dynamization) to induce adaptive remodeling of the bone and potentially accelerate healing. In the canine tibia osteotomy model, dynamization was shown to have a beneficial effect on fracture healing when performed after 6 weeks.[34]

Free-form

Free-form fixators are a type of external fixator that substitutes the metal connecting bars and clamps of KE-type fixators with acrylic or epoxy putty (Epoxy ESF putty, Jorgensen Laboratories, Loveland, CO) molded into a cylindrical shape over the pin ends. Acrylic connecting bars can be made by molding doughy acrylic (Formatray, Kerr, Romulus, MI) over the pin ends, or by syringing the acrylic (Jet Denture Repair Acrylic, Lang Dental, Wheeling, IL) into a tubular mold pierced over the external pin ends (Fig. 32.2). Examples of acrylics that can be used include custom impression tray material (Formatray, Kerr, Romulus, MI), dental acrylic (Jet Denture Repair Acrylic, Lang Dental, Wheeling, IL), polymethyl methacrylate bone cement (Simplex P, Howmedica Osteonics, Rutherford, NJ), or hoof acrylic (Technovit, Jorgensen Laboratories, Loveland CO). Examples of suitable tubular molds include corrugated anesthetic tubing, polyvinyl chloride endotracheal tubes and silicone tubing. A complete prepackaged kit (Acrylic Pin External Fixation System (APEF), Innovative Animal Products, Rochester, MN) is available that includes acrylic, plastic tubular mold and caps for the tube ends.

Free-form fixators are easy to apply and allow the surgeon to use fixation pins of any diameter and place them in any spatial arrangement without being restricted by clamp size and linearity of the connecting bars.[26] The ability to contour the side bar to the shape of the bone provides increased axial compressive stiffness.[35] Staged disassembly for dynamization or postoperative adjustments to free-form fixators cannot be performed without cutting the acrylic column with an oscillating saw, and is a recognized disadvantage of the fixator type.[26] The prehension of food can be difficult for patients with bilateral free-form fixators that extend across the rostral midline of the maxilla or mandible.[26]

External fixator systems for distraction osteogenesis

Distraction osteogenesis (DO) is the process of gradual lengthening of bone by traction, and is a surgical procedure that can be used for treating severe deficiencies in maxillary or mandibular length.[36] Distraction osteogenesis simultaneously creates adaptive changes in the associated soft tissues (distraction histiogenesis), and provides a significant advantage over traditional osteotomy techniques when large skeletal movements are required.[36,37] Other uses of DO in oral and maxillofacial surgery are arch widening, bone transport and alveolar margin augmentation prior to implant placement. The basic components of a DO apparatus for craniofacial distraction resembles a

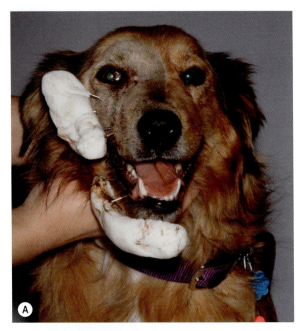

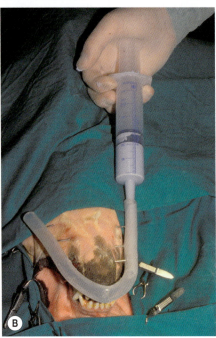

Fig. 32.2 (**A**) Acrylic external pin fixator with hand-molded acrylic connecting bars for repair of maxillary and mandibular fractures in a dog. (**B**) Acrylic external pin fixator with silicone tubing being used as a tubular mold for the syringed acrylic for repair of bilateral mandibular fractures in a dog. ((A) From Verstraete FJM, ed. *Self-assessment color review of veterinary dentistry*. London: Manson Publishing, 1999;99) ((B) From Verstraete FJM. *Maxillofacial fractures* In: Slatter DH, ed. *Textbook of small animal surgery*. 3rd ed. Philadelphia: WB Saunders, 2003;2190–2207.)

standard linear ESF device, and many of the older-model (extraoral) distraction devices can also be used for fracture fixation (Fig. 32.3). In the interest of reducing the potential for unsightly scars, most of the current DO devices used for human patients are internal devices that are placed subcutaneously or intraorally. The dog has been used extensively by human oral surgeons as a model for DO.[38–42]

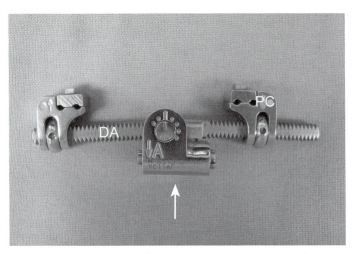

Fig. 32.3 Extraoral distractor for distraction osteogenesis. Note the similarities to a standard external pin fixator: distractor arm (DA); pin clamp (PC). The distractor body is identified with an arrow. The inset screw in the distractor body is turned to make angular adjustments to the distractor. *(Distractor courtesy of Dr SP Bartlett, Hospital of the University of Pennsylvania, Philadelphia, PA.)*

THERAPEUTIC DECISION-MAKING

Indications

Historically, it was believed that the open reduction of comminuted fractures disrupted the tenuous blood supply of the fracture fragments and increased the likelihood of resorption, sequestration and infection: the 'bag-of-bones' aphorism.[43] The technique of external pin fixation avoided direct invasion of the traumatized area, prevented stripping of the periosteum and blood supply to fracture fragments, and was the primary method of treatment for comminuted fractures. The introduction of less invasive surgical approaches and advances in bone plating systems in human oral surgery have limited the indications for external pin fixators in human patients, and even comminuted fractures are often treated with reconstruction plates and screws.[44,45]

Most maxillofacial fractures are grossly contaminated fractures that are directly exposed to the external environment through the skin, mucosa or periodontal ligament. Diffuse infection of the bone at the fracture site is a contraindication for open fracture reduction, and is an example where ESF is still the treatment of choice.[44] Despite their limited use in human oral and maxillofacial surgery, ESF devices are still widely used in veterinary medicine, which may be explained by their simplicity and low cost. Currently, the indications for ESF in maxillofacial fracture repair are mainly: grossly infected jaw fractures, fractures of atrophic edentulous jaws and severely comminuted fractures with a tenuous blood supply (Box 32.1).[44] External skeletal fixation devices are also useful for the treatment of nonunion fractures where bone grafting is necessary, corrective osteotomies and as a method of interim stabilization before jaw reconstruction.[43] Maxillofacial injuries with continuity defects may require bone grafting. These injuries often have extensive skin and mucosal lacerations. The immediate placement of bone grafts in these contaminated wounds should be avoided because of an increased risk of infection.[46] Grafts are avascular and do not have the ability to fight infection.[47] An ESF device will maintain control of the residual jaw segments until the soft tissues have healed and the defect can be grafted.[46] When jaw segments are not maintained in anatomic alignment, significant atrophy and fibrosis of the muscles of mastication may occur, making it extremely difficult to realign the fragments at the time of reconstruction.[47]

Biomechanical considerations

Pin–bone interface

Pin design, pin insertion technique, bone quality, osseous response to pin implantation and loading are factors that affect the integrity of the pin–bone interface.[48] The pin–bone interface is the weakest link of an external pin fixator system.[49] Instability at the pin–bone interface is the most common reason for fixator failure.[48] Motion is detrimental to the pin–bone interface, and can predispose to pin tract sepsis, fracture nonunion, delayed bony union and increased patient morbidity.[48,50,51] Excessive motion promotes the development of fibrous tissue over bone at the pin–bone interface.[48] Positive-profile threaded pins have greater bone-holding capacity than negative-profile threaded or smooth pins.[48] Although bone damage during pin placement is inevitable, micromechanical and thermal damage to the bone can be minimized by using fluted-tip pins, predrilling pilot holes and using low-speed drills (300 rpm or less) for pin placement.[48] Bone temperatures adjacent to the pin tract are lower for fluted-tip pins compared to trocar-tip pins.[22] Predrilled pilot holes that approximate the inner diameter of the positive-profile pin improve pin stability and reduce microstructural damage.[52] The use of high-speed drills (700 rpm or greater) for pin placement should be avoided to reduce the danger of thermal bone necrosis.[48]

Pin selection

Threaded pins have greater holding power than smooth pins and may decrease the incidence of the premature pin loosening.[50] Smooth fixation pins will conceivably cause less trauma to neurovascular structures than threaded pins if placed in the mandibular canal.[53] Larger-diameter and shorter pins are less flexible than smaller-diameter, longer pins.[35,54] Pin stiffness is directly related to the fourth power of the pin radius.[55] The largest-diameter pin possible that does not exceed 20–30% of the bone diameter should be selected.[56]

Pin placement

The patient is positioned in sternal or dorsal recumbency. Local anesthesia can be administered to the selected pin sites. Fixation pins are inserted through longitudinal percutaneous stab incisions. Longitudinal incisions are less likely to transect superficial vessels and nerves.[57] A small hemostat is used to dissect the soft tissues and expose a small area of bone. Pins may be placed exclusively by hand or power drill, or after predrilling a pilot hole with a drill bit 0.1–1 mm smaller than the diameter of the pin.[17] There are disadvantages to each technique: pin tract enlargement from wobbling with hand placement, thermal bone necrosis with power drilling and the inconvenience of the extra step associated with predrilling. Predrilling of a pilot hole at low speed (150 rpm) followed by hand placement of the pin is advocated in the current veterinary literature.[30,58]

The fixation pins that are located adjacent to the fracture line are commonly referred to as the 'mean' pins, and the second or third pins placed in each fragment are often called the 'extreme' pins.[59] By convention, the extreme rostral and caudal pins are inserted first. Pins should be placed no closer than 10 mm from the fracture line and from each other.[59] Care should be taken to avoid dental trauma when placing the pins. Temporomandibular joint range of motion should be maintained throughout treatment.[30] A minimum of two pins rostral and caudal to the fracture line is appropriate for most fractures.[43] The number of pins placed in each fragment influences the stiffness of the fixator and load distribution to the pins.[17] The addition of a third pin to each fragment will increase stability by 50% if the pins are aligned in a row, and by greater than 50% if arranged in a triangular configuration.[43] Beyond the addition of a fourth pin per fragment, the mechanical advantage is negligible.[17] Each pin should be placed in a divergent fashion and engage both cortices.[59] Angled pin placement maximizes the surface area of the pin in contact with cortical bone and increases fixator stiffness.[60] The optimum angle for pin insertion is 70° relative to the long axis of the bone.[61] If a biphasic splint is used, the long axes of the screws should diverge by approximately 5–7°.[59]

Surgical considerations

Open versus closed fracture reduction

External pin fixators for maxillofacial fracture repair are preferably placed in a closed fashion. A closed approach will avoid further disruption of the blood supply to the fracture fragments.[62] Closed reduction of a displaced mandibular fracture can often be facilitated by reestablishing the patient's preinjury occlusal relationship before attempting fixator placement. Similar to the hanging limb technique for reducing long bone fractures, restoring the patient's occlusion will help pull the bone segments into better alignment. Open reduction is occasionally necessary, and may be indicated when there is significant fracture displacement, if debridement is indicated, with autogenous bone grafting or if the fixator is used as an ancillary device.[30,62]

CLINICAL APPLICATIONS OF EXTERNAL SKELETAL FIXATION

Fractures of the mandible

In human oral and maxillofacial surgery, mandibular fracture repair by external pin fixation is synonymous with the Joe Hall Morris biphasic splint (Bi-Phase External Fixation System, W. Lorenz Surgical, Jacksonville, FL) (Fig. 32.4).[44] The biphasic nature of the splint refers to the two-part procedure required for its installation, fracture reduction with specialized screws and a reduction apparatus, followed by anatomic alignment and fixation with an acrylic bar to connect the screws.[11] The screws for the Morris splint are too long for the mandibles of small dogs and cats, and can only be used in dogs with sufficient mandibular thickness to accommodate the length of screw, generally dogs greater than 12–15 kg.[11]

Mandibular fractures in dogs occur most commonly in the premolar region.[63,64] External pin fixators can be used for both unilateral and

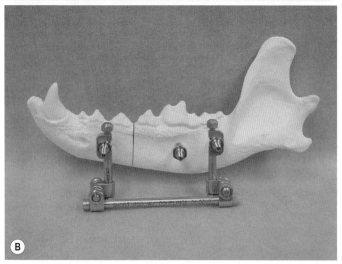

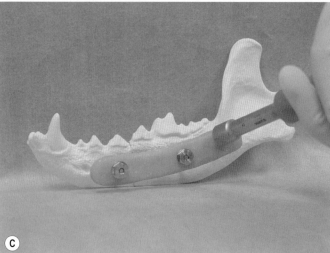

Fig. 32.4 Joe Hall Morris biphasic splint (Bi-Phase External Fixation System, W. Lorenz Surgical, Jacksonville, FL) demonstrated on a mandibular model. (**A**) Titanium self-drilling screws (left to right): short (42 mm), medium (51 mm) and long (64 mm). (**B**) Phase I: fracture reduction with primary mechanical splint (screw holding assembly and rod). (**C**) Phase II: secondary splint (acrylic bar) replaces primary mechanical splint.

bilateral fractures of the body of the mandible (Figs 32.5 and 32.6A, B).[65] For most mandibular fractures, at least two fixation pins should be inserted on either side of the fracture. The tooth roots and the mandibular canal should be avoided.[11] External pin fixation of mandibular fractures is largely limited to fractures of the mandibular body.[3] Pin placement can be difficult in caudally located mandibular fractures where bone thickness is inadequate, and mandibular fractures rostral to the third premolar teeth where there is insufficient space for the placement of multiple pins.[3] An alternative technique for rostral mandibular fractures has been described that uses a single intraoral interdental full-pin in lieu of multiple fixation pins.[66] The single intraoral pin is anchored to the mandibular canine teeth using a figure-of-eight wire and a bridge of acrylic between the canine and incisor teeth (Fig. 32.7).[66] The rigidity of this technique has been tested on a mandibular fracture gap model where osteotomies were performed between the third and fourth premolar teeth, and has been shown to be as stiff as fixator configurations containing two or four additional pins in the rostral fracture fragments.[66] The natural dental interlock between the maxilla and mandible resists torsional forces, and imparts the necessary additional stability to the fracture repair that would not have been sufficiently addressed with a single intraoral full-pin alone.[66]

Another alternative, the Gunning splint (also see Ch. 29), utilizes an indirectly fabricated acrylic or composite intraoral splint, or in humans a patient's dentures, secured to the mandible (or maxilla) with circumferential wires.[67] This type of splint is ideally suited for the repair of mandibular fractures in edentulous patients or those with mixed dentition, either as a sole method of fixation or to augment another form of fixation. In humans, Gunning splints are traditionally combined with maxillomandibular fixation or elastics to establish and maintain occlusion.[67]

Fractures of the maxilla

Fractures of the maxilla are less common than mandibular fractures and often are not sufficiently displaced to warrant surgical repair.[53] In contemporary trauma surgery practice, even severely comminuted and unstable maxillary fractures are optimally treated with open reduction and miniplate osteosynthesis. External fixation can be used as an alternative technique to plate osteosynthesis where cost is a factor, but enough maxilla must be available caudal to the fracture to allow placement of a sufficient number of pins.[65] After pre-injury occlusion is obtained with one of the previously described temporary MMF techniques, the pins are driven percutaneously through non-tooth-bearing portions of the maxillary bones and across the nasal cavity.[68] Long-term nasal problems from the transmaxillary placement of the pins are usually not significant.[65]

Other

A nonunion of a mandibular fracture can occur when diseased teeth in the fracture line are not extracted prior to fixator placement.[26] Nonunions of mandibular fractures have traditionally been treated by autogenous cancellous bone grafting, but can also be effectively treated by bone transport with distraction osteogenesis. The dog has been used as a successful model for segmental mandibular regeneration by bone transport, and good long-term results have been reported.[38,39] Bone transport is the gradual movement of a free segment of bone (transport disk) across an osseous defect.[69] A transport disk of no less than 15 mm is created from the caudal bone segment through an extraoral approach. The gingival tissues are not perforated during the corticotomy, and the contents of the mandibular canal are preserved. The pins for the external fixator are placed through separate

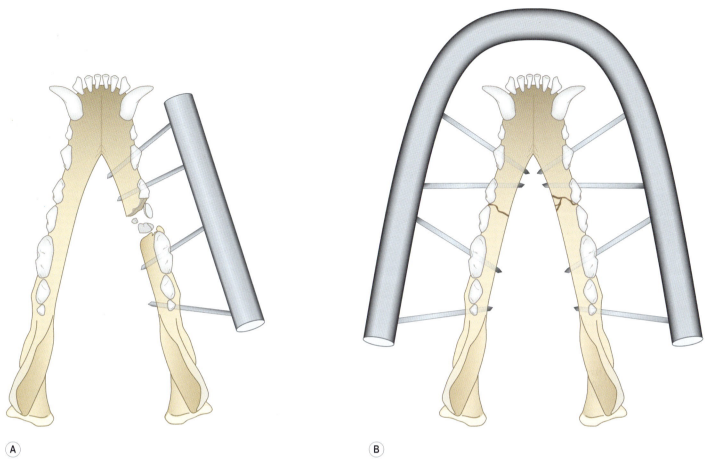

(A) (B)

Fig. 32.5 Line drawings of type I free-form fixators used for the repair of (**A**) a unilateral fracture of the body of the mandible with a substantial missing fragment and (**B**) bilateral fractures of the mandibular bodies.

stab incisions, and a minimum of two pins are placed in the transport disk to achieve rotational stability. After formation of a reparative callus (5–7 days), the disk is transported at a rate of 1 mm per day until it reaches its docking site. Upon completion of bone transport, the transported and targeted bone segments are fused by compression forces.[69] Compression forces applied to the bone segments results in transformational osteogenesis with necrosis of the pathologic tissues, resorption, remodeling and fusion of the bone segments.[69] Bone transport uses the original mandible as a template, and maintains the size and shape of the original mandible in the neomandible.[70] The local soft tissues (gingiva, buccal and lingual sulcus) are also recreated with bone transport.[70]

POSTOPERATIVE CARE AND ASSESSMENT

Aftercare

It is common practice for external pin fixators to be wrapped to prevent injury to the client (e.g., pin impalement), to avoid pin ends snagging on objects in the environment and to minimize movement between the skin and pins. Clinical movement at the pin site will disrupt the chemotactic gradient used by phagocytes to target bacteria at the pin site, predisposing to bacterial proliferation, sepsis and chronic drainage at the pin sites.[58] For obvious reasons, external pin fixation devices placed in the maxilla or mandible cannot be similarly wrapped without causing significant irritation to the patient.

A reasonable compromise to a circumferential bandage is to place gauze sponges between the skin and the fixator. The gauze sponges should initially be changed on a daily basis, and the pin sites cleansed daily with a suitable antiseptic scrub (chlorhexidine gluconate or povidone-iodine) to lessen soft tissue inflammation. Inflammation of the soft tissues surrounding pins has been shown to increase patient morbidity.[57] The frequency of bandage changes can be decreased as the pin sites heal and with development of bacteriostatic granulation tissue at the pin sites. The patient should be rechecked twice weekly for the first 2 weeks, and then weekly until fixator removal, which is usually at 6 weeks.[59]

Radiography

Postoperative radiographs should be obtained to document pin placement and fracture reduction. Bone healing is assessed radiographically at 6 weeks, unless clinical signs would indicate possible complications sooner. Follow-up radiographs are best obtained under general anesthesia and should be evaluated from a minimum of two directions if plain films are used or in the sagittal plane if computed tomography is available.

Fixator removal

External fixators should be removed at the earliest evidence of complete bony union.[71] The recommended time to ESF removal in dogs and cats is 6 weeks.[53] The status of repair and bone consolidation can

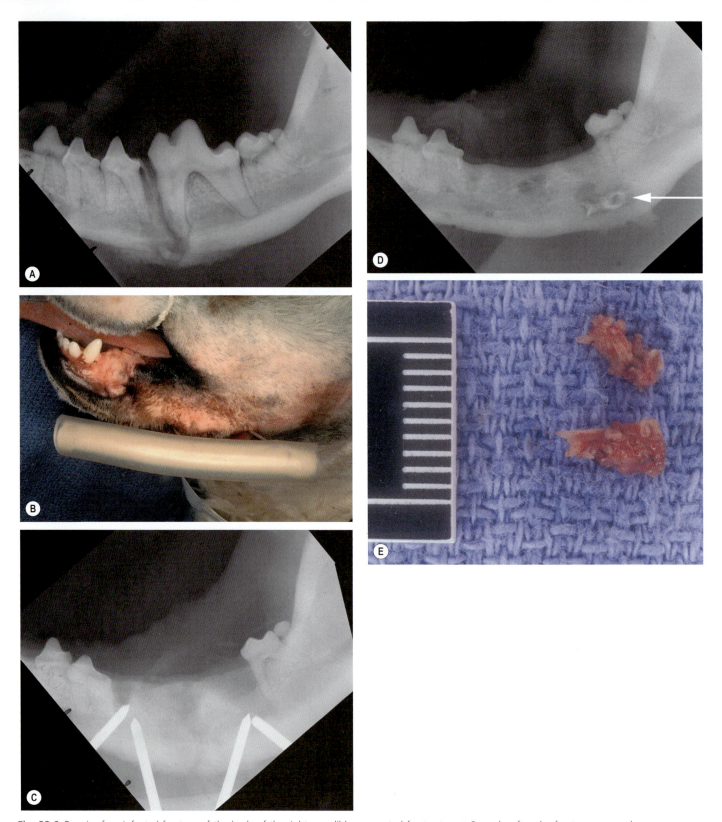

Fig. 32.6 Repair of an infected fracture of the body of the right mandible, presented for treatment 2 weeks after the fracture occurred: (**A**) Preoperative radiograph. (**B**) Repair using an acrylic external fixator. (**C**) Two-week follow-up radiograph illustrating pin placement; note that the two teeth involved in the fracture line have been extracted. (**D**) Radiograph obtained 14 weeks postoperatively and following fixator removal, showing a ring sequestrum (*arrow*) at the most caudal pin hole. (**E**) The surgically removed ring sequestrum fragments.

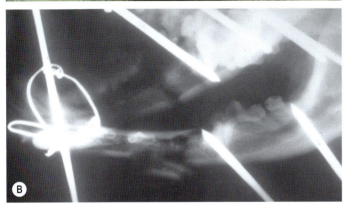

Fig. 32.7 (**A**) Clinical picture and (**B**) accompanying radiograph of the intraoral interdental full-pin technique for repair of rostral mandibular fractures. A medium centrally threaded 3.2-mm pin was secured to the distal aspect of the mandibular canine teeth with a figure-of-eight 18-gauge wire. Polymethyl methacrylate was applied over the wire and between the canine teeth for additional stability. *(Photographs courtesy of Dr. MM Smith.)*

be manually assessed following careful disassembly of the connecting bar and clamps or after sectioning of the acrylic between the pins adjacent to the fracture line. If healing is inadequate the connecting bar and clamps can be readily reassembled or rejoined with additional acrylic. At the time of definitive removal, acrylic columns can be notched and cut with an oscillating saw, and the pieces of acrylic attached to the pins can be used as handles for removal of the pins.[28] Alternatively, the pins can be backed out using a pin chuck.[72]

COMPLICATIONS

The most common complication of external pin fixation is necrosis of bone directly adjacent to the pin tract (pin tract osteomyelitis).[73] Radiographically, a ring-shaped zone of osteolysis (ring sequestrum) with variable periosteal new bone formation and osteosclerosis may appear around the pin tract (see Fig. 32.6C, D).[74] A ring sequestrum is best visualized on a radiograph where the primary X-ray beam is directed parallel to the pin tract.[75] Excessive heat build-up or thermal necrosis of the bone at the pin insertion site is a major predisposing factor in the development of pin tract osteomyelitis.[74] The use of power drills for pin placement and cortical placement of the pin may increase the risk of thermal necrosis.[74,76] Thermal damage to the soft tissues and bone can also result from the exothermic reaction of polymethyl methacrylates used for acrylic connecting columns.[77,78] The potential for thermal damage can be minimized by using the smallest-diameter acrylic column (i.e., least amount of acrylic) possible without sacrificing fixator strength and by positioning the acrylic column no less than 10 mm from the patient's body surface during curing of the acrylic.[77,78] Increasing the distance between the connecting bar and the skin decreases the axial compression stiffness of the fixator, particularly for unilateral frames, and should be kept to a minimum.[35] The use of saline-soaked gauze sponges between the patient and the acrylic, or a constant saline drip at the pin–acrylic interface during curing of the acrylic can also be used to decrease the malignant transfer of heat to bone and soft tissues.[28,77] Mobility at the pin site as a result of suboptimal pin placement technique or inadequate patient restriction can also predispose to pin tract infection. Most cases of pin tract osteomyelitis can be treated conservatively with antimicrobial therapy and local wound management, and usually does not adversely affect outcome.[74,79] A ring sequestrum should be surgically removed (see Fig. 32.6D).

Other potential complications of external pin fixation include pin breakage, pin pull-out, pin loosening, fracture and secondary dental disease. Pin breakage, pull-out and loosening are device failures, and are almost always the result of technical error or insufficient patient restriction.[79] Stress points in acrylic connecting bars are created where air has become entrapped in the acrylic mass.[66] Air bubbles can be minimized by maintaining contact of the mixing tip with the extruded acrylic during filling of the tube. Fractures can occur when fixation pins are placed in osteoporotic bone or when pin selection is inappropriate and exceeds more than 20% of the bone diameter.[74] Tooth roots and their neurovascular supply may be violated during pin placement and can result in periodontal or endodontic complications, nerve injury and hemorrhage. Tooth impaction may occur if a developing tooth bud is injured.[80] The applied knowledge of cross-sectional anatomy and the use of drill guides and tissue protectors can minimize the risk of iatrogenic injury to nerves and blood vessels.[79] External scarring is unavoidable with this technique.[46]

REFERENCES

1. Ochs MW, Tucker MR. Management of facial fractures. In: Peterson LJ, Ellis III E, Hupp JR, et al, editors. Contemporary oral and maxillofacial surgery. 4th ed. St. Louis, MO: Mosby Inc; 2003. p. 527–58.
2. Cooper J, Rojer CL, Rosenfeld PA. Management of mandibular fractures using biphasic pins and mandibular splints. Laryngoscope 1982;92:1042–8.
3. Davidson JR, Bauer MS. Fractures of the mandible and maxilla. Vet Clin North Am Small Anim Pract 1992;22:109–19.
4. Verstraete FJM, Ligthelm AJ. Dental trauma caused by screws in internal fixation of mandibular osteotomies in the dog. Vet Comp Orthop Traumatol 1992;5: 104–8.
5. Robins GM, Read RA. The use of a transfixation splint to stabilize a bilateral mandibular fracture in a dog. J Small Anim Pract 1981;22:759–68.

6. Haynes HH. Treating fractures by skeletal fixation of the individual bone. South Med J 1939;32:720–4.

7. Stader O. A preliminary announcement of a new method of treating fractures. North Am Vet 1937;18:37–8.

8. Armistead MM. Unusual management of mandibular fracture in a dog. J Am Vet Med Assoc 1947;111:110–11.

9. Ehmer E. Bone pinning in fractures in small animals. J Am Vet Med Assoc 1947;110:14.

10. Morris JH. Biphase connector, external skeletal splint for reduction and fixation of mandibular fractures. Oral Surg Oral Med Oral Pathol 1949;2:1382–98.

11. Greenwood KM, Creagh Jr GB. Bi-Phase external skeletal splint of mandibular fractures in dogs. Vet Surg 1980;9:128–34.

12. Weigel JP, Dorn AS, Chase DC, et al. The use of the biphase external fixation splint for repair of canine mandibular fractures. J Am Anim Hosp Assoc 1981;17:547–54.

13. Becker E. Ein Instrumentarium zur perkutanen Osteosynthese und extrakutanen Überbrückung mit Kunststoffe. Zentralbl Veterinärmed 1957;4:205–42.

14. Becker E. Ein Instrumentarium zur extracutanen Osteosynthese bei Unterkieferfrakturen unter Verwendung plastischer Kunststoffe. Der Chirurg 1958;29:63–7.

15. Michelet FX, Deymes J, Dessus B. Osteosynthesis with miniaturized screwed plates in maxillo-facial surgery. J Maxillofac Surg 1973;1:79–84.

16. Champy M, Lodde JP, Schmitt R, et al. Mandibular osteosynthesis by miniature screwed plates via a buccal approach. J Maxillofac Surg 1978;6:14–21.

17. Fossum TW, Hedlund CS, Hulse DA, et al. Fundamentals of orthopedic surgery and fracture management. In: Fossum TW, Hedlund CS, Hulse DL, et al, editors. Small animal surgery. 2nd ed. St. Louis, MO: Mosby Inc; 2002. p. 821–900.

18. Anderson MA, Palmer RH, Aron DN. Improving pin selection and insertion technique for external skeletal fixation. Compend Contin Educ Pract Vet 1997; 19:485–93.

19. Palmer RH, Aron DN. Ellis pin complications in seven dogs. Vet Surg 1990;19:440–5.

20. Egger EL, Histand M, Blass CE, et al. Effect of fixation pin insertion on the bone-pin interface. Vet Surg 1986;15:246–52.

21. Bennett RA, Egger EL, Histand M, et al. Comparison of the strength and holding power of 4 pin designs for use with half pin (type I) external skeletal fixation. Vet Surg 1987;16:207–11.

22. Marti JM, Roe SC. Biomechanical comparison of the trocar tip point and the hollow ground tip point for smooth external skeletal fixation pins. Vet Surg 1998;27:423–8.

23. DeCamp CE, Brinker WO, Soutas-Little RW. Porous titanium-surfaced pins for external skeletal fixation. J Am Anim Hosp Assoc 1988;24:295–300.

24. Roe SC, Keo T. Epoxy putty for free-form external skeletal fixators. Vet Surg 1997; 26:472–7.

25. Stork CK, Canivet P, Baidak AA, et al. Evaluation of a nontoxic rigid polymer as connecting bar in external skeletal fixators. Vet Surg 2003;32:262–8.

26. Ross JT, Matthiesen DT. The use of multiple pin and methylmethacrylate external fixation for the treatment of orthopaedic injuries in the dog and cat. Vet Comp Orthop Traumatol 1993;6:115–21.

27. Willer RL, Egger EL, Histand MB. Comparison of stainless steel versus acrylic for the connecting bar of external skeletal fixators. J Am Anim Hosp Assoc 1991; 27:541–8.

28. Okrasinski EB, Pardo AD, Graehler RA. Biomechanical evaluation of acrylic external skeletal fixation in dogs and cats. J Am Vet Med Assoc 1991;199:1590–3.

29. Johnson AL, DeCamp CE. External skeletal fixation. Linear fixators. Vet Clin North Am Small Anim Pract 1999;29:1135–52.

30. Marcellin-Little DJ. External skeletal fixation. In: Slatter DH, editor. Textbook of small animal surgery. 3rd ed. Philadelphia, PA: WB Saunders Co; 2003. p. 1818–34.

31. Wu JJ, Shyr HS, Chao EY, et al. Comparison of osteotomy healing under external fixation devices with different stiffness characteristics. J Bone Joint Surg Am 1984;66:1258–64.

32. Kraus KH, Wotton HM. Effect of clamp type on type II external fixator stiffness. Vet Comp Orthop Traumatol 1999;12:178–82.

33. Kraus KH, Toombs JP, Ness MG. The Securos external fixation system. In: Kraus KH, Toombs JP, Ness MG, editors. External fixation in small animal practice. Oxford, UK: Blackwell Science Ltd; 2003. p. 43–52.

34. Egger EL, Gottsauner-Wolf F, Palmer J, et al. Effects of axial dynamization on bone healing. J Trauma 1993;34:185–92.

35. Bouvy BM, Markel MD, Chelikani S, et al. Ex vivo biomechanics of Kirschner–Ehmer external skeletal fixation applied to canine tibiae. Vet Surg 1993;22:194–207.

36. Samchukov ML, Cope JB, Cherkashin AM. Introduction to distraction osteogenesis. In: Samchukov ML, Cope JB, Cherkashin AM, editors. Craniofacial distraction osteogenesis. St. Louis, MO: Mosby Inc; 2001. p. 3–16.

37. Tucker MR, Ochs MW. Correction of dentofacial deformities. In: Peterson LJ, Ellis III E, Hupp JR, et al, editors. Contemporary oral and maxillofacial surgery. 4th ed. St. Louis, MO: Mosby Inc; 2003. p. 560–602.

38. Costantino PD, Shybut G, Friedman CD, et al. Segmental mandibular regeneration by distraction osteogenesis. An experimental study. Arch Otolaryngol Head Neck Surg 1990;116:535–45.

39. Costantino PD, Friedman CD, Shindo ML, et al. Experimental mandibular regrowth by distraction osteogenesis. Long-term results. Arch Otolaryngol Head Neck Surg 1993;119:511–16.

40. Block MS, Daire J, Stover J, et al. Changes in the inferior alveolar nerve following mandibular lengthening in the dog using distraction osteogenesis. J Oral Maxillofac Surg 1993;51:652–60.

41. Makarov MR, Harper RP, Cope JB, et al. Evaluation of inferior alveolar nerve function during distraction osteogenesis in the dog. J Oral Maxillofac Surg 1998;56:1417–23; discussion 1424–5.

42. Block MS, Chang A, Crawford C. Mandibular alveolar ridge augmentation in the dog using distraction osteogenesis. J Oral Maxillofac Surg 1996;54:309–14.

43. Seldin EB. Operative management of mandibular fractures. In: Keith DA, editor. Atlas of oral and maxillofacial surgery. Philadelphia, PA: WB Saunders Co; 1992. p. 257–84.

44. Spina AM, Marciani RD. Mandibular fractures. In: Fonseca RJ, editor. Oral and maxillofacial surgery. Philadelphia, PA: WB Saunders Co; 2000. p. 85–135.

45. Ellis III E, Muniz O, Anand K. Treatment considerations for comminuted mandibular fractures. J Oral Maxillofac Surg 2003;61:861–70.

46. Hilger PA. Rigid internal and external fixation of mandibular fractures. In: Foster CA, Sherman JE, editors. Surgery of facial bone fractures. New York: Churchill Livingstone Inc; 1987. p. 195–211.

47. Ellis III E. Surgical reconstruction of jaw defects. In: Peterson LJ, E. Ellis III E, Hupp JR, et al, editors. Contemporary oral and maxillofacial surgery. 4th ed. St. Louis, MO: Mosby Inc; 2003. p. 646–59.

48. Clary EM, Roe SC. Enhancing external skeletal fixation pin performance: consideration of the pin–bone interface. Vet Comp Orthop Traumatol 1995; 8:1–8.

49. Toombs JP. Principles of external skeletal fixation using the Kirschner–Ehmer splint. Semin Vet Med Surg (Small Anim) 1991; 6:68–74.

50. Aron DN, Toombs JP, Hollingsworth SC. Primary treatment of severe fractures by external fixation: threaded pins compared with smooth pins. J Am Anim Hosp Assoc 1986;22:659–70.

51. Anderson MA, Mann FA, Wagner-Mann C, et al. A comparison of non-threaded, enhanced threaded, and Ellis fixation pins used in type I external skeletal fixators in dogs. Vet Surg 1993;22:482–9.

52. Clary EM, Roe SC. In vitro biomechanical and histological assessment of pilot hole diameter for positive-profile external skeletal fixation pins in canine tibiae. Vet Surg 1996;25:453–62.

53. Verstraete FJM. Maxillofacial fractures. In: Slatter DH, editor. Textbook of small animal surgery. 3rd ed. Philadelphia, PA: WB Saunders Co, 2003;2190–207.

54. Muir P, Johnson K, Markel MD. Area moment of inertia for comparison of implant cross-sectional geometry and bending stiffness. Vet Comp Orthop Traumatol 1995;8:146–52.

55. Palmer RH, Hulse DA, Hyman WA, et al. Principles of bone healing and biomechanics of external skeletal fixation. Vet Clin North Am Small Anim Pract 1992;22:45–68.

56. Edgerton BC, An KN, Morrey BF. Torsional strength reduction due to cortical defects in bone. J Orthop Res 1990;8:851–5.

57. Aron DN, Toombs JP. Updated principles of external skeletal fixation. *Compend* Contin Educ Pract Vet 1994;6:845–58.

58. Aron DN, Dewey CW. Application and postoperative management of external skeletal fixators. Vet Clin North Am Small Anim Pract 1992;22:69–97.

59. Morris JH, Hipp BR. Biphasic pin fixation. In: Williams JL, editor. Rowe and Williams' maxillofacial injuries. 2nd ed. Edinburgh, UK: Churchill Livingstone; 1994. p. 329–40.

60. Gumbs JM, Brinker WO, DeCamp CE, et al. Comparison of acute and chronic pull-out resistance of pins used with the external skeletal fixator (Kirschner splint). J Am Anim Hosp Assoc 1988;24: 231–4.

61. Brinker WO, Verstraete MC, Soutas-Little RW. Stiffness studies on various

configurations and types of external fixators. J Am Anim Hosp Assoc 1986; 21:801–8.

62. Kraus KH, Toombs JP, Ness MG. Fracture reduction. In: Kraus KH, Toombs JP, Ness MG, editors. External fixation in small animal practice. Oxford, UK: Blackwell Science Ltd; 2003. p. 27–32.

63. Phillips IR. A survey of bone fractures in the dog and cat. J Small Anim Pract 1979;20:661–74.

64. Umphlet RC, Johnson AL. Mandibular fractures in the dog. A retrospective study of 157 cases. Vet Surg 1990;19:272–5.

65. Tomlinson JL, Constantinescu GM. Acrylic external skeletal fixation of fractures. *Compend* Contin Educ Pract Vet 1991;13: 235–40.

66. Cook WT, Smith MM, Markel MD, et al. Influence of an interdental full pin on stability of an acrylic external fixator for rostral mandibular fractures in dogs. Am J Vet Res 2001;62:576–80.

67. Stacey DH, Doyle JF, Mount DL, et al. Management of mandibular fractures. Plast Reconstr Surg 2006;117:48e–60e.

68. Stambaugh JE, Nunamaker DM. External skeletal fixation of comminuted maxillary fractures in dogs. Vet Surg 1982;11: 72–6.

69. Samchukov ML, Cope JB, Cherkashin AM. Basic principles of bone transport. In: Samchukov ML, Cope JB, Cherkashin AM, editors. Craniofacial distraction osteogenesis. St. Louis, MO: Mosby Inc; 2001. p. 349–57.

70. Stucki-McCormick SU, Fox RM, Bruder RB, et al. Craniofacial bone transport. In: Samchukov ML, Cope JB, Cherkashin AM, editors. Craniofacial distraction osteogenesis. St. Louis, MO: Mosby Inc; 2001. p. 358–67.

71. Smith MM, Kern DA. Skull trauma and mandibular fractures. Vet Clin North Am Small Anim Pract 1995;25:1127–48.

72. Brinker WO, Flo GL. Principles and application of external skeletal fixation. Vet Clin North Am 1975;5:197–208.

73. Séguin B, Harari J, Wood RD, et al. Bone fracture and sequestration as complications of external skeletal fixation. J Small Anim Pract 1997;38:81–4.

74. Kantrowitz B, Smeak D, Vannini R. Radiographic appearance of ring sequestrum with pin tract osteomyelitis in the dog. J Am Anim Hosp Assoc 1988;24: 461–5.

75. Nguyen VD, London J, Cone III RO. Ring sequestrum: radiographic characteristics of skeletal fixation pin-tract osteomyelitis. Radiology 1986;158:129–31.

76. Green SA, Ripley MJ. Chronic osteomyelitis in pin tracks. J Bone Joint Surg Am 1984;66:1092–8.

77. Williams N, Tomlinson JL, Hahn AW, et al. Heat conduction of fixator pins with polymethylmethacrylate external fixation. Vet Comp Orthop Traumatol 1997;10: 153–9.

78. Martinez SA, Arnoczky SP, Flo GL, et al. Dissipation of heat during polymerization of acrylics used for external skeletal fixator connecting bars. Vet Surg 1997;26:290–4.

79. Kraus KH, Toombs JP, Ness MG. Complications. In: Kraus KH, Toombs JP, Ness MG, editors. External skeletal fixation in small animal practice. Oxford, UK: Blackwell Science Ltd; 2003. p. 88–99.

80. Suei Y, Mallick PC, Nagasaki T, et al. Radiographic evaluation of the fate of developing tooth buds on the fracture line of mandibular fractures. J Oral Maxillofac Surg 2006;64:94–9.

Chapter 33

Fractures and luxations involving the temporomandibular joint

Gary C. Lantz & Frank J.M. Verstraete

DEFINITIONS

A *dislocation* is a temporary displacement of bone from its normal position in a joint.[1] A complete dislocation in which the articular surfaces of a joint are separated is referred to as a *luxation*. A *subluxation* is a partial or incomplete dislocation. *Ankylosis* is defined as an abnormal immobility of a joint from a fibrous or bony union due to disease, injury, or a surgical procedure.[1,2]

CLINICAL PRESENTATION

History and physical findings

Temporomandibular joint (TMJ) fractures and luxations occur as a result of trauma.[3–6] They are often seen in combination with other maxillofacial injuries, especially in the cat.[7] A complete physical examination including assessment of cranial nerves is performed to search for other injuries secondary to trauma. The most common finding with TMJ subluxation, luxation or fracture is an inability to completely close the mouth. Subluxation usually does not result in malocclusion but luxation does result in malocclusion. Unilateral rostral luxation results in shifting of the mandible toward the side opposite the luxation. Unilateral caudal luxation results in shifting of the mandible toward the side of luxation. Bilateral rostral luxation results in slight rostral protrusion of the mandible. A fracture involving the TMJ may or may not result in malocclusion, depending on the degree of displacement. Fractures of the mandibular ramus and coronoid process commonly cause malocclusion. Radiographic confirmation of suspected mandibular injuries is essential.

Oral examination

Initial oral examination without anesthesia is typically limited to evaluation of occlusion and observation of the animal's ability or inability to open and close its mouth. A complete oral examination requires anesthesia. After anesthetic induction, an oral examination is performed looking for oral wounds and open fractures. The mandibles and maxillas are gently palpated. The mandibles are manipulated. Palpable crepitus suggests fracture, and gentle pressure will usually allow mouth closure. Malocclusion and inability to close the mouth by manipulation suggests TMJ luxation. The oral examination is combined with the diagnostic imaging of the skull as more than one maxillofacial injury may be present.

ANESTHETIC CONSIDERATIONS

Pre-anesthesia evaluation

A pre-anesthesia database should consist of physical examination, complete blood count, serum biochemistry profile and urinalysis. Thoracic radiographs, abdominal ultrasound, and an electrocardiogram are obtained for all patients because of the traumatic nature of the condition. The patient is completely evaluated to determine the presence of additional injuries before the induction of anesthesia. After oral examination, diagnostic skull radiographs and/or computed tomography scanning are performed and the injuries addressed. Repair of concurrent mandibular fractures may require endotracheal tube placement by pharyngotomy to allow intraoperative evaluation of occlusion (see Ch. 57). The pharyngotomy is performed on the side opposite to the involved TMJ. If both TMJs are involved, then a temporary tracheostomy may be needed for intubation.

DIAGNOSTIC IMAGING

Radiographic findings

The radiographic anatomy and patient positioning for TMJ radiographs have been described.[7–11] Skull radiographs include ventrodorsal or dorsoventral, laterolateral and open-mouth projections. Right and left lateral oblique projections are made to isolate each TMJ. Radiographic findings may include evidence of TMJ fracture, luxation or a

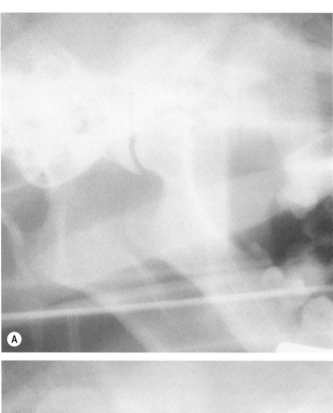

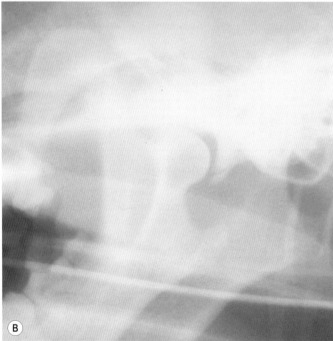

Fig. 33.1 Lateral oblique radiographic projections showing (**A**) normal temporomandibular joint compared to (**B**) the slightly widened joint space of the subluxated joint with fracture of the retroarticular process.

combination.[7,11] A widened TM joint space suggests subluxation (Fig. 33.1A, B). With luxation, the mandibular condyle is displaced from the mandibular fossa, most commonly in a rostrodorsal direction.[6] Luxation may be unilateral or bilateral with rostral or caudal displacement (Fig. 33.2A–C). Temporomandibular joint fractures are most easily seen in the ventrodorsal, dorsoventral and oblique radiographic projections. Fractures may include the condylar process (mandibular neck and head) and the mandibular fossa region of the temporal bone (Fig. 33.3A–C). Luxation in a caudal direction is typically associated

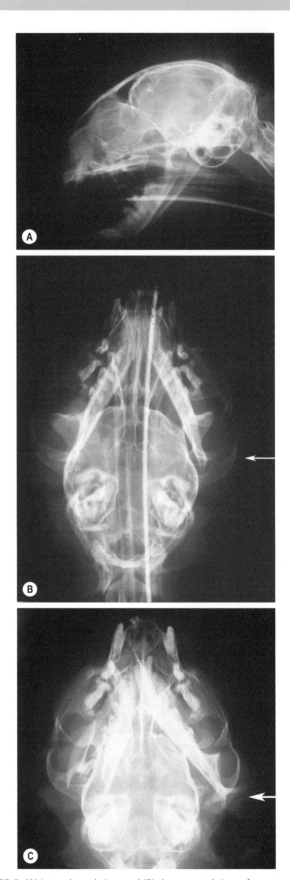

Fig. 33.2 (**A**) Laterolateral view and (**B**) dorsoventral view of a rostrodorsal luxation of the temporomandibular joint (*arrow*). (**C**) Dorsoventral view of a comminuted mandibular fracture, symphyseal separation and caudal luxation of the temporomandibular joint (*arrow*).

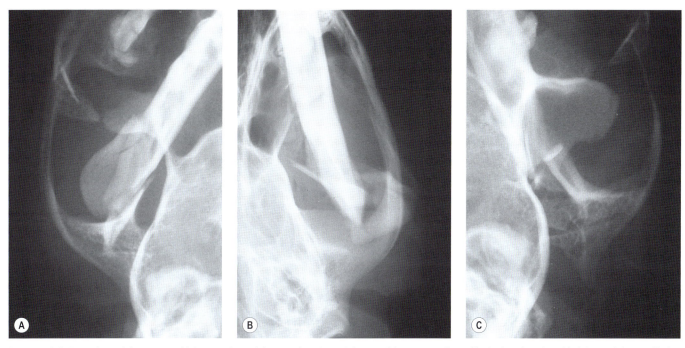

Fig. 33.3 (**A**) Comminuted fracture and (**B**) comminuted fracture/luxation of the condylar process (mandibular head and neck). (**C**) Caudal mandibular fracture with fracture of the mandibular fossa.

with a fracture of the retroarticular process.[7,11] Temporomandibular joint fractures often occur with other maxillofacial fractures. On the ventrodorsal and dorsoventral projections, the mandible may be shifted to one side.

Computed tomography

Computed tomographical anatomy of the canine and feline TMJ has been described.[8,11] This imaging modality may allow detection of subtle anatomic abnormalities and a comparison between both joints of one patient. A rostral–caudal 'view' of the TMJ is provided without superimposed structures and may aid in the diagnosis of certain TMJ fractures that may not be readily apparent on conventional radiographic projections. Tridimensional reconstruction based on thin slices is especially useful.[12]

SURGICAL ANATOMY[13,14]

The anatomy and function of the TMJ are described in Chapter 55. The head of the mandibular condylar process articulates in the mandibular fossa of the temporal bone (Fig. 33.4). This synovial joint has a joint capsule that extends between the articular cartilages and fibrocartilaginous disk separating the articular surfaces. The lateral aspect of the joint capsule is strengthened by the lateral ligament. In comparison with the dog, the feline TMJ has a closer congruity and the structure of the feline mandibular symphysis allows less independent movement of the mandibles.[15]

The lateral aspect of the joint is covered by the masseter muscle (Fig. 33.5A, B). The facial nerve is located caudal–ventral to the joint and its branch, the palpebral nerve, courses along the dorsal border of the zygomatic arch. The maxillary artery and origin of the inferior alveolar and caudal deep temporal arteries lie ventromedial to the condylar process. The mandibular branch of the trigeminal nerve lies medial to the process. The auriculotemporal nerve passes

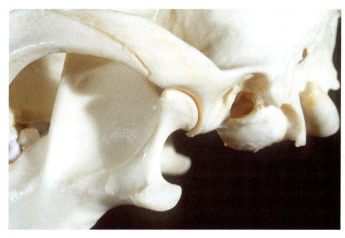

Fig. 33.4 The temporomandibular joint: normal relationship of the condylar process (mandibular head and neck) and mandibular fossa.

immediately caudal to the retroarticular process of the temporal bone. The lateral pterygoid muscle inserts on the medial aspect of the condylar process. The masticatory nerve lies immediately rostral to the TMJ.

THERAPEUTIC DECISION-MAKING

Differential diagnoses

Differential diagnoses include conditions that result in acute or chronic inability to completely close the mouth. These include traumatic TMJ subluxation or luxation, mandibular fracture, TMJ dysplasia, oral foreign body, periodontal disease resulting in extrusion of a tooth with subsequent malocclusion, and trigeminal neuropraxia.

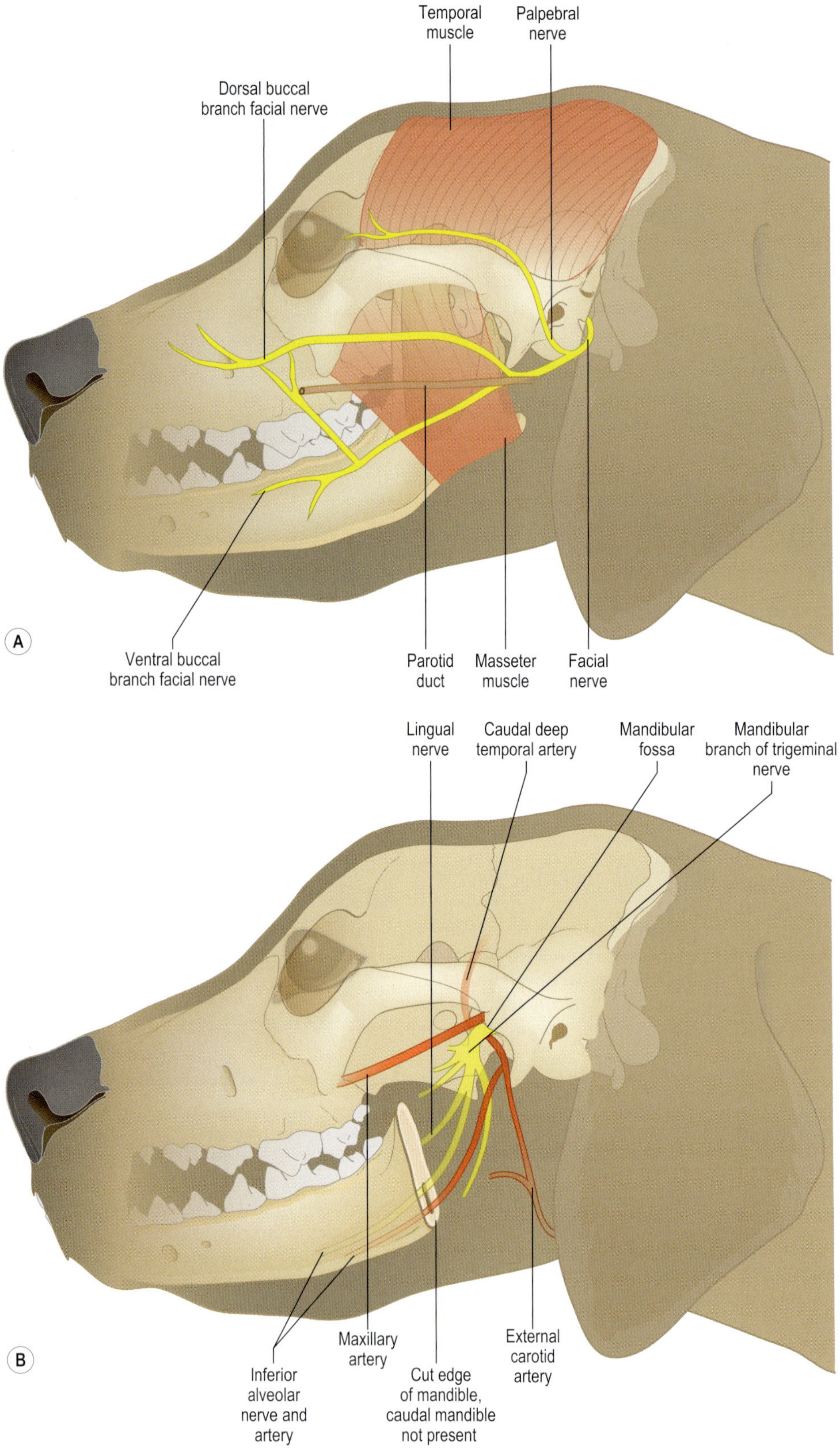

Temporal
muscle

Palpebral
nerve

Dorsal buccal
branch facial nerve

(A)

Ventral buccal
branch facial nerve

Parotid
duct

Masseter
muscle

Facial
nerve

Lingual
nerve

Caudal deep
temporal artery

Mandibular
fossa

Mandibular
branch of trigeminal
nerve

(B)

Inferior
alveolar
nerve and
artery

Maxillary
artery

Cut edge
of mandible,
caudal mandible
not present

External
carotid
artery

Fig. 33.5 Surgical anatomy (**A**) lateral and (**B**) medial to the temporomandibular joint.

Closed versus open reduction of subluxations and luxations

Subluxation of the TMJ requires no specific treatment other than soft foods and restriction of oral activity during healing. Reduction of TMJ luxations is attempted using closed techniques. Reduction of a chronic luxation is difficult or impossible due to organized fibrous tissue that fills the joint space. Therefore, closed reduction should be attempted as soon as possible after the injury occurred. Open reduction or condylectomy is considered for nonreducible luxation and recurrent luxation.

Nonsurgical versus surgical treatment of condylar and pericondylar fractures

The indications for surgical treatment versus nonsurgical treatment of condylar and pericondylar fractures are summarized in Figure 33.6. The condylar process may be fractured in a sagittal or transverse plane, or the fracture may be subcondylar. Pericondylar fractures include fractures of the retroarticular process, mandibular fossa, and zygomatic process of the squamous part of the temporal bone.[7]

Fractures of the condylar process treated conservatively may heal by bony union or as a pain-free and functional nonunion.[16,17] Conservative treatment of minimally displaced subcondylar and pericondylar fractures without joint surface involvement is therefore justifiable.

Comminuted and intra-articular fractures, however, are likely to result in temporomandibular joint arthrosis and possible ankylosis; the latter complication is characterized by a progressive inability to open the mouth.[2,18] It is controversial whether this justifies performing a condylectomy at the time of diagnosis of an intra-articular fracture,

or waiting for arthritic changes to develop and performing the condylectomy at that stage.[19,20]

CLOSED REDUCTION AND NONSURGICAL TECHNIQUES

Closed reduction of luxations

The most common direction of TMJ luxation is rostrodorsal, although this must be confirmed radiographically. The patient is anesthetized, intubated and placed in sternal recumbency. A fulcrum is obtained by placing a pencil or other similar softer wooden or plastic dowel transversely across the mandible at the level of the second and third molar teeth.[3,6,20,21] Larger dogs require using a larger-diameter fulcrum. Cotton-tipped applicators work well in cats. A fulcrum made of hard material may inadvertently cause tooth cusp tip fracture. The mouth is gently closed. This manipulation moves the displaced mandibular condylar process in a ventral direction. The mandible is shifted caudally toward the side of the luxation to seat the condylar process into the mandibular fossa (Fig. 33.7A–C). The mouth is gently opened and closed and observed for shifting of the jaw toward the side opposite to the luxation, indicating luxation recurrence. Ventrodorsal or dorsoventral, and lateral oblique radiographs are obtained to confirm reduction.

If the reduction was easily accomplished and maintained after manipulation of the mandible, no restriction of movement of the mandible is needed. Soft food and elimination of foreign object chewing for 5–6 weeks allows healing. A difficult reduction or recurrence of the luxation during manipulation requires placement of tape

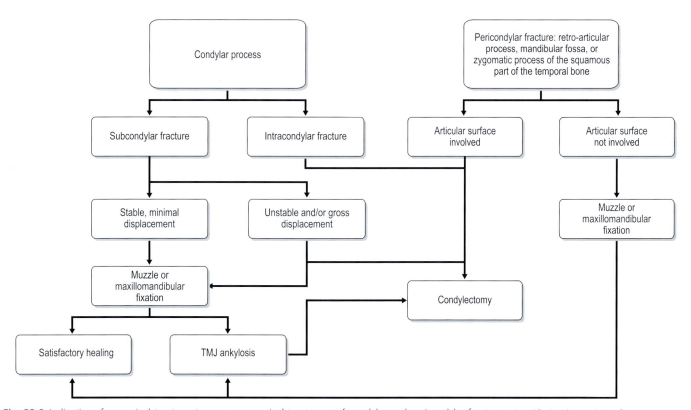

Fig. 33.6 Indications for surgical treatment *versus* nonsurgical treatment of condylar and pericondylar fractures. *(Modified with permission from: Verstraete FJM. Maxillofacial fractures. In: Holmstrom SE, Frost Fitch P, Eisner ER, eds. Veterinary dental techniques for the small animal practitioner. 3rd ed. Philadelphia: WB Saunders Co, 2004;559–600).*

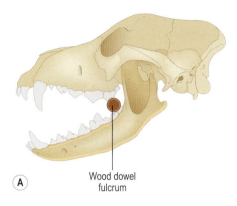

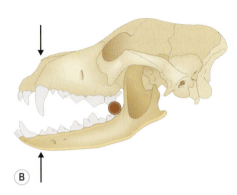

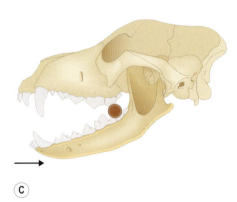

Wood dowel
fulcrum

Fig. 33.7 Closed reduction of a rostrodorsal temporomandibular luxation: (**A**) A wooden dowel fulcrum is placed transversely across the dental quadrants and the level of the caudal molars. (**B**) The mouth is gently closed bringing the displaced condylar process to the level of the mandibular fossa. (**C**) The jaw is moved caudally to reduce the luxation.

muzzle, maxillomandibular fixation (MMF) or interdental composite bonding to maintain the reduction (see Ch. 29).[22,23] Most closed reductions require one of these methods of immobilization. The bone holes for placement of MMF wires are drilled before the luxation is reduced. Mandible manipulation for placing these holes may result in recurrent luxation. A tape muzzle allows more mandibular movement than does MMF wiring or interdental bonding. Success when using the tape muzzle comes from allowing the patient only minimal mouth opening for eating and drinking and maintaining normal occlusal relationships between the distal mandibular and maxillary

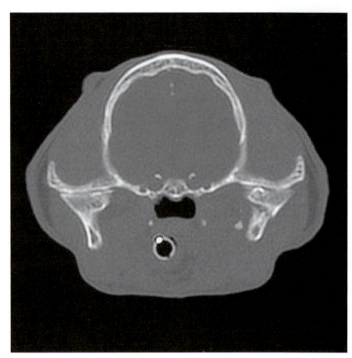

Fig. 33.8 Healing nondisplaced fracture of the neck of the condylar process.

teeth to prevent lateral displacement of the mandible. If postreduction radiographs and mandible manipulation indicate excessive TMJ laxity and recurrent luxation readily occurs, then MMF wires or interdental bonding should be considered.

Nonsurgical treatment of minimally displaced fractures

Fractures involving the TMJ commonly occur with other maxillofacial fractures or separation of the mandibular symphysis. Intra-articular fracture fragments may be stabilized by the muscles of mastication, joint capsule and joint ligaments. These fractures are difficult to rigidly stabilize with internal fixation because of the small fragment size; therefore, conservative treatment is commonly used.[20] However, damage to the articular surface and the presence of an intra-articular bone fragment has been shown experimentally to lead to TMJ ankylosis.[24] Minimally or nondisplaced fractures of the condylar process or base (Fig. 33.8) or retroarticular process (see Fig. 33.1B) are managed by feeding soft foods and elimination of other oral activity. If, after correction of other mandibular injuries, malocclusion persists that limits the ability to close the mouth or interferes with eating, then restriction of mandible movement by a tape or nylon muzzle, interdental composite splint or MMF wires is applied.[17] Minimally displaced fractures involving the caudal mandible and the TMJ require similar restriction of mandible movement (see Fig. 33.3C).

SURGICAL TECHNIQUES

Open reduction of luxations

For luxation repair, bilateral MMF wires are initially placed but not tightened. The patient is positioned in lateral recumbency for unilateral repair and in dorsal recumbency for bilateral repair. In this position the head is rotated to allow access to each TMJ. A skin incision is made along the ventral border of the caudal half of the zygomatic arch.[14] Incision and retraction of the subcutaneous tissue, platysma, zygomaticus and sphincter colli muscles exposes the ventral border of the zygomatic arch and masseter muscle. The palpebral nerve, parotid duct and masticatory nerve are avoided. The caudal half of the origin of the masseter muscle is subperiosteally elevated and the muscle retracted in a rostroventral direction. Often, the TMJ capsule has been torn and articular cartilage of the condylar process is visible. If the joint capsule is intact, it is opened with an incision parallel to the zygomatic arch.

Blood clots and tissue debris are removed from the joint space. An intact articular disk prevents postoperative ankylosis and should be left in place.[25] However, tearing or folding of the articular disk requires diskectomy. Extensive damage to articular cartilage requires condylectomy. The luxation is reduced and capsule remnants sutured together. The mouth is gently closed around the endotracheal tube and MMF wires are tightened by a nonsterile assistant. The masseteric fascia is sutured to the periosteum covering the zygomatic arch using horizontal mattress sutures. The incision is routinely closed.

Postoperative ventrodorsal and lateral oblique radiographs are made to ensure proper reduction. After extubation, the wires are further tightened as needed to close the mouth the desired amount. Although the mouth can be opened a small amount by the patient to allow eating of soft food and drinking, the wires should limit mouth opening and maintain normal occlusion.

Condylectomy[19,26]

Condylectomy is performed for nonreducible luxation, recurrent luxation or TMJ fracture with displaced bone fragments or involving the articular surface (see Fig. 33.3A, B). Displaced fractures involving the condyle are usually not reconstructed due to small fracture fragments; condylectomy is performed. In the case of fracture, all bone fragments of the condylar process and base are excised. Shredded joint capsule is excised. Osteoplasty is performed using rongeurs or bone bur as needed to remove remaining sharp bone projections and ridges. The articular disk, if undamaged, is left in place. Preservation of the articular disk reduces fibrous tissue adhesions to the region of the mandibular fossa and may be important for preserving normal postoperative range of motion.

With TMJ luxation, the joint capsule may be partially intact. The remnants of capsular insertion are removed from the condylar process by subperiosteal elevation. The condylectomy site is identified at the base of the condylar process at the level of the mandibular notch (Fig. 33.9). The ostectomy is made in a slightly rostral semilunar configuration and directed about five degrees rostromedial in order to assure

complete excision of the medial portion of the condylar process. The ostectomy is most easily made using a small bone bur; however, rongeurs, or an osteotome and mallet may be used. After ostectomy, the medial aspect of the capsule and remaining attachment of the lateral pterygoid muscle are subperiosteally elevated and removed from the condylar process. Osteoplasty is performed as needed. The articular disk, if undamaged, is left intact.

Other techniques

Luxations

Surgical stabilization of TMJ luxation has been reported.[27–29] A transarticular wire loop placed from the temporal bone to the lateral aspect of the condylar process fails to provide stabilization during healing.[27] This is due to the normal motion of the condylar process during mandibular movement (see Ch. 55).[15,30] The medial aspect of the head of the mandibular condylar process is seated firmly in the fossa during full-range mouth opening and closing. The lateral aspect of the process moves in a rostral and ventral arc during mouth opening. At maximal jaw opening, the joint capsule and lateral ligament are tense. Therefore, suture or wire used to create a lateral ligament will fail shortly after implantation due to normal motion of the lateral aspect of the condylar process. Results may improve if the jaw motion is limited during healing by tape muzzle to allow scar tissue formation around the joint; however, the ligament substitute will fail once restrictions are removed.

A temporalis muscle fascial flap has successfully been used to reconstruct the lateral aspect of the joint capsule in one dog, with a 1-year follow-up.[28] A tape muzzle was applied for 7 days and soft foods were fed for 14 days. In a cat, polyester suture material anchored by a K-wire in the mandibular condyle and a screw in the zygomatic bone was used to treat an unstable TMJ luxation, with good results on 2-year follow-up.[29]

Condylar and subcondylar fractures

Surgical correction of a subcondylar fracture using a K-wire has been mentioned in the literature, but this would probably only be feasible in a fairly large dog.[3] Wire fixation of a subcondylar fracture has been described in one cat.[31]

POSTOPERATIVE CARE AND ASSESSMENT

Immobilization

Tape or nylon muzzles, MMF wires or interdental bonding are applied with the patient extubated and in the early phase of recovery or while still under anesthesia. The patient must be observed during recovery for signs of inadequate ventilation and vomiting. In cats, placement of an esophagostomy tube is recommended, and should be performed prior to maxillomandibular fixation. Home care consists of free-choice water and feeding soft or gruel-consistency foods. Patients are not to be confined to warm environments as hyperthermia may result due to the inability to pant.

Physiotherapy

Prolonged immobilization of the TMJ is avoided as immobilization combined with healing of traumatized periarticular tissue, or pseudoarthritic tissue in the case of condylectomy, may result in limited

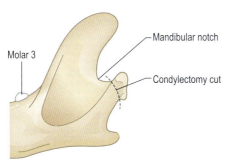

Fig. 33.9 The condylectomy site is at the base of the neck of the condylar process at the level of the mandibular notch.

Molar 3

Mandibular notch

Condylectomy cut

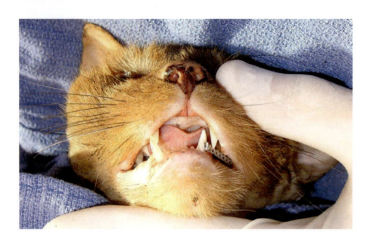

Fig. 33.10 Guided elastic traction by means of a power chain anchored to orthodontic buttons on the mandibular canine and maxillary fourth premolar teeth is used to assist the cat in closing the mouth in correct occlusion following a condylectomy.

range of mouth opening. A tape or nylon muzzle and MMF wires allow some jaw movement and interdental bonding eliminates movement. It is recommended that devices be removed and normal motion allowed by 2 weeks for luxations and TMJ fractures.[6,17,20,21] Clinical healing of fractures is determined by radiographic examination and mandible palpation and manipulation. Feeding soft food and reduced oral activity are continued for an additional 3–4 weeks during continued healing for luxation and until clinical healing of fractures. Clinical healing of fractures involving the TMJ occurs in 10–13 weeks for dogs and 4–8 weeks for cats.[4,5]

Guided elastic traction using orthodontic buttons and power chains and gentle exercise are routinely used in humans to achieve controlled protrusion of the mandible.[32] This technique can also be modified to prevent malocclusion following condylectomy in cats (Fig. 33.10).

PROGNOSIS

Conservative treatment

Results of conservative treatment for luxation and nondisplaced or minimally displaced fracture are dependent on the individual injury and postoperative patient management. Extensive soft tissue injury and/or inadequate postreduction management may result in reluxation. The lack of rigid stability at the fracture site may result in malunion or nonunion. A fibrous union may develop secondary to motion at the fracture site; however, normal mandibular function may still occur. In general, most reduced TMJ luxations and nondisplaced or minimally displaced TMJ fractures heal adequately and provide normal oral function with conservative management. Poor functional results (functionally important malocclusion, ankylosis, degenerative joint disease) can usually be corrected by mandibular condylectomy.

Condylectomy

Experimental and clinical results of unilateral and bilateral condylectomy in the dog and cat have found very good long-term functional and cosmetic results.[2,19,26,33–35]

Experimental unilateral condylectomy resulted in normal postoperative occlusion without histopathologic evidence of degenerative joint disease in the remaining joint or hypertrophy of the muscles of mastication.[19,26] Experimental bilateral condylectomy resulted in slight retrusion and lateral shift of the jaw that usually corrected itself during the healing process.[26] Fibrous connective tissue filled the condylectomy sites and was adhered to the ostectomy site and less adhered to the mandibular fossa if the articular disk was left intact. Preservation of the articular disk may reduce potential for postoperative ankylosis.[19,25,26] Maturation of this fibrous tissue reduces mandibular laxity by 4–6 postoperative weeks. Subtotal condylectomy in 2-year-old beagles, leaving the mandibular neck of the condylar process and the articular disk intact, resulted in considerable regeneration of the condylar head, including irregular articular cartilage.[36]

Clinically, malocclusion is unusual after unilateral condylectomy. Bilateral condylectomy may result in retrusion of the jaw, open bite, and some lateral shift of the jaw. Any malocclusion resulting from condylectomy is usually minimal and of no functional importance. Guided elastic traction (Fig. 33.10) may be used to assist the animal in closing the mouth in correct occlusion. Crown reduction of canine teeth may be needed with established malocclusion from bilateral condylectomy.[35] Condylectomy combined with caudal mandibulectomy may result in functionally important malocclusion and is further discussed in Chapter 46.

COMPLICATIONS

Intraoperative complications

Intraoperative hemorrhage and nerve injury may occur during dissection medial to the temporomandibular joint with inadvertent injury to large neurovascular structures in this area. This can be prevented by careful and controlled ostectomy when removing the condylar process.

Postoperative complications

Degenerative joint disease

Trauma to the TMJ that resulted in luxation or fracture and poor alignment of articular fracture fragments may result in degenerative joint disease. Clinical signs are those of oral pain and may include 'deliberate' slow chewing motion, preference for soft foods, apparent reduction of appetite with weight loss and pain on opening and closing the mouth. Crepitus may be found on mandible manipulation of the anesthetized patient. Radiographic findings may be normal or indicate irregularities of the TMJ bone structure (Fig. 33.11). Treatment with nonsteroidal antiinflammatory drugs may reduce the clinical signs. Condylectomy may ultimately be needed.

Temporomandibular joint ankylosis

Ankylosis is an immobility and consolidation of a joint resulting from fibrous or bony union due to disease, trauma (injury or surgical) or neoplasia.[1] A false ankylosis is caused by extracapsular pathology that limits normal jaw movement.[2] Causes may include fibrous adhesions between the zygomatic arch and mandible secondary to fracture,

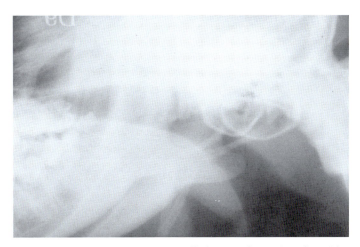

Fig. 33.11 Degenerative temporomandibular joint disease in a dog with previous condylar process fracture.

infection or neoplasia. A true ankylosis is from intracapsular pathology and fibrosis.

Clinical findings are determined by the severity of ankylosis and patient age.[2,18,33–35,37] There is an inability to completely open the mouth. Weight loss and atrophy of the muscles of mastication may be seen. Ankylosis that develops during skeletal growth results in a degree of facial deformity, indicated by unilateral or bilateral shortening of the mandible with possible lateral deviation of the mandible (Fig. 33.12A, B).[2,38]

Repeated forced opening of the jaws ('brisement forcé') combined with corticosteroid treatment is ineffective and not indicated, as reankylosis invariably occurs.[18,34] En-bloc resection of the involved bone and abnormal soft tissue is necessary to resolve the ankylosis. Endotracheal intubation may be difficult as the mouth cannot be opened adequately for conventional intubation, and may require the use of a rigid fiberscope. If necessary, a temporary tracheostomy may be performed. Resection may include condylectomy or caudal mandibulectomy, including the condylar process, with removal of zygomatic arch and interposed affected soft tissues (Fig. 33.13A–C). Fibrous connective tissue fills the excision site. Prognosis for long-term full range of mandible movement is generally good for nonmalignant etiologies provided all abnormal tissue is excised during surgery.[2,18,33–35,37]

Zygomaticomandibular ankylosis

In zygomaticomandibular ankylosis the temporomandibular joint itself may be unaffected, for example if the ankylosis occurred between the zygomatic arch and the coronoid process (Fig. 33.14).[37,39,40] This condition is occasionally seen and is also characterized by a progressive inability to open the mouth. Treatment of this type of ankylosis depends on the nature and location of the tissue interfering with the movement of the mandible, and may include resection of the coronoid process, zygomatic arch and/or osteophytes.[37,39,40] The prognosis is guarded, as the cut bony surfaces are inclined to reankylose.

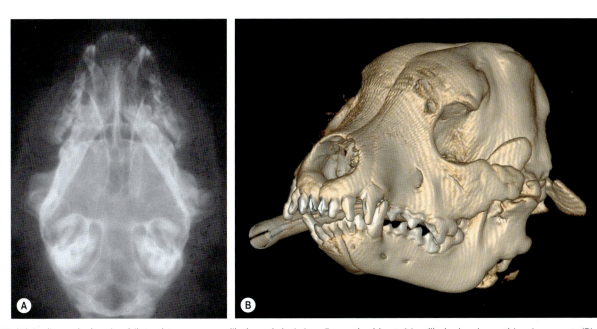

Fig. 33.12 (**A**) Radiograph showing bilateral temporomandibular ankylosis in a 5-month-old cat. Mandibular brachygnathism is present. (**B**) CT three-dimensional reconstruction of a 5.5-month-old dog showing temporomandibular joint ankylosis with resulting malocclusion, caused by a bite wound at 5 weeks of age.

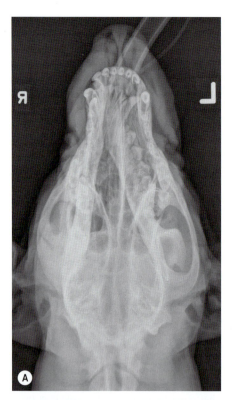

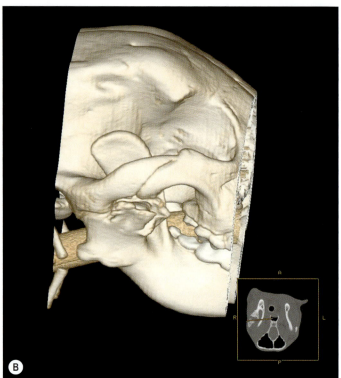

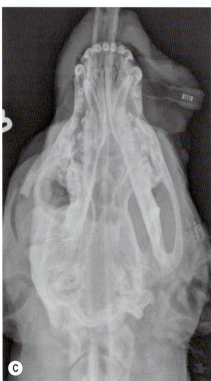

Fig. 33.13 (**A**) Radiograph showing temporomandibular joint ankylosis (R) in a dog. (**B**) CT three-dimensional reconstruction of the ankylosis showing bone proliferation. (**C**) Postoperative radiograph showing en-bloc removal of the caudal mandible including condylar process and caudal zygomatic arch.

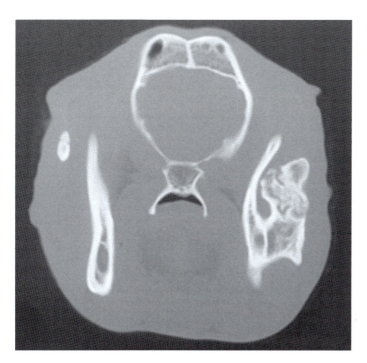

Fig. 33.14 CT image showing zygomaticomandibular ankylosis of non-neoplastic origin in a dog, with extensive new bone formation between the zygomatic arch and the ramus of the mandible.

REFERENCES

1. Venes D. Taber's cyclopedic medical dictionary. 19th ed. Philadelphia, PA: FA Davis; 2001.

2. Lantz GC. Temporomandibular joint ankylosis: surgical correction of three cases. J Am Anim Hosp Assoc 1985;21: 173–7.

3. Piermattei DL, Flo GL, DeCamp CE. Fractures and luxations of the mandible and maxilla. In: Piermattei DL, Flo GL, DeCamp CE, editors. Brinker, Piermattei, and Flo's handbook of small animal orthopedics and fracture repair. 4th ed. Philadelphia, PA: Elsevier – Saunders; 2006. p. 717–36.

4. Umphlet RC, Johnson AL. Mandibular fractures in the dog. A retrospective study of 157 cases. Vet Surg 1990;19:272–5.

5. Umphlet RC, Johnson AL. Mandibular fractures in the cat. A retrospective study. Vet Surg 1988;17:333–7.

6. Schulz K. Diseases of the joints. In: Fossum TW, editor. Small animal surgery. 3rd ed. St. Louis, MO: Mosby; 2007. p. 1143–315.

7. Ticer J, Spencer CP. Injury of the feline temporomandibular joint: radiographic signs. Vet Radiol 1978;19:146–56.

8. Kealy JK, McAllister H. The skull and vertebral column. In: Diagnostic radiology and ultrasonography of the dog and cat. 4th ed. St. Louis, MO: Elsevier Saunders; 2005. p. 387–476.

9. Schebitz H, Wilkens H. Atlas of radiographic anatomy of the dog and cat. 4th ed. Berlin: Verlag P Parey; 1986.

10. Dickie AM, Sullivan M. The effect of obliquity on the radiographic appearance of the temporomandibular joint in dogs. Vet Radiol Ultrasound 2001;42:205–17.

11. Schwarz T, Weller R, Dickie AM, et al. Imaging of the canine and feline temporomandibular joint: a review. Vet Radiol Ultrasound 2002;43:85–97.

12. Maas CPHJ, Theyse LFH. Temporomandibular joint ankylosis in cats and dogs – a report of 10 cases. Vet Comp Orthop Traumatol 2007;20: 192–7.

13. Evans HE. Miller's anatomy of the dog. 3rd ed. Philadelphia, PA: WB Saunders Co; 1993.

14. Piermattei DL, Johnson KA. The head. In: Piermattei DL, Johnson KA, editors. An atlas of surgical approaches to the bones and joints of the dog and cat. 4th ed. Philadelphia, PA: Elsevier – Saunders; 2004. p. 33–45.

15. Caporn TM. Traumatic temporomandibular joint luxation – comparative anatomy of the temporomandibular joint. Vet Comp Orthop Traumatol 1995;8:63–5.

16. Chambers JN. Principles of management of mandibular fractures in the dog and cat. J Vet Orthop 1981;2:26–36.

17. Salisbury SK, Cantwell HD. Conservative management of fractures of the mandibular condyloid process in three cats and one dog. J Am Vet Med Assoc 1989;194:85–7.

18. Sullivan M. Temporomandibular ankylosis in the cat. J Small Anim Pract 1989;30: 401–5.

19. Lantz GC, Cantwell HD, VanVleet JF, et al. Unilateral mandibular condylectomy: experimental and clinical results. J Am Anim Hosp Assoc 1982;18:883–90.

20. Verstraete FJM. Maxillofacial fractures. In: Slatter DH, editor. Textbook of small animal surgery. 3rd ed. Philadelphia, PA: WB Saunders Co; 2003. p. 2190–207.

21. Renegar WR. Axial skeletal fractures. In: Whittick WG, editor. Canine orthopedics. 2nd ed. Philadelphia, PA: Lea & Febiger; 1990. p. 308–56.

22. Lantz GC. Interarcade wiring as a method of fixation for selected mandibular injuries. J Am Anim Hosp Assoc 1981;17: 599–603.

23. Bennett JW, Kapatkin AS, Manfra Marretta S. Dental composite for the fixation of mandibular fractures and luxations in 11 cats and 6 dogs. Vet Surg 1994;23:190–4.

24. Miyamoto H, Kurita K, Ogi N, et al. The effect of an intra-articular bone fragment in the genesis of temporomandibular joint ankylosis. Int J Oral Maxillofac Surg 2000;29:290–5.

25. Miyamoto H, Kurita K, Ogi N, et al. The role of the disk in sheep temporomandibular joint ankylosis. Oral Surg Oral Med Oral Pathol Oral Radiol Endod 1999;88:151–8.

26. Tomlinson J, Presnell KR. Mandibular condylectomy – effects in normal dogs. Vet Surg 1983;12:148–54.

27. Knecht CD, Schiller AG. Head and nose. In: Archibald J, editor. Canine surgery. 2nd ed. Santa Barbara, CA: American Veterinary Publications; 1974. p. 171–92.

28. Peterson SL, Gourley IM. Temporal muscle fascial flap for temporomandibular joint luxation in a dog. J Am Anim Hosp Assoc 1989;25:186–8.

29. Caporn TM. Traumatic temporomandibular joint luxation in a cat and treatment by condylar tethering. Vet Comp Orthop Traumatol 1995;8:66–70.

30. Scapino RP. The third joint of the canine jaw. J Morphol 1965;116:23–50.

31. Leighton RL. Treatment of a subcondylar fracture of the mandible in a cat by open reduction and wire fixation. Feline Pract 1979;9:30–6.

32. Hwang K, Park JH, Lee HJ. Miniplate fixation of high condylar fracture and postoperative exercise regimen. J Craniofac Surg 2005;16:113–6.

33. Anderson MA, Orsini PG, Harvey CE. Temporomandibular ankylosis: treatment by unilateral condylectomy in two dogs and two cats. J Vet Dent 1996;13:23–5.

34. Meomartino L, Fatone G, Brunetti A, et al. Temporomandibular ankylosis in the cat: a review of seven cases. J Small Anim Pract 1999;40:7–10.

35. Eisner ER. Bilateral mandibular condylectomy in a cat. J Vet Dent 1995;12:23–6.

36. Miyamoto H, Shigematsu H, Suzuki S, et al. Regeneration of mandibular condyle following unilateral condylectomy in canines. J Craniomaxillofac Surg 2004;32:296–302.

37. Okumura M, Kadosawa T, Fujinaga T. Surgical correction of temporomandibular joint ankylosis in two cats. Aust Vet J 1999;77:24–7.

38. Oztan HY, Ulusal BG, Aytemiz C. The role of trauma on temporomandibular joint ankylosis and mandibular growth retardation: an experimental study. J Craniofac Surg 2004;15:274–82.

39. Bennett D, Campbell JR. Mechanical interference with lower jaw movement as a complication of skull fractures. J Small Anim Pract 1976;17:747–51.

40. van Ee RT, Pechman RD. False ankylosis of the temporomandibular joint in a cat. J Am Vet Med Assoc 1987;191:979–80.

Chapter 34

Maxillofacial fracture complications

Sandra Manfra Marretta

DEFINITIONS

Bone sequestrum: a non-vital piece of bone that has become separated from vital bone

Delayed union: a fracture that has not healed in the expected time when compared with other similar fractures (type, location) treated similarly in comparable patients[1]

Malocclusion: a deviation from normal occlusion, which may result in a physiologically unacceptable contact of opposing teeth

Malunion: healed fractures in which anatomic bone alignment was not achieved or maintained during healing[2]

Nonunion: an ununited fracture in which, without surgical intervention, eventual union is highly unlikely because the fracture healing process has ceased[1]

Oronasal fistula: an abnormal communication between the oral cavity and the nasal cavity

Osteomyelitis: an inflammatory process of the bone marrow, cortex and possibly the periosteum[3]

PREOPERATIVE CONCERNS

Dogs and cats with maxillofacial fracture complications should be evaluated for nutritional complications, aspiration pneumonia, secondary rhinitis and traumatic malocclusion preoperatively.

THERAPEUTIC DECISION-MAKING

Fracture complications can occur in dogs and cats following traumatic maxillofacial injuries. Accurate preoperative assessment and adherence to basic principles in the management of maxillofacial fractures and selection of appropriate techniques for repair of these fractures can help minimize complications (see Ch. 25).[4–6]

Diligent postoperative evaluation of maxillofacial fractures is imperative for the early detection of maxillofacial fracture complications to help ensure appropriate and timely management of these cases. Complete evaluation of patients suspected of having maxillofacial fracture complications includes: a complete history, physical examination, hematologic testing, a thorough oral examination under anesthesia and radiographic evaluation including skull, dental, and thoracic radiographs. Additional imaging modalities may be required including: abdominal ultrasound, computed tomography, magnetic resonance imaging, and scintigraphy.

MAXILLOFACIAL FRACTURE COMPLICATIONS

Age-related complications

Juvenile patients

Maxillofacial trauma in juvenile patients provides a unique set of potential complications, including interference with future growth and development, resulting in facial deformity and damage to unerupted permanent teeth.[7,8]

A conservative approach rather than an open reduction is generally recommended in juvenile patients to minimize these risks. Open reduction of maxillofacial fractures in young patients generally is not required because fractures in these patients are frequently greenstick fractures that can be effectively managed with closed reduction and short-term stabilization with tape or nylon muzzles. Open reduction in young patients with maxillofacial fractures is more likely to have a negative effect on growth potential because of the additional disruption of the periosteum and soft tissue that is associated with the placement of bone plates, screws or wires and is therefore generally not recommended.[7]

Maxillofacial trauma in young dogs and cats can damage unerupted teeth. A wide variety of potential complications may be associated with trauma to unerupted teeth. These potential complications range from minor insignificant complications including enamel hypoplasia to more significant problems including resorption, impaction, dentigerous cyst formation and pulpal necrosis.[9] Following maxillofacial trauma in young dogs and cats, it is important to periodically reevaluate the fracture site for evidence of damage to tooth buds. Periodic

DOI: 10.1016/B978-0-7020-4618-6.00034-8

Complications related to implants

Implant exposure, loosening, and migration and implant failure

Implant exposure can occur following internal reduction and fixation of maxillofacial fractures. In an experimental study, mandibular osteotomies between the third and fourth premolars in dogs were repaired with conventional plates and screws; erosion of the alveolar mucosa occurred in 10 of the 15 dogs with subsequent gingivitis, periodontitis and severe bone loss.[21] In a clinical study, maxillofacial miniplates were used for repair of mandibular and maxillary fractures in 15 dogs and 3 cats.[22] These implants were utilized in the fixation of 11 caudal (junction of the ramus with the mandibular body) and 2 rostral mandibular fractures, 4 maxillary fractures, and 2 zygomatic arch fractures. The results in this study were excellent except in one case of a rostral mandibular fracture in which soft tissue dehiscence and loss of fixation occurred, necessitating the performance of a rostral mandibulectomy. These studies suggest that there may be an increased risk of implant exposure when bone plates are utilized in the repair of rostral and mid-mandibular body fracture. Implant exposure may also occur on the lingual aspect over the sharp screw tips, especially if screws that are slightly too long are used.

When using intraosseous wiring techniques, bending over the knot may decrease the tension somewhat, but is usually indicated in order to prevent undue soft tissue irritation and subsequent exposure because of the sharp protruding ends of the wire.

Implant loosening, migration and failure can occur following internal reduction and fixation of maxillofacial fractures. Inappropriate use or technical errors can contribute to implant loosening, migration and failure. Intraosseous wire applied too loosely allows micromotion of the bone fragments and results in resorption of bone (Fig. 34.3).[1] Wires placed in or migrated into a fracture line interfere with the formation of a bridging callus.[1] Fracture healing may occur in the presence of micromotion but healing will be delayed. When there is significant motion at the fracture site due to implant loosening, migration or failure, the implant should be tightened or replaced to achieve stability at the fracture site. An external fixation device may be beneficial in achieving additional stability in these cases.

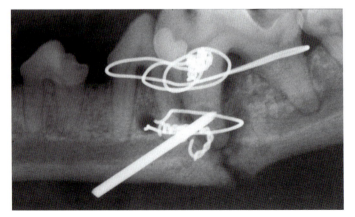

Fig. 34.3 A misplaced pin causing trauma to the mesial root of the first molar tooth. Loose wires have resulted in motion between the bone fragments and resorption of bone. Healing is not occurring because of the diseased tooth in the fracture site and the unstable fixation.

Healing complications

Factors that influence normal healing of maxillofacial fractures include the age of the animal, the degree of stability at the fracture site, the size of bony defects at the fracture site, the location of the fracture site, the integrity of soft tissues, the vascular supply at the fracture site, and foreign material located within the fracture site. All of these factors must be evaluated when assessing maxillofacial fracture healing complications. Potential maxillofacial fracture healing complications include delayed union, nonunion, and malunion.

Delayed union and nonunion

The major cause of delayed union and nonunion is inadequate fracture stability. Other factors that may contribute to the development of delayed union or nonunion include: vascular impairment, large fracture gaps, interposed soft tissues, infection and inappropriate use of skeletal implants.[1] Teeth in the fracture line can also delay or prevent healing, particularly if they are diseased or loose.[4,23]

Nonunions have been classified in the Weber-Cech classification as viable (hypervascular) or nonviable (avascular) nonunions.[1,24] Viable nonunions are further subclassified as hypertrophic, slightly hypertrophic, or oligotrophic, depending on the amount of callus present at the fracture site with hypertrophic nonunions having an abundant hypervascularized callus while oligotrophic nonunions are devoid of visible callus.[1,24] Nonviable nonunions are subclassified as dystrophic, necrotic, defect or atrophic.[1,24] Dystrophic nonunions have an intermediate fragment that has healed to one fracture fragment but is incapable of bridging the gap to the second major fragment. Necrotic nonunions have avascular or poorly vascularized fragments that eventually die. Defect nonunions are associated with the loss of a large section of bone at the fracture site. Atrophic nonunions may be the final result of the other three types of nonviable nonunions. Oligotrophic and atrophic nonunions seem to occur most commonly in the mandible.

In cases of delayed union, as long as implants remain stable and there are signs of progressive bone activity on sequential radiographs, as evidenced by increasing density of fracture lines, there is no immediate need for additional surgical intervention.[2] When loose or migrating implants are present in delayed union or nonunion, these implants should be removed, the fracture site should be stabilized and cancellous bone grafts should be applied.[2] Factors other than instability at the fracture site should also be addressed when attempting to prevent or treat delayed union and nonunion.

Vascular impairment can often be prevented by preserving vascularity to the fracture site. Extensive stripping of soft tissue from fracture fragments should be avoided to prevent vascular comprise to the underlying bone. Preservation of the integrity of soft tissue surrounding rostral mandibular fragments is particularly important for bone viability and for the prognosis of fracture union because revascularization of fracture fragments does not occur across the intraosseous portion of the symphysis, but occurs by formation of a transient extraosseous blood supply.[4,25] When selecting a fixation technique for maxillofacial fracture repair, a technique that is as minimally invasive as possible to achieve appropriate reduction and stabilization should be chosen to reduce the risk of vascular impairment. In cases in which severe vascular impairment results in bone necrosis, a mandibulectomy may be necessary (Fig. 34.4).

Large fracture gaps can usually be managed with external fixation devices and placement of a cancellous bone graft in the defect. Care should be taken not to interpose soft tissue in these fracture gaps since this will delay or prevent fracture healing. It is also important to remove diseased teeth from a fracture site prior to fixation since diseased teeth in the fracture site may result in a delayed or nonunion.[4]

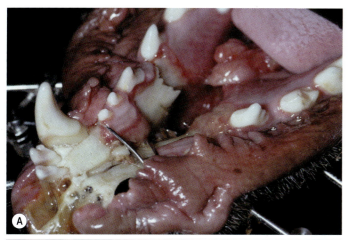

corrective osteotomy in severe cases or judicious selective extraction of maloccluding teeth caused by the malunion.

Infectious complications

Wound infection

Wound infection can occur as a complication of maxillofacial fractures. The rate of wound infection following maxillofacial trauma is significantly less than other areas of the body. The well-vascularized tissue in this area may confer an advantage on the host's ability to prevent an infection in the presence of large numbers of bacteria.[25]

Local wound changes that indicate a developing infection include redness, increased heat, pain and localized edema.[26] An elevation in body temperature may also be present. Progression of the wound infection results in purulent discharge from the incision site.

Management of wound infections following maxillofacial trauma includes several treatment modalities. Cellulitis should be treated with broad-spectrum antibiotics. Once a localized abscess becomes evident, the wound should be prepared for aseptic surgery and the sutures overlying the infected wound should be removed as needed to provide adequate drainage. Samples should be obtained for aerobic and anaerobic culture and sensitivity testing. In severe wound infections the wound should be thoroughly debrided, flushed with sterile saline and covered with wet-to-dry dressings twice daily to assist in wound debridement. In minor wound infections the wound may be closed after thorough debridement; closed suction drainage may be indicated in selected cases. A broad-spectrum antibiotic should be administered and adjusted when results of bacterial culture and sensitivity testing are available.

Osteomyelitis and bone sequestra

Osteomyelitis or bone sequestra following jaw fracture repair may be associated with diseased teeth or root tips, exposed alveolar bone or operator-induced osseous necrosis.[4]

In humans, the incidence of mandibular osteomyelitis is significantly greater than osteomyelitis of the maxilla following maxillofacial trauma. Clinical experience indicates that this is also true in small animals. The reason for this dispariety may be that the endochondral bone of the mandible is structurally similar to the long bones of the body, which are more susceptible to osteomyelitis.[26] The intramembranous bone of the maxilla has less medullary tissue, thinner cortical plates, and a more extensive blood supply than the mandible.[26] These factors all permit an infection in the maxilla to be more easily disseminated into the surrounding tissue than infection in the mandible, thereby helping to prevent maxillary osteomyelitis.

Risk factors associated with the development of post-traumatic osteomyelitis following mandibular fractures have been reported in humans (Box 34.1).[26] These risk factors can be applied to small animal patients.

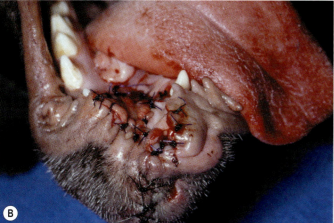

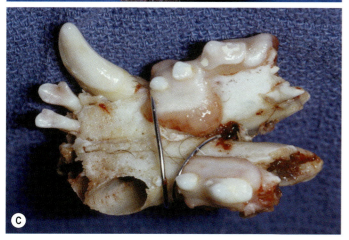

Fig. 34.4 (**A**) Bone necrosis of the rostral mandible 6 days following mandibular fracture. (**B**) A rostral mandibulectomy has been performed to remove the necrotic bone. (**C**) The necrotic bone fragment.

Malunion

Malunion is a significant complication that may be associated with maxillofacial fractures. Careful attention to proper dental occlusion during fracture fixation can help prevent malunion. Utilization of pharyngotomy endotracheal intubation during fixation will help prevent inaccurate reduction and subsequent malunion.

Severe malunion that results in significantly impaired function including inability to close the mouth or a severe deformity requires surgical intervention. Treatment of severe malunion may include

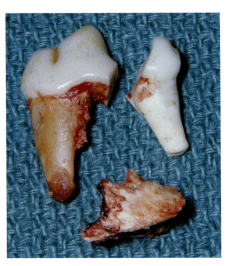

Fig. 34.5 Mandibular first molar tooth and bone sequestrum removed from a nonhealing painful mandibular fracture site 6 weeks after repair. Healing occurred rapidly following their removal and stabilization with a tape muzzle.

The treatment of osteomyelitis associated with maxillofacial fractures includes both a surgical and medical approach. The fracture site should be thoroughly assessed for adequate stability. If implants are not providing adequate stability they should be removed and/or supplemented with an alternative method of stabilization. External fixation devices are often helpful in providing stabilization without significant loss of blood supply to the surrounding soft tissues and bone.

In addition to stabilizing the fracture it is also important to remove all nonvital tissue, including bone sequestra and diseased or loose teeth (Fig. 34.5). Specimens of infected bone should be obtained for aerobic and anaerobic bacterial culture and sensitivity testing. Broad-spectrum bactericidal antibiotic therapy should be instituted and should be modified based on culture results and clinical response. Appropriate antibiotics should be administered for a minimum of 4–6 weeks.

Complications related to teeth

Several maxillofacial fracture complications are related to the teeth, including malocclusion and dental trauma. Recognition of these complications early in the course of treatment will permit timely management of these problems and decrease the post-traumatic recovery period.

Malocclusion

Malocclusion can be a serious postoperative complication in jaw fracture management. Failure to properly align fracture segments, particularly in caudal mandibular fractures, results in significant deviation of the rostral mandibular segment. In severe cases, the patient may not be able to properly close the mouth because of traumatically occluding maxillary and mandibular cheek teeth. If occlusion is not carefully assessed during fracture fixation, serious malocclusion may not be recognized until the immediate postoperative recovery period. In these cases, it becomes necessary to immediately reanesthetize the patient and place a pharyngotomy endotracheal tube to permit intraoperative assessment of occlusion during the proper realignment and stabilization of the fracture segments.

In less severe cases of malocclusion secondary to maxillofacial fracture repair there may be traumatic occlusion between a few teeth. These cases may be treated as previously described or by selective extraction of maloccluding teeth. Selective extraction of maloccluding teeth can permit the patient to close the mouth postoperatively in poorly reduced fracture fixations but is considered a significant compromise for poor surgical technique.[8]

Dental pathology

Maxillofacial fracture complications that may be related to dental pathology include periodontal, endodontic, and iatrogenic pathologic conditions.

As described above, pre-existing severe periodontal disease may predispose geriatric small-breed dogs to pathologic fractures.[4,11] Severe endodontic pathology can potentially predispose patients to pathologic mandibular fractures; however, endodontic pathology of this magnitude is rarely encountered.

Pathologic fractures through severe periodontic or endodontic lesions can be very difficult to treat because of poor bone quality. Initial treatment includes extraction of the diseased tooth from the fracture site, debridement and flushing of the fracture site, placement of a cancellous bone graft in the alveolus of the fracture, closure of the gingiva over the alveolus and application of a tape muzzle until a fibrous union occurs. A broad-spectrum antibiotic should also be administered perioperatively and for several weeks postoperatively. Alternatively, an external fixation device or bone plate in conjunction with a cancellous bone graft and antibiotics may be utilized; however, poor bone quality in these cases predisposes to implant failure. A salvage procedure involving bilateral segmental mandibulectomies with bilateral advancement of the commissures of the lips can be performed to manage bilateral pathologic fractures through the alveoli of the mandibular first molar teeth.[8] (Fig. 34.6A–F). This procedure should be reserved for severe cases in which bony union is highly unlikely.

Prognostic factors affecting teeth in the line of mandibular fractures have been previously reviewed.[23] The decision to retain or extract a tooth located in a fracture site should be based on multiple criteria. Timing is a critical factor and if treatment can be initiated early then the teeth can often be retained. Removal of teeth from a fracture line can adversely affect the operator's ability to achieve anatomic reduction and fracture stability; therefore, teeth should be retained if possible. Guidelines for the decision-making process concerning the management of teeth in fracture sites have previously been reviewed (see Ch. 25).[23]

The long-term prognosis for teeth affected by maxillofacial fractures depends on the location of the fracture line in relationship to the periodontal ligament. The fracture line with the most guarded long-term dental prognosis is a fracture that extends from the gingival margin along the root surface to the apex of the tooth. This fracture line creates a communication between the apical area of the tooth and the oral cavity. It has been recommended that a tooth associated with this type of fracture be either extracted or hemisected.[23]

Retention of healthy teeth in a fracture line can help reduce the frequency of postoperative complications and help facilitate anatomic reduction of the fracture. However, it is important to monitor for evidence of endodontic and periodontic lesions during and following fracture healing. This monitoring process should include periodontal probing and radiographic evaluation. Postoperative complications should be treated with endodontic therapy, periodontal therapy, hemisection or extraction.

Iatrogenic dental lesions may be associated with maxillofacial fracture repair. These injuries are most often associated with placement of screws during application of bone plates and inappropriately

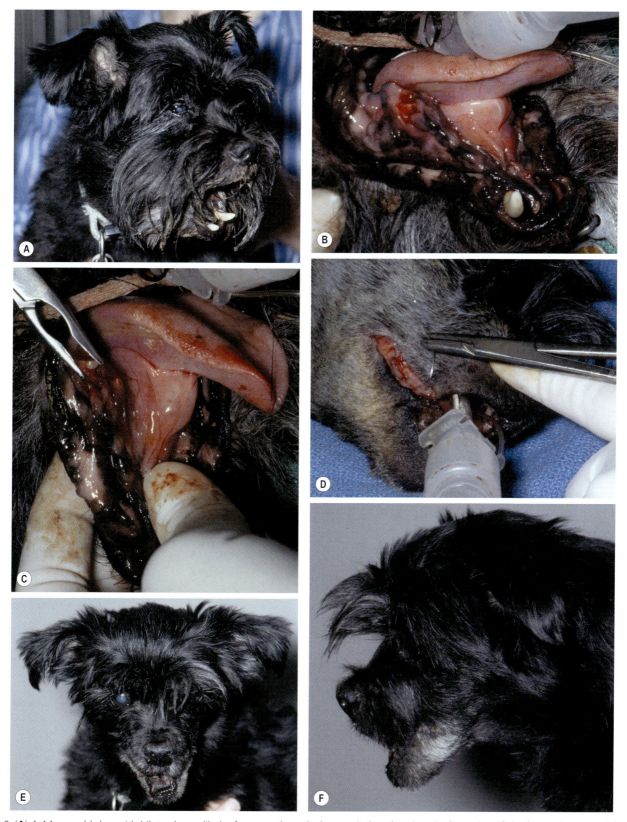

Fig. 34.6 (**A**) A 14-year-old dog with bilateral mandibular fractures through deep periodontal pockets in the region of the first molar teeth. (**B**) Open fracture site in the region of the extracted first molar tooth. (**C**) The sharp ends of the fracture fragments are removed with a rongeur prior to flushing and closure of the gingiva. (**D**) Bilateral advancement of the commissures of the lips is achieved by excising the lip margins to the level of the canine teeth and suturing the oral mucosa and skin in two layers. (**E**) Postoperative view of bilateral cheiloplasty. (**F**) Lateral view of bilateral cheiloplasty.

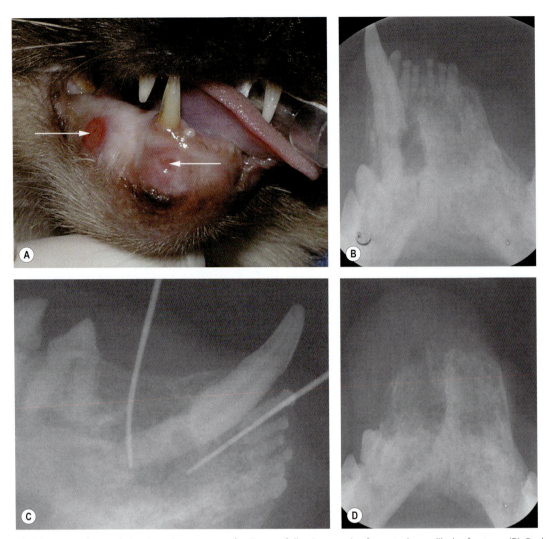

Fig. 34.7 (**A**) Two draining tracts (*arrows*) that have been present for 7 years following repair of a rostral mandibular fracture. (**B**) Occlusal radiograph showing severe osteolysis at the right mandibular canine tooth. (**C**) Lateral radiograph showing gutta-percha points placed in the draining tracts. (**D**) Postoperative radiograph following extraction of the canine and all incisor teeth; note the moth-eaten appearance of the rostral mandible, suggestive of osteomyelitis.

placed pins during the application of external fixation devices (Figs 34.7 and 34.8). In an experimental study where osteotomies of the body of the mandible in 15 dogs were repaired with plates and screws, 32.5% of the screws were found to have caused pulpal damage, suggesting that it is difficult to place bone plates on the canine mandible without traumatizing the teeth.[21] It is also difficult to place an external fixation device at the rostral mandible without traumatizing the teeth.

Trauma to the pulp or periapical tissues with either screws or pins will result in endodontic lesions necessitating removal of the implant and either endodontic therapy or extraction of the iatrogenically traumatized tooth (Fig. 34.8).

Complications associated with extensive callus formation

Extensive callus formation following maxillofacial trauma may result in an inability to open the mouth. This inability following maxillofacial fractures may be associated with excessive callus formation around the temporomandibular joint or between the zygomatic arch and the coronoid process of the mandible. Computed tomography may be utilized to help localize these lesions. Excessive callus formation

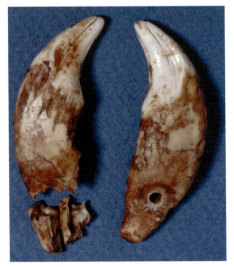

Fig. 34.8 Teeth extracted from a dog because of a 3-year history of cutaneous draining tracts located ventral to the apices of the canine teeth following repair of a rostral mandibular fracture with an external fixation device. Note the holes in the roots of both mandibular canine teeth.

around the temporomandibular joint can be treated with a condylectomy. Adhesions between the zygomatic arch and the coronoid process should be treated with surgical removal of part of the zygomatic arch; in some cases a coronoidectomy and condylectomy may also be necessary. Postoperative physical therapy and antiinflammatory drugs may help decrease the recurrence of clinical signs (see Ch. 33).

of infection in the immediate perioperative period and as needed, based on clinical signs, since infections secondary to maxillofacial complications can occur months to years following maxillofacial fractures. Maxillofacial fractures should be radiographically reevaluated 6 weeks postoperatively and as needed to assess proper healing. If progressive inability to open the mouth occurs, a CT scan of the skull is recommended.

POSTOPERATIVE CARE AND ASSESSMENT

Diligent postoperative care and assessment are important parts of the management of maxillofacial complications. Maxillofacial trauma patients may develop multiple complications. Early recognition of these problems utilizing frequent oral examinations, serial dental radiographic studies and special imaging modalities such as computed tomography and magnetic resonance imaging will help facilitate early detection of maxillofacial fracture complications.

Immediately following maxillofacial fracture repair patients should be evaluated for malocclusion. Patients should be monitored for signs

PROGNOSIS

The prognosis for most maxillofacial fracture complications is good to excellent. The prognosis for return to normal function is guarded for geriatric patients with severe bone loss, in patients with large oronasal fistulas, in patients with bilateral nasal obstruction and in patients with established skeletal malocclusion. Selection and proper application of appropriate fixation techniques can help minimize complications. Early detection of complications and timely administration of appropriate treatment will also improve the prognosis in animals with maxillofacial trauma.

REFERENCES

1. Kaderly RE. Delayed union, nonunion and malunion. In: Slatter DH, editor. Textbook of small animal surgery. 2nd ed. Philadelphia, PA: WB Saunders; 1993. p. 1676–85.

2. Johnson AL, Hulse DA. Fundamentals of orthopedic surgery and fracture management. In: Fossum TW, editor. Small animal surgery. 2nd ed. St. Louis, MO: Mosby; 2002. p. 821–900.

3. Johnson AL, Hulse DA. Other diseases of bones and joints. In: Fossum TW, editor. Small animal surgery. 2nd ed. St. Louis, MO: Mosby; 2002. p. 1168–91.

4. Manfra Marretta S, Schrader SC, Matthiesen DT. Problems associated with the management and treatment of jaw fractures. Probl Vet Med 1990; 2:220–47.

5. Chambers JN. Principles of management of mandibular fractures in the dog and cat. J Vet Orthop 1981;2:26–36.

6. Weigel JP. Trauma to oral structures. In: Harvey CE, editor. Veterinary dentistry. Philadelphia, PA: WB Saunders; 1985. p. 140–55.

7. Blakely GH, Ruiz RL, Turvey TA. Management of facial fractures in the growing patient. In: Fonseca RJ, Walker RV, Betts NJ, et al, editors. Oral and maxillofacial trauma. 2nd ed. Philadelphia, PA: WB Saunders; 1997. p. 1003–43.

8. Manfra Marretta S. Maxillofacial surgery. Vet Clin North Amer Small Anim Pract 1998;28:1285–96.

9. Manfra Marretta S, Patnaik AK, Schloss AJ, et al. An iatrogenic dentigerous cyst in a dog. J Vet Dent 1989;6:11–12.

10. Scott RF. Oral and maxillofacial trauma in the geriatric patient. In: Fonseca RJ, Walker RV, Betts NJ, et al, editors. Oral and maxillofacial trauma. 2nd ed. Philadelphia, PA: WB Saunders; 1997. p. 1044–72.

11. Manfra Marretta S. The common and uncommon clinical presentations and treatment of periodontal disease. Semin Vet Med Surg 1987;2:230–40.

12. Harvey CE, Emily PP. Oral surgery. In: Harvey CE, Emily PP, editors. Small animal dentistry. St Louis, MO: Mosby; 1993. p. 312–77.

13. Romback DM, Quinn PD. Trauma to the temporomandibular joint region. In: Fonseca RJ, Walker RV, Betts NJ, et al, editors. Oral and maxillofacial trauma. 2nd ed. Philadelphia, PA: WB Saunders; 1997. p. 527–70.

14. Helfrick JF. Early assessment and treatment planning in the maxillofacial trauma patient. In: Fonseca RJ, Walker RV, Betts NJ, et al, editors. Oral and maxillofacial trauma. 2nd edn. Philadelphia, PA: WB Saunders; 1997. p. 364–90.

15. Manfra Marretta S, Grove TK, Grillo JF. Split palatal U-flap: A new technique for repair of caudal hard palate defects. J Vet Dent 1991;8:5–8.

16. Robertson JJ, Dean PW. Repair of a traumatically induced oronasal fistula in a cat with a rostral tongue flap. Vet Surg 1987;16:164.

17. Smith MM. Island palatal mucoperiosteal flap for repair of oronasal fistula in a dog. J Vet Dent 2001;18:127–9.

18. Powers MP, Beck BW, Fonseca RJ. Management of soft tissue injuries. In:

Fonseca RJ, Walker RV, Betts NJ, et al, editors. Oral and maxillofacial trauma. 2nd ed. Philadelphia, PA: WB Saunders; 1997. p. 792–854.

19. Nelson AW. Upper respiratory system. In: Slatter DH, editor. Textbook of small animal surgery. 2nd ed. Philadelphia, PA: WB Saunders; 1993. p. 733–76.

20. Coolman BR, Manfra Marretta S, McKiernan BC, et al. Choanal atresia and secondary nasopharyngeal stenosis in a dog. J Am Anim Hosp Assoc 1998;34: 497–501.

21. Verstraete FJM, Ligthelm AJ. Dental trauma caused by screws in internal fixation of mandibular osteotomies in the dog. Vet Comp Orthop Traumatol 1992;5:104–8.

22. Boudrieau RJ, Kudisch M. Miniplate fixation for repair of mandibular and maxillary fractures in 15 dogs and 3 cats. Vet Surg 1996;25:277–91.

23. Schloss AJ, Manfra Marretta S. Prognostic factors affecting teeth in the line of mandibular fractures. J Vet Dent 1990;7: 7–9.

24. Weber BG, Cech O. Pseudoarthorosis – pathophysiology, biomechanics, therapy, results. Bern, Switzerland: Hans Huber Publishers; 1976. p. 40–4.

25. Roush JK, Wilson JW. Healing of mandibular body osteotomies after plate and intramedullary pin fixation. Vet Surg 1989;18:190–6.

26. Lieblich SE, Topazian RG. Infection in the patient with maxillofacial trauma. In: Fonseca RJ, Walker RV, Betts NJ, et al, editors. Oral and maxillofacial trauma. 2nd ed. Philadelphia, PA: WB Saunders; 1997. p. 1248–73.

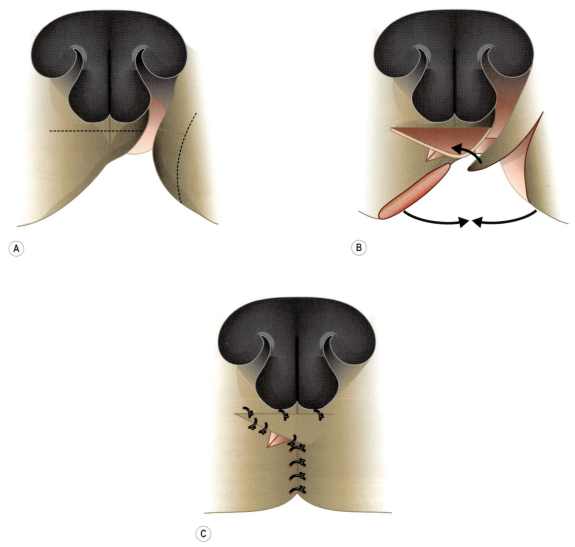

Fig. 36.4 The incisions utilized in the repair of a cleft lip include a perpendicular incision across the philtrum and a triangular-shaped pedicle flap on the lateral side of the cleft (**A**). The triangular pedicle flap is rotated across the cleft (**B**) and is sutured in place (**C**).

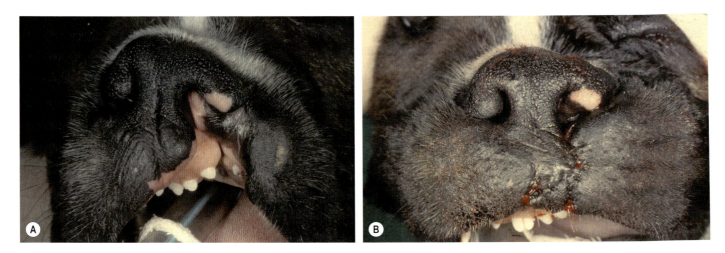

Fig. 36.5 Preoperative (**A**) and postoperative (**B**) view of a cleft lip repaired using a modification of the technique illustrated in Fig. 36.4. Important cosmetic aspects include facial symmetry, a straight philtrum and a smooth, continuous lip contour.

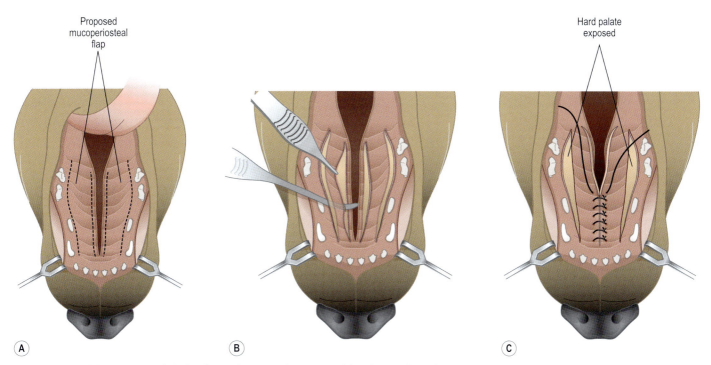

Proposed mucoperiosteal flap

Hard palate exposed

(A)   (B)   (C)

Fig. 36.6 A medially repositioned double-flap technique is demonstrated for closure of a cleft in the hard palate utilizing a midline appositional closure.

Cleft hard palate repair

Two basic techniques have been described in the veterinary literature for the repair of congenital hard palatal defects including the medially repositioned double-flap technique and the overlapping-flap technique.[1,11,13,14] In addition, selected human reconstructive techniques may be indicated for selected cases.

von Langenbeck technique

The medially repositioned double-flap technique involves creation of bilateral releasing incisions approximately 2 mm palatal and parallel to the maxillary teeth. The epithelial margins of the cleft are tangentially excised. The mucoperiosteum is undermined bilaterally on both sides of the defect, carefully avoiding laceration of the palatine arteries as they exit the major palatine foramina medial to the maxillary fourth premolar teeth. The flaps are repositioned medially and sutured over the defect (Fig. 36.6A–C).

The overlapping-flap technique is generally preferred for repair of midline hard palatal defects because this technique is associated with less tension on the suture line, the suture line is not located directly over the defect, and the area of opposing connective tissue is larger, which results in a stronger repair.[11]

Overlapping-flap technique

The overlapping-flap technique is initiated by making an incision the length of the palatal defect on the patient's right side 2–3 mm palatal to the maxillary teeth. Perpendicular incisions are made at the rostral and caudal ends of this incision extending to the cleft (Fig. 36.7A). The caudal incision should be preplanned so that it lies over the hard palate and not through the soft palate to prevent creation of an

oronasal fistula. A blunt-tipped periosteal elevator is used to elevate the mucoperiosteal layer, carefully avoiding the palatine artery as it exits the major palatine foramen approximately halfway between the midline and the maxillary fourth premolar tooth. When elevating in the area overlying the palatine fissure, a partial-thickness elevation is recommended so that the deepest layer remains with the bone, thereby preventing exposure of the palatine fissure and formation of an iatrogenic oronasal fistula. Care must also be taken when elevating this flap not to penetrate the medial edge of the cleft where the oral mucosa is confluent with the nasal mucosa.

A second incision is made in the mucoperiosteum on the left side of the patient's cleft along the entire length of the defect, perpendicular to the cleft margin, thereby separating the nasal from the oral mucoperiosteum. The oral mucoperiosteum is elevated approximately 8–10 mm away from the cleft margin along the entire length of the defect.

The mucoperiosteal flap from the right side of the defect is hinged or folded over the defect and positioned between the hard palate and the mucoperiosteal flap on the left side of the cleft (see Fig. 36.5B). The hinged flap should cover the defect and overlap beneath the opposite mucoperiosteal flap approximately 6 mm without tension. In very wide defects, a secondary releasing incision 2–3 mm palatal to the left dental quadrant may be required to permit adequate overlap without tension. The hinged flap is sutured in place using multiple simple interrupted horizontal or vertical mattress sutures using 3–0 or 4–0 monofilament absorbable suture material. These sutures should be preplaced from caudal to rostral and tagged temporarily with hemostats. Following placement of all sutures, the sutures are tied from caudal to rostral (Fig. 36.7C & Fig. 36.8A, B). The defect created by the raised hinged flap is allowed to heal by second intention and usually takes 3–4 weeks to completely granulate and reepithelialize (Fig. 36.8C).

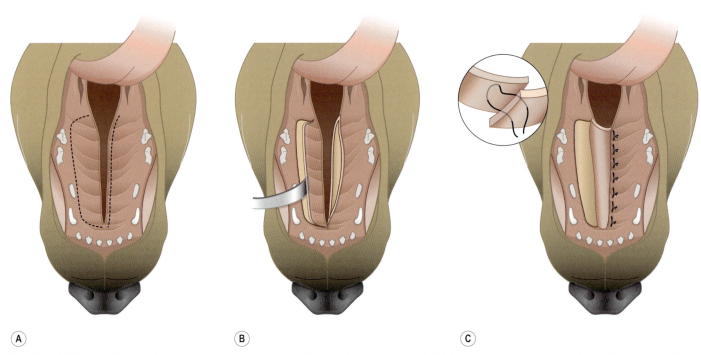

Fig. 36.7 (**A**) The incision sites for utilization of the overlapping-flap technique for repair of cleft hard palatal defects are depicted. (**B**) A periosteal elevator is used to elevate the flaps. (**C**) The large flap is reflected 180° and laid beneath the mucosa on the opposite side of the flap and sutured in place with multiple simple interrupted horizontal mattress sutures.

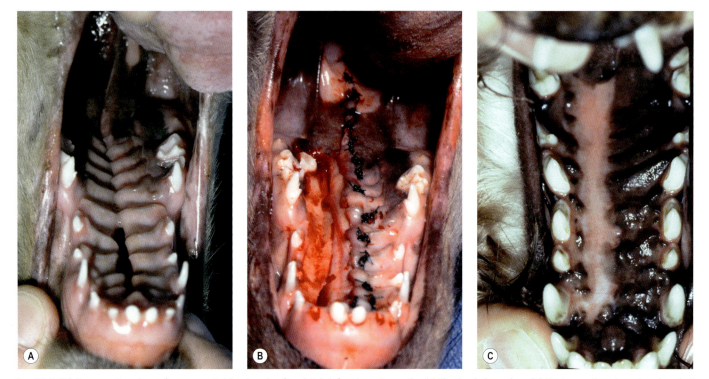

Fig. 36.8 (**A**) Preoperative view of a congenital hard and soft palatal defect in a 4-month-old Shetland sheepdog. (**B**) Postoperative view showing that the hard palatal defect has been repaired utilizing the overlapping-flap technique while the soft palatal defect has been repaired with a double-layer appositional technique. (**C**) Appearance 6 weeks following surgical repair of a similar palatal defect; note the reepithelialization of the denuded bone.

Cleft soft palate repair

Midline soft palatal defects commonly accompany hard palatal defects.[14] Soft palatal defects may occur in the absence of hard palatal defects; however, they are more frequently identified when hard palatal defects are present.[15] Midline clefts of the soft palate are most commonly seen and are located medial to the palatine muscles.[16] Unilateral or bilateral congenital defects of the soft palate occur less commonly and are located lateral to the palatine muscle.[16]

Double-layer appositional technique

Narrow midline clefts of the soft palate can be corrected utilizing a double-layer appositional technique as long as no tension is created during closure of the defect (Fig. 35.8B). The double-flap appositional technique has been previously described.[1,11,13] This technique is initiated by making an incision along the medial margin of the soft palatal defect on each side to the level of the middle or caudal aspect of the tonsils. A blunt-ended tenotomy scissors (Miltex, Lake Success, IL) or small Metzenbaum scissors (Hu-Friedy Instrument Co, Chicago, IL) are used to bluntly separate the soft palatal tissue, forming dorsal and ventral flaps on each side. Apposition of the dorsal flaps results in apposition of the nasal epithelial edges. Closure of this layer should be directed from caudal to cranial utilizing 4–0 monofilament absorbable sutures in a simple interrupted pattern so that the knots are located in the nasopharynx. Some surgeons recommend apposition of the palatal muscle and connective tissue with a simple continuous suture pattern[1] while other surgeons recommend not closing this layer since excessive suture material may predispose to the formation of scar tissue within the muscle tissue of the palate and impede healing.[17] A compromise may include closure of the muscular layer with a very fine monofilament absorbable suture material using a continuous pattern. The ventral flaps are sutured in a simple interrupted pattern with the knots located in the oral cavity to oppose the oral epithelium. Verification of the proper length of the repaired soft palate is confirmed following temporary extubation of the patient. Ideally the caudal edge of the repaired soft palate should be located somewhere between the level of the middle to the caudal aspect of the tonsils and just touch the tip of the epiglottis. If tension is present along the suture line, partial-thickness lateral relief incisions can be made. These partial-thickness relief incisions, when required, are made in the oral mucosa from the lingual aspect of the last molar tooth to near the level of the tip of the soft palate (Fig. 36.9A–C).[1]

Bilateral overlapping single-pedicle flap technique

An alternative technique has been described for the repair of midline soft palatal defects, called the bilateral overlapping mucosal single-pedicle flap technique. Surgical correction using this technique is technically more challenging and may not be necessary in most cases. The reported benefits of the bilateral overlapping single-pedicle flap technique over the simple double-layer apposition technique for correction of soft palatal defects is that in the overlapping technique, each layer is supported by an underlying layer of intact mucosa, as the suture lines are offset and, by placing the suture lines laterally, the technique also minimizes the effect of the pull of the palatine muscles on the incision line.[18]

Repair of soft palatal defects utilizing the bilateral overlapping single-pedicle flaps is performed by creating a nasal mucosal flap on one side of the defect and an oral mucosal flap on the other side of the defect, undermining the flaps to develop bilateral single-pedicle flaps with their bases on the edge of the cleft. The nasal mucosal flap is reflected into the oral cavity and the oral mucosal flap is rotated into the nasal cavity. The flaps are sutured in place with a simple interrupted pattern using fine absorbable suture material (Fig. 36.10A–C).[18]

Repair of unilateral hypoplasia of the soft palate

Unilateral defects of the soft palate occur infrequently. Several reports have described the recognition and successful treatment of these defects.[16,19,20] Dogs with unilateral clefts of the soft palate are presented primarily because of rhinitis.

A relatively simple two-layer technique can be utilized in the closure of unilateral clefts of the soft palate where sufficient soft palatal tissue exists. This technique is similar to the two-layer closure of midline palatal defects except for the location of the defect.[19] The patient is placed in dorsal recumbency, the upper jaw is taped to the surgical table and the lower jaw and endotracheal tube are suspended from an anesthetic screen or fluid stands. Following surgical preparation of the soft palate, three stay sutures are placed around the cleft, one at the rostral border and one at the caudal end of each side of the soft palatal defect. Tension is placed on the edges of the defect with the previously placed stay sutures and a small incision is made in the edge of the cleft using a #11 scalpel blade. The margins of the defect are separated into dorsal and ventral components using blunt-ended tenotomy scissors (Miltex, Lake Success, IL). The cleft is closed from caudal to cranial in two layers utilizing a simple continuous pattern using fine absorbable suture material in the nasal mucosa. Suturing of the defect should be accomplished with relatively large bites and the sutures should be snug but should not strangulate the tissue.[19] The oral mucosa is apposed in a similar manner. The knots for each layer should be placed on the epithelial surface to prevent burying excessive suture material.

Large unilateral clefts that are difficult to appose without tension may require a more complex reconstruction technique such as the use of buccal mucosal flaps, which have also been recommended for the surgical correction of hypoplastic soft palates.[16]

Bilateral hypoplasia of the soft palate

Animals with hypoplastic soft palates with bilateral soft palatal defects have significantly shortened soft palates. Oropharyngeal examination in these patients typically reveals a near absence of the soft palate with a small uvula-like projection that extends from the mid-caudal aspect of the hard palate (Fig. 36.11A, B).

Various recommendations have been made concerning the most appropriate treatment for hypoplasia or congenital absence of the soft palate, ranging from surgical correction to euthanasia.[11,15,16,21] Normal compensatory mechanisms, proper dietary management combined with surgery if necessary, may permit these patients to lead a relatively normal life.[21]

Various surgical techniques have been utilized in the treatment of congenital absence of the soft palate. One technique involves the bilateral removal of the tonsils with creation of dorsal and ventral pharyngeal flaps bilaterally, incision of the edges of the uvula-like structure, and suturing of the pharyngeal flaps to the uvula-like structure using a two-layer, simple interrupted pattern with fine absorbable monofilament suture material.[21]

Buccal mucosal flaps for the correction of hypoplastic soft palatal defects have been recommended.[16] This technique involves creation of bilateral buccal mucosal flaps based at the palatoglossal fold, at the caudal end of the hard palate. The buccal flaps are carefully undermined to prevent damage to the deep facial vein. The free edge of the soft palatal remnant and the mucosa of the pharyngeal walls are

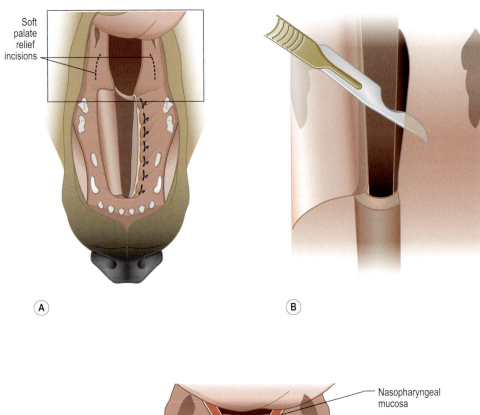

(A)

(B)

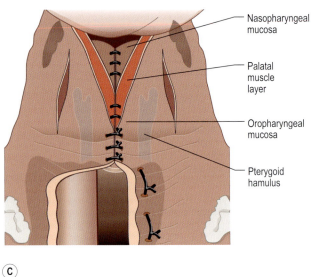

Nasopharyngeal mucosa

Palatal muscle layer

Oropharyngeal mucosa

Pterygoid hamulus

(C)

Fig. 36.9 (**A**) Closure of midline soft palatal defects should begin with partial-thickness relief incisions, if needed, to prevent tension on the incision line. (**B**) Incisions are made along the edges of the soft palatal defect to produce dorsal and ventral flaps. (**C**) The palatal defect is closed in 2 or 3 layers.

incised to create both dorsal (nasal) and ventral (oral) mucosal free edges. The first buccal flap is rotated so that the mucosal surface of the flap faces dorsally to become the floor of the nasopharynx and is sutured rostrally to the nasal mucosal free edge of the soft palate and laterally to the dorsal free mucosal edge of the pharyngeal wall. The second buccal flap on the opposite side is elevated as previously described. This flap is rotated across the defect so that the mucosal surface faces the oral cavity to become the mucosal surface of the oropharynx. The flap is sutured to the oral mucosal free edge of the pharyngeal wall of the pharynx and to the first flap laterally and to

the soft palate remnant rostrally along the oral mucosal free edge. The caudal aspects of the two flaps are sutured together. A simple interrupted pattern using fine absorbable suture material on a cutting needle has been recommended for this procedure.[16]

An alternative technique for repair of a hypoplastic soft palate that had been unsuccessfully treated multiple times has been reported in one dog.[22] This technique involved a free muscle transfer of the M. latissimus dorsi and accompanying thoracodorsal artery and vein with microvascular anastomosis. Unfortunately, this technique was also unsuccessful and the dog was euthanized.

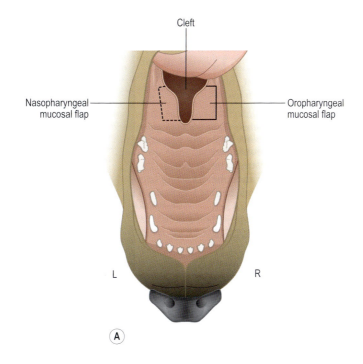

Cleft

Nasopharyngeal mucosal flap

Oropharyngeal mucosal flap

L   R

(A)

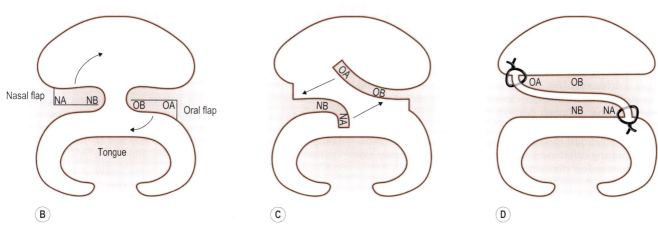

Nasal flap NA NB   OB OA Oral flap

Tongue

(B)

OA OB

NB NA

(C)

OA OB

NB NA

(D)

Fig. 36.10 Bilateral overlapping mucosal single-pedicle flaps for correction of soft palatal defects are harvested from nasal and oral mucosal flaps (**A**,**B**), which are rotated 180° (**C**) and sutured in position (**D**) to close the defect.

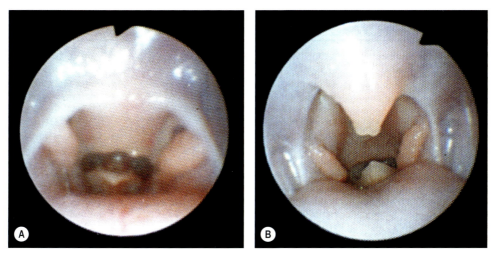

(A)   (B)

Fig. 36.11 (**A**) Endoscopic view of a normal soft palate in a 6-week-old Shetland sheepdog. (**B**) Endoscopic view of a severely hypoplastic soft palate in a littermate, presented because of bilateral mucopurulent nasal discharge; note the uvula-like projection extending caudally in the middle of the hypoplastic soft palate.

Chapter 37

Repair of acquired palatal defects

Sandra Manfra Marretta

DEFINITIONS

Acquired oronasal fistula: an abnormal communication between the oral and nasal cavities caused by trauma or disease, or following unsuccessful cleft palate repair[1]

Advancement flap: a mucoperiosteal pedicle flap that is advanced along its long axis

Double-layer palatal flap: two separate flaps that are utilized in the closure of an oronasal fistula in two overlapping layers

Island palatal flap: a palatal flap incorporating the major palatine artery with complete separation of the flap from the surrounding palatal mucoperiosteal tissues so that the flap is an island of tissue that can be freely rotated around the major palatine artery[2]

Split palatal U-flap: bilateral transposition flaps in which each pedicle is based on the location of the major palatine artery

Tongue flap: flap based on a portion of the tongue used for closure of palatal defects

Transposition palatal flap: a mucoperiosteal pedicle flap that is rotated on its basis to cover a palatal defect

Vestibular mucosal flap: a pedicle mucosal flap with associated underlying connective tissue harvested from the alveolar mucosa and the buccal mucosa of the lip or cheek

PREOPERATIVE CONCERNS

Prior to surgical treatment of acquired palatal defects, the overall clinical status of the patient should be thoroughly evaluated and appropriately treated. Following stabilization of the patient, the acquired palatal defect should be thoroughly evaluated to determine the underlying cause and the full extent of the lesion and the condition of the tissue surrounding the defect. Acquired palatal defects may be caused by bite wounds, blunt head trauma, electrical burns, gunshot wounds, foreign body penetration and pressure necrosis (Figs 37.1 and 37.2). Other causes of acquired palatal defects include periodontal disease, tooth extraction, neoplasia, radiation necrosis or dehiscence of a surgical wound (see Chs 45 and 53). Diagnostic imaging (oral radiography and computed tomography) and rhinoscopy may assist in the diagnosis and management of acquired palatal defects caused by foreign body penetration. A preoperative incisional biopsy, diagnostic imaging and thoracic radiographs are recommended in all palatal defects that may be associated with a neoplastic process.

When the viability of the tissue surrounding the palatal defect cannot be predicted, delay in closure of the defect may be warranted. Alternative forms of alimentation should be considered including esophagostomy and gastrostomy tubes (see Ch. 5) in animals in which surgical repair of the defect must be delayed.

ANESTHETIC CONSIDERATIONS

Following adequate stabilization of patients with acquired palatal defects, each patient should be anesthetized with an appropriate anesthetic protocol based on the individual's clinical status. A guarded endotracheal tube is recommended for intubation to prevent kinking of the tube during the surgical procedure. Patients with acquired palatal defects should be positioned in either dorsal or lateral recumbency, based on the location of the defect, with the endotracheal tube firmly secured to the mandible.

SURGICAL ANATOMY

The incisive, maxillary and palatine bones form the roof of the mouth. The palatine fissures, two large openings in the incisive bones, are located at the level of the canine teeth and can be palpated as soft areas in the rostral aspect of the palate bilaterally (see Fig. 36.1).

The caudal aspect of the hard palate is located just caudal to the maxillary second molar teeth where it merges with the rostral aspect of the soft palate. The caudal aspect of the soft palate normally just touches the tip of the epiglottis.

The major palatine arteries are the main arteries to the mucoperiosteum of the hard palate. These vessels pass through the caudal

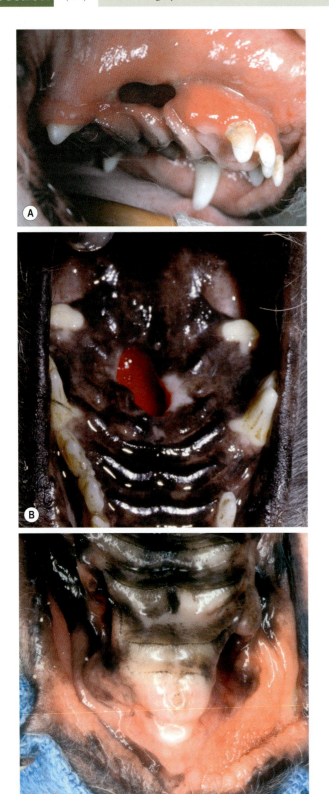

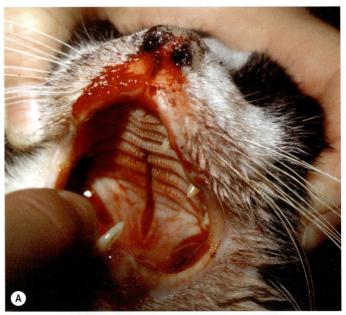

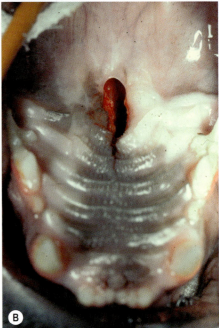

Fig. 37.2 Acquired oronasal fistulas in cats: (**A**) Acute traumatic defect of the caudal palate – note the bilateral hemorrhagic nasal discharge. (**B**) Chronic oronasal fistula resulting from a similar lesion that was left to heal by second intention but failed to do so.

Fig. 37.1 Acquired oronasal fistulas in dogs: (**A**) Oronasal fistula following the forceful extraction of the right maxillary canine tooth. (**B**) Palatal defect caused by the prolonged retention of a foreign body wedged between the maxillary fourth premolar teeth, which resulted in pressure necrosis of the underlying palate. (**C**) Bilateral oronasal fistulas and tooth loss due to severe periodontitis of the maxillary canine teeth.

palatine foramina bilaterally and course rostrally in the shallow palatine grooves on the surface of the hard palate (see Fig. 36.1). The infraorbital vessels and nerves exit through the infraorbital foramina located rostral to the mesiobuccal root apex of the maxillary fourth premolar teeth and course cranially.

SPECIAL INSTRUMENTS AND MATERIALS

A Bard-Parker # 3 long scalpel handle with a # 15 scalpel blade can be used to incise mucosa in patients with acquired palatal defects. A blunt-tipped, curved Freer periosteal elevator (Miltex, Lake Success,

NY) can be used for elevating the mucoperiosteal layer from the hard palate. A smaller periosteal elevator (e.g., 24G periosteal elevator (Hu-Friedy Mfg. Co., Chicago, IL)) can be used for elevating the attached gingiva from the underlying bone during flap procedures in small patients. A small curved tipped Metzenbaum scissors (Hu-Friedy Mfg. Co., Chicago, IL) can be used for blunt dissection of the vestibular mucosal flaps into two layers.

THERAPEUTIC DECISION-MAKING

Prior to surgical repair of acquired palatal defects it is important to carefully decide what therapeutic plan is likely to be most successful in a particular type of defect. Therapeutic decision-making in these cases is usually based on the cause, the size and location of the defect and whether or not there has been any prior surgical intervention. The best chance of success for repair of palatal defects is with the first surgical procedure; therefore, appropriate treatment planning is crucial. Various single-layer surgical techniques can be used to repair acquired palatal defects, including vestibular flaps, transposition flaps, advancement flaps, tongue flaps, split palatal U-flaps and island palatal flaps.[1-10] Double-layer techniques including vestibular and reflected palatal flaps can also be utilized. In general, the technique that provides the largest flap with no tension and an adequate blood supply is recommended.

SURGICAL TECHNIQUES

Primary closure of a midline palatal fracture/separation[11]

This injury is often seen in cats (Fig. 37.2A, and also see Ch. 25). Narrow defects may heal without surgical treatment. Alternatively, and if the defect is wide, this injury can easily and effectively be managed by soft tissue debridement and approximating the displaced bony structures by gentle digital pressure, followed by primary closure of the torn palatal soft tissues in a simple interrupted pattern (Fig. 37.3). Flushing and suctioning the nasal cavity is indicated if large blood clots are present. Provided the patient is stable, the benefit of this initial management may outweigh the risk inherent in leaving this injury to heal by second intention. Occasionally, this healing does not take place and a persistent oronasal fistula results (Fig. 37.2B); the latter condition is far more difficult to manage.

Single-layer techniques

Vestibular flaps

Vestibular flaps can be utilized for repair of marginal palatal defects in edentulous regions.[6] These flaps are recommended in the repair of oronasal fistulas secondary to periodontal disease and for closure of large palatal defects associated with partial maxillectomy procedures.[6]

Prior to closure of chronic oronasal fistulas, the edges of the fistula must be thoroughly debrided along the entire epithelial margin. This can be accomplished by excising a 3-mm rim of tissue from the entire edge of the fistula to produce a healthy bleeding circumferential margin (Fig. 37.4A). Two divergent incisions are then made in the mucosa beginning at the mesial and distal aspect of the fistula through the attached gingiva, across the mucogingival junction, and extending into the alveolar mucosa. A periosteal elevator is used to gently elevate

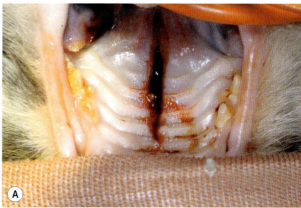
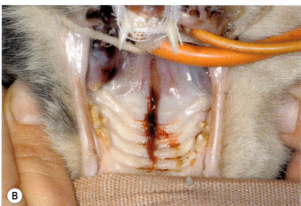
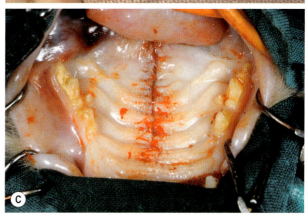

Fig. 37.3 Primary closure of a traumatic cleft of the hard palate in a cat: (**A**) Soft tissue debridement. (**B**) Approximation of the displaced bony structures by gentle digital pressure. (**C**) Primary closure of the torn palatal soft tissues in a simple interrupted pattern. (*A and C from: Verstraete FJM. Maxillofacial fractures. In: Slatter DG ed.* Textbook of small animal surgery. *3rd ed. Philadelphia: WB Saunders; 2003:2190–2207.*)

the mucoperiosteal flap from the underlying bone. The inelastic innermost layer of the flap, the periosteal layer, may be incised along the entire inner aspect of the base of the flap; this results in a more elastic, mobile flap. Prior to closure the flap should be tested for any evidence of potential tension at the surgical site. If there is any evidence of tension along the proposed suture line, additional periosteal releasing, extension of the mesial and distal incisions and additional undermining may be necessary prior to closure of the flap. Reduction in the height of the alveolar margin bone with an osteoplasty bur may also be beneficial in reducing tension on the flap. Once a tensionless

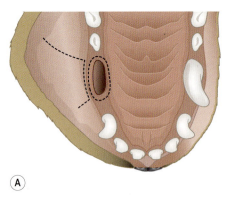
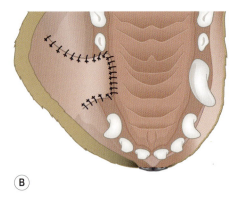

Fig. 37.4 Single-layer vestibular flap: (**A**) The rim of mucosa is excised from the margins of the fistula and the proposed incision line for the vestibular flap is illustrated. (**B**) The vestibular flap is advanced over the defect and sutured in place.

closure is insured, the flap is then sutured in place with fine monofilament absorbable suture material in a simple interrupted pattern (Fig. 37.4B). The corners of the flap should be sutured first, followed by closure of the palatal and gingival margins. Sutures are then alternately placed in the mesial and distal aspects of the flap, progressing from the gingival margin to the most apical portion of the flap.

Vestibular flaps that are used to close surgical sites following extensive maxillectomy procedures often require extensive undermining to prevent tension on the incision line. The vestibular mucosal flaps are created by undermining the mucosa and submucosa from the edge of the maxillectomy site toward the mucocutaneous junction of the lip until the flap can be brought into apposition with the subperiosteally elevated edge of the hard palate mucoperiosteum without tension. The vestibular flaps are sutured in position using a two-layer interrupted suture pattern using monofilament absorbable suture material. The initial or deep layer should be placed so that the knots are located in the nasal cavity and the more superficial layer should be placed so that the knots are located in the oral cavity.

Transposition flaps

Transposition flaps are recommended for small, circular defects, especially defects located in the hard palate lateral to the midline and rostral to the maxillary fourth premolar tooth.[4,6,9] The palatal mucoperiosteal tissues contain less elastic tissue, thereby offering very limited pliability of these flaps when compared to vestibular flaps; however, the palatal tissue is keratinized and thicker than the unkeratinized alveolar and buccal tissue, providing increased strength in palatal flaps.[3,9] In addition, procedures involving palatal transposition flaps do not affect the depth of the vestibulum.[3] Transposition flaps can also be raised from the soft palate, in which case they are split-thickness.

These flaps should be designed significantly larger than the defect to be covered. Initially a 2–3-mm rim of tissue is tangentially excised from the entire edge of the fistula to produce a healthy, bleeding nonepithelialized margin. The transposition flap is created by making a U-shaped incision with one arm of the U adjacent to the defect, leaving the caudal aspect of the base of the flap intact. The removal of a small triangular segment (known as a Bürow's triangle) of mucoperiosteal tissue from the caudal aspect of the lesser curvature of the flap can facilitate adaptation of the flap over the palatal defect without kinking of the rotated redundant palatal tissue.[3] When creating the rostral aspect of the U-shaped flap, the major palatine artery will be encountered and must be ligated rostrally. The flap should be carefully raised with the major palatine artery, using a curved Freer periosteal elevator (Miltex, Lake Success, NY) to avoid traumatizing the major

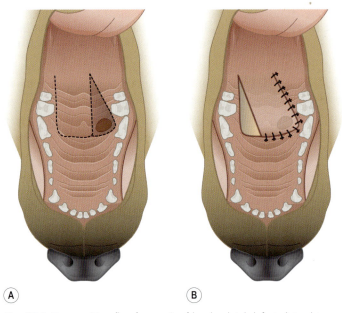

Fig. 37.5 Transposition flap for repair of hard palatal defects lateral to the midline: (**A**) shaded area represents proposed site for removal of perifistula palatal mucosa to permit rotation of proposed flap. (**B**) Transposition flap sutured in place over palatal defect.

palatine artery as it courses along the palate rostrally and enters onto the surface of the palate through the major palatine foramen approximately halfway between the midline of the hard palate and the maxillary fourth premolar tooth. The flap is transposed to cover the defect and sutured in place with simple interrupted sutures. Because there is no soft tissue to secure the flap on the donor side, it is recommended that small holes be predrilled in the hard palate with a small K-wire to allow placement of sutures to secure the flap along the donor side of the fistula repair.[9] Care should be taken when creating these holes so that they remain small and will be covered by the transposed flap to help prevent the formation of small iatrogenic fistulas. The flap is transposed to cover the defect and sutures are preplaced between the inner layer of the flap and the predrilled holes in the palate while avoiding the major palatine artery. The flap is sutured in place using monofilament absorbable suture material in a simple interrupted pattern. The exposed palatal bone of the donor site is allowed to heal by second intention (Fig. 37.5).

Advancement flaps

Advancement flaps are recommended for repair of wide caudal palatal defects that cross the midline. As with any palatal defect, a 2–3-mm section of mucosa is tangentially excised from the perimeter of the defect. A large mucoperiosteal flap is created caudal to the defect to include part of the soft palate so that sufficient tissue can be advanced rostrally to prevent tension on the suture line.[4,5] The flap is sutured over the defect using a monofilament absorbable suture material in a simple interrupted pattern (Fig. 37.6).

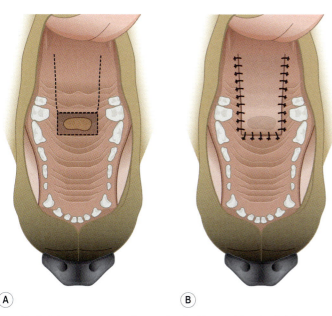

Fig. 37.6 Advancement flap for repair of wide caudal palatal defects that cross the midline: (**A**) shaded area represents proposed site for removal of perifistula palatal mucosa to permit advancement of proposed flap. (**B**) Advancement flap sutured in place over palatal defect.

Partial-thickness transposition flaps

Partial-thickness transposition flaps can be utilized in the closure of palatal defects located in the area between the hard and soft palate.[9] The mucosa around the fistula is denuded of epithelium. The oral mucosa of the soft palate is incised with a #15 scalpel blade and a partial-thickness U-shaped flap of adequate length is elevated with a combination of blunt and sharp dissection using a blunt-tipped tenotomy scissors (Hu-Friedy Mfg. Co., Chicago, IL). The flap is rotated over the defect and any mucosal surface that will lie beneath the transposed flap must be debrided to remove the epithelial layer. The flap is sutured in position using monofilament absorbable suture material in a simple interrupted pattern and the donor site is allowed to heal by second intention.

Tongue flaps

Tongue flaps have been recommended for the repair of large rostral palatal defects.[11] However, because of the high incidence of dehiscence associated with tongue flaps in animals, alternative techniques are preferred whenever possible.[4,6,7] The initial phase of this procedure involves debridement of the edges of the palatal defect and excision of the edges of the rostral, rostrolateral and dorsal mucosal edges of the tongue. The tongue should then be rotated 180 degrees on its long axis so that the dorsal aspect of the tongue still faces intraorally when placed in the palatal defect and sutured beneath the elevated palatine mucosa using a simple interrupted suture pattern (Fig. 37.7). Maxillomandibular fixation (see Ch. 29) for 4 weeks postoperatively with a gap of 3 mm between the incisors, and feeding a blended diet through a pharyngostomy or esophagostomy tube has been recommended.[11] The tongue pedicle is amputated in successive stages over a 4-week period to stimulate vascularization and sufficient tongue is left with the palate to close the palatal defect without tension.

Split palatal U-flap

The split palatal U-flap has been utilized for the repair of central hard palatal defects located approximately at the level of the fourth premolar teeth.[8] This surgical procedure is initiated with tangential excision

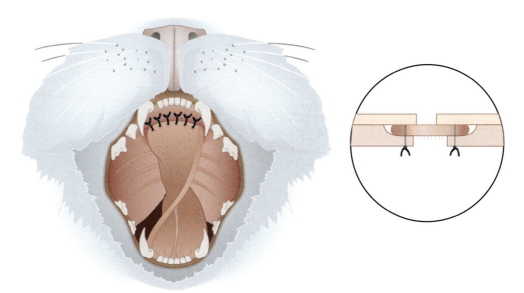

Fig. 37.7 Following debridement of the rostral edges of the tongue, the tongue is rotated 180° on its axis into the large rostral palatal defect and sutured in place beneath the elevated palatal mucosa. Other methods of repair of large rostral palatal defects are preferred, and this procedure should be considered only if other alternatives are not feasible.

of the epithelial margin of the palatal defect with a # 15 scalpel blade. A large, full-thickness, U-shaped, mucoperiosteal flap is created rostral to the defect. When creating the rostral aspect of the U-shaped flap, the major palatine arteries will be encountered bilaterally and must be ligated at the rostral aspect of the incision. The flap must be carefully elevated using a curved Freer periosteal elevator to avoid traumatizing the major palatine arteries bilaterally as they course along the palate rostrally and enter onto the surface of the palate through the major palatine foramina, approximately 10 mm palatal to the maxillary fourth premolar teeth. Gentle intermittent lifting of the flap from the underlying bone during periosteal elevation can help provide visualization of the major palatine arteries as they exit the major palatine foramina, and will help prevent inadvertent laceration of these vessels.

Following subperiosteal elevation of the U-shaped flap, the flap is incised along the midline using a # 15 scalpel blade. This divides the large U-flap into two equally-sized flaps, with a major palatine artery entering the base of each flap providing each flap with an excellent blood supply. One side of the hemisected U-flap is rotated 90 degrees over the palatal defect. The medial aspect of the flap is sutured to the caudal aspect of the palatal defect with monofilament absorbable suture material in a simple interrupted pattern. The second side of the hemisected U-flap is rotated 90 degrees, transposed rostral to the previously rotated flap and sutured in place using a simple interrupted suture pattern (Fig. 37.8). Small holes may be predrilled in the palate rostral to the palatal defect using small K-wires in an area of the palate that will be covered by the second flap to help hold the flap in apposition with the hard palate rostrally. This is performed by preplacing sutures through the small predrilled holes in the palate and passing the suture split thickness through the palatal side of the second flap. The exposed bone at the donor site is allowed to heal by second intention and will generally reepithelialize within 1 month.

Island palatal flap

A variation of the split palatal U-flap, the island palatal flap, has been described for use in the repair of a caudal palatal defect which occurred following an extensive caudal maxillectomy procedure.[2]

Caudal palatal defects in these types of cases are often located in areas that are deficient in local mucoperiosteal tissue, with local perifistula tissues having tension at the time of initial repair, or subsequent to wound contraction.[2] The island palatal flap in this previously reported case was harvested from the side of the palate that had remained intact following the previously-performed caudal maxillectomy procedure. An island palatal flap is created by making a large, full-thickness, U-shaped flap positioned over the maxilla with the base of the flap located caudal to the major palatine foramen. The mucoperiosteum is gently raised to avoid traumatizing the major palatine artery during its course along the hard palate and where it enters through the major palatine foramen, approximately halfway between the midline and the maxillary fourth premolar tooth. The final caudal incision is made through the base of the flap at the level of the maxillary first molar tooth to complete the harvesting of the island palatal mucoperiosteal flap. All flap incisions are full-thickness, thereby isolating the attachments of the island palatal mucoperiosteal flap to the major palatine neurovascular pedicle.[2] The margins of the fistula are debrided, and the island palatal mucoperiosteal flap is rotated into the defect and sutured in place with monofilament absorbable suture material in a simple interrupted pattern (Fig. 37.9). The portion of the rotated palatal flap bordering the denuded, rostrally located donor site is not sutured and the donor site is left to heal with granulation tissue and reepithelialization. The island palatal mucoperiosteal flap can be utilized in the repair of defects in the caudal oral cavity within a 180 degree rotation arc of the ipsilateral major palatine foramen.[2]

Double-layer techniques

Various double-layer closure techniques utilizing local tissues have been described.[3–5,9,12–14] Double-layer flap techniques include two separate flaps that may be used to close chronic or recurrent oronasal fistulas. The initial flap is used to provide a mucosal surface for the nasal passage and a vascularized support for the oral graft. The second flap is placed over the first flap and provides the oral mucosal surface for the repair. There are unique benefits associated with the use of double-layer and single-layer flaps. The double-layer flaps oppose a much larger area of connective tissue, which results in a stronger

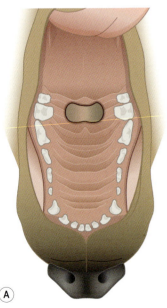
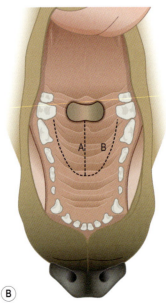
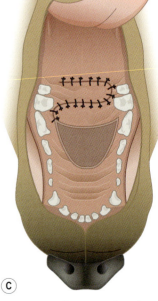

(A)　　　　　(B)　　　　　(C)

Fig. 37.8 Split palatal U-flap: (**A**) Central hard palatal defect. (**B**) Proposed incision lines for creation of split U-flap. (**C**) Split U-flap sutured in place over defect.

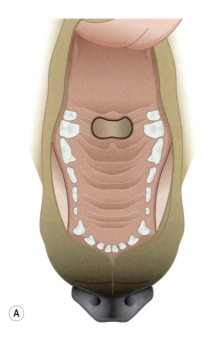
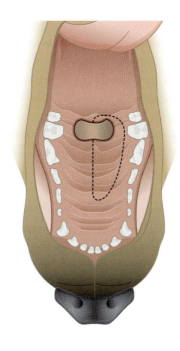
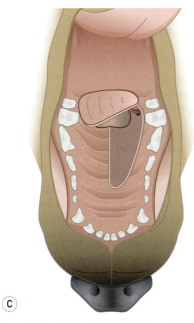
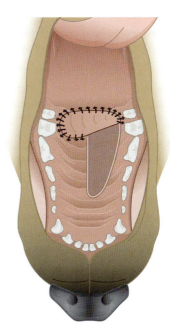

Fig. 37.9 Island palatal flap: (**A**) Caudal hard palatal defect. (**B**) The rim of mucosa is excised from the margins of the fistula; the proposed incision lines for creation of an island palatal flap are illustrated. (**C**) The island palatal flap has been raised – note the neurovascular pedicle. (**D**) Island palatal flap sutured in place over defect.

repair.[4] The disadvantages of the double-layer flap techniques are that they are more technically challenging to perform, and increase the time required to perform the surgical procedure.[3]

Vestibular-mucosal/perifistula/hard palatal flaps

Three anatomic sites for flap development for closure of chronic oronasal fistulas secondary to chronic periodontal disease of the maxillary canine tooth have been described.[13,14] These three sites include:

(1) the mucosa of the periphery of the fistula, (2) the alveolar and buccal mucosa, and (3) the hard palate mucosa or mucoperiosteum.[13] Two of three sites may be combined to repair chronic oronasal fistulas.

The repair of chronic oronasal fistulas utilizing a combination of the mucosa of the periphery of the fistula and a buccal mucosal flap is initiated by making a circular incision in the perifistula mucosa at an appropriate distance from the defect to provide sufficient length to permit primary closure over the defect. A wedge of tissue is removed

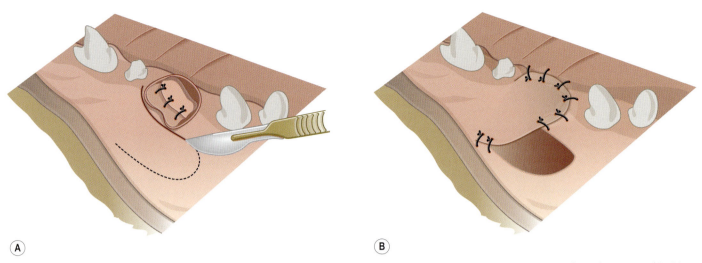

Fig. 37.10 Double-layer flap: (**A**) The perifistula oral mucosa has been elevated and rotated into the defect and sutured in place; the proposed incision line for the vestibular mucosal flap is illustrated. (**B**) The second flap is sutured over the submucosal surface of the perifistula flap.

from the mesial and distal aspects of the perifistula circumferential incision. The remaining perifistula tissue is carefully elevated with a small feline periosteal elevator leaving the nasal mucosal edges of the flaps intact. The flaps are hinged into the defect from each side and sutured in place with 5–0 or 6–0 absorbable sutures in a simple interrupted pattern to provide a mucosal surface facing the nasal cavity.

The vestibular mucosal flap is created from the mucosa lateral to the oronasal fistula. The incision for the vestibular flap should extend rostral to the oronasal fistula to provide a flap of sufficient length and width to cover the defect created by the perifistula flaps. The vestibular flap is elevated in a plane that is superficial to the branches of the buccal and infraorbital nerves to prevent excessive hemorrhaging and nerve dysfunction secondary to transection of these neurovascular structures.[13] The vestibular flap is then rotated over the submucosal surface of the perifistula flaps and sutured in place with 4–0 monofilament absorbable suture material in a simple interrupted pattern. The donor site for the vestibular flap may be closed primarily if this can be accomplished without resulting in tension on the surgical site, or alternatively it may be allowed to heal by contraction and reepithelialization (Fig. 37.10).

The repair of chronic oronasal fistulas utilizing a combination of hard palatal mucosa and vestibular mucosal flaps is initiated by making a U-shaped, partial-thickness incision in the hard palate mucosa, palatal to the oronasal fistula, of sufficient size to adequately cover the oronasal fistula without tension. The flap is gently elevated to the edge of the fistula, leaving the mucosa of the base of the flap intact. The vestibular mucosal flap is then incised and elevated opposite the oronasal fistula, leaving a rim of perifistula tissue to serve as a suture location for the transposed, hard palate mucosal flap. Prior to suturing the palatal flap to the perifistula tissue, the superficial mucosal layer of the perifistula tissue is removed with a diamond bur to prevent complications that might result from buried epithelium. The palatal flap is then hinged into the defect with the mucosal surface of the flap directed towards the nasal cavity and sutured in place with 5–0 monofilament absorbable suture in a simple interrupted pattern. The vestibular flap is then transposed over the palatal flap site and donor site (if this can be accomplished without resulting in tension on the vestibular flap), or alternatively transposed to cover only the submucosa of the palatal flap, allowing the palatal donor site to heal by contraction and reepithelialization. The vestibular flap is sutured

in place with 4–0 or 5–0 monofilament absorbable sutures in a simple interrupted pattern (Fig. 37.11).

Miscellaneous techniques

Myoperitoneal microvascular free flaps

Myoperitoneal microvascular free flaps have been reported in the reconstruction of large acquired palatal defects in dogs in which multiple operations using local tissue flaps were unsuccessful.[15,16]

Utilization of a myoperitoneal microvascular free flap involves the harvesting of the myoperitoneal flap from the body wall. The myoperitoneal flap may be based on the right cranial abdominal artery and vein and the cranial portion of the transversus abdominis muscle[15] or the caudal epigastric artery and vein and the rectus abdominis muscle.[16] Following isolation of the infraorbital artery and the superior labial vein and preparation of the palatal wound bed by incision of the palatine mucosa along the border of the oronasal fistula, microvascular techniques are utilized to perform the anastomosis. Following anastomosis of the vessels, the edges of the myoperitoneal flap are sutured under the elevated edges of the palatine mucosa using a combination of vest-over-pants sutures and a simple interrupted pattern.

Obturators

Closure of large palatal defects may be difficult to achieve using autogenous tissue. In cases in which repeated attempts to close large palatal defects are unsuccessful, prosthetic appliances may be used to cover these defects.

In humans, various alloplastic materials have been used in the construction of obturators including gold foil, gold plate, tantalum plate, soft polymethyl methacrylate and lyophilized collagen.[3] Various types of obturators have been used in the treatment of large acquired palatal defects in dogs and cats including permanent and removable, acrylic, Silastic and metal obturators (Fig. 37.12).[4,17–20]

Direct fabrication of prosthetic acrylic obturators has been described;[17] however, most obturators are fabricated in a dental laboratory, necessitating two anesthetic episodes. During the initial anesthetic episode an impression of both mandibles is obtained using alginate

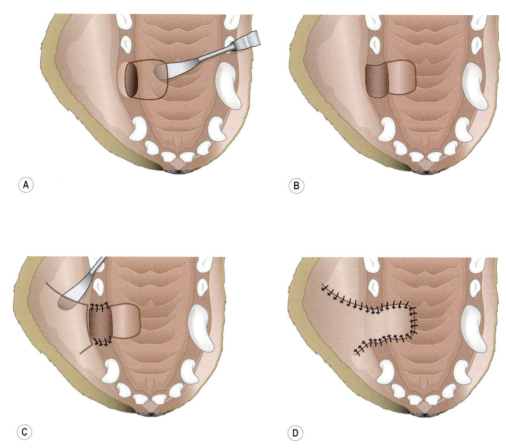

Fig. 37.11 Double-layer flap: (**A**) The mucosa palatal to the fistula is elevated with a periosteal elevator. (**B**) The palatal flap is hinged over the defect. (**C**) The palatal flap has been sutured in place and the vestibular flap is elevated. (**D**) The vestibular flap is sutured over the palatal flap and donor site.

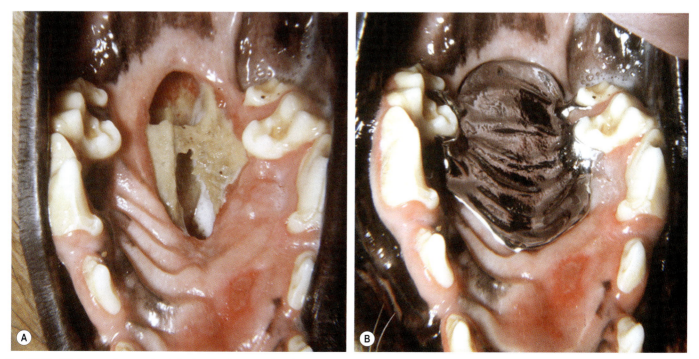

Fig. 37.12 (**A**) Osteoradionecrosis of the hard palate in a dog following radiation therapy of a fibrosarcoma. (**B**) Palliative treatment with a stainless steel obturator following debridement. *(Photograph courtesy of Dr. G.V. Ling, University of California, Davis.)*

and vinyl polysiloxane impressions of the maxillas and the defects are obtained using custom-made impression trays.[18] The impressions, along with clinical photographs of the palatal defect, are submitted to a dental laboratory. Stone models are made and used to construct the obturator. During a second anesthetic episode the obturator is positioned into the defect and appropriately secured, based on the design of the obturator.

Obturators requiring wire components for coronal attachment may not be useful in cats because of the morphologic features of their premolar and molar teeth.[19] A nasal septal button designed for repair of nasal septal perforations in humans has been used to successfully treat a large oronasal fistula in a cat.[19] The intranasal portion of the 30-mm Silastic button (Xomed-Treace, Jacksonville, FL) can be trimmed to fit into the defect. The use of this button should be considered for obturation of 7- to 25-mm oronasal fistulas in small animals that cannot be closed with autogenous tissue.[19]

POSTOPERATIVE CARE AND ASSESSMENT

Administration of a broad-spectrum antibiotic is recommended for 10–14 days postoperatively, especially in cases with persistent rhinitis.[13] Intravenous fluids should be administered until the patient begins eating and drinking, which is usually within 24 hours after surgery. Oral intake should begin with a blended diet for 2 weeks followed by the slow conversion to a soft diet for an additional 4 weeks. Placement of a pharyngostomy, esophagostomy or gastrostomy tube may be considered in patients that refuse oral intake; however, alternative methods to routine oral intake are usually not required in most cases. Chew toys and other hard objects should be withheld for a minimum of 6 weeks. The surgical sites should be reevaluated at 2 and 6 weeks postoperatively.

Sedation or anesthesia may be required to thoroughly assess the surgical repair.

COMPLICATIONS

The most common complication associated with repair of acquired palatal defects is dehiscence. This complication can be minimized by performing tension-free closures, gentle intraoperative tissue handling, maintaining an adequate blood supply to the flap, providing adequate bony support of the suture line and application of appropriate suturing techniques.

Surgical intervention for treatment of dehiscence following the initial attempt to repair the acquired palatal defect should be delayed for about 6 weeks because tissues are friable following dehiscence. This delay in surgery will help delineate the full extent of dehiscence and permit the tissues to revascularize and regain strength.[1]

PROGNOSIS

The prognosis is excellent for most animals following the repair of acquired palatal defects. Most acquired palatal defects can be closed surgically if the client is willing to persist with repeated procedures. Large inoperable palatal defects have a guarded to poor prognosis. Utilization of free flaps and obturators should be considered in the management of large inoperable acquired palatal defects. Long-term use of obturators in animals may result in enlargement of the palatal defect secondary to chronic inflammation caused by the obturators, and chronic rhinitis because of leakage around the obturators into the nasal cavity.

REFERENCES

1. Hedlund CS. Surgery of the oral cavity and oropharynx. In: Fossum TW, editor. Small animal surgery. 2nd ed. St. Louis, MO: Mosby; 2002. p. 274–306.
2. Smith MM. Island palatal mucoperiosteal flap for repair of oronasal fistula in a dog. J Vet Dent 2001;18:127–9.
3. Awang MN. Closure of oroantral fistula. Int J Oral Maxillofac Surg 1988;17:110–5.
4. Harvey CE, Emily PP. Oral surgery. In: Harvey CE, Emily PP, editors. Small animal dentistry. St. Louis, MO: Mosby; 1993. p. 312–77.
5. Harvey CE. Palate defects in dogs and cats. Compend Cont Educ Pract Vet 1987;9:404–18.
6. Manfra Marretta S. Maxillofacial surgery. Vet Clin North Am Small Anim Pract 1998;28:1285–96.
7. Manfra Marretta S. Palatal defects. In: Harari J, editor. Small animal surgery secrets. Philadelphia, PA: Hanley & Belfus, Inc; 2000. p. 347–50.
8. Manfra Marretta S, Grove TK, Grillo JF. Split palatal U-flap: A new technique for repair of caudal hard palate defects. J Vet Dent 1991;8(1):5–8.
9. Pope ER, Constantinescu GM. Oral cavity. In: Bojrab MJ, Ellison GW, Slocum B, editors. Current techniques in small animal surgery. 4th ed. Baltimore, MD: Williams & Wilkins; 1998. p. 113–42.
10. Robertson JJ, Dean PW. Repair of a traumatically induced oronasal fistula in a cat with a rostral tongue flap. Vet Surg 1987;16:164–6.
11. Verstraete FJM. Maxillofacial fractures. In: Slatter DG, editor. Textbook of small animal surgery. 3rd ed. Philadelphia, PA: WB Saunders; 2003. p. 2190–207.
12. Manfra Marretta S. Dentistry and diseases of the oropharynx. In: Birchard SJ, Sherding RG, editors. Saunders manual of small animal practice. 2nd ed. Philadelphia, PA: WB Saunders; 2000. p. 702–25.
13. Smith MM. Oronasal fistula repair. Clin Tech Small Anim Pract 2000;15:243–50.
14. Nelson AW. Upper respiratory system. In: Slatter DH, editor. Textbook of small animal surgery. 2nd ed. Philadelphia, PA: WB Saunders; 1993. p. 733–76.
15. Degner DA, Lanz OI, Walshaw R. Myoperitoneal microvascular free flaps in dogs: an anatomical study and a clinical case report. Vet Surg 1996;25:463–70.
16. Lanz OI. Free tissue transfer of the rectus abdominis myoperitoneal flap for oral reconstruction in a dog. J Vet Dent 2001;18:187–92.
17. Coles BH, Underwood LC. Repair of the traumatic oronasal fistula in the cat with a prosthetic acrylic implant. Vet Rec 1988;122:359–60.
18. Hale FA, Sylvestre AM, Miller C. The use of a prosthetic appliance to manage a large palatal defect in a dog. J Vet Dent 1997;14:61–4.
19. Smith MM, Rockfill AD. Prosthodontic appliance for repair of an oronasal fistula in a cat. J Am Vet Med Assoc 1996;208:1410–12.
20. Thoday KL, Charlton DA, Graham-Jones O, et al. The successful use of a prosthesis in the correction of a palatal defect in a dog. J Small Anim Pract 1975;16:487–94.

Chapter | 38 |

Clinical staging and biopsy of maxillofacial tumors

Boaz Arzi & Frank J.M. Verstraete

GENERAL CONSIDERATIONS

Malignant neoplasms of the oral cavity represent approximately 6% of all canine tumors;[1] the incidence is lower in cats.[2] A variety of neoplastic lesions occur, including both odontogenic and nonodontogenic tumor types. Non-neoplastic masses such as gingival hyperplasia and infectious conditions may be confused with oral tumors. Conversely, oral neoplasms may present as nonhealing, ulcerated lesions instead of 'typical' prominent masses.[3] Oral tumors frequently go unnoticed by the animal's owner until the tumor reaches an advanced stage of development; it is therefore important to make an accurate assessment of the extent and nature of the condition at the first time of presentation.[4]

If the patient allows, the tumor should be carefully inspected and palpated. The size and location of the tumor, the presence of any ulceration, necrosis, and any abnormal mobility of the teeth are important findings and should be recorded. Fixation of the tumor to underlying tissues suggests bone infiltration; this possibility should be further investigated radiographically. The regional lymph nodes are palpated to evaluate their size, shape, consistency and fixation to underlying tissues. Irregular enlargement, and especially lack of mobility, is highly suggestive of lymph node involvement. However, lymph node metastasis may be present without palpable enlargement. Finally, the patient is thoroughly examined by means of inspection, palpation, auscultation, thoracic radiographs and abdominal ultrasound to detect any signs of distant metastasis.

Neoplasms are diseases each with their own course, and each tumor in each patient has its own characteristics.[5] The development and course of a tumor are determined by many factors associated with the neoplasm and the host.[5] One of the purposes for the classification and staging of a tumor is planning and evaluation of treatment options. Neoplasms can be classified in several ways, including clinical investigation into the extent of the disease (clinical staging), classification of the host and illness, histologic diagnosis, histologic grading and prognostic significance. The expected biologic behavior of an oral tumor also depends on the species in which it occurs and the location in the oral cavity.[5] Understanding the biologic behavior enables the clinician to select the method of treatment indicated and to inform the client correctly.

CLINICAL STAGING

Due to a historical lack of agreement in categorizing malignancies and their therapeutic results in humans, a clinical staging system was adopted by the International Union Against Cancer.[5] The stage of disease at the time of diagnosis may be a reflection of not only the rate of growth and extension of the tumor, but also on the type and tumor–host relationship. The term 'stage' does not imply a regular progression from stage 1 to 4; rather, stages are arbitrary divisions often related to prognosis and treatment.[5]

The TNM-system was adopted by the World Health Organization–Collaborating Center for Comparative Oncology and is basically the same as the CTNM staging of human cancers.[5,6] These systems are based on the assessments of:

1. The extent of the primary tumor – T
2. The involvement of the regional lymph node – N
3. The absence or presence of distant metastases – M

The addition of numbers to these components (e.g., T_1, T_2, T_3) indicates the extent of the neoplasm or involvement. Site-specific clinical staging according to the TNM system is shown in Tables 38.1–38.3.[6]

Primary tumor

T_0 means that no primary tumor has been detected. T_1, T_2 and T_3 indicate an increasing degree of extent of the primary tumor. T_x means that it is impossible to fully determine the extent of the primary tumor. T_{is} is reserved for carcinoma in situ (early carcinoma with the absence of invasion of the surrounding tissue).[5] The tumor extent is commonly based on three features: the depth on invasion, surface spread and size. Tumor size is determined by the amounts of vital and necrotic tumor tissue, secretion product, cystic structures, stroma and inflammatory reaction. Inflammation can often be found around and in the tumor and may cause a false impression of the tumor size and invasion to adjacent tissues.[5]

Table 38.1 Clinical staging of tumor of the lips (TNM)[6]

T Primary Tumor
T_{is} Preinvasive carcinoma (carcinoma in situ)
T_0 No evidence of tumor
T_1 Tumor <20 mm maximum diameter, superficial or exophytic
T_2 Tumor <20 mm maximum diameter, with minimal invasion in depth
T_3 Tumor >20 mm diameter with deep invasion irrespective of size
T_4 Tumor invading bone

N Regional Lymph node (RLN): superficial cervical, mandibular and parotid
N_0 No evidence of RLN involvement
N_1 Movable ipsilateral nodes
    N_{1a} Nodes not considered to contain growth [histologically (–)]
    N_{1b} Nodes considered to contain growth [histologically (+)]
N_2 Movable contralateral or bilateral nodes
    N_{2a} Nodes not considered to contain growth [histologically (–)]
    N_{2b} Nodes considered to contain growth [histologically (+)]
N_3 Fixed node

M Distant metastasis
M_0 No evidence of distant metastasis
M_1 Distant metastasis (including distant nodes)

Table 38.2 Clinical staging of tumors of the oral cavity (TNM)[6]

T Primary Tumor
T_{is} Preinvasive carcinoma (carcinoma in situ)
T_0 No evidence of tumor
T_1 Tumor <20 mm maximum diameter
    T_{1a} Without bone invasion
    T_{1b} With bone invasion
T_2 Tumor 20–40 mm maximum diameter
    T_{2a} Without bone invasion
    T_{2b} With bone invasion
T_3 Tumor >40 mm diameter
    T_{3a} Without bone invasion
    T_{3b} With bone invasion

N Regional Lymph node (RLN): superficial cervical, mandibular and parotid
N_0 No evidence of RLN involvement
N_1 Movable ipsilateral nodes
    N_{1a} Nodes not considered to contain growth [histologically (–)]
    N_{1b} Nodes considered to contain growth [histologically (+)]
N_2 Movable contralateral or bilateral nodes
    N_{2a} Nodes not considered to contain growth [histologically (–)]
    N_{2b} Nodes considered to contain growth [histologically (+)]
N_3 Fixed node

M Distant metastasis
M_0 No evidence of distant metastasis
M_1 Distant metastasis (including distant nodes)

Table 38.3 Clinical staging of tumors of the oropharynx (TNM)[6]

T Primary Tumor
T_{is} Preinvasive carcinoma (carcinoma in situ)
T_0 No evidence of tumor
T_1 Tumor superficial or exophytic
    T_{1a} Without systemic signs
    T_{1b} With systemic signs
T_2 Tumor with invasion of tonsil only
    T_{2a} Without systemic signs
    T_{2b} With systemic signs
T_3 Tumor with invasion of surrounding tissue
    T_{3a} Without systemic signs
    T_{3b} With systemic signs

N Regional Lymph node (RLN): superficial cervical, mandibular and parotid
N_0 No evidence of RLN involvement
N_1 Movable ipsilateral nodes
    N_{1a} Nodes not considered to contain growth [histologically (–)]
    N_{1b} Nodes considered to contain growth [histologically (+)]
N_2 Movable contralateral or bilateral nodes
    N_{2a} Nodes not considered to contain growth [histologically (–)]
    N_{2b} Nodes considered to contain growth [histologically (+)]
N_3 Fixed node

M Distant metastasis
M_0 No evidence of distant metastasis
M_1 Distant metastasis (including distant nodes)

caudal mandibular lesions, to evaluate possible temporomandibular joint involvement. Magnetic resonance imaging and ultrasound can be useful for visualizing tumors with deep soft tissue infiltration and for lymph nodes.[3]

The radiologic findings associated with oral tumors are often subtle and non-specific. Careful and systematic evaluation of radiographs, using specific radiologic descriptors, may make it possible to associate different patterns with certain tumor types, and/or suggest a benign or malignant (aggressive) lesion.[8,9] However, with the exception of odontomas, the type of tumor cannot be determined based on radiographs, and biopsy is always required for definitive diagnosis. It is equally important to match the radiologic findings with the clinical features and location of the tumor, and, following biopsy, with the histopathological findings.[3]

Bone involvement may be evidenced by varying degrees of bone resorption and/or new bone formation. It is generally accepted that bone lysis only becomes evident radiographically when more than 40% of the cortical bone has been demineralized; radiographs therefore usually underestimate the extent of the tumor.[1] However, the presence of bone lysis is an indication of advanced bone infiltration, which influences the therapeutic plan. Good diagnostic imaging is especially important in correctly planning a surgical procedure.

Regional lymph nodes

The staging value of lymph nodes (N) may be assessed by palpation that consists of size, mobility versus fixation, firmness, single versus multiple nodes, ipsilateral–contralateral, and bilateral distribution. Size of the node is important; however, it is not a strong enough criterion to indicate ascending order of progression because an enlarged lymph node is not necessarily due to metastasis (e.g., reactive lymph node).[5,10] In one study, only 17% of palpably enlarged mandibular lymph nodes in dogs and cats with oral tumors were found to contain metastases.[11] Mobility versus fixation is a more important

Diagnostic imaging of oral tumors

Radiography forms an integral part of assessing the tumor characteristics, in particular the extent of the tumor and the presence of bone involvement.[3] Intraoral dental radiographs and extraoral skull radiographs are generally indicated in cases of suspected oral neoplasia. Other advanced diagnostic imaging techniques may be indicated in selected cases.[7] Tumors located in the maxilla often necessitate computed tomography (CT) to visualize the intranasal and/or periorbital extent of the tumor. Computed tomography is also indicated with consideration than size, because loss of mobility may be an indicator of invasion of the lymph node capsule by the neoplasm, which has been found to be associated with a poor prognosis.[10]

Regional lymph node filter function has traditionally been assumed to be crucial in the prevention of the systemic spread of malignant cells shed from the primary neoplasm.[12,13] However, in a multitude of clinical studies, prophylactic removal of such regional lymph nodes did not improve the cure rate compared with the observation of these nodes.[14,15] In addition, laboratory studies indicate that lymph node filter function may be neither complete nor effective, and that many lymphatic and lymphaticovenous shunts exist that bypass regional lymph nodes and allow both lymphatic and hematogenous dissemination of malignant cells.[12,13] Therefore, lymph node metastases should be regarded as indicators but not governors of survival in cancer. The timing of the clinical appearance of regional lymph node metastases and their number are, in most cases, excellent indicators of the biologic behavior of the primary cancer.[12,13]

Distant metastasis

The absence or presence of distant metastases is designated by the letter M, where M_0 indicates absence and M_1 indicates presence of distant metastasis. Metastatic involvement of the abdominal cavity is best assessed by abdominal ultrasound, which is currently considered the standard of care. Another diagnostic tool that may become available in the future is ultrasound with contrast media. Preliminary research suggests that this modality detects more lesions and may be better at differentiating benign and malignant lesions than ultrasound without contrast.[16-18] Computerized tomography (CT), with and without contrast, and magnetic resonance imaging (MRI) are excellent alternatives; however, they require general anesthesia, take more time, and are more expensive than ultrasound. CT has been found to be significantly more sensitive than thoracic radiographs for detecting soft tissue nodules.[19] Only 9% of CT-detected pulmonary nodules are identified on thoracic radiographs.[19] The lower size threshold is approximately 1 mm to detect pulmonary nodules on CT images and 7–9 mm to reliably detect nodules on radiographs. Therefore, thoracic CT should be considered in any patient with neoplasia that has potential for pulmonary metastasis, particularly when accurate characterization of the extent and distribution of pulmonary metastasis affects therapeutic planning.[19]

HISTOPATHOLOGIC STAGING

Principles of oral and maxillofacial biopsy

Proper management of a patient with an oral tumor starts with accurate diagnosis.[20] The current gold standard for definitive diagnosis is histopathologic assessment of a tissue biopsy from the lesion. Although biopsy frequently demands relatively few technical skills, the decisions related to the performance of the biopsy require considerable thought and experience.[21] Without appropriate planning and execution, biopsies may lead to adverse effects on patient prognosis and on treatment options. Poorly performed biopsies, poorly placed incisions, and biopsy complications can considerably compromise the local management of bone and soft tissue tumors.[21,22] In addition to accurate histopathologic diagnosis, which depends on the clinician performing an appropriate biopsy and providing adequate clinical information, the diagnosis depends on the pathologist correctly interpreting the biopsy results. In order to carry out the biopsy appropriately, the surgeon should ensure that adequate diagnostic and staging studies were performed. These studies include clinical, laboratory, and radiologic assessments to provide the surgeon with knowledge of the extent of the tumor as well as its systemic involvement.[21,23] Since biopsy has potential prognostic and therapeutic consequences, it is recommended that it should be undertaken by the surgeon who plans to carry out the definitive treatment.[21,23]

Developing the biopsy strategy

Ideally, the management of oral tumors involves a multidisciplinary approach.[21] In addition to the surgeon, radiologists and pathologists should play a role in the planning of the diagnostic and staging strategy prior to biopsy. Depending on the suspected differential diagnosis, pre-biopsy consultation may also include radiation oncologists, medical oncologists and field-specific surgical specialists.[21] For example, a patient with a clinically extensive maxillary tumor that is not amenable to surgical resection may be prepared for radiation treatment during the diagnostic stages (e.g., molding of a custom-fitted mask for radiotherapy during the same anesthetic episode as CT imaging).

The mainstay of planning the biopsy sites relies on diagnostic imaging. A conventional radiograph of a soft tissue mass does not usually provide any diagnostic information.[21,24] In addition, the maxillofacial region has complex structures and therefore is difficult to accurately evaluate, especially in the presence of oral or maxillofacial tumors. Therefore, the gold standard of biopsy planning should include advanced diagnostic imaging such as CT, with and without contrast (Fig. 38.1), and possibly MRI (Fig. 38.2). In the oral and maxillofacial region, CT is preferred due to its ability to demonstrate the extent of bone involvement in finer detail.[25] However, in selected cases with a soft tissue mass that may invade other structures (e.g., tongue base tumor), MRI may be beneficial.

When obtaining CT images, 0.5–1.0-mm CT sections provide more information than 3.0- or 5.0-mm sections. In addition, three-dimensional reconstruction images from 0.5- or 1.0-mm sections provide a better platform for biopsy and treatment planning. The diagnostic value of CT and MRI is especially beneficial for lesions involving the hard and soft palate. In these locations, incorrect selection of the biopsy site may lead to permanent oronasal communication and associated morbidity. Moreover, CT is also extremely useful in evaluating masses at the caudal mandible, in the area of the coronoid process and the temporomandibular joint (TMJ).[3]

In addition to CT and/or MRI, it is recommended to obtain dental radiographs of the area involved, as these will demonstrate the extent of involvement of adjacent teeth and alveolar bone associated with the mass.[3,26,27]

An appropriate biopsy contains tissue that is representative of the most severe or significant change in the lesion. Achieving this involves three key factors: selection of the biopsy site, the procedure used to collect the samples, and proper submission of the biopsy sample.[20] An oral tumor, especially a large mass, often varies in disease severity from one part of the lesion to another. For example, a lesion may have early invasive squamous cell carcinoma in one part and dysplasia in another.[20,28] As a rule, an appropriate biopsy should include tissue from the worst part of the lesion.[20] However, the worst part of a lesion may not be readily apparent from its clinical and radiographic appearance; therefore, the collection of multiple biopsies is recommended.[20] For example, for a 40-mm lesion, obtaining two biopsies from representative areas or those with different clinical appearance is justified. The biopsies should always remain within the lesion: obtaining adjacent normal-appearing tissue for comparison, as recommended for dermatologic lesions, is contraindicated.[29] The biopsy track also should not transect a normal anatomical musculoskeletal compartment in order to reach a compartment that is affected by neoplasia, so that it will not be necessary to remove both compartments at the

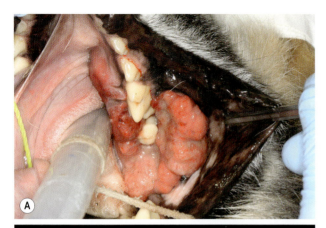

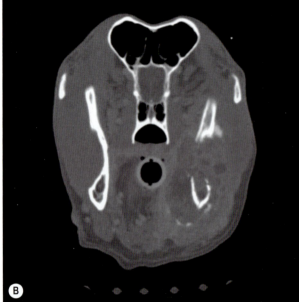

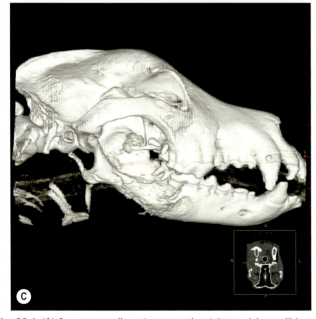

Fig. 38.1 (A) Squamous cell carcinoma at the right caudal mandible of a 12-year-old German shepherd dog (with the patient in dorsal recumbency). (B) Note the severe bony destruction demonstrated by CT and (C) the tridimensionally reconstructed image.

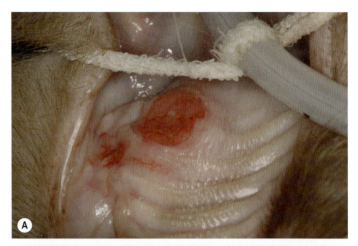

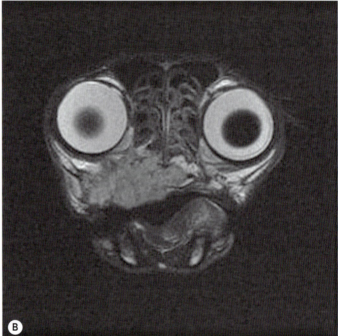

Fig. 38.2 (A) Squamous cell carcinoma at the hard palate of a 14-year-old cat (with the cat in dorsal recumbency). (B) Note the severe infiltration of the tumor into the nasal cavity and the ventral aspect of the left orbit as demonstrated by the MRI image.

time of the definitive procedure.[21] Also, because infection may be misinterpreted clinically as a tumor, or the reverse, it is often advisable to obtain additional specimens for aerobic, anaerobic, and fungal cultures and sensitivity.[30]

Open and closed biopsy

In a closed biopsy procedure, no incision is required and the tissue specimen is obtained by skin or mucosal puncture, most commonly with a needle.[21] An open biopsy, which requires incision, has been the most common and conventional method. In an open biopsy, the surgeon can obtain a relatively large amount of tissue for diagnosis.[21] The larger tissue specimen may help the pathologist to make a more accurate diagnosis. An open biopsy also decreases the likelihood that the surgeon will make a sampling error.[21,23] However, the risk, complications and consequences of poor biopsy placement increase with open biopsy compared to closed. In addition, open biopsy is more likely to result in hematoma, tumor cell spillage, operative infection, and, if bone is entered, iatrogenic fracture.[21] Nevertheless, open biopsy is the method of choice in oral and maxillofacial biopsies,[21] because aspiration of oral tumors, particularly those which derive from connective tissue, usually results in collection of too few cells to provide an accurate diagnosis.[31] Similarly, 'impression smears' and scraping the tumor tissue usually do not provide an adequate sample for interpretation.[31] In addition, basic histopathologic diagnostic methods may not be sufficient for determining the diagnosis, and immunohistochemical studies will be needed in many cases to differentiate among many types of malignancies. In these cases, procurement of a large biopsy specimen initially will avoid the need for rebiopsy.

For soft tissue lesions, closed biopsy may reduce the cost of biopsy and the time required for diagnosis.[32] Fine needle aspiration of soft tissue masses can be carried out with a relatively small needle (0.7 mm in diameter).[21,32,33] The reported diagnostic accuracy in nonoral masses for determining malignancy is 90%.[32,33] However, the accuracy rate is lower for determination of a specific tumor type, or histological grade, because of limited tissue volume obtained and the loss of tissue architecture. Fine needle aspiration may be useful in the determination of local recurrence of soft tissue tumors and spread to lymph nodes.[21] With the use of the Tru-cut needle biopsy system, it is possible to obtain a limited amount of tissue from the lesion with the original architecture preserved.[21] The reported accuracy in nonoral tumors is 96%.[34,35] However, because the amount of tissue retrieved is limited, the disposition of the material must be planned carefully before the tissue is processed, preferably by a pathologist experienced in oral pathology.[21] It should be emphasized that despite the high degrees of accuracy reported (in nonoral lesions), a nondiagnostic closed biopsy should not be interpreted as a reassurance that no tumor exists, as the sample may be from normal adjacent tissue, superficial inflammatory tissue, or from a pseudocapsule surrounding the tumor.[21]

Open biopsy procedures

An open biopsy may be incisional or excisional. Incisional biopsy is most common and is the procedure of choice for open biopsy of most tumors.[21] The decision to perform a primary excision of a mass is complex. As a general rule, if the mass is small, pedunculated and its complete removal will not affect the treatment options, excisional biopsy can be attempted. However, excisional biopsy of a large or deep mass may cause extensive tumor contamination at the time of biopsy and can subsequently limit treatment options.[21]

Soft tissue biopsy

A number of biopsy techniques are available for soft tissue biopsy, including scalpel, punch biopsy, laser and electrosurgery.[20] For biopsy of mucosal lesions, the use of laser or electrosurgery should be avoided, as these techniques produce a coagulation artifact that jeopardizes histologic interpretation of the specimen.[20] They are also more traumatic to the mucous membranes, and are associated with higher tissue morbidity and suture dehiscence.

Prior to biopsy, administration of local anesthesia is recommended, either as a regional block (such as infraorbital, inferior alveolar or mental blocks), or local infiltration administered to the area adjacent to the biopsy site (not directly into the biopsy site, to avoid distortion artifacts in the specimen).[20]

Punch biopsy (Fig. 38.3) has been shown to produce fewer artifacts then scalpel biopsy and is considered by the authors to be the method of choice to obtain biopsy specimens from oral soft tissue masses.[36] Ideally, biopsies of the mucosa should be at least 3 mm in diameter.[20] Since biopsies shrink after formalin fixation, punch biopsies 4–6 mm in diameter are recommended.[20] The depth should be at least 2 mm.

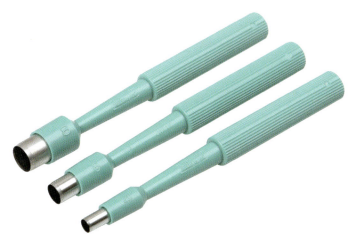

Fig. 38.3 Biopsy punch instruments used for biopsy of soft tissues in 4 mm, 6 mm, and 8 mm diameter (from bottom to top).

However, for some malignancies, deeper biopsies such as 4–5 mm are needed.[20] The bevel of the cutting edge can be measured and used as a depth guide. The punch should be gently inserted into the lesion with a rotating motion to facilitate cutting the tissue. Once an appropriate depth has been reached, the punch can be gently tilted to the sides to facilitate the removal of the sample ('scooping'). Alternatively, tissue forceps and a scalpel may be used to remove the biopsy sample. If possible, the biopsy site should be sutured with 5–0 or 4–0 poliglecaprone 25 (Monocryl™) in a simple interrupted pattern to achieve hemostasis. If suturing is not possible, the biopsy site should be left open, and hemostasis can be achieved by applying digital pressure with sterile wet gauze. In some cases that use of absorbable hemostatic agents may be used.

Hard tissue biopsy

When selecting the site for an incisional biopsy of a hard tissue mass, the clinician should assess the radiographs and CT images to locate the least differentiated or least mineralized portion of the mass, because this is usually the most representative portion.[21] The authors use two methods for biopsy of hard tissue mass: an appropriate size osteotome (e.g., 4 mm, 6 mm, or 8 mm) and mallet (Fig. 38.4), and Michele trephine (Fig. 38.5). Neither technique has been reported to be superior. However, Michele trephine is more prone to produce crushing artifacts of the specimens.

Osteotome technique

Once the tissue to be biopsied is identified, the osteotome should be placed at the desired biopsy site. Then, a 100-g mallet is used to drive in the osteotome in gentle, rapid strokes until the desired depth has been achieved. A second incision should be made 5 mm away, at an angle to the first incision in the same manner, creating a wedge-shaped biopsy specimen. Once the two incisions have been made, the surgeon should gently wiggle the osteotome until the sample detaches from the underlying tissue. A tissue forceps can then be used to remove the specimen, which should be in a wedge shape. The depth of the biopsy depends on the size of the mass. Care must be taken not to create an iatrogenic fracture, especially when wiggling the osteotome.

Michele trephine technique[37]

Once the mass is exposed, the trephine is placed at the desired location. It is held with one hand while the other hand helps secure it in place. The trephine is guided downward with slight pressure with a

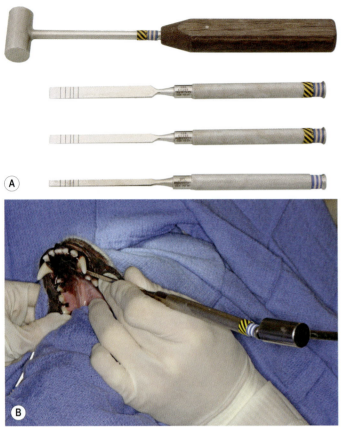

Fig. 38.4 (**A**) 100-g mallet and osteotomes (8 mm, 6 mm, and 4 mm, from top to bottom, respectively) used for biopsy of hard tissue masses. (**B**) Intraoral biopsy at the right mandible of a dog using 100-g mallet and 4-mm osteotome.

slight twisting action, which leads the trephine into the mass. Once the proper depth has been achieved, the trephine is rocked gently and then removed. The operator can then use the stylet, inserting it into the trephine with gentle pressure, to remove the specimen, which should be in a cylindrical shape.

Tissue handling and submission of the specimen

Hard tissue specimens should be placed immediately in a 10% neutral buffered formalin fixative. Soft tissue samples obtained with a punch biopsy should be placed on a piece of clear paper with the connective tissue surface facing down for 1 minute to ensure that the sample stays flat and to prevent it from curling during fixation, and to orient it properly for histologic examination.[20] The sample is then placed in a 10% neutral buffered formalin fixative. To avoid improper fixation or autolysis, the volume of fixative should be at least 20 times the volume of the sample.[20] No other fixative should replace the formalin. Alcohol, surface disinfectant, local anesthesia solution or mouth rinse cannot fix the tissue properly for adequate histologic analysis.[20] The biopsy specimen should always be accompanied by pertinent clinical information, including a detailed description of the mass and its radiographic appearance, preferably accompanied by a clinical color image to facilitate the clinical–pathologic correlation.[38] If other imaging was performed, details of those findings should also be included. If multiple lesions were biopsied, each sample should be submitted separately and labeled accordingly. A close rapport between the pathologist

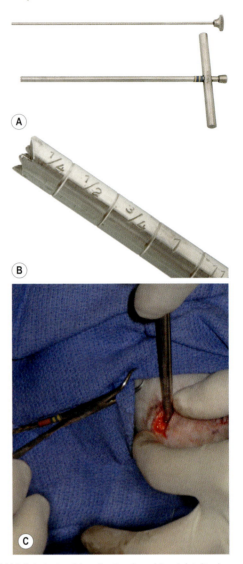

Fig. 38.5 (**A**) Michele trephine (*bottom*) and its stylet (*top*) used for biopsy of hard tissue masses. (**B**) The tip of the Michele trephine; note the serrated conformation of the tip and the $\frac{1}{4}$-inch increments marks. (**C**) Extraoral biopsy at the left mandible using Michele trephine.

and surgeon facilitates communication, streamlining the diagnosis and management of oral lesions.

Frozen sections

The development of the cryostat in the late 1950s led to the use of frozen section in most human hospitals[39] and some veterinary hospitals. The delay between procurement of a biopsy specimen and receipt of the results is difficult for both the client and the clinician. It is therefore desirable to make a definitive diagnosis from the initial biopsy as quickly as possible, and to avoid repeated anesthetic episodes for rebiopsy if the first sample is not diagnostic. Obtaining an intraoperative frozen section may ensure that diagnostic tissue has been obtained, thus avoiding repeat biopsy.[40] Analysis of a frozen section can be of great value to the surgeon, but both the surgeon and pathologist should agree that such a test only be used when interpretation can provide information of immediate or ultimate value in patient management.[39] In addition, the clinician should be aware that tissue examination using frozen samples is much more difficult than when using fixed tissue. Therefore, some of the tissue should be saved for permanent and definitive microscopic examination, and the final decision regarding definitive treatment should be made after an assessment of the fixed tissue.[39]

POSTOPERATIVE CONSIDERATIONS

The biopsy of an oral lesion is a relatively minor operation, performed under general anesthesia accompanied by local anesthesia. However, this procedure is associated with pain and swelling. The human literature describes maximum pain intensity 2 hours following a biopsy, and swelling that peaks between 6 and 48 hours after biopsy.[41] There is considerable reduction in pain after the third day post surgery, and from this point onward the pain decrease gradually during the course of the week.[41] Therefore, it is highly recommended to follow a biopsy procedure with appropriate analgesia for 3–7 days and to recommend a soft diet and avoidance of chew toys or treats for the same time period.

REFERENCES

1. Liptak JM, Withrow SJ. Oral tumors. In: Withrow SJ, Vail DM, editors. Withrow & MacEwen's small animal clinical oncology. 4th ed. Philadelphia, PA: Elsevier – Saunders; 2007. p. 455–75.

2. Stebbins KE, Morse CC, Goldschmidt MH. Feline oral neoplasia: a ten-year survey. Vet Pathol 1989;26:121–8.

3. Verstraete FJ. Mandibulectomy and maxillectomy. Vet Clin North Am Small Anim Pract 2005;35:1009–39.

4. Oakes MG, Lewis DD, Hedlund CS, et al. Canine oral neoplasia. Compend Cont Educ Pract Vet 1993;15:90–104.

5. Misdorp W. The impact of pathology on the study and treatment of cancer. In: Theilen GH, Madewell BR, editor. Veterinary cancer medicine. 2nd ed. Philadelphia, PA: Lea & Febiger; 1987. p. 53–70.

6. Owen LN. TNM classification of tumours in domestic animals. Geneva: World Health Organization; 1980.

7. Salisbury SK. Maxillectomy and mandibulectomy. In: Slatter DH, editor. Textbook of small animal surgery. 3rd ed. Philadelphia, PA: W.B. Saunders; 2003. p. 561–72.

8. Wood RE. Malignant diseases of the jaws. In: White SC, Pharoah MJ, editors. Oral radiology – principles and interpretation. 5th ed. St. Louis, MO: Mosby; 2004. p. 458–84.

9. Miles DA, Kaugars GE, Van Dis M, et al. Oral and maxillofacial radiology: radiologic pathologic correlations. 1st ed. Philadelphia, PA: WB Saunders; 1991.

10. Parodi AL, Misdorp W, Mialot JP, et al. Intratumoral BCG and Corynebacterium parvum therapy of canine mammary tumours before radical mastectomy. Cancer Immunol Immunother 1983; 15:172–7.

11. Herring ES, Smith MM, Robertson JL. Lymph node staging of oral and maxillofacial neoplasms in 31 dogs and cats. J Vet Dent 2002;19:122–6.

12. Cady B. Regional lymph node metastases, a singular manifestation of the process of clinical metastases in cancer: contemporary animal research and clinical reports suggest unifying concepts. Cancer Treat Res 2007;135:185–201.

13. Cady B. Lymph node metastases. Indicators, but not governors of survival. Arch Surg 1984;119:1067–72.

14. Gervasoni Jr JE, Taneja C, Chung MA, et al. Biologic and clinical significance of lymphadenectomy. Surg Clin North Am 2000;80:1631–73.

15. Taneja C, Cady B. Decreasing role of lymphatic system surgery in surgical oncology. J Surg Oncol 2005;89:61–6.

16. Volta A, Gnudi G, Manfredi S, et al. The use of contrast-enhanced ultrasound with a second generation contrast medium: preliminary report in the dog. Vet Res Commun 2009;33(Suppl 1):221–3.

17. Ivancic M, Long F, Seiler GS. Contrast harmonic ultrasonography of splenic masses and associated liver nodules in dogs. J Am Vet Med Assoc 2009;234:88–94.

18. O'Brien RT. Improved detection of metastatic hepatic hemangiosarcoma nodules with contrast ultrasound in three dogs. Vet Radiol Ultrasound 2007;48: 146–8.

19. Nemanic S, London CA, Wisner ER. Comparison of thoracic radiographs and single breath-hold helical CT for detection of pulmonary nodules in dogs with metastatic neoplasia. J Vet Intern Med 2006;20:508–15.

20. Poh CF, Ng S, Berean KW, et al. Biopsy and histopathologic diagnosis of oral premalignant and malignant lesions. J Can Dent Assoc 2008;74:283–8.

21. Simon MA, Biermann JS. Biopsy of bone and soft-tissue lesions. J Bone Joint Surg Am 1993;75:616–21.

22. Rougraff BT, Aboulafia A, Biermann JS, et al. Biopsy of soft tissue masses: evidence-based medicine for the musculoskeletal tumor society. Clin Orthop Relat Res 2009;467:2783–91.

23. Simon MA. Biopsy of musculoskeletal tumors. J Bone Joint Surg Am 1982; 64:1253–7.

24. Rydholm A, Berg NO. Size, site and clinical incidence of lipoma. Factors in the differential diagnosis of lipoma and sarcoma. Acta Orthop Scand 1983;54: 929–34.

25. Bar-Am Y, Pollard RE, Kass PH, et al. The diagnostic yield of conventional radiographs and computed tomography in dogs and cats with maxillofacial trauma. Vet Surg 2008;37:294–9.

26. Verstraete FJ, Kass PH, Terpak CH. Diagnostic value of full-mouth radiography in cats. Am J Vet Res 1998;59:692–5.

27. Verstraete FJ, Kass PH, Terpak CH. Diagnostic value of full-mouth radiography in dogs. Am J Vet Res 1998;59:686–91.

28. Lumerman H, Freedman P, Kerpel S. Oral epithelial dysplasia and the development of invasive squamous cell carcinoma. Oral Surg Oral Med Oral Pathol Oral Radiol Endod 1995;79:321–9.

29. Gilson SD, Stone EA. Principles of oncologic surgery. Compend Cont Educ Pract Vet 1990;12:827–38.

30. Kapatkin AS, Marretta SM, Patnaik AK, et al. Mandibular swellings in cats: prospective study of 24 cats. J Am Anim Hosp Assoc 1991;27:575–80.

31. Zinkl JG. Cytodiagnosis. In: Theilen GH, Madewell BR, editor. Veterinary cancer medicine. 2nd ed. Philadelphia, PA: Lea & Febiger; 1987. p. 71–84.

32. Wedin R, Bauer HC, Skoog L, et al. Cytological diagnosis of skeletal lesions. Fine-needle aspiration biopsy in 110 tumours. J Bone Joint Surg Br 2000; 82:673–8.

33. Kreicbergs A, Bauer HC, Brosjo O, et al. Cytological diagnosis of bone tumours. J Bone Joint Surg Br 1996;78:258–63.

34. Ball AB, Fisher C, Pittam M, et al. Diagnosis of soft tissue tumours by Tru-Cut biopsy. Br J Surg 1990;77: 756–8.

35. Kissin MW, Fisher C, Carter RL, et al. Value of Tru-cut biopsy in the diagnosis of soft tissue tumours. Br J Surg 1986;73: 742–4.

36. Moule I, Parsons PA, Irvine GH. Avoiding artefacts in oral biopsies: the punch biopsy versus the incisional biopsy. Br J Oral Maxillofac Surg 1995;33: 244–7.

37. Michele AA, Krueger FJ. Surgical approach to the vertebral body. J Bone Joint Surg Am 1949;31A:873–8.

38. Ethunandan M, Downie IP. Digital photographs of excised lesions: an aid to histopathology reports. Br J Oral Maxillofac Surg 2008;46: 251–2.

39. McCoy JM. Pathology of the oral and maxillofacial region: diagnostic and surgical considerations. In: Braun TW, Carlson ER, Marciani RD, editors. Oral and maxillofacial surgery. 2nd ed. St. Louis, MO: Elsevier; 2009. p. 413–7.

40. Ashford RU, McCarthy SW, Scolyer RA, et al. Surgical biopsy with intra-operative frozen section. An accurate and cost-effective method for diagnosis of musculoskeletal sarcomas. J Bone Joint Surg Br 2006;88:1207–11.

41. Camacho-Alonso F, Lopez-Jornet P. Study of pain and swelling after oral mucosal biopsy. Br J Oral Maxillofac Surg 2008; 46:301–3.

Chapter | 39 |

Clinical–pathologic correlations

Joseph A. Regezi & Frank J.M. Verstraete

CLINICAL–PATHOLOGIC CORRELATIONS

When historical data and physical signs associated with an oral condition are not clinically diagnostic, microscopic evaluation is generally required. Definitive diagnosis is usually apparent from histopathologic features, although results may occasionally be equivocal and subject to more than one interpretation. Additional special or immunohistochemical stains may help resolve these difficult cases. Importantly, correlation of clinical and pathologic features can be of considerable benefit. That is, the putative diagnosis should correlate or be consistent with the expected patient age, anatomic site, species and breed. For example, a diagnosis of canine acanthomatous ameloblastoma would be highly unlikely in a cat, and likewise, a diagnosis of feline inductive odontogenic tumor would be inappropriate for a dog. Among the limited number of oral diseases occurring in dogs and cats, some diseases seem to be relatively restricted to one species or the other (Table 39.1). Other situations in which clinical–pathologic correlations are important are when the pathologist overinterprets the histopathology (e.g., fibrosarcoma for a focal fibrous hyperplasia, or squamous cell carcinoma for acanthomatous ameloblastoma), or underinterprets the histopathology (e.g., peripheral ossifying fibroma for low-grade osteosarcoma). Accurate and complete historical and clinical data can be of immense help to the pathologist in biopsy interpretation. Clinical–pathologic correlation is essential for definitive diagnosis, particularly in difficult and equivocal cases.

The clinician who has a working knowledge of histopathology will be better able to correlate microscopy with clinical features, and to ultimately determine definitive diagnosis. This knowledge also gives the clinician an appreciation of underlying disease processes and an edge in clinical interpretation. Cellular and tissue changes are reflected in presenting appearances, giving the knowledgeable clinician, who is aware of these correlations, greater skill in developing a rational differential diagnosis and diagnostic plan. The cases discussed below serve to illustrate the importance of clinical correlation, differential diagnosis and appreciation of histopathology.

Case 1

A 5-year-old golden retriever was presented with a 40×50-mm swelling of the incisive part of the mandible (Fig. 39.1A). The lesion was the same color as the surrounding tissue and was covered by intact epithelium. A radiograph showed resorption of subjacent bone (Fig. 39.1B). The exact duration of the lesion was unknown, but it had recently been growing rapidly. Believed to represent a gingival soft tissue tumor, a clinical differential diagnosis was developed that included connective tissue neoplasm, acanthomatous ameloblastoma and squamous cell carcinoma. A connective tissue neoplasm was favored because the latter two lesions both characteristically exhibit irregular ulcerated surfaces even though they can present with similar architectural features in this site (Figs 39.2 and 39.3). Note that the example of squamous cell carcinoma in Figure 39.3 lies rostral to a lobulated focal fibrous hyperplasia lesion with intact epithelium.

A biopsy of the lesion showed a bland spindle cell proliferation with a modest collagenous background (Fig. 39.1C). The pattern was predominantly haphazard, although some fascicular areas were seen. Few inflammatory cells were present. Spindle cell nuclei were uniform and no mitotic figures were found. A microscopic diagnosis of spindle cell proliferation, consistent with either fibrous hyperplasia or low-grade fibrosarcoma was made. Clinical–pathologic correlation however favored low-grade fibrosarcoma.[1]

As a group, gingival fibrous connective lesions are the most common tumors in dogs (see Table 39.1).[2] The histopathology of well-differentiated spindle cell lesions can be particularly deceptive, a feature characteristic of both animal and human tumors. Their bland microscopy can often belie their clinical behavior. Clinically aggressive low-grade fibrosarcomas and fibromatoses can be difficult to separate from some cellular fibrous hyperplasias, making clinical correlation critical.[1] In this particular case, an important aspect of the clinical–pathologic correlation was the awareness that this variant of fibrosarcoma is known to occur in large-breed dogs (mostly golden retrievers).[1] Clinically, this tumor presents as a rapidly enlarging swelling of the jaw, covered by intact epithelium, contrary to the typical oral fibrosarcoma. The histopathological findings of well-differentiated spindle

© 2012 Elsevier Ltd
DOI: 10.1016/B978-0-7020-4618-6.00039-7

Table 39.1 Oral diseases in dogs and cats: summary of biopsy specimens from the University of California – Davis Dentistry & Oral Surgery Service (1995–2001)

	Dogs	Cats
Inflammatory/hyperimmune	**(25%)**	**(53%)**
Gingivitis/gingival hyperplasia	33	10
Ulcerative gingivitis/stomatitis	19	17
Periodontitis	3	2
Mucositis (stomatitis)	21	18
Eosinophilic granuloma	3	2
Osteomyelitis	7	8
Pulpitis	3	0
Hyperplasias	**(31%)**	**(9%)**
Pyogenic granuloma	2	2
Peripheral fibroma/fibrous hyperplasia	59	6
Peripheral ossifying fibroma	45	0
Peripheral giant cell granuloma	3	0
Papilloma	2	1
Lymphoid hyperplasia	3	1
Cysts	**(3%)**	**(2%)**
Periapical cyst/granuloma, abscess	6	1
Dentigerous cyst	2	0
Lymphoepithelial cyst	0	1
Gingival cyst	2	0
Benign neoplasms	**(4%)**	**(1%)**
Adenoma (salivary)	2	0
Granular cell tumor	3	0
Plasmacytoma	4	0
Lipoma	1	0
Fibromatosis	2	0
Osteoma/osteochondroma	1	1
Benign odontogenic tumors	**(13%)**	**(3%)**
Canine acanthomatous ameloblastoma	39	0
Central ameloblastoma	2	0
Amyloid producing odontogenic tumor	1	2
Myxoma	1	0
Odontoma	5	0
Feline inductive odontogenic tumor	0	1

Table 39.1 Oral diseases in dogs and cats: summary of biopsy specimens from the University of California – Davis Dentistry & Oral Surgery Service (1995–2001)—cont'd

	Dogs	Cats
Malignant neoplasms	**(25%)**	**(32%)**
Squamous cell carcinoma	21	20
Papillary squamous cell carcinoma	4	0
Verrucous carcinoma	1	1
Fibrosarcoma	16	1
Rhabdomyosarcoma	1	0
Osteosarcoma	8	2
Mast cell tumor	2	3
Giant cell tumor (central)	2	0
Melanoma	26	0
Lymphoma	2	3
Adenocarcinoma	1	1
Metastatic adenocarcinoma/carcinoma	0	2
Sarcoma NOS	5	1
	n=363	n=107

cells and rare or no mitotic figures suggest a fibroma or a well-differentiated fibrosarcoma, which is in contrast with the tumor's rapid growth, invasion and metastatic potential. Treatment should be dictated more by biologic behavior than microscopy in such cases.

Case 2

A 1-year-old cat was presented with a lobular submucosal swelling of the left rostral maxilla (Fig. 39.4A, B). The lesion involved the alveolar process and was covered by intact epithelium. Radiographically, a loculated maxillary lucency was evident. The cortex was expanded and discontinuous. The duration of the lesion was unknown. There were no other physical signs or systemic problems. Because of the destructive nature of the lesion, and probable intrabony origin, the differential diagnosis included odontogenic tumor, osteosarcoma and possibly squamous cell carcinoma. Although the surface of the lesion was intact, squamous cell carcinoma was included because of the destructive nature of the lesion. Typical for this species is that the extent of bone involvement is often much greater than is anticipated from the clinical appearance of the lesion.[3] Also, surface ulceration with squamous cell carcinoma in cats may be very discrete; however, a squamous cell carcinoma in a 1-year-old cat would be most unusual.[3,4]

On biopsy, a poorly circumscribed, predominantly epithelial odontogenic lesion was evident (Fig. 39.4C). Nests, strands and a reticulum of odontogenic epithelium with peripheral palisades surrounded focal areas of myxoid connective tissue. A diagnosis of feline inductive odontogenic tumor was made.[5] Ameloblastoma was ruled out because of the prominent myxoid component of the lesion.[6] This diagnosis correlated well with the reported age of the patient, location and clinical presentation.

The feline inductive odontogenic tumor is a relatively rare mixed epithelial/mesenchymal odontogenic tumor, which is unique to cats

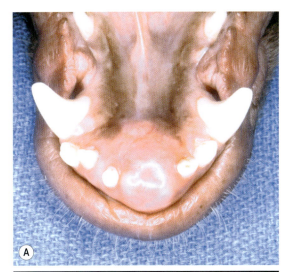

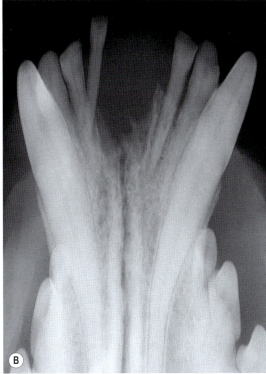

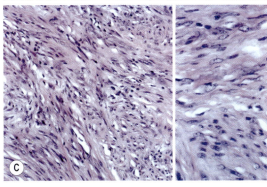

Fig. 39.1 (**A**) Histologically low-grade, biologically high-grade fibrosarcoma of the mandible in a 5-year-old golden retriever. (**B**) Corresponding radiograph shows geographic bone resorption. (**C**) Corresponding photomicrograph shows well-differentiated fibroblasts in a fascicular pattern (hematoxylin and eosin, ×100 and ×250).

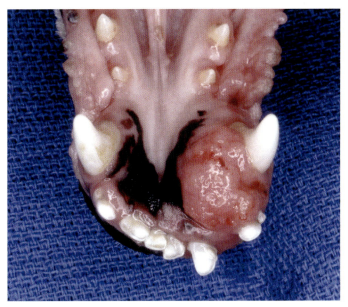

Fig. 39.2 Canine acanthomatous ameloblastoma of the mandible.

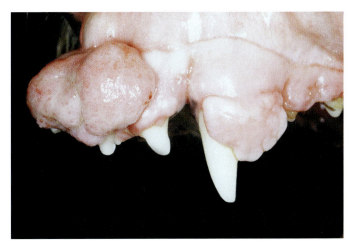

Fig. 39.3 Squamous cell carcinoma of the incisive bone and rostral maxilla, and focal fibrous hyperplasia on the buccal aspect of the canine tooth. *(From Verstraete FJM. Dental pathology and microbiology. In: Slatter DH, ed. Textbook of small animal surgery. 2nd ed. Philadelphia: W.B. Saunders, 1993;2316–2326.)*

under the age of 3 years, has some resemblance to ameloblastic fibroma in humans. However, the biologic behavior of feline inductive tumor, through its capacity for local infiltration, appears to be more aggressive than the ameloblastic fibroma.[5,7]

Case 3

A 12-year-old Lhasa apso was presented with a gingival mass associated with the right mandibular second and third premolar teeth (Fig. 39.5A). The lesion, which was the same color as surrounding tissue, bled upon physical examination. Only slight erosion of the subjacent alveolar bone was noted on radiographic examination. Based upon apparent origin from gingival soft tissues, clinical differential diagnosis included peripheral (ossifying) fibroma, canine acanthomatous ameloblastoma, squamous cell carcinoma and other nonodontogenic tumor types.

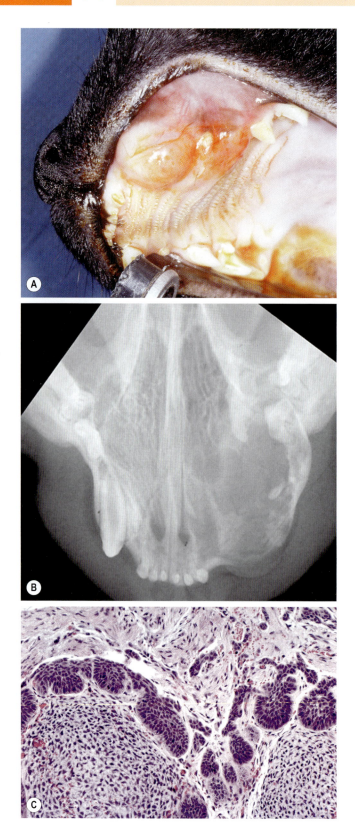

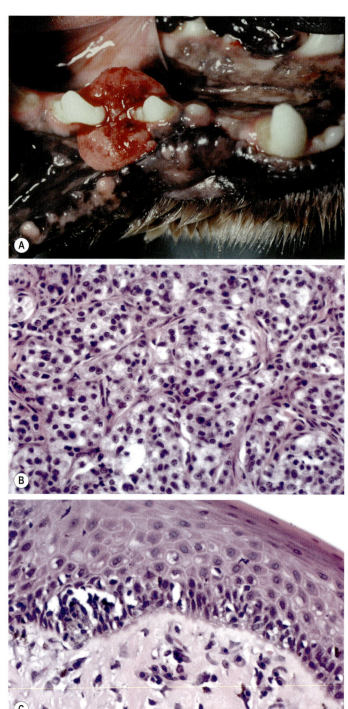

Fig. 39.5 (**A**) Melanoma of the body of the mandible in a 12-year-old dog. (**B**) Corresponding photomicrograph shows nested polygonal tumor cells in an area in which no melanin is apparent (hematoxylin and eosin, ×250) (**C**), High-magnification photomicrograph illustrates lateral tumor spread at the epithelium–connective tissue interface in both a nested and single-cell pattern (hematoxylin and eosin, ×250).

Fig. 39.4 (**A**) Feline inductive odontogenic tumor in a 1-year-old cat. (**B**) Corresponding radiograph (see text); (**C**) Surgical specimen shows 'budding' odontogenic epithelium surrounding primitive-appearing connective tissue. Note supporting connective tissue (no inductive change) above (hematoxylin and eosin, ×100). (**A** *and* **B** *from Self-Assessment Colour Review of Veterinary Dentistry, edited by Frank Verstraete. Manson Publishing Ltd, London, 1999.*)

Biopsy showed submucosa expanded by a dense cellular proliferation of polygonal cells (Fig. 39.5B). Most of the tumor cells had clear cytoplasm, and a few contained melanin. A diagnosis of melanoma was made. Immunohistochemistry using antibody Melan A could be used for histologic confirmation if necessary, although amelanotic lesions may be nonreactive. Alternatively, anti-S-100 protein could be used for confirmation, although it is less specific and less sensitive than Melan A.

This relatively common oral malignancy of dogs has a poor prognosis. It is seen in older animals, and the gingiva is the most common intraoral site.[8] Histologically, a number of different patterns can be seen (spindle, nested, clear cell, amelanotic). Of note is the occasional appearance of lateral tumor spread at the epithelial connective tissue interface (Fig. 39.5C). In these cases, wide excision is necessary to reduce the risk of recurrence. There are some interesting comparisons between animal and human oral melanomas. Human oral melanomas are typically adult lesions that have a strong predilection for the gingiva and palate. They also may exhibit a preinvasive lateral spread, and their prognosis is poor. Oral melanomas have a much poorer prognosis than cutaneous lesions in both dogs and humans.

REFERENCES

1. Ciekot PA, Powers BE, Withrow SJ, et al. Histologically low-grade, yet biologically high-grade, fibrosarcomas of the mandible and maxilla in dogs: 25 cases (1982–1991). J Am Vet Med Assoc 1994;204:610–15.

2. Oakes MG, Lewis DD, Hedlund CS, et al. Canine oral neoplasia. Compend Cont Educ Pract Vet 1993;15:90–104.

3. Postorino Reeves NC, Turrel JM, Withrow SJ. Oral squamous cell carcinoma in the cat. J Am Anim Hosp Assoc 1993;29:438–41.

4. Stebbins KE, Morse CC, Goldschmidt MH. Feline oral neoplasia: a ten-year survey. Vet Pathol 1989;26:121–8.

5. Gardner DG, Dubielzig RR. Feline inductive odontogenic tumor (inductive fibroameloblastoma)–a tumor unique to cats. J Oral Pathol Med 1995;24:185–90.

6. Gardner DG. Ameloblastomas in cats: a critical evaluation of the literature and the addition of one example. J Oral Pathol Med 1998;27:39–42.

7. Beatty JA, Charles JA, Malik R, et al. Feline inductive odontogenic tumour in a Burmese cat. Aust Vet J 2000;78:452–5.

8. Ramos-Vara JA, Beissenherz ME, Miller MA, et al. Retrospective study of 338 canine oral melanomas with clinical, histologic, and immunohistochemical review of 129 cases. Vet Pathol 2000;37:597–608.

Chapter 40

Clinical behavior of nonodontogenic tumors

Margaret C. McEntee

GENERAL CONSIDERATIONS

Incidence

Dogs

Many studies have been done to determine the incidence of oral tumors in dogs and cats, although few studies have been performed in recent years. In 1968, the incidence rate for oral and pharyngeal tumors reported to a central animal neoplasm registry was 20.4 per 100 000 dogs or 5.4% of all canine tumors.[1] The annual incidence rate of oropharyngeal tumors in dogs seen at 13 colleges of veterinary medicine in the United States and Canada from 1964 to 1974 was determined to be 129.8 per 100 000 dogs.[2] In a more recent study conducted on insured dogs in the United Kingdom (1997–1998) the annual incidence rate for oropharyngeal tumors was 112 per 100 000 dogs.[3] Specific tumor types (and annual incidence rates) included 'epulis' (47/100 000 dogs), malignant melanoma (MM) (13/100 000 dogs), and 'other' (52/100 000 dogs).[3] A compilation of information from 12 colleges of veterinary medicine analyzed the relative risk and frequency of tumors in dogs.[4] In dogs the oral cavity was the fifth most common site of tumor involvement after skin, mammary, digestive and hemolymphatic systems.[4] In a large case series of oropharyngeal cancer in dogs the most common tumor was oral melanoma followed by squamous cell carcinoma (SCC) and then fibrosarcoma (FS).[2]

Cats

The incidence rate for oral and pharyngeal tumors reported to a central animal neoplasm registry was 11.6 per 100 000 cats, or 7.4% of all feline tumors.[1] The annual incidence rate of oropharyngeal tumors in cats seen at 13 colleges of veterinary medicine in the United States and Canada from 1964 to 1974 was determined to be 45.4 cases per 100 000 cats.[2] In a 1952–1967 case series of tumors in cats, the third most common site of involvement was found to be the gingiva, with oropharyngeal tumors accounting for 10.6% of cases.[5] The most common tumor was SCC, which most commonly involved the gingiva or tongue.[5] In another feline study, tumors of the oral cavity also represented the third most common site of tumor involvement, after the hemolymphatic system and skin, and 68% of the oral tumors were malignant.[4] In a 10-year survey of tumors in cats, oral tumors represented 10.0% of all tumors; 89.0% of the oral tumors were malignant.[6]

Signalment

There is variation between studies as to the breeds reported to be at risk for the development of oral tumors, although cocker spaniels and German shepherd dogs have been cited in a number of studies. In a study of oral and pharyngeal tumors in dogs in 1951–1962, the only breed at risk was the cocker spaniel, with a significantly higher rate of oral melanomas (80.2 per 10 000).[7] In the same study there was also a predominance of males among the dogs with MM (79.7%) and tonsillar SCC (74.0%).[7] The specific rate for all types of oral cancer was 41.3 per 10 000 for males and 24.0 per 10 000 for females. The average age for all dogs with oropharyngeal tumors was 9.8 years, the oldest mean age was in dogs with melanoma (10.7 years) and the youngest mean age in dogs with FS (7.9 years).[7]

German shepherd dogs have a greater risk of developing oropharyngeal tumors.[1] Dogs and cats have a marked increase in tumor rates after 8–9 years of age.[1]

There are reports on the greater risk for the development of oral tumors in males versus females. In one study, male dogs had a significantly greater risk of developing FS and MM than female dogs.[2] In another survey, male dogs had a 2.4 times greater risk of developing oropharyngeal malignant neoplasia than females, whereas tumor rates were similar in male and female cats.[1]

In a large series of dogs with oropharyngeal cancer, it was determined that the German shorthaired pointer, Weimaraner, golden retriever, boxer and cocker spaniel had a significantly higher risk of developing oral tumors, and dachshunds and beagles had a significantly lower risk.[2] In another major study of dogs with malignant oral and pharyngeal tumors, there were 41 different breeds represented but mixed-breed dogs, cocker spaniels, poodles and German shepherd dogs accounted for 60.0% of the cases but only 44.0% of the hospital population.[8] Smaller breeds tended to develop MM and tonsillar SCC, while the larger breed dogs had more FS and nontonsillar SCC.[8]

In a study of 338 oral MM cases, Anatolian sheepdog, cocker spaniel, Gordon setter, mixed breed dogs, chow chow, golden retriever,

© 2012 Elsevier Ltd
DOI: 10.1016/B978-0-7020-4618-6.00040-3

Pekingese/poodle cross and miniature poodle breeds were significantly overrepresented, whereas boxer and German shepherd dogs were underrepresented.[9] Ages ranged from 1 to 19 years (mean 11.4 years) and there was no apparent sex predilection.[9]

Etiology and risk factors

There have been reports on the increased relative risk for the development of oral tumors in males versus females. In one survey of oropharyngeal tumors, male dogs had a significantly greater risk of developing FS and MM than female dogs,[2] confirming the results of a previous study by the same author that male dogs had a 2.4 times greater relative risk of developing oral and pharyngeal cancer than females.[1]

The apparent prevalence of tonsillar SCC in dogs that live in urban industrialized regions as opposed to rural environments may be due to increased exposure to environmental carcinogens. In a study of dogs that were presented to a veterinary hospital in a rural area, there were significantly fewer tonsillar SCC diagnosed than expected.[10]

A survey and comparison to previous reports assessed the variation in prevalence of oropharyngeal tumors in dogs over time and by location.[11] The authors determined that the differences in tumor prevalence between locations (USA, England and Australia) were entirely due to the proportion of tonsillar SCC.[11] There was not a significant difference in overall percentages for MM, nontonsillar SCC and FS. The difference in prevalence of canine tonsillar carcinoma suggests that atmospheric carcinogens play a role in carcinogenesis.

A study in cats with oral SCC identified some environmental and lifestyle risk factors.[12] Cats that wear flea collars had five times increased risk of developing oral SCC. Other significant associations included canned food diet (3.6 times increased risk), canned tuna fish diet (>4-fold increase), and exposure to household environmental tobacco smoke (twofold increase, not significant).[12] Another study further supported the relationship between oral SCC and exposure to household environmental tobacco smoke, and furthermore implicated p53 as a potential site for carcinogen-related mutation, with cats exposed to smoke 4.5 times more likely to overexpress p53 based on evaluation of tumor biopsy samples.[13]

Canine oral papillomavirus is known to be involved in the development of oral papillomas in dogs. Furthermore, it is thought that there can be progression of viral papillomas to carcinomas in dogs.[14] Papillomavirus has been identified in biopsy samples from dogs with oral SCC.[15] In an investigation of 20 oral SCC in cats, a papillomavirus was detected in one cat, which does not support a causal association between viral infection and development of feline oral SCC.[16]

COX-1 and COX-2 overexpression has been demonstrated in both feline[17] and canine[18] oral SCC, suggesting that it may have a role in the pathogenesis of this disease.

There is a higher prevalence of MM in certain purebred dogs, which supports the supposition that there is a genetic basis for the development of this tumor. It appears that alterations of tumor suppressor genes and protooncogenes, with resultant disruption of cell cycle control, contributes to both the development and progression of MM in dogs.[19]

Oral osteosarcomas (OS) have been reported to develop secondary to exposure to ionizing radiation, a known carcinogen.[20,21]

SQUAMOUS CELL CARCINOMA

In a survey of dogs with oropharyngeal tumors, SCC was the second most frequently diagnosed oral tumor (24.5 %), and sites of involvement included gingiva, tonsil, oral mucosa, lip and palate (Fig. 40.1).[2]

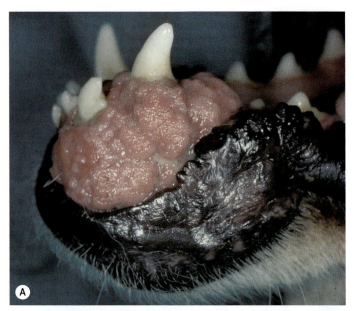

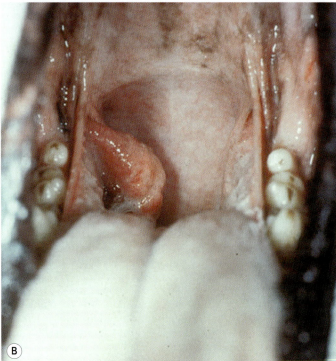

Fig. 40.1 (**A**) Gingival squamous cell carcinoma affecting the rostral mandible in a dog, which was treated by bilateral rostral mandibulectomy. (**B**) Tonsillar squamous cell carcinoma in a dog.

In another study of dogs with oropharyngeal tumors, 41.5 % were SCC, with the two most common sites of involvement being the tonsils or gingiva.[22] Other sites of involvement included the palate, pharynx and tongue.[22] The mean age of dogs with gingival SCC was 8.4 years; no sex or breed predilection was noted.[22] The tumors were described as typically reddened, friable and vascular.[22] The clinical history frequently included tooth extraction with subsequent tumor growth at the extraction site.[22] Of the 22 dogs with gingival SCC, three had ipsilateral mandibular lymphadenopathy suggestive of metastasis, and one had pulmonary metastasis.[22]

In a survey of malignant oral and pharyngeal tumors in dogs, the most common tumor was SCC (39.9 %); approximately half were nontonsillar in origin.[8] The median age for dogs with nontonsillar SCC was 9 years (range 1.2–14 years).[8] Of the total 164 dogs with oral SCC, the sites of involvement included tonsil (80), gingiva (68), labial mucosa (7), tongue (7), and 1 each for buccal mucosa and hard palate.[8] One of the 35 dogs that had thoracic radiographs had evidence of pulmonary metastasis.[8] Skull radiographs made in 27 dogs showed evidence of bone invasion in 21 dogs, primarily osteolysis.[8] Of 11 necropsied dogs with nontonsillar SCC, five had regional lymph node metastasis and four had distant metastasis.[8] The metastatic rate for rostral oral SCC is low and occurs late in the disease course, whereas a high metastatic rate is encountered for tumors in the caudal oral cavity, most notably tonsillar SCC.

Mandibular/maxillary squamous cell carcinoma in dogs

Surgical resection typically requires a partial mandibulectomy or maxillectomy. Determination of the extent of the disease radiographically or based on computed tomography imaging aids in surgical planning. Long-term control is possible with aggressive local resection of oral SCC. In a report of 24 dogs that underwent partial mandibulectomy for SCC, the median disease-free interval was 26 months with a 91% 1-year survival.[23] Two of the 24 dogs (8.3%) had local recurrence and metastasis with a survival time of 6 and 18 months. One dog developed only metastasis and had a 33-month survival, for an overall metastatic rate of 12.5%.[23] Nineteen dogs underwent either maxillectomy or mandibulectomy for oral SCC. The local recurrence rate was 5.0%; metastatic rate was 11.0% and the 1-year survival was 84.0%.[24]

There have been a number of reports that document the efficacy of radiation therapy in the treatment of canine oral SCC. A retrospective study of dogs with nontonsillar SCC evaluated prognostic factors for survival following orthovoltage radiation therapy.[25] Dogs with rostral tumors had significantly longer mean survival (28.1 months) than dogs with caudal tumors (10 months), or dogs with tumors that extended from rostral to caudal (1.7 months).[25] The mean survival for dogs ≤6 years old was 39 months versus 9.8 months for dogs older than 6 years.[25] Local tumor recurrence had a negative effect on mean survival, with a survival of 7.1 months in dogs with recurrence versus 28.8 months in dogs without recurrence.[25] In another study, dogs that received radiation treatment for oral SCC had a median disease-free interval (DFI) of 365 days and a median disease-free survival (DFS) of 450 days.[26] The median DFI and DFS were significantly shorter in dogs older than 9 years (210 days and 315 days, respectively) compared to dogs <9 years (470 days and 1080 days, respectively).[26] Age as a prognostic variable is likely a reflection of the longer life expectancy in younger dogs when dealing with a radioresponsive tumor.[26]

Progression-free survival (PFS) time and rate were reported for dogs with oral SCC treated with [60]Cobalt photons.[27] Mean PFS time by stage was 68 months for T1 (<20 mm maximum diameter), 47.7 months for T2 (20–40 mm diameter), and 25.4 months for T3 (>40 mm diameter).[27] Overall the mean and median PFS times were 51.3 and 36 months, respectively.[27]

Piroxicam has been used in dogs with oral SCC.[28] There has been documented expression of cyclooxygenase-2 (Cox-2) in oral (gingival, tonsillar) SCC in dogs supporting the use of a Cox-2 inhibitor.[29] The overall response rate was 17.6% in a group of 17 dogs with measurable disease treated with piroxicam at a dose of 0.3 mg/kg orally once daily.[28] Five dogs (29.4%) had stable disease with a median time to failure of 102 days (range 59–858 days).[28]

Cisplatin in combination with piroxicam has been used in a phase I/II trial with 5 of 9 dogs with oral SCC having a response to therapy (complete response in 2 dogs, partial response in 3 dogs).[30] Renal toxicity was encountered and careful monitoring is recommended with this drug combination.

Lingual/sublingual squamous cell carcinoma in dogs

The most common tumor identified in a retrospective study of 57 dogs with tongue tumors was SCC (21; 36.8%).[31] In a study of 1196 dogs with lingual lesions, 54% had neoplasia with SCC (113 dogs) the second most common tumor (18% of tumors) after MM.[32] The median age of dogs with lingual SCC was 9 years (range 4–12 years).[32] White dogs represented 43.0%, and poodles comprised 28.6% of the cases.[31] Females of all breeds and poodles, Labrador retrievers and samoyeds were more likely to have SCC, based on one large retrospective study.[32] The tumors typically exhibited bilaterally symmetrical involvement (61.9%), diffusely infiltrated the thickness of the tongue (52.4%), and involved the rostral two-thirds of the tongue (85.7%). Three of the 21 dogs had regional lymph node metastasis. Five of the 21 dogs did not receive any treatment and were euthanized within 1 month.[31] Five dogs were treated with surgery alone with survival times of 0.5, 2, 8, 36 and 39 months. Eleven dogs were treated with radiation therapy alone (6), radiation plus hyperthermia (3), surgery, radiation and hyperthermia (1), or radiation therapy and cisplatin (1). Survival times in dogs treated with radiation alone or combination therapy ranged from 0.5 to 26 months (median 4 months).[31] Of the 16 dogs that received some form of treatment for the lingual SCC only 4 (25.0%) had local tumor control; 6 dogs developed regional and/or distant metastasis.[31]

In a review of 10 dogs with lingual SCC, 3 had a white coat color.[33] The most common presenting signs were excessive drooling and oral bleeding. Eight of the 10 dogs received treatment. All 8 dogs had surgery with removal of 40–60% of the tongue, mitoxantrone in 3 dogs, and radiation therapy in 2 dogs.[33] The metastatic rate was 37.5%. The prognosis for survival was poor in dogs with high-grade tumors (characterized by lack of keratinization, poor differentiation, high mitotic rate and local invasion); only 1 of 4 dogs lived longer than 6 months.[33] A good functional outcome has been associated with major glossectomy in dogs.[34]

Tonsillar squamous cell carcinoma in dogs

A 15-year retrospective survey of 364 oropharyngeal tumors in dogs in London included 117 tonsillar SCC (32.1%).[35] The ages of dogs with tonsillar SCC ranged from 2 to 14.5 years (tended to occur in dogs 8 or 9 years of age). Regional and/or distant metastasis was identified in 61.1% of dogs with lymph node metastasis to both ipsilateral and contralateral lymph nodes.[35] Clinical signs include dysphagia, cervical mass, dyspnea, anorexia, coughing, drooling, cervical pain, change in voice and bleeding from the mouth.[22] Dogs with tonsillar SCC can be presented with enlarged metastatic regional lymph nodes and silent primary tumors.[22] In one study, 28 of 29 dogs (96.6%) had lymph node metastasis to the mandibular lymph nodes (24; ipsilateral in 23 as well as contralateral in 8; and only contralateral in 1), and retropharyngeal lymph nodes (8).[22] Metastasis to the thyroid gland was detected in 8 dogs.[22] Seventeen of 29 dogs were necropsied and other sites of metastasis included lung, liver, spleen, pericardium and heart, ribs, kidney, cranial mediastinal and pancreatic lymph node.[22]

Tonsillar SCC has a higher rate of metastasis than gingival tumors, presumably due to the fact that tonsils are richly supplied with efferent lymphatics that drain to the ipsilateral as well as contralateral mandibular and retropharyngeal lymph nodes.[22]

In a study of 80 dogs with tonsillar SCC, the median age was 10 years (range 2.5–17 years).[8] The male to female ratio was 1.5 : 1.[8] The tumors ranged in size from nearly microscopic to bulky exophytic tumors.[8] Of the 24 dogs that had thoracic radiographs, 2 (8.3%) had pulmonary metastasis.[8] Of 48 dogs necropsied 11 had local disease (5 had bilateral tonsillar tumors), 17 had regional lymph node metastasis, and 20 had distant metastasis.[8]

A retrospective study of canine tonsillar SCC documented the response to surgery and irradiation.[36] Eight dogs were irradiated with [60]Cobalt photons.[36] Survival time ranged from 44 to 631 days (median 110 days).[36] None of the 8 dogs had metastasis past the regional lymph nodes at initial presentation, but 6 of 7 dogs evaluated ultimately developed distant metastasis.

A study evaluated the effect of adjuvant chemotherapy versus combined chemotherapy (doxorubicin and cisplatin) and radiation therapy in 22 dogs with advanced-stage tonsillar carcinoma.[37] The overall response in 16 dogs treated with adjuvant chemotherapy was poor, with survival times ranging from 30 to 180 days (median 105 days). The range in survival time for 6 dogs treated with combination chemotherapy and radiation was 90 to 665 days (median 270 days), and 5 had a complete response.[37]

Surgical resection followed by coarse fractionated radiotherapy (9 Gy once a week for 4 weeks) and carboplatin (300 mg/m^2) in 4 dogs or carboplatin alone in 1 dog with tonsillar SCC resulted in a median survival of 211 days with two dogs alive at 826 and 1628 days.[38]

Papillary squamous cell carcinoma of young dogs

There is a distinct entity of papillary SCC that occurs in young dogs that may be associated with papillomavirus.[39–41] In a report of 3 dogs that presented for papillary SCC the ages were 2, 2 and 5 months. The tumors appear locally aggressive with underlying bone lysis (Fig. 40.2). The dogs responded well to a combination of surgery and orthovoltage radiotherapy, with no evidence of disease at 10, 32 and 39 months.[39] There have been no reports of metastasis in dogs with papillary SCC.

Mandibular/maxillary squamous cell carcinoma in cats

In two surveys of oropharyngeal tumors in cats the most frequently diagnosed tumor was SCC, representing 61–64% of the oral tumors.[2] In a review of 58 cats with tumors involving bone, the most common diagnosis was SCC, including 12 mandibular and 12 maxillary SCC, and regional lymph node metastasis was detected in 2 cats.[42] In one study, age ranged from 3 to 21 years (mean 12.5 years).[6] On presentation most cats have enlargement of the affected bone or facial asymmetry, gingival ulceration and difficulty eating (Fig. 40.3A). Other clinical signs include halitosis, loose teeth, excessive salivation, oral bleeding, and exophthalmos in cats with maxillary tumors.[43] In one report, all cats had bone lysis radiographically, and most had new bone formation (Fig. 40.3B).[42] In another report of 52 cats with oral SCC, 73.1% had marked osteolysis on radiographs with minimal new bone formation; and 46.2% had more extensive disease based on radiographs than physical examination.[44]

Cats with oral SCC are typically diagnosed late and the response to therapy is poor. It is not uncommon for cats to present with a palpable or visible enlargement of the mandible or maxilla and a history of recent dental treatment. There is no appreciable difference in clinical signs at presentation in cats with malignant mandibular tumors as opposed to cats with benign lesions including dental disease and

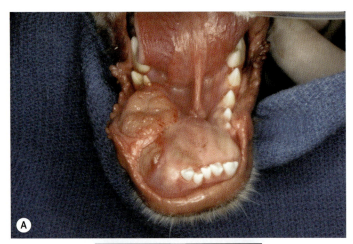

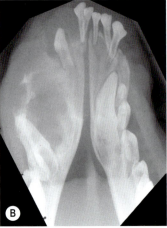

Fig. 40.2 Papillary squamous cell carcinoma in a 5-month-old dog: (**A**) Clinical appearance. (**B**) Radiograph illustrating extensive bony involvement.

osteomyelitis.[43] In a study of cats with mandibular swellings only 50.0% had a tumor, and osteomyelitis could not be differentiated from cancer, based on radiographic appearance.[43] In a study of 18 cats with oral SCC (sublingual/lingual 7, maxilla 5, buccal mucosa 4, mandible 4, pharyngeal 2, soft palate mucosa 1, and lip 1) common CT imaging features included marked heterogeneous contrast enhancement, osteolysis and extension of maxillary masses most often affected the orbit (5).[45] Although CT imaging assisted in identification of extent of disease and regional lymph node enlargement, the results did not correlate with survival time; treatment varied but the overall median survival time was 60 days.[45]

Five cats with mandibular SCC that underwent mandibulectomy had a median survival of 6 months (range 4–12 months).[46] One cat developed local recurrence and 1 cat had documented lymph node metastasis.[46] The mean and median survival time for 7 cats that underwent surgical resection of oral SCC was 2.1 and 1.5 months, respectively.[44] In a study of 42 cats with oral tumors treated with mandibulectomy with a subset also receiving radiation therapy and/or chemotherapy, cats with SCC (21) had a significantly shorter survival time than cats with FS or OS.[47] However, cats with mandibular SCC had relatively long-term control and survival with a progression-free and survival rate at 1 year of 51% and 43%, and at 2 years of 34% and 43%, respectively.[47]

Oral SCC in cats is often advanced at presentation, and therapy is palliative in intent. In a series of 54 cats with oral SCC that received only nonsteroidal antiinflammatory drugs, antibiotics, steroids or no

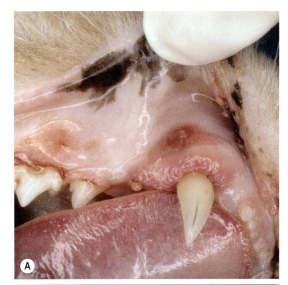

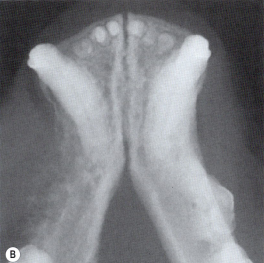

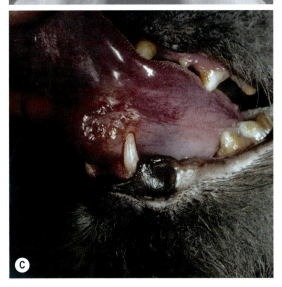

Fig. 40.3 (**A**) Squamous cell carcinoma of the maxilla in a cat, clinically presenting as a discrete swelling of the maxilla and superficial ulceration overlying the canine tooth. (**B**) Radiograph of a squamous cell carcinoma of the mandible in a cat illustrating the extensive bony involvement. (**C**) Sublingual squamous cell carcinoma in a cat.

treatment, the median survival time was 44 days, with a 1-year survival of 9.5% with an apparent longer survival in those cats that received nonsteroidal antiinflammatory drugs.[48] A phase I clinical trial of intravenous carboplatin in 59 cats included 16 cats with oral SCC of which there were no complete responses and one partial response.[49] Seven cats with advanced oral SCC were irradiated with a linear accelerator; only 4 of the 7 cats completed treatment.[50] Survival ranged from 36 to 97 days and the authors concluded that, due to the relative lack of palliation of clinical signs, radiation in this setting is not efficacious.[50]

Eleven cats with oral SCC (4 lingual, 7 mandible or maxilla) were treated with a combination of radiation therapy and intravenous mitoxantrone.[51] Of the 11 cats there were 8 complete responses and 1 partial response. The remission time for the cats with a complete response ranged 28–485 days with a median of 170 days. The partial response duration was 60 days.[51] Eight cats with advanced nonresectable oral SCC (sublingual in 4, mandibular in 2, maxillary in 2) were treated with a combination of low-dose gemcitabine and palliative radiation therapy with 2 complete and 4 partial responses, a median duration of remission of 42.5 days, and an overall median survival time of 111.5 days.[52]

Improved responses can be seen with combination therapy including aggressive local resection and radiation therapy. In a report of 7 cats treated with mandibulectomy and postoperative radiation therapy, the median survival time was 14 months.[53] Six of the 7 cats were euthanized due to recurrence, with a median disease-free interval of 11 months.[53]

In a retrospective study of 52 cats with oral SCC the cats ranged in age from 2.5 to 18 years (median 12 years).[44] Radiographic examination of the primary tumor revealed marked osteolysis with minimal new bone formation in 73.1%. Tumor location included the tonsil, tongue or pharynx (22), the mandible or maxilla (28) and the palate (2). Treatment entailed a number of different modalities including surgery alone (7), radiation therapy (24), radiation plus chemotherapy (11) or radiation combined with local hyperthermia (10).[44] Survival time ranged from 1 to 15 months with an overall median survival of 2 months, with no significant difference in survival based on treatment modality.[44]

Cyclooxygenase inhibitors may represent another option for the management of feline oral SCC.[54]

Lingual/sublingual squamous cell carcinoma in cats

In one report, 61.2% of cats with oral tumors had SCC and most occurred sublingually although a specific percentage was not given.[6] Careful evaluation of the oral cavity with examination under the tongue as well as palpation of the tongue will provide information on location and extent of disease (Fig. 40.3C). Tumor extension into the musculature of the tongue is firm on palpation and will cause rigidity and decreased mobility of the tongue. Imaging modalities that clearly show soft tissue changes are indicated in these cases (see Ch. 38).

Eighteen cats with nonresectable oral SCC including 8 cats with lingual tumors were treated with a lipophilic cisplatin analog, which was shown to be ineffective, with a median survival of 59.8 days and acute toxicity that would limit clinical utility.[55]

Five cats with nonresectable oral SCC were treated every 3 weeks with a combination of doxorubicin and cyclophosphamide.[56] There was only 1 partial response. Survival time in the cat with a partial response was 90 days, and ranged from 15 to 60 days in the other 4 cats.[56]

Nine cats (4 lingual, 3 mandibular, 1 tonsillar and 1 buccal) treated with an accelerated radiation protocol had a median overall survival of 86 days.[57] Notably, the median survival of 6 cats that had a partial response was 60 days, and for 3 cats that had a complete response was 298 days.[57]

Overall feline oral SCC, but most notably lingual and sublingual SCC, represents a locally aggressive tumor that is difficult to treat. Death is usually due to local disease progression and euthanasia. Palliative measures including nonsteroidal antiinflammatory drugs and feeding tubes can provide short-term supportive care but definitive therapy is typically unsuccessful in effecting a durable response.

Tonsillar squamous cell carcinoma in cats

Tonsillar SCC is very uncommon in cats.[5] Of four cats with tonsillar SCC that underwent partial or complete tumor removal, the survival times were 2–14 weeks and all were euthanized due to local recurrence and metastasis.[58]

MALIGNANT MELANOMA

Malignant melanoma in dogs

Malignant melanoma is the most common[59] or second most common malignant oral tumor in dogs.[8,22] Males are predisposed, with a male to female ratio of 3 : 1 to 6 : 1, and mean age of 10.5–12 years.[8,22,59] In one report one-third of the tumors occurred in cocker spaniels and otherwise tended to occur in dogs with heavily pigmented oral mucosa.[22] The majority of MM involve the gingiva. In one report two dogs had tumor involving both the upper and lower surfaces of the opposing gingivae, which signifies either tumor spread or multicentric disease.[22] Other sites of involvement include the labial mucosa, palate, buccal mucosa and tongue (see Fig. 39.5). Melanomas of the lip that arise from mucous membranes typically have a better prognosis than gingival tumors but are more aggressive than tumors arising from haired skin. Of 32 dogs with lip MM with histologic features of malignancy, 22 were dead due to tumor within a year, and 10 were tumor-free for at least 1 year.[60] Melanomas are firm, grayish or brownish black, rapidly enlarge, develop ulceration, hemorrhage and metastasis within weeks or months.[59]

A report of 64 dogs with 69 histologically well-differentiated melanocytic neoplasms involving the mucous membranes of the lips and oral cavity underwent surgery alone.[61] Sixty-one of 64 (95%) were alive at the end of the study or died of other causes, with a mean survival of 23.4 months, and a median survival of 34 months after surgery.[61] There were five dogs in total that either died of tumor-related causes or had recurrent tumors, and all had tumors in the oral cavity.

Twenty-three of 43 dogs with oral MM in one report were necropsied and 74.0% had regional lymph node metastasis and 65.0% had pulmonary metastasis.[22] Other sites of metastasis reported include brain, meninges, pituitary gland, striated muscle, pleura, pericardium, heart, prostate, pancreas, adrenal glands, liver, kidney, spleen, ileum, omentum, mediastinal lymph nodes, thyroid, prostate, salivary gland, stomach, testis and eyes.[8,22] Six of eight dogs with buccal or labial MM had metastasis to the tonsils.[22] There can be variable pigmentation of the primary and metastatic lesions, although the majority of dogs have pigmented primary and metastatic lesions.[22] It should be noted that there is not necessarily a relationship between regional lymph node size and presence of metastasis. In a study of 100 dogs with oral MM, 53% had evidence of regional lymph node metastasis, with 70% having enlarged mandibular lymph nodes and 30% had normal-sized lymph nodes.[62] The miliary pattern of metastasis sometimes seen with oral MM may impede radiographic detection of pulmonary metastasis.

A recent study of 338 canine oral MM with clinical, histologic and immunohistochemical review of 129 cases provided some insights.[9] Diagnosis can be impeded by the variable pigmentation, tumors ranging from highly pigmented to nonpigmented. Additionally there is variable microscopic appearance of cells. There are three main categories based on microscopic features of the predominant cell type including polygonal (epithelioid), spindle and mixed (epithelioid and spindle) cells. The distribution by cell type in 129 oral MM was 20.9% epithelioid, 34.1% spindle, and 41.9% mixed.[9] However, this varies, as in a study of 70 oral MM 66% were epithelioid, 7% spindle, and 24% mixed.[63] There was a difference in survival based on the mitotic index but it was not statistically significant.[9] Vascular invasion was apparent in only eight (6.5%) cases. Complete excision was documented histologically in only eight of 122 (6.5%) cases. The average postsurgical survival time was 173 days. The most common tumor location was the gingiva with 53.3% involving either the labial mucosa or mandibular gingiva. Less common sites of involvement included the cheeks, palate/pharynx, tongue, maxillary gingiva and tonsils.[9] A number of different immunohistochemical stains were used to identify 129 oral MM. Antibodies against vimentin, S-100 protein, neuron-specific enolase and Melan A stained 129 (100%), 98 (76.0%), 115 (89.1%), and 118 (91.5%) MM, respectively.[9] It was concluded that Melan A is a specific and sensitive marker for canine MM. Vimentin yielded a higher percentage of positive samples but is a marker for mesenchymal versus epithelial cells and provides only a preliminary categorization. In one study, the best prognostic model for predicting outcome was based on nuclear atypia in MM.[63] In this study, the median survival time was 147 days with a median time to recurrence or metastasis of 78 days.[63]

Osteocartilaginous differentiation in oral melanomas is rare but has been reported.[64,65] In a review of 10 dogs with this feature it was determined that they have a similar clinical course to other MM in the oral cavity.[64]

A retrospective study was done to evaluate a staging system including assessment of tumor size, location and mitotic index in comparison to the WHO staging system for canine oral MM.[66] Based on the alternative staging system, tumors smaller than 8 cm³, on the rostral mandible or caudal maxilla, and/or having a mitotic index ≤3 had a significantly longer remission duration and survival regardless of the treatment modality.[66] Radical resection effected the longest remission and survival times, and this was independent of whether or not the surgical margins were clean.[66]

There have been studies in dogs on the role of immunotherapy for MM. Eighty-nine dogs with malignant oral MM were treated by surgical excision alone (47) or surgery and *Corynebacterium parvum* immunotherapy (42).[67] There was no difference in survival between the two treatment groups; although in dogs with advanced-stage disease there was a statistically significant difference between surgery alone and combination therapy.[67] Dogs with stage I disease (tumor diameter <20 mm) had a statistically significant longer survival regardless of therapy given. Stage I dogs had a median survival of 511 days, compared to 160 and 168 days for stage II (tumor 20–40 mm in diameter, no other evidence of disease) and stage III (tumor >40 mm or any size with lymph node metastasis, lymph node positive, no distant metastasis) dogs, respectively.[67]

Liposome-encapsulated muramyl tripeptide-phosphatidylethanol-amine (L-MTP-PE) alone and in combination with recombinant canine granulocyte macrophage colony-stimulating factor (rcGM-CSF) was evaluated in dogs following surgery.[68] A total of 98 dogs with oral MM were entered into two randomized, double-blind, surgical adjuvant trials. Therapy had no effect on survival in advanced-stage disease, but L-MTP-PE was shown to prolong survival in dogs with early-stage disease with a median survival of 622 days.[68] There was no demonstrable difference in survival based on the extent of surgery and whether it was a simple or radical resection, indicating that the primary concern is metastasis.[68]

Gene therapy has been evaluated in the management of canine oral MM. Twenty-six dogs with MM (20 oral) were treated with a lipid-complexed plasmid DNA encoding staphylococcal enterotoxin B and either GM-CSF or IL-2.[69] The overall response rate was 46.2% (12 of 26 dogs had a partial or complete response); and in these dogs a decrease in tumor size usually occurred within 10 weeks. The median survival of the 9 stage III dogs that completed the 12-week induction phase of therapy was 66 weeks,[69] compared to a median survival of 15 weeks for stage III dogs in another study treated with surgery alone.[67]

The most recent advancement in the treatment of canine MM has been the development and clinical application of a xenogeneic DNA vaccine which has been FDA approved (conditional license) for use in dogs.[70–73] Dogs that gain the greatest benefit from xenogeneic DNA vaccination with tyrosinase family members are those with loco-regionally controlled MM that are vaccinated.[71] For 33 dogs with stage II–III disease across the xenogeneic vaccine studies performed, the median survival time was 569 days.[71]

In a report of 27 dogs with MM (25 located in the oral cavity) treated with intravenous carboplatin, 12 (44.4%) had regional lymph node metastasis, and 7 (25.9%) had pulmonary metastasis.[74] There was an overall response rate of 28.0%, with 1 complete response, 6 partial responses, and 18 had stable disease.[74]

Eleven dogs with oral MM were treated with a combination of cisplatin and oral piroxicam, with two out of the 11 dogs having a complete response to therapy for an overall response rate of 18%.[30] A synergistic response is possible with this drug combination but it is important to closely monitor renal function, as both drugs can be nephrotoxic.

A total of 38 dogs with oral MM were treated with [60]Cobalt photons. The overall mean progression-free survival (PFS) was 18.8 months (median 7.9 months).[27] The 1- and 3-year PFS rates were 36.4% and 20.2%, respectively. There was a significant difference in prognosis based on tumor stage with a mean (and median) PFS time by stage of 38 months (T1, median 18.8 months), 11.7 months (T2, median 6 months), and 12 months (T3, median 6.7 months).[27]

Palliative radiation protocols are frequently used for oral MM and there is information to support this, with MM being typically more responsive to coarsely fractionated radiation protocols with larger doses per fraction (e.g., 6 or 8 Gy per fraction). Eighteen dogs with oral MM irradiated with [60]Cobalt photons received 8 Gy/fraction on days 0, 7 and 21 for a total dose of 24 Gy.[75] There were 9 (52.9%) complete responses and 5 (29.4%) partial responses.[75] The median survival time was 7.9 months. Tumor response and survival were not significantly affected by tumor site, stage or prior surgical excision.

In another study 36 dogs with oral MM treated with external beam radiation therapy received four fractions of 9 Gy/fraction once weekly (total dose 36 Gy).[76] Twenty-four dogs had previous surgery, but 34 dogs had macroscopic disease at the time of radiation therapy. Responses included a complete response in 25 (69%), partial response in 9 (25.0%) and stable disease in two dogs (5.5%). Survival time ranged from 5 to 213 weeks, with a median survival time for dogs with a complete response of 37 weeks (range 5–213), and 20 weeks (range 10–38) in dogs with a partial response.[76] There was also a significant difference in survival based on tumor size, with a median survival of 86 weeks in dogs with tumors <5 cm[3], 16 weeks in dogs with tumors 5–15 cm[3], and 20.5 weeks in dogs with tumors >15 cm[3].[76]

A retrospective study of 140 dogs with oral MM compared three different radiation protocols (9 Gy×4 fractions; 10 Gy×3 fractions; >45 Gy, 2–4 Gy×12–19 fractions). There was no difference in response based on radiation protocol but, on multivariate analysis rostral tumor sublocation, lack of bone lysis on skull imaging and

microscopic tumor burden were joint predictors of time to first event and survival.[77] The overall median survival was 7 months.[77] Dogs with no risk factors had a longer median survival time (21 months) than dogs with one (11 months), two (5 months) or three (3 months) risk factors.[77]

The efficacy of a hypofractionated radiation protocol in conjunction with platinum-based chemotherapy was evaluated in 39 dogs.[78] The radiation protocol was 6 Gy once weekly for six consecutive weeks using either [60]Cobalt or a linear accelerator. Sixty minutes prior to each radiation treatment the dogs received low-dose cisplatin or carboplatin as a radiation sensitizer. Fifteen percent of the dogs had local recurrence with a median time to recurrence of 139 days.[78] Fifty-one percent of the dogs developed metastasis with a median time of 311 days (range 24–2163 days). The overall median survival was 363 days.[78] In another study that evaluated a hypofractionated radiation protocol (4 weekly fractions of 9 Gy) alone (13 dogs) to the primary and any lymph node metastases or in combination with full-dose carboplatin chemotherapy (15 dogs), there was no survival benefit with the addition of chemotherapy or alteration in the number of dogs dying due to metastases.[79] The median survival time for radiation alone was 307 days, and with combination radiation and carboplatin chemotherapy 286 days.[79]

Oral MM most commonly involve the oral cavity, gingiva or mucocutaneous junctions. Rarely, MM will occur on the tongue.[31,80,81] However, in a study of 1196 dogs with lingual lesions, neoplasia comprised 54% of the lesions and the most common tumor was MM (23% of tumors) with chow chows and Shar-Peis at increased risk.[32] Additionally, dogs with lingual MM were older (mean 11.1 years) and MM occurred more frequently in large-breed dogs.[32] In a retrospective study of 57 dogs with tongue tumors, seven were diagnosed with MM.[31] At presentation, five dogs had only local disease, one had regional lymph node involvement, and one had regional lymph node and pulmonary metastasis. The MM most commonly was on the dorsum of the tongue (71.4%), and involved the caudal third of the tongue (57.1%). Treatment included none (1), surgery (4), surgery and chemotherapy (DTIC) and immunotherapy (BCG) (1), and combination radiation therapy and hyperthermia (1).[31] Survival times ranged from 2 to 45 months (median 11 months).[31]

Malignant melanoma in cats

Melanomas are uncommon in cats, with ocular and cutaneous sites more common than the oral cavity (Fig. 40.4).[82,83] Only 3 out of 371 cats with oral tumors were diagnosed with MM (1 palate, 2 gingiva).[6] In a review of 39 cats with MM the most common site of involvement was ocular, with only 4 oral tumors.[84]

Twenty-nine cats were diagnosed with MM, including 19 ocular, 5 oral and 5 dermal MM.[85] Of the cats with oral MM the mean age was 12 years (range 8–16 years), and there were 4 females and 1 male. Tumor location included maxilla (3), palate (1), and mandible (1). Four of the cats with oral MM were euthanized at 1–135 days (mean 61 days) and all had metastasis.[85]

In a retrospective study from 1991–1999 the databases of four veterinary college diagnostic laboratories and/or teaching hospitals were searched to identify cases of feline nonocular MM.[86] Twenty-three MM were identified, with 3 oral cavity (maxilla), and 20 dermal.[86] The cats with oral tumors were 10–12 years old. Two of the tumors were malignant based on histopathology and 1 was benign. There were 2 epithelioid and 1 spindle-type tumors. One cat presented for local recurrence and had pulmonary metastasis 6 months after surgical excision of the primary, and was treated with carboplatin, then taxol, with an overall survival of 365 days. The other two cats were both treated with radiation therapy, and chemotherapy in one. The cat treated with radiation alone had progressive disease despite therapy.[86]

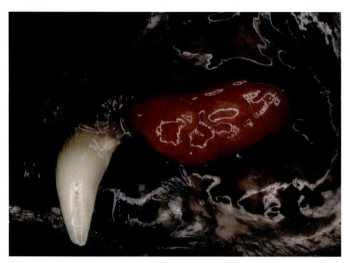

Fig. 40.4 A malignant melanoma in a cat, a rare occurrence in this species.

Five cats with oral MM were treated with palliative radiation therapy.[87] Three of the 5 cats had a documented response (1 complete response, 2 partial responses) but all cats were euthanized due to progressive disease. The median survival time was 146 days (range 66–224 days).[87]

FIBROSARCOMA

Mandibular/maxillary fibrosarcoma

Based on two surveys totaling 910 dogs with oropharyngeal tumors, the third most common tumor was FS representing 17.7% of oral tumors.[2,8] In a report of 76 dogs with oral FS the median age was 8 years (range 0.5–15 years), 25% were less than 5 years of age; and all were large-breed dogs.[8] Sites of involvement for oral FS included gingiva (66), hard palate (5), labial mucosa (3), and 1 each for soft palate and tongue.[8] Of the 40 dogs that had thoracic radiographs at diagnosis, 4 (10.0%) had pulmonary metastasis.[8] Of 31 dogs with gingival tumors that had skull radiographs made, 21 (67.7%) had evidence of bone invasion, primarily osteolysis (Fig. 40.5).[8] Of a group of 26 dogs with oral FS necropsied 3 had regional lymph node involvement and 6 had distant metastasis (lung in 6, and brain in 1).[8]

In a retrospective study of 57 dogs with tongue tumors, there was one FS.[31] A mixed-breed dog with a T2aN0M0 tumor was irradiated and subsequently euthanized at 2 months due to local recurrence.[31]

In two surveys of oral tumors in cats, FS represented the second most common oral tumor representing 12.9% and 22.0% of the oral tumors.[2,6] Age of the cats ranged from 1 to 21 years (mean 10.3 years).[6] The FS arose from the submucosal stroma and were accompanied by local tissue destruction and invasion of skeletal muscle and bone; no predilection site was noted (Fig. 40.5C).[6]

Surgery alone for oral FS results in a relatively high local recurrence rate. In a group of 14 dogs with oral FS that underwent mandibulectomy or maxillectomy the 1-year survival rate was 50.0%; 36.0% had local recurrence and 14.0% had documented metastasis.[24] In a report of 19 dogs that had mandibulectomy for oral FS the 1-year survival rate was 50.0%, and the median disease-free survival was 10.6 months.[23] Twelve of the 19 dogs had recurrence and/or metastasis (9 dogs had local recurrence; 1 dog had metastasis; 2 dogs had local recurrence and metastasis).[23]

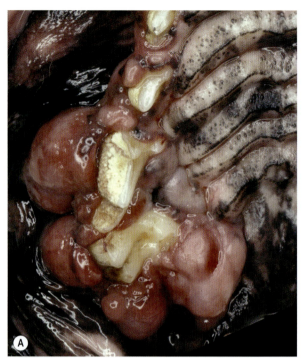

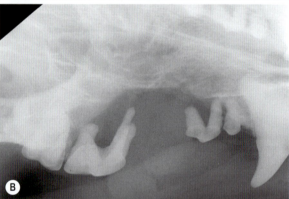

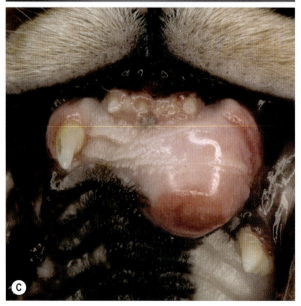

Fig. 40.5 (**A**) Fibrosarcoma of the maxilla in a dog. (**B**) Radiograph of a fibrosarcoma of the maxilla showing extensive osteolysis. (**C**) Fibrosarcoma of the left rostral maxilla and hard palate in a cat.

It has been thought that radiation therapy is ineffective in the management of oral FS in dogs, based on a report of a mean time to local tumor regrowth of 3.9 months after orthovoltage radiotherapy, with a mean survival of 6.8 months.[88] Soft tissue sarcomas at other sites have been shown to be amenable to combination surgery and radiation therapy. The 17 dogs in the report of irradiation of oral FS had gross disease and would be less likely to respond to radiation therapy alone.[88] However, in a more recent report, 31 dogs with macroscopic oral soft tissue sarcomas were treated with either curative intent (20 dogs; median total dose 52.5 Gy) or palliative intent (11 dogs; 3×8 Gy or 5×6 Gy) with comparable overall survival of 331 and 310 days, respectively.[89]

A report on 28 dogs with oral FS treated with radiation therapy reported an overall mean and median PFS of 29.7 months, and 26.2 months, respectively.[27] A poorer prognosis was associated with higher stage. The mean (and median) PFS by T stage was 53 months (T1, median 45 months), 30 months (T2, median 31 months), and 12.6 months (T3, median 7.1 months).[27] The overall 1- and 3-year PFS rates were 76.2% and 39.8%, respectively.[27]

In a report of postoperative radiation therapy for soft tissue sarcomas in 35 dogs, seven dogs had oral FS.[90] The median survival for dogs with oral soft tissue sarcomas was significantly less (1.5 years) compared to other sites (6.2 years).[90]

Six cats underwent mandibulectomy alone (five cats) or in combination with chemotherapy (one cat) for mandibular FS with a 1–2-year survival rate and progression-free rate of 67%.[47]

Histologically low-grade, biologically high-grade fibrosarcoma

Histologically low-grade yet biologically high-grade FS of the mandible and maxilla is a distinct histopathologic entity that has been identified in dogs (see Fig. 39.1).[91] The histopathologic appearance is compatible with benign fibrous connective tissue but the biologic behavior indicates otherwise, with 72.7% of dogs evaluated found to have underlying bone lysis.[91] Additionally, 12.0% ultimately developed pulmonary metastasis and 20.0% regional lymph node metastasis. The most common breed appears to be golden retrievers, representing 52.0% of the dogs in one study.[91] Age at presentation ranged from 3–13 years (median 8 years).[91] In five dogs that were treated with radiation alone, the mean survival time was 12 months.[91] Mean survival time in three dogs treated with a combination of radiation therapy and hyperthermia was 16 months.[91] Smaller numbers of dogs were treated with other types of therapy alone or in combination, with variable results, but overall the most successful approaches that prolonged survival entailed the use of surgery, with or without radiation therapy or hyperthermia. The importance of recognizing this lesion cannot be over emphasized, and aggressive local therapy is indicated to effect local control. This is a metastatic tumor as well in a subset of dogs, and systemic therapy should be considered, although information is lacking on efficacy.

BONE TUMORS

Osteosarcoma

Osteosarcoma occurs more commonly in the appendicular than axial skeleton.[92–94] Of 394 dogs with bone lesions, the most common tumor was OS (183; 46.5%), and 26.7% of the OS involved the axial skeleton, of which 14 (7.6%) involved the skull (Fig. 40.6A).[94] In a report of 144 dogs with OS, 118 involved the appendicular skeleton and only 7 of the 26 axial OS involved the skull.[92] A retrospective study of 116

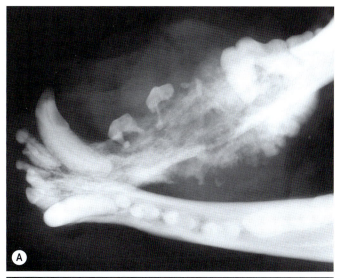
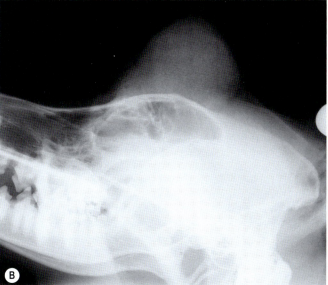
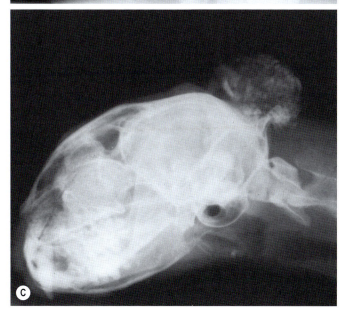

Fig. 40.6 (**A**) Osteosarcoma of the mandible in a dog. (**B**) Multilobular osteochondrosarcoma in a dog. (**C**) Multilobular osteochondrosarcoma in a cat.

dogs with axial skeletal OS determined that the most common sites of involvement were the mandible and maxilla.[93] There were 31 tumors in the mandible, 26 maxilla, 17 vertebral, 14 cranium, 12 rib, 10 nasal/paranasal sinus, and 6 pelvic tumors.[93] The majority of axial OS occurred in medium- and large-breed dogs, and most of the dogs were middle-aged or older. Thoracic radiographs were available from 19 of the dogs with mandibular tumors; one had pulmonary metastasis. None of the 11 dogs with maxillary tumors that had thoracic radiographs had pulmonary metastasis. Treatment varied, including none, maxillectomy or mandibulectomy versus local excision; some dogs received chemotherapy and one dog was irradiated. The median survival for all dogs with axial OS that underwent surgical resection (38) was 22 weeks with a 1- and 2-year survival of 26.3% and 18.4%, respectively.[93] The majority (79.6%) died or were euthanized due to the primary tumor, with metastasis the cause of death in 7.4%.[93]

A retrospective study of 45 dogs with axial OS included 12 mandibular and 7 maxillary tumors.[95] Favorable prognostic variables identified included tumors of the mandible, complete surgical excision and smaller dogs. The median survival was 223 days for dogs with complete excision and 87 days for dogs with incomplete excision.[95] The median survival for 12 dogs with mandibular tumors was 165 days as compared to 105 days for all other sites combined. There was no significant difference in survival based on whether or not the dogs received cisplatin chemotherapy.[95]

In a retrospective study over a 12-year period of 51 dogs with mandibular OS, the overall 1-year survival rate was 59.3%, 71% in dogs treated with surgery alone.[96] The median overall survival time was 17.6 months. The 1-year overall DFS rate was 48.2% with a median overall DFI of 9.5 months. Treatment included partial mandibulectomy (32), partial mandibulectomy and chemotherapy (10), partial mandibulectomy and radiation therapy (3), partial mandibulectomy, radiation therapy, and chemotherapy (4), and radiation therapy alone (2).[96] The majority of dogs that were treated with chemotherapy received intravenous cisplatin. The mean age was 9.5 years (range 3–15 years), mean body weight was 27.8 kg (range 6.4–53.2 kg), and the male to female ratio was 1:1.8. The local recurrence rate for the dogs treated surgically (32) was 28%, and the metastasis rate was 28.1%. No conclusions could be made regarding the role of adjuvant therapy.[96]

In a retrospective study of 22 large-breed dogs with axial skeleton OS (including four maxillary and three mandibular tumors) the metastatic rate was 46% and the overall median survival for all dogs was 137 days.[97] Dogs treated with a definitive versus a palliative radiation therapy protocol experienced a significantly longer survival time of 265 days as opposed to 76 days.[97]

Ninety dogs with stage III OS (mandible in one dog, maxilla in one dog) that received a variety of different treatments (NSAIDs, surgery, chemotherapy, radiation therapy) had an overall median survival time of 76 days.[98] It was noted that dogs that had bone metastasis as opposed to soft tissue metastasis, and those treated palliatively with radiation and chemotherapy, had the longest survival times.[98]

In a report of 22 cats with OS 15 involved the appendicular skeleton and 7 the axial skeleton including 1 on the mandible, 1 on the maxilla, and 2 on the rest of the skull.[99] Radiographically, in all 7 cats with axial tumors there was a significant amount of periosteal new bone formation. Of the 22 cats only 1 cat with an appendicular tumor had documented pulmonary metastasis.[99] The 4 cats with skull tumors were treated surgically with resultant incomplete excision; 1 received radiation therapy postoperatively and lived for 16 months prior to being euthanized for recurrence; and the remaining 3 cats with skull OS died within 3 months postoperatively due to recurrence or progression.[99] The overall median survival for cats with axial OS was 5.5 months.[99]

In a review of 58 cats with tumors involving bone there were 19 OS, 11 of which were axial in origin, and of these there was 1 mandibular, 1 palatine and 1 maxillary OS.[42] In a series of 24 primary bone tumors the most common tumor was OS (19 cats) with only 1 mandibular OS.[100] In a recent review of 145 cats with OS there were only 3 cats with oral OS.[101]

Mandibulectomy alone or in combination with radiation (1 cat) or chemotherapy (1 cat) in 6 cats with mandibular OS was associated with a 1–3-year survival rate and progression-free rate of 83%.[47]

Multilobular osteochondrosarcoma

Multilobular osteochondrosarcoma (MLO) is a relatively uncommon tumor in dogs, rare in cats, and typically involves the flat bones of the cranium (Fig. 40.6B, C).[102–104] In a report of 39 dogs with MLO, sites of involvement included maxilla (11), mandible (14), calvarium (14), and 1 each at various other sites.[103] The most common presenting complaint was firm, fixed mass (54%), and other signs included swelling, pain, exophthalmos or neurologic signs.[103] There were 20 males and 19 females. The ages ranged between 4–17 years (median 8 years). Body weight ranged from 8.2 to 69.4 kg (median 29 kg). MLO has a stippled appearance on radiographs due to the multilobular arrangement of osseous, cartilaginous tissue or both surrounded by mesenchymal stroma. CT and MRI appearance of MLO have also been described and provide more detailed information on the extent of the disease for surgical planning.[105,106] Twenty-five dogs were treated with surgery alone and nine with surgery combined with adjuvant therapy. Adjuvant therapy included implantation of cisplatin-impregnated open cell polylactic acid (OPLA-PT), radiation therapy, and intravenous cisplatin.[103] The effect of adjuvant therapy on outcome could not be ascertained. Of the dogs treated, 47% had local tumor recurrence, and 56% had documented metastasis.[103] The median time to recurrence was 797 days, median time to metastasis was 542 days, and median survival was 797 days (range 28–1670 days).[103] Four dogs had metastasis at the time of initial presentation. Outcome was affected by histological grade (criteria included borders, size of lobules, organization, mitotic figures, cellular pleomorphism and presence of necrosis), surgical margins and tumor location. Metastasis occurred in 7 of 9 (77.8%) grade III tumors, 9 of 15 (60.0%) grade II tumors, and 3 of 10 (30.0%) grade I tumors.[103] Dogs with grade II and III tumors had significantly shorter times to metastasis. The local recurrence rate was higher in dogs with high-grade tumors. The local recurrence rate was 77.8% for grade III, 46.7% for grade II and 30.0% for grade I tumors. Median time to local recurrence in dogs with complete margins was not reached at 1332 days with 8 of 19 (42%) having recurrence. Median time to local recurrence for incomplete margins was 320 days with 10 of 13 (76.9%) having recurrence.[103] Median survival time for dogs with mandibular tumors was 1487 days compared to 528 days for other sites.[103]

OTHER NONODONTOGENIC TUMOR TYPES

Undifferentiated malignant tumor of young dogs

Undifferentiated malignant tumor of the oral cavity is a distinct clinical entity that has been identified in young dogs, with only six cases identified over a 15-year period.[107] All were less than 2 years of age with a range of 6 to 22 months.[107] Five of the six dogs had an ill-defined soft gray–tan, hemorrhagic mass involving the maxillary premolar and molar regions; and one dog had involvement of the soft palate. The tumors were locally aggressive and had variable extension of the tumor into the maxillary, nasal and orbital tissues, and in some into the brain. Necropsy of five dogs revealed diffuse metastasis in four, and liver metastasis in one. The most common sites of metastasis were lymph nodes, lung, liver, heart, kidney and brain. Electron microscopy and immunohistochemistry did not reveal any characteristics that would indicate that these tumors were epithelial or mesenchymal in origin, hence the diagnosis of undifferentiated malignant tumor.[107] Surgery was the only treatment attempted with an average survival of 22 days (range 2–60 days).[107]

Extramedullary plasmacytoma

Extramedullary plasmacytomas arise outside of bone, are typically mucocutaneous in location and occur most commonly in the mouth, on the feet or trunk and in the ears (Fig. 40.7A).[108,109] In a report of 136 dogs with extramedullary plasmacytomas 31 (22.8%) occurred in the oral cavity and locations included gingiva (17), tongue (12) and 1 each involved the hard palate and oropharynx.[109] In a report of 75 dogs with mucocutaneous plasmacytomas 17 (22.7%) were located in the mouth.[108] Only 2 of the 17 dogs with tumors in the mouth had radiographs made and 1 had evidence of underlying bone lysis. In a study of 46 dogs with cutaneous plasmacytomas, the second most common site of involvement was the lip (23.9%).[110] Cutaneous plasmacytomas are typically small (mean diameter 8 mm), broad-based, spherical or dome-shaped and hairless.[110]

In a retrospective study, 16 of 302 (5.2%) dogs with oral tumors had extramedullary plasmacytomas representing 28.5% of all EMP over a 10-year period.[111] Tumor location included: lingual (4), rostral mandible (7), maxilla/hard palate (3), buccal surface of upper lip (1) and extensive disease (1). Treatment included none (3), surgery with local recurrence (7) with a median time to recurrence of 50 days (range 23–690 days), and a few had chemotherapy and/or radiation therapy. At the time of the study, 5 were alive and 11 had died with a median survival of 474 days (range 37–2906 days).[111]

The primary mode of therapy is surgical excision and the majority of dogs have long-term local control.[108,109] The local recurrence rate as well as distant failure is low.[109] It has been noted that gingival tumors have the highest rate of local recurrence (4/17 in one study) presumably due to the difficulty in obtaining wide margins although partial maxillectomy or mandibulectomy may be successful.[109] There is limited information on the efficacy of treatment for plasmacytomas with either chemotherapy or radiation therapy. Plasmacytomas are considered to be radiation-sensitive; however, data are lacking on the efficacy of radiation therapy in canine oral plasmacytomas.

Oral lymphoma

In a study of 130 dogs with oropharyngeal tumors, six had primary oral lymphoma.[22] The sites of involvement included tonsils and cervical lymph nodes, membrana nictitans and soft palate, gingiva, buccal mucosa, and pharynx, tongue and epiglottis.[22]

Epitheliotropic lymphoma in dogs can involve the gingiva and/or lips at the mucocutaneous junction (Fig. 40.7B). Radiation therapy has been used in the management of the local disease in the oral cavity in addition to systemic chemotherapy, although detailed information is lacking on response to therapy.

Eleven (2.9%) out of a total of 371 cats with oral tumors had oral lymphoma, and there were also two with tonsillar lymphoma.[6] The appearance of oral lymphoma was described as single or multiple raised submucosal masses composed of unencapsulated sheets of neoplastic lymphoid cells. Of the 13 cats, 7 tumors were lymphoblastic and 6 were lymphocytic. The overlying gingival was often ulcerated with secondary chronic inflammation and necrosis.[6]

In a report on the use of lomustine in 17 cats with lymphoma, 2 cats had oral lymphoma, 1 had a partial response and 1 had progressive disease.[112] Radiation therapy alone or in combination with chemotherapy has been used in cats with lymphoma, with 1 cat with maxillary lymphoma having a complete response (survival 47 weeks) and 1 cat with a mandibular lymphoma having a partial response (survival 9 weeks).[113]

Miscellaneous tumor types

Merkel cell tumor

Neuroendocrine (Merkel) cell tumors of the canine oral cavity are rare. Merkel cells occur in the epidermis in close association with nerve endings and have been reported to occur in the oral mucosa. Merkel cells are part of the neuroendocrine system and function as mechanoreceptors. Although typically dermal in origin, there is a report of four dogs with oral Merkel cell tumors.[114] The dogs ranged in age from 7 to 9 years, 3 of the tumors were located on the gingiva, 1 caused lysis of underlying bone, and 1 was located on the lip. Cutaneous Merkel cell tumors are clinically benign in behavior, and the oral tumors were considered benign as well. Three dogs underwent surgical excision which was curative and the fourth dog was treated with radiation and was tumor-free for 18 months.[114]

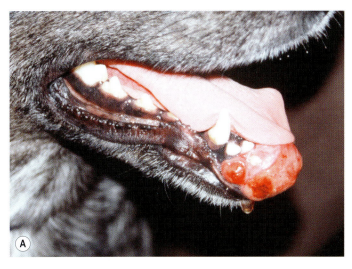

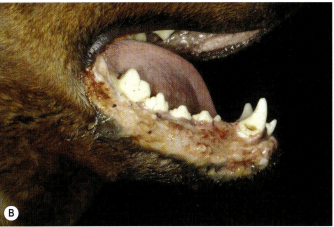

Fig. 40.7 (**A**) Extramedullary plasmacytoma of the rostral mandible in a dog. (**B**) Oral lymphoma affecting the lower lips in a dog.

397

Mast cell tumor

In 130 dogs with oropharyngeal tumors there was one dog with a mast cell tumor of the buccal mucosa.[22] In 155 dogs with malignant oropharyngeal tumors 9 mast cell tumors were identified that involved the upper lip (6), gingiva or buccal mucosa (2), and hard palate (1).[59]

In a retrospective review of a total of 57 canine tongue tumors there were five dogs with mast cell tumors.[31] The dogs ranged in age from 3 to 10 years. Treatment was mainly surgical. The longest survival time was 16 months and local disease control was only achieved in one of the five dogs.[31]

Three oral mast cell tumors were diagnosed out of 371 cats with oral tumors. One cat had a mast cell tumor arising from the soft palate, and two had tumors at the mucocutaneous junction of the lips.[6] The ages ranged from 3 to 8 years with a mean of 5.3 years.[6] There is a case report of a 9-year-old cat with a sublingual mast cell tumor that was responsive to lomustine with a complete remission noted after the third of six doses.[115]

Granular cell myoblastoma

In a review of the literature of dogs with oral granular cell myoblastoma, sites of occurrence included tongue (8), lip (1) and larynx (1).[116] Age ranged from 2.5 to 13 years (mean 8.9 years). There was no breed or sex predilection. Additionally, there was no evidence of either tumor recurrence or metastasis after surgery.[116]

In a retrospective study of 57 dogs with tongue tumors there were seven dogs diagnosed with granular cell myoblastoma.[31] Ages ranged from 7 to 15 years, and there was no apparent sex predilection. One dog had diffuse involvement of the tongue, 5 tumors occurred on the dorsal, and 1 on the ventral surface.[31] Six of the 7 dogs had early stage disease (T1aN0M0). Treatment entailed surgery alone. Survival times ranged from 2 to 72 months. One dog died with metastatic disease, and only one dog did not have local tumor control.[31]

Hemangiosarcoma

In a survey of 469 oropharyngeal tumors in dogs there were six hemangiosarcomas (1.3%).[2] In a compilation of 130 dogs with oropharyngeal tumors there were two dogs identified with oral hemangiosarcoma of the gingiva.[22]

Three out of 57 dogs with lingual tumors were diagnosed with hemangiosarcoma.[24] Treatment included none, surgery, and surgery combined with chemotherapy, with survival times of up to 8 months.[31] In another report, 38 of 646 dogs with lingual tumors had hemangiosarcoma, which was the third most common tumor, and it was noted that Border collies were 11.8 times as likely to be diagnosed with this tumor as opposed to other breeds.[32]

In a retrospective study of 395 neoplasms from 372 cats there were two cats with oral hemangiosarcoma; one involved the gingiva and one the palate.[5] In a retrospective study of 53 cats with hemangiosarcoma, two involved the gingiva.[117] Both cats had surgery with incomplete resection and no other adjunctive therapy.

PAPILLOMATOSIS

In a retrospective study that included 146 dogs with benign oropharyngeal mass lesions, papillomatosis represented 24 (16.4%) of the tumors.[59]

Oral papillomas can be solitary but are often multiple cauliflower-like growths that may have frond-like projections (Fig. 40.8). This tumor occurs most commonly in young dogs. Canine oral papillomatosis virus (COPV) is contagious from one dog to another, but is

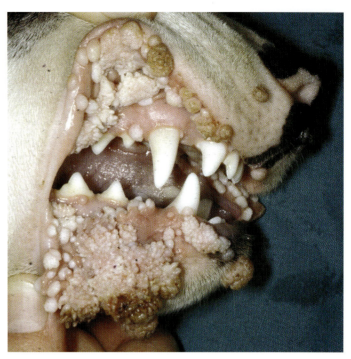

Fig. 40.8 Extensive oral papillomatosis in a dog.

species-specific. Experimentally induced canine oral papillomas routinely undergo incubation periods of 4–8 weeks, rapid growth and expansion, followed by spontaneous immune-mediated regression within an additional 4–8 weeks.[118] Treatment in clinical cases is usually not necessary as the lesions will typically regress spontaneously. Excisional surgery, laser surgery or cryosurgery may be indicated in dogs that have multiple lesions that are causing difficulty eating. However, immune-compromised dogs tend to show persistent and florid lesions that are refractory to therapy.[119–121] Autogenous vaccinations prepared from homogenized papillomas have been found to induce regression of the lesions in a number of species including the dog.[121–123] There is increased interest in developing an effective prophylactic vaccine in order to reduce the occurrence of genital papillomas in humans, and COPV is often used as a model in developing vaccines.[124] Inactivated papilloma extract[125] and recombinant vaccinations consisting of viral coat proteins[124] have been reported as a prophylaxis of canine oral papillomatosis. In one case report, a recombinant vaccination was used therapeutically and led to resolution of persistent, florid oral papillomatosis in a young dog.[126]

In a retrospective study of 395 neoplasms from 372 cats there was one oral papilloma of the tongue; no other details were provided.[5] In a more recent report there were a total of seven domestic cats that had papillomas, five involved haired skin and two had lingual tumors.[127] The two cats with lingual papillomas were 6 months and 9 years of age.[127] The oral tumors were described as multifocal, small, soft, light-pink, oval, slightly raised flat, sessile lesions, less than 10 mm in diameter on the ventral lingual surface.[127] The tumors were all positive for papillomavirus antigens by immunohistochemistry.[127]

SALIVARY GLAND TUMORS

The histological classification of salivary gland tumors in humans includes adenomas, carcinomas, nonepithelial tumors and malignant lymphoma (arising from lymphoid tissue associated with salivary glands).[128] The adenomas include a number of subtypes, the most common being the pleomorphic adenoma, and ductal papilloma and cystadenoma. The carcinomas comprise the different types of adenocarcinoma, ductal carcinoma, SCC and mucoepidermoid carcinoma.[128] Salivary gland tumors are relatively rare in the dog and cat, and not all types have been recognized. Salivary gland tumors arise most commonly in the major salivary glands, but can occur in minor accessory salivary gland tissue present throughout the oral cavity. In a search of 87 392 biopsy records, there were a total of 245 cases (0.3%) in which salivary gland tissue was evaluated from 160 dogs and 85 cats, and 30.2% of these were malignant neoplasms.[129] Malignant salivary gland tumors included salivary gland adenocarcinoma or carcinoma (36 dogs, 31 cats), salivary adenocarcinoma in dispersed accessory salivary tissue of the oral submucosa and tongue (two dogs, two cats), and malignant mixed salivary gland tumor (three dogs).[129] The mandibular gland was most frequently involved with the parotid gland second.[129] A case report of a cat documented bilateral involvement of the mandibular salivary glands with metastasis to the regional lymph nodes, soft palate, laryngopharynx and lung.[130] Benign tumors of the salivary glands included salivary gland adenoma/cystadenoma (two cats), and accessory papillary adenoma (one cat).[129]

In a search of 35 609 canine pathology submissions, there were 140 (0.4%) submissions of salivary gland tissue.[131] Forty-three of these (31%) were neoplastic.[131] The majority were adenocarcinomas (23) and carcinomas (15), but there were also malignant mixed tumors (2), metastatic lymphomas (2), and 1 OS.[131] Other tumors that have been reported to involve salivary glands in dogs include mast cell tumor,[132] infiltrative lipomas[133,134] and malignant myoepithelioma.[135]

A retrospective review of medical records from an academic institution from 1975 to 1986 revealed 81 dogs and 57 cats with salivary gland tumors.[136] The incidence of salivary gland tumors diagnosed over this period was 0.17%.[136] Tumor types in 81 dogs included adenocarcinoma (48), carcinoma (13), mixed salivary gland tumor (8), adenoma (5), SCC (2), FS (1), mast cell tumor (1) and unspecified histologic type (3).[136] The median age of dogs was 10 years (range 2–16 years).[136] Tumors in 57 cats included adenocarcinoma (45), carcinoma (6), SCC (2), adenoma (2), mixed salivary gland tumor (1) and unspecified histologic type (1).[136] The median age of cats was 10 years (range 0.2–16 years).[136] Signs on presentation include nonpainful slowly enlarging mass, dysphagia, anorexia and pain on opening the mouth.[136] In a report of three dogs that had either cytoreductive surgery or biopsy only, survival times ranged from 1 to 4 months.[136] Two cats that underwent surgical resection of salivary gland tumors survived 6 and 7 months, both cats had regional lymph node metastasis at initial diagnosis, and one later developed pulmonary metastasis.[136] A cat with an oncocytoma of the mandibular salivary gland was alive with no evidence of disease 28 months postoperatively.[137]

There is limited information on therapy other than surgery for salivary gland tumors. Orthovoltage radiation therapy was used successfully postoperatively in three dogs with parotid gland adenocarcinomas.[138] Survival time in one dog was 40 months and the other two dogs were alive with no evidence of disease at 12 and 25 months.[138]

There is a report on treatment of salivary gland tumors in dogs and cats that utilized various combinations of surgery, chemotherapy and radiation therapy.[139] There were a total of seven out of 24 dogs and five out of 30 cats treated with megavoltage radiation therapy. The overall median survival time for all dogs was 550 days, and the surgery and chemotherapy group had shorter survival times compared to surgery alone or surgery and radiation therapy.[139] A cat with a malignant mixed tumor in the right mandibular salivary gland underwent surgical resection and postoperative orthovoltage radiation therapy.[140] Local recurrence and pulmonary metastasis were detected within 7 weeks after surgery, treatment was stopped, and the cat died 1 month later.[140]

Salivary gland adenocarcinomas were diagnosed in seven out of a total of 372 cats diagnosed with neoplasia, and involved the parotid gland in six, and the mandibular gland in one cat.[5]

Salivary gland adenocarcinoma in the oral cavity was diagnosed in eight cats out of a total of 371 cats all with oral tumors.[6] All of the salivary gland adenocarcinomas were located in the lower gingival or buccal submucosa.[6]

A review of archival material from 35 cats with salivary gland tumors revealed five cats with salivary duct carcinomas.[141] Tumor location in four cats included parotid gland, and minor salivary gland tissue from the oral cavity, soft palate, and cheek. The ages ranged from 7 to 13 years with a median of 8, and there were four females and one male.[141] Two cats had evidence of metastasis but complete case information was not available.

In a report of 30 cats with salivary gland tumors, none of the cats were Siamese or Siamese-cross; there was a 2 : 1 predilection for males; and the median age was 12 years (range 7–22 years).[139] The most common histopathological diagnosis was simple adenocarcinoma; other tumor types included ductular adenocarcinoma, complex adenocarcinoma, solid carcinoma, SCC, acinic cell carcinoma and mucoepidermoid carcinoma.[139] Presence of a mass was the most common presenting complaint. Other clinical signs included halitosis, weight loss and dysphagia.[139] The mandibular gland was most commonly affected (59%) followed by the parotid gland.[139] Various treatment modalities were utilized with an overall median survival of 516 days with no difference in survival based on treatment type.[139]

REFERENCES

1. Dorn CR, Taylor DON, Schneider R, et al. Survey of animal neoplasms in Alameda and Contra Costa counties, California. II. Cancer morbidity in dogs and cats from Alameda county. J Natl Cancer Inst 1968;40:307–18.

2. Dorn CR, Priester WA. Epidemiologic analysis of oral and pharyngeal cancer in dogs, cats, horses, and cattle. J Am Vet Med Assoc 1976;169:1202–6.

3. Dobson JM, Samuel S, Milstein H, et al. Canine neoplasia in the UK: estimates of incidence rates from a population of insured dogs. J Small Anim Pract 2002; 43:240–6.

4. Priester WA, Mantel N. Occurrence of tumors in domestic animals. Data from 12 United States and Canadian colleges of veterinary medicine. J Nat Cancer Inst 1971;47:1333–44.

5. Engle GC, Brodey RS. A retrospective study of 395 feline neoplasms. J Am Anim Hosp Assoc 1969;5:21–31.

6. Stebbins KE, Morse CC, Goldschmidt MH. Feline oral neoplasia: a ten-year survey. Vet Pathol 1989;26:121–8.

7. Cohen D, Brodey RS, Chen SM. Epidemiologic aspects of oral and pharyngeal neoplasms of the dog. Am J Vet Res 1964;25:1776–9.

8. Todoroff RJ, Brodey RS. Oral and pharyngeal neoplasia in the dog: a retrospective survey of 361 cases. J Am Vet Med Assoc 1979;175: 567–71.

9. Ramos-Vara JA, Beissenherz ME, Miller MA, et al. Retrospective study of 338 canine oral melanomas with clinical, histologic, and immunohistochemical

review of 129 cases. Vet Pathol 2000; 37:597–608.

10. Ragland WL, Gorham JR. Tonsillar carcinoma in rural dogs. Nature 1967; 214:925–6.

11. Bostock DE, Curtis R. Comparison of canine oropharyngeal malignancy in various geographical locations. Vet Rec 1984;114:341–2.

12. Bertone ER, Snyder LA, Moore AS. Environmental and lifestyle risk factors for oral squamous cell carcinoma in domestic cats. J Vet Intern Med 2003; 17:557–62.

13. Snyder LA, Bertone ER, Jakowski RM, et al. p53 expression and environmental tobacco smoke exposure in feline oral squamous cell carcinoma. Vet Pathol 2004;41:209–14.

14. Teifke JP, Lohr CV, Shirasawa H. Detection of canine oral papillomavirus-DNA in canine oral squamous cell carcinoma and p53 overexpressing skin papillomas of the dog using the polymerase chain reaction and non-radioactive in situ hybridization. Vet Microbiol 1998;60:119–30.

15. Zaugg N, Nespeca G, Hauser B, et al. Detection of novel papillomaviruses in canine mucosal, cutaneous and in situ squamous cell carcinomas. Vet Dermatol 2005;16:290–8.

16. Munday JS, Howe L, French A, et al. Detection of papillomaviral DNA sequences in a feline oral squamous cell carcinoma. Res Vet Science 2009;86: 359–61.

17. Hayes A, Scase T, Miller J, et al. Cox-1 and Cox-2 expression in feline oral squamous cell carcinoma. J Comp Path 2006;135:93–9.

18. Mohammed SI, Khan KNM, Sellers RS, et al. Expression of cyclooxygenase-1 and 2 in naturally-occurring canine cancer. Prostaglandins Leukot Essent Fatty Acids 2004;70:479–83.

19. Modiano JF, Ritt MG, Wojcieszyn J. The molecular basis of canine melanoma: pathogenesis and trends in diagnosis and therapy. J Vet Intern Med 1999;13: 163–74.

20. Thrall DE, Goldschmidt MH, Evans SM, et al. Bone sarcoma following orthovoltage radiotherapy in two dogs. Vet Radiol 1983;24:169–73.

21. McChesney Gillette S, Gillette EL, Powers BE, et al. Radiation-induced osteosarcomas in dogs after external beam or intraoperative radiation therapy. Cancer Res 1990;50:54–7.

22. Brodey RS. A clinical and pathologic study of 130 neoplasms of the mouth and pharynx in the dog. Am J Vet Res 1960;21:787–812.

23. Kosovsky JK, Matthiesen DT, Manfra Marretta S, et al. Results of partial mandibulectomy for the treatment of oral tumors in 142 dogs. Vet Surg 1991;20:397–401.

24. White RAS. Mandibulectomy and maxillectomy in the dog: long term survival in 100 cases. J Small Anim Pract 1991;32:69–74.

25. Evans SM, Shofer F. Canine oral nontonsillar squamous cell carcinoma. Prognostic factors for recurrence and survival following orthovoltage radiation therapy. Vet Radiol 1988;29:133–7.

26. LaDue-Miller T, Price GS, Page RL, et al. Radiotherapy of canine non-tonsillar squamous cell carcinoma. Vet Radiol Ultrasound 1996;37:74–7.

27. Théon AP, Rodriguez C, Madewell BR. Analysis of prognostic factors and patterns of failure in dogs with malignant oral tumors treated with megavoltage irradiation. J Am Vet Med Assoc 1997; 210:778–84.

28. Schmidt BR, Glickman NW, DeNicola DB, et al. Evaluation of piroxicam for the treatment of oral squamous cell carcinoma in dogs. J Am Vet Med Assoc 2001;218:1783–6.

29. de Almeida EMP, Phiche C, Sirous J, et al. Expression of cyclo-oxygenase-2 in naturally occurring squamous cell carcinomas in dogs. J Histochem Cytochem 2001;49:867–75.

30. Boria PA, Murry DJ, Bennett PF, et al. Evaluation of cisplatin combined with piroxicam for the treatment of oral malignant melanoma and oral squamous cell carcinoma in dogs. J Am Vet Med Assoc 2004;224:388–94.

31. Beck ER, Withrow SJ, McChesney AE, et al. Canine tongue tumors: a retrospective review of 57 cases. J Am Anim Hosp Assoc 1986;22:525–32.

32. Dennis MM, Ehrhart N, Duncan CG, et al. Frequency of and risk factors associated with lingual lesions in dogs: 1,196 cases (1995–2004). J Am Vet Med Assoc 2006;228:1533–7.

33. Carpenter LG, Withrow SJ, Powers BE, et al. Squamous cell carcinoma of the tongue in 10 dogs. J Am Anim Hosp Assoc 1993;29:17–24.

34. Dvorak LD, Beaver DP, Ellison GW, et al. Major glossectomy in dogs: a case series and proposed classification system. J Am Anim Hosp Assoc 2004;40:331–7.

35. Cotchin E. Some tumours of dogs and cats of comparative veterinary and human interest. Vet Rec 1959;71: 1040–54.

36. MacMillan R, Withrow SJ, Gillette EL. Surgery and regional irradiation for treatment of canine tonsillar squamous cell carcinoma: retrospective review of eight cases. J Am Anim Hosp 1982; 18:311–14.

37. Brooks MB, Matus RE, Leifer CE, et al. Chemotherapy versus chemotherapy plus radiotherapy in the treatment of tonsillar squamous cell carcinoma in the dog. J Vet Intern Med 1988;2:206–11.

38. Murphy S, Hayes A, Adams V, et al. Role of carboplatin in multi-modality

treatment of canine tonsillar squamous cell carcinoma – a case series of five dogs. J Small Anim Pract 2006;47: 216–20.

39. Ogilvie GK, Sundberg JP, O'Banion K, et al. Papillary squamous cell carcinoma in three young dogs. J Am Vet Med Assoc 1988;192:933–6.

40. Stapleton BL, Barrus JM. Papillary squamous cell carcinoma in a young dog. J Vet Dent 1996;13:65–8.

41. Lownie JF, Altini M, Austin JC, et al. Verrucous carcinoma presenting in the maxilla of a dog. J Am Anim Hosp Assoc 1981;17:315–19.

42. Quigley PJ, Leedale AH. Tumors involving bone in the domestic cat: a review of fifty-eight cases. Vet Pathol 1983;20:670–86.

43. Kapatkin AS, Manfra Marretta S, Patnaik AK, et al. Mandibular swellings in cats: prospective study of 24 cats. J Am Anim Hosp Assoc 1991;27:575–80.

44. Postorino Reeves NC, Turrel JM, Withrow SJ. Oral squamous cell carcinoma in the cat. J Am Anim Hosp Assoc 1993;29: 438–41.

45. Gendler A, Lewis JR, Reetz JA, et al. Computed tomographic features of oral squamous cell carcinoma in cats: 18 cases (2002–2008). J Am Vet Med Assoc 2010;236:319–25.

46. Bradley RL, MacEwen EG, Loar AS. Mandibular resection for removal of oral tumors in 30 dogs and 6 cats. J Am Vet Med Assoc 1984;184:460–3.

47. Northrup NC, Selting KA, Rassnick KM, et al. Outcomes of cats with oral tumors treated with mandibulectomy: 42 cases. J Am Anim Hosp Assoc 2006;42: 350–60.

48. Hayes AM, Adams VJ, Scase TJ, et al. Survival of 54 cats with oral squamous cell carcinoma in United Kingdom general practice. J Small Anim Pract 2007;48:394–9.

49. Kisseberth WC, Vail DM, Yaissle J, et al. Phase I clinical evaluation of carboplatin in tumor-bearing cats: a veterinary cooperative oncology group study. J Vet Intern Med 2008;22:83–8.

50. Bregazzi VS, LaRue SM, Powers BE, et al. Response of feline oral squamous cell carcinoma to palliative radiation therapy. Vet Radiol Ultrasound 2001;42:77–9.

51. Ogilvie GK, Moore AS, Obradovich JE, et al. Toxicoses and efficacy associated with administration of mitoxantrone to cats with malignant tumors. J Am Vet Med Assoc 1993;202:1839–44.

52. Jones PD, de Lorimier LP, Kitchell BE, et al. Gemcitabine as a radiosensitizer for nonresectable feline oral squamous cell carcinoma. J Am Anim Hosp Assoc 2003;39:463–7.

53. Hutson CA, Willauer CC, Walder EJ, et al. Treatment of mandibular squamous cell carcinoma in cats by use of mandibulectomy and radiotherapy: seven

cases (1987–1989). J Am Vet Med Assoc 1992;201:777–81.

54. DiBernardi L, Doré M, Davis JA, et al. Study of feline oral squamous cell carcinoma: potential target for cyclooxygenase inhibitor treatment. Prostaglandins Leukot Essent Fatty Acids 2007;76:245–50.

55. Fox LE, Rosenthal RC, King RR, et al. Use of cis-bis-neodecanoato-trans-R,R-1,2-diaminocyclohexane platinum (II), a liposomal cisplatin analogue, in cats with oral squamous cell carcinoma. Am J Vet Res 2000;61:791–5.

56. Mauldin GN, Matus RE, Patnaik AK, et al. Efficacy and toxicity of doxorubicin and cyclophosphamide of selected malignant tumors in 23 cats. J Vet Intern Med 1988;2:60–5.

57. Fidel JL, Sellon RK, Houston RK, et al. A nine-day accelerated radiation protocol for feline squamous cell carcinoma. Vet Radiol Ultrasound 2007;48:482–5.

58. Bostock DE. The prognosis in cats bearing squamous cell carcinoma. J Small Anim Pract 1972;13:119–25.

59. Gorlin RJ, Barron CN, Chaudhry AP, et al. The oral and pharyngeal pathology of domestic animals. A study of 487 cases. Am J Vet Res 1959;20:1032–61.

60. Schultheiss PC. Histologic features and clinical outcomes of melanomas of lip, haired skin, and nail bed locations of dogs. J Vet Diagn Invest 2006;18:422–5.

61. Esplin DG. Survival of dogs following surgical excision of histologically well-differentiated melanocytic neoplasms of the mucous membranes of the oral cavity. Vet Pathol 2008;45:889–96.

62. Williams LE, Packer RA. Association between lymph node size and metastasis in dogs with oral malignant melanoma: 100 cases (1987–2001). J Am Vet Med Assoc 2003;222:1234–6.

63. Spangler WL, Kass PH. The histologic and epidemiologic bases for prognostic considerations in canine melanocytic neoplasia. Vet Pathol 2006;43:136–49.

64. Sanchez J, Ramirez GA, Buendia AJ, et al. Immunohistochemical characterization and evaluation of prognostic factors in canine oral melanomas with osteocartilaginous differentiation. Vet Pathol 2007;44:676–82.

65. Ellis AE, Harmon BG, Miller DL, et al. Gingival osteogenic melanoma in two dogs. J Vet Diagn Invest 2010;22:147–52.

66. Hahn KA, DeNicola DB, Richardson RC, et al. Canine oral malignant melanoma: prognostic utility of an alternative staging system. J Small Anim Pract 1994;35:251–6.

67. MacEwen EG, Patnaik AK, Harvey HJ, et al. Canine oral melanoma: comparison of surgery versus surgery plus Corynebacterium parvum. Cancer Invest 1986;4:347–402.

68. MacEwen EG, Kurzman ID, Vail DM, et al. Adjuvant therapy for melanoma in dogs: results of randomized clinical trials using surgery, liposome-encapsulated muramyl tripeptide, and granulocyte macrophage colony-stimulating factor. Clin Cancer Res 1999;5:4249–58.

69. Dow SW, Elmslie RE, Wilson AP, et al. In vivo tumor transfection with superantigen plus cytokine genes induces tumor regression and prolongs survival in dogs with malignant melanoma. J Clin Invest 1998;101:2406–14.

70. Bergman PJ. Canine oral melanoma. Clin Tech Small Anim Pract 2007;22:55–60.

71. Bergman PJ, Camps-Palau MA, McKnight JA, et al. Development of a xenogeneic DNA vaccine program for canine malignant melanoma at the Animal Medical Center. Vaccine 2006;24:4582–5.

72. Bergman PJ, McKnight J, Novosad A, et al. Long-term survival of dogs with advanced malignant melanoma after DNA vaccination with xenogeneic human tyrosinase: a phase I trial. Clin Cancer Res 2003;9:1284–90.

73. Liao JCF, Gregor P, Wolchok JD, et al. Vaccination with tyrosinase DNA induces antibody responses in dogs with advanced melanoma. Cancer Immunity 2006;6:8–17.

74. Rassnick KM, Ruslander DM, Cotter SM, et al. Use of carboplatin for treatment of dogs with malignant melanoma: 27 cases (1989–2000). J Am Vet Med Assoc 2001;218:1444–8.

75. Bateman KE, Catton PA, Pennock PW, et al. 0-7-21 radiation therapy for the treatment of canine oral melanoma. J Vet Intern Med 1994;8:267–72.

76. Blackwood L, Dobson JM. Radiotherapy of oral malignant melanomas in dogs. J Am Vet Med Assoc 1996;209:98–102.

77. Proulx DR, Ruslander DM, Dodge RK, et al. A retrospective analysis of 140 dogs with oral melanoma treated with external beam radiation. Vet Radiol Ultrasound 2003;44:352–9.

78. Freeman KP, Hahn KA, Harris FD, et al. Treatment of dogs with oral melanoma by hypofractionated radiation therapy and platinum-based chemotherapy (1987–1997). J Vet Intern Med 2003;17:96–101.

79. Murphy S, Hayes AM, Blackwood L, et al. Oral malignant melanoma – the effect of coarse fractionation radiotherapy alone or with adjuvant carboplatin therapy. Vet Comp Oncol 2005;3:222–9.

80. Mulligan RM. Melanoblastic tumors in the dog. Am J Vet Res 1961;22:345–51.

81. Carpenter JW, Novilla MN, Griffing WJ. Metastasis of a malignant amelanotic lingual melanoma in a dog. J Am Anim Hosp Assoc 1980;16:685–9.

82. Patnaik AK, Liu SK, Hurvitz AI, et al. Nonhematopoietic neoplasms in cats. J Natl Cancer Inst 1975;54:855–60.

83. Ramos-Vara JA, Miller MA, Johnson GC, et al. Melan A and S100 protein immunohistochemistry in feline melanomas: 48 cases. Vet Pathol 2002;39:127–32.

84. Carpenter JL, Andrews LK, Holzworth J. Tumors and tumor-like lesions. In: Holzworth J, editor. Diseases of the Cat. Medicine and Surgery. Philadelphia, PA: WB Saunders; 1987. p. 407–596.

85. Patnaik AK, Mooney S. Feline melanoma: a comparative study of ocular, oral, and dermal neoplasms. Vet Pathol 1988;25:105–12.

86. Luna LD, Higginbotham ML, Henry CJ, et al. Feline non-ocular melanoma: a retrospective study of 23 cases (1991–1999). J Feline Med Surg 2000;1:173–81.

87. Farrelly J, Denman DL, Hohenhaus AE, et al. A retrospective analysis of hypofractionated radiation therapy for the treatment of oral melanoma in five cats. Vet Rad Ultrasound 2003;45:91–3.

88. Thrall DE. Orthovoltage radiotherapy of oral fibrosarcomas in dogs. J Am Vet Med Assoc 1981;179:159–62.

89. Poirier VJ, Bley CR, Roos M, et al. Efficacy of radiation therapy for the treatment of macroscopic canine oral soft tissue sarcoma. In Vivo 2006;20:415–19.

90. Forrest LJ, Chun R, Adams WM, et al. Postoperative radiotherapy for canine soft tissue sarcomas. J Vet Intern Med 2000;14:578–82.

91. Ciekot PA, Powers BE, Withrow SJ, et al. Histologically low-grade, yet biologically high-grade, fibrosarcomas of the mandible and maxilla in dogs: 25 cases (1982–1991). J Am Vet Med Assoc 1994;204:610–15.

92. Misdorp W, Hart AAM. Some prognostic and epidemiologic factors in canine osteosarcoma. J Natl Cancer Inst 1979;62:537–45.

93. Heyman SJ, Diefenderfer DL, Goldschmidt MH, et al. Canine axial skeletal osteosarcoma. A retrospective study of 116 cases (1986 to 1989). Vet Surg 1992;21:304–10.

94. Liu SK, Dorfman HD, Hurvitz AI, et al. Primary and secondary bone tumours in the dog. J Small Anim Pract 1977;18:313–26.

95. Hammer AS, Weeren FR, Weisbrode SE, et al. Prognostic factors in dogs with osteosarcomas of the flat or irregular bones. J Am Anim Hosp Assoc 1995;31:321–6.

96. Straw RC, Powers BE, Klausner J, et al. Canine mandibular osteosarcoma: 51 cases (1980–1992). J Am Anim Hosp Assoc 1996;32:257–62.

97. Dickerson ME, Page RL, LaDue TA, et al. Retrospective analysis of axial skeleton osteosarcoma in 22 large-breed dogs. J Vet Intern Med 2001;15:120–4.

98. Boston SE, Ehrhart NP, Dernell WS, et al. Evaluation of survival time in dogs with

stage III osteosarcoma that undergo treatment: 90 cases (1985–2004). J Am Vet Med Assoc 2006;228:1905–8.

99. Bitetto WV, Patnaik AK, Schrader SC, et al. Osteosarcoma in cats: 22 cases (1974–1984). J Am Vet Med Assoc 1987;190:91–3.

100. Liu SK, Dorfman HD, Patnaik AK. Primary and secondary bone tumours in the cat. J Small Anim Pract 1974;15: 141–56.

101. Heldmann E, Anderson MA, Wagner-Mann C. Feline osteosarcoma: 145 cases (1990–1995). J Am Anim Hosp Assoc 2000;36:518–21.

102. Straw RC, LeCouteur RA, Powers BE, et al. Multilobular osteochondrosarcoma of the canine skull: 16 cases (1978–1988). J Am Vet Med Assoc 1989;195: 1764–1769.

103. Dernell WS, Straw RC, Cooper MF, et al. Multilobular osteochondrosarcoma in 39 dogs: 1979–1993. J Am Anim Hosp Assoc 1998;34:11–18.

104. Morton D. Chondrosarcoma arising from multilobular chondroma in a cat. J Am Vet Med Assoc 1985;186:804–6.

105. Hathcock JT, Newton JC. Computed tomographic characteristics of multilobular tumor of bone involving the cranium in 7 dogs and zygomatic arch in 2 dogs. Vet Radiol Ultrasound 2000;41:214–17.

106. Lipsitz D, Levitski RE, Berry WL. Magnetic resonance imaging features of multilobular osteochondrosarcoma in 3 dogs. Vet Radiol Ultrasound 2001;42: 14–19.

107. Patnaik AK, Lieberman PH, Erlandson RA, et al. A clinicopathologic and ultrastructural study of undifferentiated malignant tumors of the oral cavity in dogs. Vet Pathol 1986;23:170–5.

108. Rackich PM, Latimer KS, Weiss R, et al. Mucocutaneous plasmacytomas in dogs: 75 cases (1980–1987). J Am Vet Med Assoc 1989;194:803–10.

109. Clark GN, Berg J, Engler SJ, et al. Extramedullary plasmacytomas in dogs: results of surgical excision in 131 cases. J Am Anim Hosp Assoc 1992;28:105–11.

110. Baer KE, Patnaik AK, Gilbertson SR, et al. Cutaneous plasmacytomas in dogs: a morphologic and immunohistochemical study. Vet Pathol 1989;26:216–21.

111. Wright ZM, Rogers KS, Mansell J. Survival data for canine oral extramedullary plasmacytomas: a retrospective analysis (1996–2006). J Am Anim Hosp Assoc 2008;44:75–81.

112. Rassnick KM, Gieger TL, Williams LE, et al. Phase I evaluation of CCNU (lomustine) in tumor-bearing cats. J Vet Intern Med 2001;15:196–9.

113. Elmslie RE, Ogilvie GK, Gillette EL, et al. Radiotherapy with and without chemotherapy for localized lymphoma in 10 cats. Vet Radiol 1991;32:277–80.

114. Whiteley LA, Leininger JR. Neuroendocrine (merkel) cell tumors of the canine oral cavity. Vet Pathol 1987; 24:570–2.

115. Wright ZM, Chretin JD. Diagnosis and treatment of a feline oral mast cell tumor. J Fel Med Surg 2006;8:285–9.

116. Turk MAM, Johnson GC, Gallina AM, et al. Canine granular cell tumor (myoblastoma): a report of four cases and review of the literature. J Small Anim Pract 1983;24:637–45.

117. Johannes CM, Henry CJ, Turnquist SE, et al. Hemangiosarcoma in cats: 53 cases (1992–2002). J Am Vet Med Assoc 2007;231:1851–6.

118. Nicholls PK, Klaunberg BA, Moore RA, et al. Naturally occurring, nonregressing canine oral papillomavirus infection: host immunity, virus characterization, and experimental infection. Virology 1999;265:365–74.

119. Bredal WP, Thoresen SI, Rimstad E, et al. Diagnosis and clinical course of canine oral papillomavirus infection. J Small Anim Pract 1996;37:138–42.

120. Le Net JL, Orth G, Sundberg JP, et al. Multiple pigmented cutaneous papules associated with a novel canine papillomavirus in an immunosuppressed dog. Vet Pathol 1997;34:8–14.

121. Sundberg JP, Smith EK, Herron AJ, et al. Involvement of canine oral papillomavirus in generalized oral and cutaneous verrucosis in a Chinese Shar-Pei dog. Vet Pathol 1994;31:183–7.

122. Jarrett WF, O'Neil BW, Gaukroger JM, et al. Studies on vaccination against papillomaviruses: a comparison of purified virus, tumour extract and transformed cells in prophylactic vaccination. Vet Rec 1990;126:449–52.

123. Jarrett WF, O'Neil BW, Gaukroger JM, et al. Studies on vaccination against papillomaviruses: the immunity after infection and vaccination with bovine papillomaviruses of different types. Vet Rec 1990;126:473–5.

124. Suzich JA, Ghim SJ, Palmer-Hill FJ, et al. Systemic immunization with papillomavirus L1 protein completely prevents the development of viral mucosal papillomas. Proc Natl Acad Sci USA 1995;92:11553–7.

125. Bell JA, Sundberg JP, Ghim SJ, et al. A formalin-inactivated vaccine protects against mucosal papillomavirus infection: a canine model. Pathobiology 1994;62: 194–8.

126. Kuntsi-Vaattovaara H, Verstraete FJM, Newsome JT, et al. Resolution of persistent oral papillomatosis in a dog after treatment with a recombinant canine oral papillomavirus vaccine. Vet Comp Oncol 2003;1:57–63.

127. Sundberg JP, Van Ranst M, Montali R, et al. Feline papillomas and papillomaviruses. Vet Pathol 2000;37:1–10.

128. Seifert G. Histological typing of salivary gland tumours. 2nd ed. New York: Springer Verlag; 1991.

129. Spangler WL, Culbertson MR. Salivary gland disease in dogs and cats: 245 cases (1985–1988). J Am Vet Med Assoc 1991;198:465–9.

130. Mazzullo G, Sfacteria A, Iannelli N, et al. Carcinoma of the submandibular salivary glands with multiple metastases in a cat. Vet Clin Pathol 2005;34:61–4.

131. Thomsen BV, Myers RK. Extraskeletal osteosarcoma of the mandibular salivary gland in a dog. Vet Pathol 1999;36:71–3.

132. Carberry CA, Flanders JA, Anderson WI, et al. Mast cell tumor in the mandibular salivary gland in a dog. Cornell Vet 1987;77:362–6.

133. Stubbs WP, Voges AK, Shiroma JT, et al. What is your diagnosis? Infiltrative lipoma with chronic salivary duct obstruction. J Am Vet Med Assoc 1996; 209:55–6.

134. Bindseil E, Madsen JS. Lipomatosis causing tumour-like swelling of a mandibular salivary gland in a dog. Vet Rec 1997;140:583–4.

135. Faustino AM, Pereira PD. A salivary malignant myoepithelioma in a dog. The Vet Journal 2007;173:223–6.

136. Carberry CA, Flanders JA, Harvey HJ, et al. Salivary gland tumors in dogs and cats: a literature review and case review. J Am Anim Hosp Assoc 1988; 24:561–7.

137. Brocks BA, Peeters ME, Kimpfler S. Oncocytoma in the mandibular salivary gland of a cat. J Feline Med and Surg 2008;10:188–91.

138. Evans SM, Thrall DE. Postoperative orthovoltage radiation therapy of parotid salivary gland adenocarcinoma in three dogs. J Am Anim Hosp Assoc 1983; 182:993–4.

139. Hammer A, Getzy D, Ogilvie G, et al. Salivary gland neoplasia in the dog and cat: survival times and prognostic factors. J Am Anim Hosp Assoc 2001;37: 478–82.

140. Kim H, Nakaichi M, Itamoto K, et al. Malignant mixed tumor in the salivary gland of a cat. J Vet Sci 2008;9:331–3.

141. Sozmen M, Brown PJ, Eveson JW. Salivary duct carcinoma in five cats. J Comp Pathol 1999;121:311–19.

Chapter | **41** |

Clinical behavior of odontogenic tumors

Thomas P. Chamberlain & Milinda J. Lommer

GENERAL CONSIDERATIONS

Odontogenic tumors (OT) arise from remnants of the embryonic tissues destined to develop into teeth and associated structures.[1,2] They originate from remnants of odontogenic epithelium (rests of Malassez and rests of Serres located within the periodontal ligament stroma and gingiva, respectively), odontogenic mesenchyme, or a combination of the cellular elements that comprise the tooth-forming apparatus.[2–4] Clinical behavior ranges from hamartoma-like proliferations to benign and invasive neoplasms.[1,2] Table 41.1 lists odontogenic tumors according to their behavior and potential for recurrence. Although the etiology and pathogenesis remain unknown, fundamental knowledge of odontogenesis is important to understanding the categorization and biologic behavior of these neoplasms.[3] Histologically, OT may mimic some stage of the developing tooth bud.[4] There may be soft tissues of the dental organ or dental pulp, or they may contain hard tissue elements of enamel, dentin, and/or cementum.[1,2]

With the exception of the canine peripheral odontogenic fibroma (formerly fibromatous epulis) and canine acanthomatous ameloblastoma (formerly acanthomatous epulis), OT are considered uncommon in animals.[4,5] The most detailed information on OT is obtained from human studies; however, this knowledge is not always transferable to companion animals and it must be appreciated that incidence, morphology and biological behavior variations occur between different species.[4]

Although there are several studies addressing the incidence of oral and odontogenic tumors in animals, there have been no recent additions to the literature.[5–12] The actual incidence is unknown because of confusion over nomenclature (tissue of origin) and the fact that many clinicians do not routinely submit specimens for histopathological identification.[4,13] Gingival enlargements are often considered simply as hyperplastic or inflammatory lesions and not submitted for definitive diagnosis.[3,14] A bias is, therefore, incorporated into studies based on archival material.[13]

Historically, OT have fallen under the heading of *'epulides' (singular epulis)*. The term 'epulis' has no specific histopathologic connotation and is a clinical designation for any localized, exophytic swelling on the gingiva.[13,15,16] The term is still commonly utilized and is a source of confusion, as several different pathologic entities are categorized as epulides. Generally, epulides can be divided into three groups: (1) reactive lesions; (2) odontogenic tumors and cysts; and (3) nonodontogenic tumors (typically malignant).[15] It is erroneous to consider all epulides as benign and inconsequential. In dogs, many epulides are actually OT and their true nature as such should be determined histologically by pathologists with formal training in the pathology of odontogenic tumors and cysts.[13] Differential diagnosis of odontogenic tumors is presented in Table 41.2.

Since the mid-1950s, there has been an evolution in the systems used to categorize OT in humans and in animals. Originally, OT classification was based upon differences in the so-called 'reciprocal inductive phenomena' noted in normal odontogenesis and in the pathogenesis of many OT.[17,18] This original system was based on the reciprocal inductive effect of the odontogenic epithelium on adjacent connective tissue (the internal enamel epithelium induces adjacent mesenchymal cells of the dental papilla to differentiate into odontoblasts, which form dentin. The dentin then induces the internal enamel epithelium to differentiate into ameloblasts).[4] Although this system was easier to comprehend, it was incomplete and confusing because not all OT have inductive properties and some are largely mesenchymal in origin.[4,5,12,19,20] Ensuing classification advances utilized the tissue of origin as the basis for distinguishing OT. The three

Table 41.1 Biologic classification of odontogenic tumors	
Benign, little recurrence potential Odontoma	**Benign, locally aggressive** Central ameloblastoma Acanthomatous ameloblastoma Amyloid-producing odontogenic tumor Feline inductive odontogenic tumor
Benign, some recurrence potential Peripheral odontogenic fibroma	**Malignant*** Ameloblastic fibro-odontoma Odontogenic myxoma Ameloblastic carcinoma
* Malignant odontogenic tumors are extremely rare in dogs and cats	

© 2012 Elsevier Ltd
DOI: 10.1016/B978-0-7020-4618-6.00041-5

Table 41.2 Differential diagnosis of odontogenic tumors

Localized gingival enlargements

Reactive lesions
Focal fibrous hyperplasia
Pyogenic granuloma
Peripheral giant cell granuloma
Reactive exostosis
Odontogenic tumors
Peripheral odontogenic fibroma
Canine acanthomatous ameloblastoma
Central ameloblastoma
Odontoma
Odontogenic cysts
Dentigerous cyst
Odontogenic keratocyst (keratocystic odontogenic tumor)
Nonodontogenic tumors (see Ch. 40)

Gross swellings with distortion of bone

Odontogenic tumors
Peripheral odontogenic fibroma
Canine acanthomatous ameloblastoma
Central ameloblastoma
Odontoma
Odontogenic cysts
Dentigerous cyst
Odontogenic keratocyst (keratocystic odontogenic tumor)
Nonodontogenic tumors (see Ch. 40)

Osteolytic and cystic lesions

Odontogenic tumors
Central ameloblastoma
Amyloid-producing odontogenic tumor
Odontogenic cysts
Radicular cyst
Dentigerous cyst
Odontogenic keratocyst (keratocystic odontogenic tumor)

resulting groups are: (1) those consisting of odontogenic epithelium *without* odontogenic mesenchyme; (2) tumors arising from odontogenic epithelium and mesenchymal cells, with or without dental hard tissue formation; and (3) those consisting primarily of mesenchyme, with or without odontogenic epithelium.[2,4,19,20] In 1998, it was noted that major enamel matrix proteins (amelogenins) were expressed by some naturally occurring animal and human OT and may provide a new approach to typing OT.[21] In 2002, a revision was suggested to the World Health Organization's 1992 typing of OT.[19,22] Inclusion of immunochemistry and molecular biology methodologies was recommended.[19,23] These revisions were adopted in 2005.[24] Although traditional histopathology remains the gold standard for diagnosis, future advancements in OT classification schemes are likely to be based upon genetic, molecular biologic and immunochemical criteria.[21,25]

EPITHELIAL TUMORS

Ameloblastoma

Ameloblastoma is an epithelial tumor that originates from remnants of the dental organ (rests of Malessez), dental lamina, cells of epithelial origin lining odontogenic cysts or possibly from basal epithelial cells of the oral mucosa.[5,12–14,26] It is a noninductive (no effect on surrounding mesenchyme) tumor described in many domestic species, and occurs in the tooth-bearing areas of the mandible, maxilla and incisive bone.[4–6,12,14–16,27,28] Because there is no production of enamel or dentin, it remains a soft tissue tumor and is considered the least differentiated of the epithelial OT.[3,5,12] In spite of a benign appearance histologically in animals, ameloblastoma typically is a locally invasive, slowly growing neoplasm that does not metastasize.[4,12,15,26] The stimulus for neoplastic transformation of odontogenic epithelium is unknown; however, some of the molecular pathogenesis of ameloblastoma has been elucidated and includes overexpression of several proteins including tumor necrosis factor alpha, anti-apoptotic proteins and other molecules that appear to enhance the proliferative and invasive properties of this tumor.[29–31] Because ameloblastoma may have a variety of histologic patterns, variants and subtypes are defined.[5,18,28] The differentiation between subtypes is of importance when treatment modalities are considered.[19] Hypercalcemia of malignancy has been associated with ameloblastoma in dogs, horses and humans.[32–34]

Central (or intraosseous) ameloblastoma

Clinical features

The central ameloblastoma is a relatively uncommon odontogenic tumor in dogs.[4,5] It usually manifests as a gross swelling with distortion of bone; however, the presenting complaint may be notable tooth displacement or malocclusion.[2] Because it is usually painless, with slow expansion, patients may be asymptomatic.[4,26] Central ameloblastoma most often appears radiographically as an osteolytic, unilocular or multilocular cystic lesion around tooth roots, with well-defined, sclerotic margins (Fig. 41.1).[2,3,15] Jaw expansion with

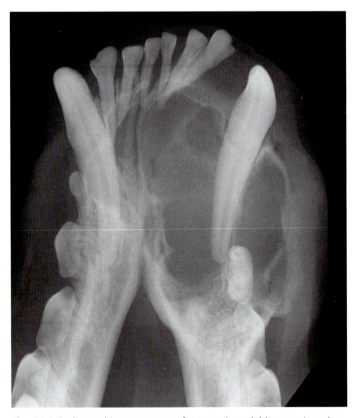

Fig. 41.1 Radiographic appearance of a central ameloblastoma in a dog. *(From Self-Assessment Colour Review of Veterinary Dentistry, edited by Frank Verstraete. Manson Publishing Ltd, London, 1999.)*

or without cortical thinning is usually apparent.[2,15] In cats, amelo-blastoma is considered rare and is sometimes confused with other more common types of odontogenic tumors in this species.[28] Two histologic variants have been reported in cats: a follicular pattern similar to that in humans, and a keratinizing pattern similar to that in dogs.[28]

Histopathology

The classical histological appearance of an ameloblastoma includes palisading of columnar basal epithelial cells perpendicular to the basement membrane, polarization of basal cell nuclei away from the basement membrane (reverse polarization) and hyperchromatic nuclei. Stellate reticulum may or may not be present focally.[4,5,12,14,35] Ameloblastoma in the dog may have a prominent feature of the central cells undergoing varying degrees of keratinization with subse-quent calcification of the keratin.[35] This is referred to as keratinizing ameloblastoma.[35,36]

Treatment recommendations

Wide surgical excision (mandibulectomy or maxillectomy) is the treat-ment of choice.[12] In a survey of 12 dogs with central or keratinizing ameloblastomas, local recurrence was noted in two of two patients who were treated with local nonaggressive surgery (curettage only) and three of four patients treated with radiation therapy and for whom follow-up information was available.[36] Conversely, three of three patients who were treated with radical surgical excision remained tumor-free with follow-up of up to 28 months.[36]

Prognosis

Wide surgical excision is considered curative.[12,36]

Canine acanthomatous ameloblastoma

The second common histologic variant of ameloblastoma found in dogs is the canine acanthomatous ameloblastoma (CAA). In two feline surveys, no acanthomatous ameloblastoma was diagnosed.[6,7] In previous classification schemes, this was called acanthomatous epulis and was distinguished biologically and histologically from other types of epulides by their tendency to infiltrate cancellous bone.[4,16,24] The acanthomatous epulis was later recognized as a type of ameloblast-oma and termed a peripheral ameloblastoma.[13] The term peripheral ameloblastoma was later replaced by canine acanthomatous amelo-blastoma, to differentiate it from the peripheral ameloblastoma in humans, which is a noninvasive tumor type.[37] Acanthomatous amelo-blastoma also arises from remnants of odontogenic epithelium located in the gingiva (rests of Serres) in the tooth-bearing areas of the jaws.[16,24] Although CAA is generally accepted as arising from gin-gival epithelium, it may also arise intraosseously and then break out of bone.[37]

Clinical features

Acanthomatous ameloblastoma typically appears as an exophytic gingival mass with an irregular surface (Fig. 41.2A). It is considered to be a benign tumor with invasive properties into surrounding bone. The infiltration of bone distinguishes the CAA from central ameloblastoma.[24] The radiographic pattern is dominated by bony infiltration, alveolar bone resorption and tooth displacement (Fig. 41.2B).[3,13]

Histopathology

Histologically, CAA is composed of islands and sheets of mature cells that are clearly squamous epithelium.[13,37] The connective tissue com-ponent is typically of low to moderate cellularity; however, the stroma

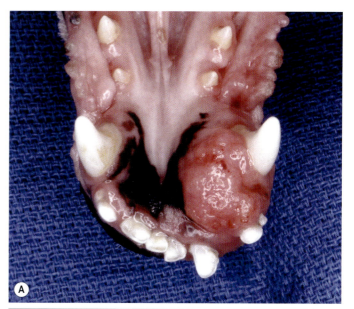

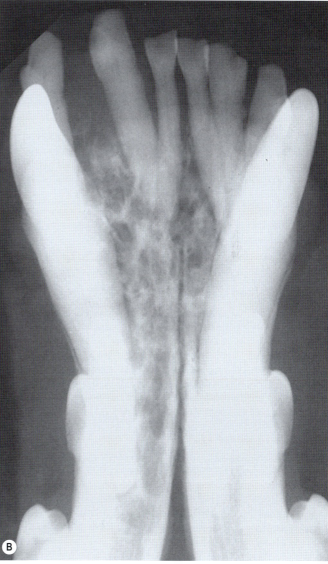

Fig. 41.2 (**A**) Clinical and (**B**) radiographic appearance of an acanthomatous ameloblastoma in a dog.

may be variable, similar to the dense connective tissue of the gingiva, fibroblastic connective tissue of the periodontal ligament or the loose connective tissue of bone marrow.[13,37] The epithelial islands and sheets are each bounded by a row of palisading cells with reverse nuclear polarization, and infiltration in the underlying bone is evident in most cases.[13]

Treatment recommendations

Because acanthomatous ameloblastoma is locally aggressive and invades bone, curative surgical treatment requires en bloc excision of the tumor and at least 1 cm of normal-appearing tissue.[38] This is typically achieved by performing partial mandibulectomy or maxillectomy.[3] Radiation therapy is also an option, and good results have been reported.[39–42] However, there is significant risk of osteoradionecrosis,[42,43] which can lead to permanent oronasal fistula formation. In addition, malignant tumor formation has been reported in up to 18% of previously irradiated sites.[41,43,44] Therefore, wide surgical excision is considered the treatment of choice for acanthomatous ameloblastoma.[38]

Prognosis

If the tumor is completely excised, the prognosis is excellent. Following wide local excision, one author reported a 1-year survival rate of 100% among 25 dogs,[38] while another study reported a 97% 1-year survival rate among 42 dogs.[45] In the latter, excision was incomplete in one dog, resulting in local recurrence of the tumor.[45]

Amyloid-producing odontogenic tumor

This OT type is rare in dogs and cats and presents as an 'epulis' on either jaw in patients between 8 to 13 years old.[16,46] It has been previously referred to in the veterinary literature as a calcifying epithelial odontogenic tumor, although it has been determined not to be equivalent to the human calcifying epithelial odontogenic tumor.[12,46,47]

Clinical features

Amyloid-producing odontogenic tumor (APOT) appears as a gingival enlargement which grows by expansion. It is locally invasive but not metastatic.[47] It often has a cystic appearance on radiographs (Fig. 41.3).

Histopathology

Histologically, APOT is a very cellular epithelial tumor. It bears some resemblance to an ameloblastoma: the epithelium in some areas exhibits palisading of the basal cells, reverse polarization of nuclei, stellate reticulum and collagenous matrix are variable focal findings.[16,37] Amyloid (Congo red stain) which tends to calcify may be present in some parts of the tumor.[16] Any epithelial tumor of the jaws that exhibits amyloid should be suspected of being odontogenic in origin.[4]

Treatment recommendations

Although metastasis has not been observed, local recurrence may occur after incomplete excision.[5,48] Radiation therapy has reportedly been successful in preventing recurrence in one cat after incomplete surgical excision.[49] One author reports no evidence of local recurrence after marginal excision in one dog and two cats, with follow-up ranging from 7 to 19 months.[50] However, for definitive treatment, wide excision is recommended.

Prognosis

Complete excision is considered curative.[51]

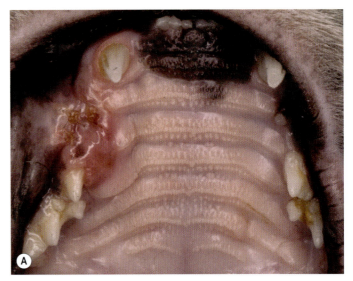

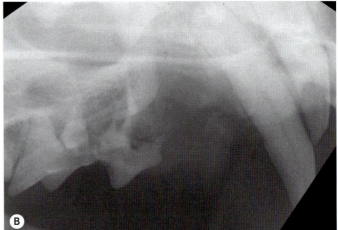

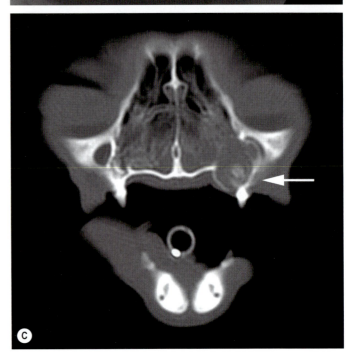

Fig. 41.3 (**A**) Clinical, (**B**) radiographic and (**C**) computed tomographic appearance of an amyloid-producing odontogenic tumor in a cat.

Feline inductive odontogenic tumor

Clinical features

This tumor type is unique to young cats (usually 8 to 18 months).[3,7,15,52,53] It was originally described as inductive fibroameloblastoma.[7] Feline inductive odontogenic tumor (FIOT) is a raised submucosal soft tissue mass typically located on the rostral maxilla (Fig. 41.4).[15,52,53]

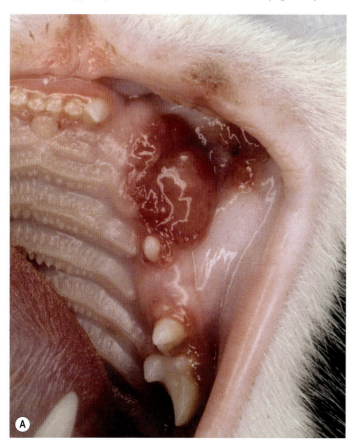

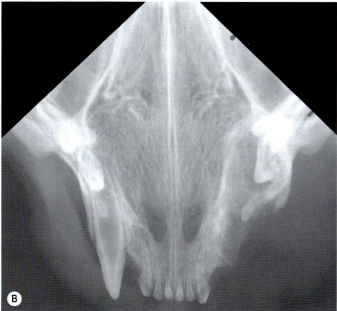

Fig. 41.4 (A) Clinical and (**B**) radiographic appearance of a feline-inductive odontogenic tumor. Note the absence of the left maxillary canine tooth in the region of the tumor, a hallmark of this tumor type.

The tumor may be locally invasive, but metastasis has not been recorded.[3,15]

Histopathology

This tumor is characterized histologically by multifocal formations of spherical condensations of fibroblastic connective tissue associated with islands of odontogenic epithelium dispersed throughout the connective tissue stroma.[52,53] The ameloblastic-type epithelial cells may appear arranged around a dental pulp-like stroma of ectomesenchymal tissue.[7,52]

Treatment recommendations

Wide surgical excision is the treatment of choice. Radiation therapy has reportedly been successful in preventing recurrence in one cat after incomplete surgical excision.[49]

Prognosis

The biologic behavior of FIOT appears to be similar to that of other locally invasive but benign odontogenic neoplasms: wide surgical excision is considered curative, with local recurrence expected after incomplete excision.[52,53]

MESENCHYMAL TUMORS

Peripheral odontogenic fibroma

Many of the tumors previously described as fibromatous and ossifying epulides have been reclassified as peripheral odontogenic fibroma (POF).[13,16]

Clinical features

Peripheral odontogenic fibroma is a slowly growing, benign neoplasm that is common in the dog and uncommon in the cat.[5–7,13,16] Surface epithelium appears normal, and radiographic features vary according to the presence and amount of mineralized products (Fig. 41.5).[13]

Histopathology

Histologically, POF is characterized by a low-grade neoplastic proliferation of fibroblastic connective tissue of variable cellularity in which a variety of bone, osteoid, dentinoid (dentin-like) or even cementum-like material is present (Fig. 41.6). Isolated islands or strands of proliferative odontogenic epithelium are found in close association with foci of hard tissues, suggesting induction.[7,13,16]

Treatment recommendations

Definitive treatment typically requires en bloc resection of the mass and underlying bone. In one survey including 17 dogs with peripheral odontogenic fibromas which were marginally excised (i.e., without including the underlying bone), three of the tumors recurred.[14] En bloc resection has been reported to result in tumor-free margins and local cure in two cases which had previously recurred following radiation therapy[54] or marginal excision.[55]

Prognosis

Incomplete excision and local recurrence can result in difficulty with prehension and mastication; one author reported mortality secondary to malnutrition following recurrence of an incompletely excised 'ossifying epulis.'[56] Complete excision, which may be achieved with en bloc resection of the mass and underlying bone, is considered curative.

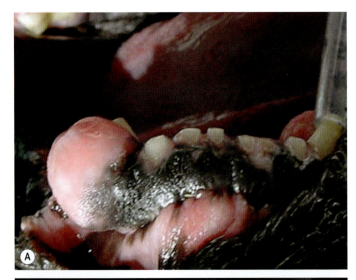

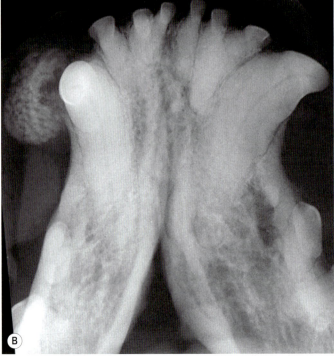

Fig. 41.5 (**A**) Clinical and (**B**) radiographic appearance of a peripheral odontogenic fibroma adjacent to right mandibular canine tooth in a dog.

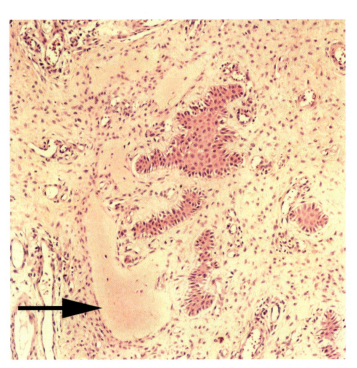

Fig. 41.6 Histopathologic appearance of a peripheral odontogenic fibroma. Note the foci of mineralization, the largest of which is marked with an arrow.

MIXED (MESENCHYMAL AND EPITHELIAL) TUMORS

Odontoma

Odontomas are benign inductive tumors diagnosed in young dogs and cats, generally appearing at 6 to 18 months of age.[4,5,12,18,57–61] They are the most common OT in humans and may be associated with an unerupted tooth, a dentigerous cyst, or attached to an otherwise normal tooth.[3,4] Because odontoma contains well-differentiated cells, it is characterized by the simultaneous occurrence of a composite of soft and hard dental tissues (enamel, dentin, cementum, dental

papilla) of both epithelial and mesenchymal origin.[2,4,5] Odontoma may be considered a non-neoplastic hamartoma.[4] Hamartoma is a tumor-like malformation derived from local cellular hyperactivity, and is composed of excessive cells and tissues (native to a part) which arise during development.[62,63] The dental tissues in odontomas may or may not exhibit a normal relation to one another. An odontoma in which rudimentary tooth-like structures are present indicates advanced cellular differentiation and is referred to as a *compound* odontoma. An odontoma in which the conglomerate of dental tissues is disorderly, bearing no resemblance to a tooth, is called a *complex* odontoma.[3–5,12] The radiological appearance is typical: either a sharply defined mass of calcified material surrounded by a narrow radiolucent band (complex odontoma), or a variable number of tooth-like structures (compound odontoma) are present.[3] If identified in its early stages, the lesion may be primarily radiolucent with focal areas of opacifying hard dental tissue.[2] Complex odontomas appear as opaque amorphous masses while compound odontomas appear as numerous tiny tooth-like structures in a focal area (Fig. 41.7).[2] The term ameloblastic odontoma is occasionally encountered in the veterinary literature, and represents an ameloblastoma with focal differentiation into an odontoma.[4,5,12] Because odontomas are not true neoplasms, marginal excision and/or curettage to remove the abnormal material may be curative.

MALIGNANT ODONTOGENIC TUMORS

Malignant odontogenic tumors are considered extremely rare; however, several have been reported in the dog.[64–66] As with nonodontogenic malignant tumors, it is advisable to consult with an oncologist prior to determining a treatment plan (see Ch. 40).

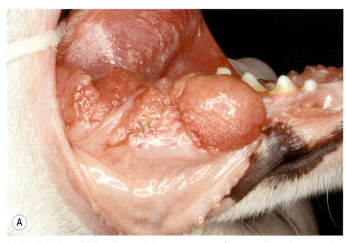
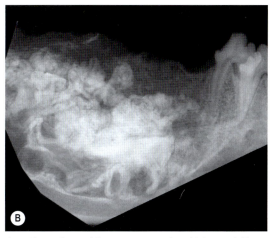

Fig. 41.7 (**A**) Clinical and (**B**) radiographic appearance of a complex odontoma in a dog. The radiographic appearance of multiple tooth-like structures is pathognomonic.

REACTIVE LESIONS

Reactive lesions are non-neoplastic gingival enlargements that are commonly grouped under the previously noted nondescript classification of *Epulides*. Reactive lesions include focal fibrous hyperplasia, pyogenic granuloma, peripheral giant cell granuloma and reactive exostosis.[13,15,16,67–69] Marginal excision of these lesions, without inclusion of adjacent normal tissue, is generally sufficient, as local recurrence is uncommon. Further discussion of reactive lesions is found in Chapter 42.

REFERENCES

1. Eversole LR, Tomich CE, Cherrick HM. Histogenesis of odontogenic tumors. Oral Surg Oral Med Oral Pathol 1971;32:569–81.
2. Regezi JA, Sciubba JJ, Jordan RK. Odontogenic Tumors. In: Oral pathology – clinical pathologic correlations. 5th ed. St. Louis, MO: Saunders Elsevier; 2008. p. 261–82.
3. Verstraete FJM. Oral pathology. In: Slatter DH, editor. Textbook of small animal surgery. 3rd ed. Philadelphia, PA: WB Saunders Co; 2003. p. 2638–51.
4. Gardner DG. An orderly approach to the study of odontogenic tumours in animals. J Comp Pathol 1992;107:427–38.
5. Poulet FM, Valentine BA, Summers BA. A survey of epithelial odontogenic tumors and cysts in dogs and cats. Vet Pathol 1992;29:369–80.
6. Colgin LM, Schulman FY, Dubielzig RR. Multiple epulides in 13 cats. Vet Pathol 2001;38:227–9.
7. Stebbins KE, Morse CC, Goldschmidt MH. Feline oral neoplasia: a ten-year survey. Vet Pathol 1989;26:121–8.
8. Todoroff RJ, Brodey RS. Oral and pharyngeal neoplasia in the dog: a retrospective survey of 361 cases. J Am Vet Med Assoc 1979;175:567–71.
9. Dorn CR, Priester WA. Epidemiologic analysis of oral and pharyngeal cancer in dogs, cats, horses, and cattle. J Am Vet Med Assoc 1976;169:1202–6.
10. Engle GC, Brodey RS. A retrospective study of 395 feline neoplasms. J Am Anim Hosp Assoc 1969;5:21–31.
11. Cohen D, Brodey RS, Chen SM. Epidemiological aspects of oral and pharyngeal neoplasms of the dog. Am J Vet Res 1964;25:1776–9.
12. Walsh KM, Denholm LJ, Cooper BJ. Epithelial odontogenic tumours in domestic animals. J Comp Pathol 1987;97:503–21.
13. Verstraete FJ, Ligthelm AJ, Weber A. The histological nature of epulides in dogs. J Comp Pathol 1992;106:169–82.
14. Bostock DE, White RAS. Classification and behaviour after surgery of canine 'epulides'. J Comp Pathol 1987;97:197–206.
15. Verstraete FJM. Self-assessment color review of veterinary dentistry. 1st ed. Ames, IA: Iowa State University Press; 1999.
16. Gardner DG. Epulides in the dog: a review. J Oral Pathol Med 1996;25: 32–7.
17. Gorlin RJ, Chaudhry A, Pindborg JJ. Odontogenic tumors – classification, histopathology, and clinical behavior in man and domesticated animals. Cancer 1961;14:73–101.
18. Pindborg JJ, Clausen F. Classification of odontogenic tumors: a suggestion. Acta Odontol Scand 1958;848–53.
19. Philipsen HP, Reichart PA. Revision of the 1992-edition of the WHO histological typing of odontogenic tumours. A suggestion. J Oral Pathol Med 2002;31: 253–8.
20. Philipsen HP, Reichart PA. Classification of odontogenic tumours. A historical review. J Oral Pathol Med 2006;35:525–9.
21. Yuasa Y, Kraegel SA, Verstraete FJM, et al. Amelogenin expression in canine oral tissues and lesions. J Comp Pathol 1998; 119:15–25.
22. Kramer IRH, Pindborg JJ, Shear M. Histological typing of odontogenic tumours. 2nd ed. Berlin & New York: Springer-Verlag; 1992.

23. Gao YH, Yang LJ, Yamaguchi A. Immunohistochemical demonstration of bone morphogenetic protein in odontogenic tumors. J Oral Pathol Med 1997;26:273–7.

24. Barnes L, Eveson JW, Reichart P, et al. World Health Organization classification of tumours – pathology and genetics of head and neck tumours. Lyon, France: IARC Press; 2005.

25. Philipsen HP, Reichart PA. Classification of odontogenic tumours. A historical review. J Oral Pathol Med 2006;35:525–9.

26. Ghandhi D, Ayoub AF, Pogrel MA, et al. Ameloblastoma: a surgeon's dilemma. J Oral Maxillofac Surg 2006;64:1010–14.

27. Verstraete FJM, Ligthelm AJ, Weber A. The histological nature of epulides in dogs. J Comp Pathol 1992;106:169–82.

28. Gardner DG. Ameloblastomas in cats: a critical evaluation of the literature and the addition of one example. J Oral Pathol Med 1998;27:39–42.

29. Kumamoto H, Ooya K. Immunohistochemical analysis of bcl-2 family proteins in benign and malignant ameloblastomas. J Oral Pathol Med 1999;28:343–9.

30. Kumamoto H. Molecular pathology of odontogenic tumors. J Oral Pathol Med 2006;35:65–74.

31. Kumamoto H, Ooya K. Expression of tumor necrosis factor alpha, TNF-related apoptosis-inducing ligand, and their associated molecules in ameloblastomas. J Oral Pathol Med 2005;34:287–94.

32. Cox DP, Muller S, Carlson GW, et al. Ameloblastic carcinoma ex ameloblastoma of the mandible with malignancy-associated hypercalcemia. Oral Surg Oral Med Oral Pathol Oral Radiol Endod 2000;90:716–22.

33. Rosol TJ, Nagode LA, Robertson JT, et al. Humoral hypercalcemia of malignancy associated with ameloblastoma in a horse. J Am Vet Med Assoc 1994;204:1930–3.

34. Inoue N, Shimojyo M, Iwai H, et al. Malignant ameloblastoma with pulmonary metastasis and hypercalcemia. Report of an autopsy case and review of the literature. Am J Clin Pathol 1988;90:474–81.

35. Gardner DG, Dubielzig RR. The histopathological features of canine keratinizing ameloblastoma. J Comp Pathol 1993;109:423–8.

36. Dubielzig RR, Thrall DE. Ameloblastoma and keratinizing ameloblastoma in dogs. Vet Pathol 1982;19:596–607.

37. Gardner DG, Baker DC. The relationship of the canine acanthomatous epulis to ameloblastoma. J Comp Pathol 1993; 108:47–55.

38. White RA, Gorman NT. Wide local excision of acanthomatous epulides in the dog. Vet Surg 1989;18:12–14.

39. Langham RF, Mostosky UV, Shirmer RG. X-ray therapy of selected odontogenic neoplasms in the dog. J Am Vet Med Assoc 1977;170:820–2.

40. Langham RF, Keahey KK, Mostosky UV, et al. Oral adamantinomas in dogs. J Am Vet Med Assoc 1965;146:474–80.

41. Thrall DE. Orthovoltage radiotherapy of acanthomatous epulides in 39 dogs. J Am Vet Med Assoc 1984;184:826–9.

42. Theon AP, Rodriguez C, Griffey S, et al. Analysis of prognostic factors and patterns of failure in dogs with periodontal tumors treated with megavoltage irradiation. J Am Vet Med Assoc 1997;210:785–8.

43. Thrall DE, Goldschmidt MH, Biery DN. Malignant tumor formation at the site of previously irradiated acanthomatous epulides in four dogs. J Am Vet Med Assoc 1981;178:127–32.

44. White RAS, Jefferies AR, Gorman NT. Sarcoma development following irradiation of acanthomatous epulis in two dogs. Vet Rec 1986;118:668.

45. Kosovsky JK, Matthiesen DT, Manfra Marretta S, et al. Results of partial mandibulectomy for the treatment of oral tumors in 142 dogs. Vet Surg 1991;20: 397–401.

46. Kuwamura M, Kanehara T, Yamate J, et al. Amyloid-producing odontogenic tumor in a Shih-Tzu dog. J Vet Med Sci 2000;62: 655–7.

47. Ohmachi T, Taniyama H, Nakade T, et al. Calcifying epithelial odontogenic tumours in small domesticated carnivores: histological, immunohistochemical and electron microscopical studies. J Comp Pathol 1996;114:305–14.

48. Gardner DG, Dubielzig RR, McGee EV. The so-called calcifying epithelial odontogenic tumour in dogs and cats (amyloid-producing odontogenic tumour). J Comp Pathol 1994;111:221–30.

49. Moore AS, Wood CA, Engler SJ, et al. Radiation therapy for long-term control of odontogenic tumours and epulis in three cats. J Feline Med Surg 2000;2: 57–60.

50. Abbott DP, Walsh K, Diters RW. Calcifying epithelial odontogenic tumours in three cats and a dog. J Comp Pathol 1986;96: 131–6.

51. Ishikawa T, Yamamoto H. Case of calcifying epithelial odontogenic tumour in a dog. J Small Anim Pract 1996; 37:597–9.

52. Gardner DG, Dubielzig RR. Feline inductive odontogenic tumor (inductive fibroameloblastoma) – a tumor unique to cats. J Oral Pathol Med 1995;24:185–90.

53. Beatty JA, Charles JA, Malik R, et al. Feline inductive odontogenic tumour in a Burmese cat. Aust Vet J 2000;78:452–5.

54. Bracker KE, Trout NJ. Use of a free cortical ulnar autograft following en bloc resection of a mandibular tumor. J Am Anim Hosp Assoc 2000;36:76–9.

55. Woodward TM. Recurrent ossifying epulis in a dog. J Vet Dent 2002;19:82–5.

56. Bjorling DE, Chambers JN, Mahaffey EA. Surgical treatment of epulides in dogs: 25 cases (1974–84). J Am Vet Med Assoc 1987;190:1315–18.

57. Eickhoff M, Seeliger F, Simon D, et al. Erupted bilateral compound odontomas in a dog. J Vet Dent 2002;19:137–43.

58. Felizzola CR, Martins MT, Stopiglia A, et al. Compound odontoma in three dogs. J Vet Dent 2003;20:79–83.

59. Frankel M. Surgical removal of an odontoma in a dog. J Vet Dent 1988; 5:21–2.

60. Hale FA, Wilcock BP. Compound odontoma in a dog. J Vet Dent 1996; 13:93–5.

61. Sowers JM, Gengler WR. Diagnosis and treatment of maxillary compound odontoma. J Vet Dent 2005;22:26–34.

62. Reichart PA, Philipsen HP. Revision der WHO-Klassifikation odontogener Tumoren von 1992. Ein Vorschlag [Revision of the 1992 edition of the WHO histological typing of odontogenic tumors. A suggestion]. Mund Kiefer Gesichtschir 2003;7:88–93.

63. Gardner DG. The concept of hamartomas: its relevance to the pathogenesis of odontogenic lesions. Oral Surg Oral Med Oral Pathol 1978;45:884–6.

64. Ueki H, Sumi A, Takaishi H, et al. Malignant ameloblastic fibro-odontoma in a dog. Vet Pathol 2004;41:183–5.

65. Meyers B, Boy SC, Steenkamp G. Diagnosis and management of odontogenic myxoma in a dog. J Vet Dent 2007;24:166–71.

66. Jimenez MA, Castejon A, San Roman F, et al. Maxillary ameloblastic carcinoma in an Alaskan Malamute. Vet Pathol 2007; 44:84–7.

67. Burstone MS, Bond E, Litt R. Familial gingival hypertrophy in the dog (boxer breed). Arch Pathol 1952;54:208–12.

68. Valentine BA, Eckhaus MA. Peripheral giant cell granuloma (giant cell epulis) in two dogs. Vet Pathol 1986;23:340–1.

69. Regezi JA. Odontogenic cysts, odontogenic tumors, fibroosseous, and giant cell lesions of the jaws. Mod Pathol 2002; 15:331–41.

Chapter | **42** |

Non-neoplastic proliferative oral lesions

Dea Bonello, Celeste G. Roy & Frank J.M. Verstraete

GINGIVAL HYPERPLASIA AND RELATED LESIONS

General considerations

A group of non-neoplastic, reactive conditions occur as tumor-like lesions of the gingiva, as a result of chronic low-grade irritation. These include generalized gingival hyperplasia, focal fibrous hyperplasia, pyogenic granuloma, peripheral giant cell granuloma, peripheral ossifying fibroma and reactive exostosis. The histological classification of these lesions may be confusing, as they present a wide variety of different cellular elements.[1] Hyperplasia implies that the enlargement is caused by an increase in number of cells.[2] In addition, enlargement of the gingiva may also be caused by an excessive accumulation of extracellular matrix proteins. In the latter case, or in the absence of a histopathological diagnosis, the terms gingival enlargement or gingival overgrowth are more appropriate.[3–6]

The clinical appearance of the different types of gingival hyperplasia is not pathognomonic.[1] They generally arise in close proximity to one or more teeth, as a pedunculated or sessile mass, and can be smooth or rough, frequently ulcerated. They show no predilection for the maxilla or the mandible. Occasionally, gingival hyperplasia can be associated with displacement of teeth, with or without radiological signs of bone lysis. Due to the inability to distinguish between them based on clinical appearance, hyperplastic lesions on the gingiva must always be biopsied, and all should be biopsied if multiple lesions are present.[7] Differential diagnoses include benign neoplastic lesions of odontogenic origin, canine acanthomatous ameloblastoma, and various malignant nonodontogenic tumors.

Disease entities

Gingival hyperplasia

Gingival hyperplasia is a proliferation of the attached gingiva, often due to a chronic inflammatory response to the bacteria in plaque, food impaction, dental malposition and dental resorptive lesions.[1,8,9] The histological appearance is characterized by proliferation of the gingival epithelium, ulceration of the sulcular epithelium, in addition to the proliferation of the connective tissue, edema and neoangiogenesis. In a later phase, the connective tissue proliferation and gingival fibrosis predominate, with less or no edema.[1,3] The gingival hyperplasia slowly progresses, if not complicated by trauma or secondary infection. Initially it involves the marginal contour of the gingiva; subsequently it evolves and it can almost completely cover the crowns of the teeth. The slowly growing painless enlargements tend to appear most commonly in areas occupied by teeth, not in edentulous areas.

These lesions can be localized, but often they are generalized, especially in breeds that are believed to have a familial tendency, such as the boxer, collie, Great Dane, Dalmatian and Doberman (Fig. 42.1A).[10] It is characterized by a slow development of enlarged, firm gingival margin, can be symmetrical or localized, and can involve one or more dental quadrants.

Drug-induced gingival enlargement

Drug-induced gingival enlargement or overgrowth occurs mainly in humans but also sporadically in dogs and cats (Fig. 42.1B).[1,4,11–15] The terms *gingival enlargement* and *gingival overgrowth* are preferred for all drug-induced gingival lesions previously termed *gingival hyperplasia* or *gingival hypertrophy*.[3–5] These older terms do not accurately reflect the histopathology of these lesions, which is characterized by excessive accumulation of extracellular matrix proteins, such as collagen, or amorphous ground substance.[4] An inflammatory infiltrate dominated by plasmacytes and thickened keratinized epithelium is typically present.

The three types of drugs that have been documented to cause gingival enlargement are phenytoin derivatives, calcium channel blockers and cyclosporine. Phenytoin is an anticonvulsant which is seen to cause gingival enlargement in human patients with a reported incidence of 50%.[1,4] Two experimental studies in cats and one clinical canine patient with phenytoin-induced gingival enlargement have been documented.[11,12,14] In humans, the extent of enlargement is dependent on the presence of concomitant inflammation and a genetic predisposition to develop lesions. The enlargement is chronic, slow growing, regrows after surgical resection, and usually regresses after the drug is discontinued.[3–5]

© 2012 Elsevier Ltd
DOI: 10.1016/B978-0-7020-4618-6.00042-7

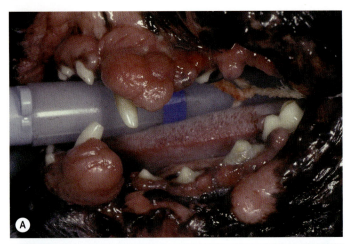

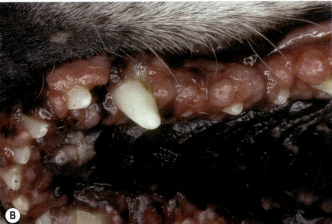

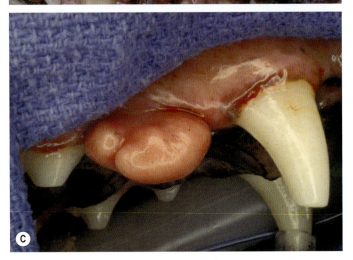

Fig. 42.1 Gingival hyperplasia and related lesions: (**A**) Generalized gingival hyperplasia in a boxer dog; (**B**) Amlodipine-induced gingival enlargement in a dog treated for hypertension; (**C**) Focal fibrous hyperplasia in a dog.

Gingival enlargement caused by calcium channel blockers, e.g., nifedipine and amlodipine, has been documented in the human and veterinary literature.[15-18] As with most drug-related lesions, the presence of the enlarged gingiva makes plaque control difficult, resulting in secondary inflammation that further complicates the condition.[3-5]

Cyclosporine, an immunosuppressive agent, causes slow-growing gingival enlargement in approximately 25% of human patients

treated.[4,5] Cyclosporine-induced enlargement is reversible following cessation of drug administration.[1,3-5] Drug-related lesions are related to the level of oral hygiene and genetic susceptibility. Excellent oral hygiene greatly reduces, but does not eliminate, the occurrence of the lesions.[4,5] Frequent routine periodontal treatment is indicated for cyclosporine-induced gingival enlargement patients.[4,5] Chlorhexidine rinses can reduce the severity of gingival enlargement and may prevent recurrence following gingivectomy.[4,5]

Focal fibrous hyperplasia

Focal fibrous hyperplasia is often referred to as a fibrous or fibromatous epulis in veterinary medicine. It is a different entity from the peripheral odontogenic fibroma, which is a benign neoplastic lesion of odontogenic origin. Focal fibrous hyperplasia is very common in dogs; in one study it was found to account for 43.5% of all 'epulis'-like lesions in dogs.[7] The clinical appearance of focal fibrous hyperplasia is not typical. It is usually a sessile lesion, smooth and pink, and not inflamed or ulcerated (Fig. 42.1C). It consists of dense fibrous connective tissue covered by stratified squamous epithelium.[1,7,19,20] If large enough, it can interfere with mastication.

Pyogenic granuloma

Pyogenic granuloma is a reactive lesion occurring at a specific site on the gingiva, as a result of a chronic low-grade irritation. It mainly consists of granulation tissue, rich in blood vessels, with a high-grade proliferation of endothelial cells and scarce collagen fibers. The superficial layers of the epithelium are usually ulcerated and inflamed.[1,3,7,9,19-22] Calcification may occur in a pyogenic granuloma.[22] It is thought to evolve into a peripheral fibroma, if left undisturbed, due to an increase of the fibrosis, a reduction of its vascular component and presence of calcification.[23] Bacteriologic culture often reveals both *Staphylococcus aureus* and *Streptococcus haemolyticus*, which are believed to be contaminants. It is common that the initiating irritation is a foreign body or small infected wound. With surgical removal of the lesions in conjunction with elimination of irritating local factors, recurrence is uncommon.[24]

Peripheral giant cell granuloma

This is a well-defined lesion, more common in humans and cats than in dogs, characterized by a lobular architecture, where a fibroblastic connective tissue surrounds different areas rich in giant cells, similar to osteoclasts.[20,25] The lesions are covered by hyper- or parakeratinized epithelium, often ulcerated. Osteoid and bone formation may be present. Clinically, peripheral giant cell granulomas appear as vascular, lobulated gingival masses. There is no breed, sex or age predilection. Recurrence following marginal excision is common in the cat.[25]

Reactive exostosis

Reactive exostosis is a focal lesion, probably of traumatic origin.[1,26] These lesions consist of compact or cancellous bone and appear as proliferations on the alveolar bone. They are of little or no clinical importance, but can be confused with an osteoma, thus biopsy is mandatory.

Therapeutic decision-making

Hyperplastic lesions on the gingiva should always be biopsied because they are often very difficult to diagnose based on clinical appearance. All must be biopsied if multiple lesions are present. Diagnosis of some oral proliferative lesions can be made by contact smear or fine needle aspirate of the mass; however, in general, an incisional biopsy is recommended for histopathological examination. The masses are usually accessible, and a specimen of appropriate size can be obtained with biopsy punch or other suitable instrument. Minimal restraint and local anesthesia are often sufficient. Radiological examination of the involved jaw is mandatory to determine the presence and the extent of bone involvement.[27]

Gingival hyperplasia often results in pseudopocket formation. These should be differentiated from true periodontal pockets, which occur due to attachment loss associated with periodontitis. The base of a pseudopocket is normally located at the level of the cemento-enamel junction and the hyperplastic soft tissue forms the walls of the pocket. Pseudopockets are removed by means of gingivectomy and gingivoplasty (see Ch. 18). These are excisional procedures that allow the restoration of the normal anatomy of the gingiva, and to facilitate oral hygiene.

In case of drug-induced gingival enlargement, discontinuation of the drug may cause cessation and possibly regression of the gingival enlargement.[4,5] If permitted, substitution with an alternative drug is preferred. If the drug is required, frequent routine periodontal treatments, as well as meticulous home care, are imperative.[4,5] Topical chlorhexidine reduces plaque build-up and bacterial load, decreasing the inflammatory stimulus for gingival enlargement.[4,5] Systemic or topical folic acid has been demonstrated to decrease gingival hyperplasia.[28] Surgical treatment (gingivectomy/gingivoplasty) is indicated for severe cases and for cases where regression does not occur following discontinuation of the drug.[4,5]

For focal fibrous hyperplasia, pyogenic granuloma and peripheral giant cell granuloma wide surgical excision is usually curative. A gingivoplasty is performed afterwards to reshape the gingival contour.

Postoperative care and assessment

It is generally not necessary to administer antibiotics unless severe secondary infection is present. Chlorhexidine gluconate gel can be applied on the gingiva during the first days postoperatively, while daily toothbrushing can be instituted as soon as the gingivectomy wounds have epithelialized (see Ch. 18).

Prognosis

Prognosis is usually good, as long as oral hygiene is maintained. Recheck examinations are to be scheduled every 3 to 6 months, combined with routine periodontal treatment as indicated. There may be long-term recurrence, at all or at specific sites. In some cases extraction of adjacent teeth may be indicated, combined with a repeat gingivectomy.[29] If periosteal reaction or exostosis is present, an osteoplasty and smoothing of the alveolar margin is indicated to prevent recurrence.

TRAUMATIC BUCCAL OR SUBLINGUAL MUCOSAL HYPERPLASIA

Pathophysiology

Self-induced oral trauma to the buccal or sublingual mucosa can result in acutely hemorrhagic mucosal lesions, or, more commonly, chronic proliferative lesions (Fig. 42.2). Lesions on the buccal mucosa are frequently confused with calcinosis circumscripta or stomatitis. Sublingual lesions can be caused by excessive barking or panting, with resultant stretching of sublingual tissues over occlusal surfaces of mandibular teeth and subsequent oral trauma.[30] Sublingual lesions can be

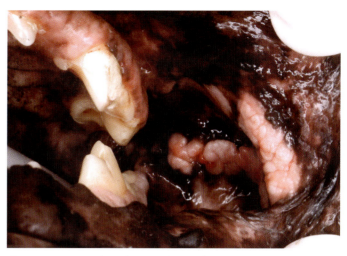

Fig. 42.2 Traumatic buccal mucosal hyperplasia in a dog. *(From Self-Assessment Colour Review of Veterinary Dentistry, edited by Frank Verstraete. Manson Publishing Ltd, London, 1999.)*

confused with eosinophilic granulomas or ranulas. The diagnosis is based on clinical presentation and histopathology.

Treatment

Full excision is not necessary unless previously biopsied lesions continue to be traumatized.[31] Traumatized tissues can be excised in a fusiform pattern, ensuring no tissue remains in the occlusal path. Surgical closure is routine, using fine monofilament absorbable material. Prognosis is good if an adequate amount of tissue is excised.[30]

PROLIFERATIVE LESIONS OF INFECTIOUS ORIGIN

Pathophysiology

Infectious agents, such as bacteria, viruses, protozoa and fungi can produce very proliferative lesions in both immunocompromised and healthy individuals.

Leishmania donovani infantum and *Leishmania tropica* can cause leishmanial stomatitis, characterized by proliferative cauliflower-like lesions on the oral mucosa. This disease is very rare in North America, although it has been reported.[32] The diagnosis is based on the identification of anti-*Leishmania* antibodies, or the demonstration of amastigotes in lymph node aspirates, bone marrow aspirates or lesion imprints.

Mycotic stomatitis caused by an opportunistic yeastlike pathogen, *Candida albicans*, is uncommon in the dog and cat. This disease is usually associated with long-term antibiotic therapy. The lesions include diffuse inflammation and ulceration of all parts of the oral cavity, most noted at the mucocutaneous junction. The lesions can be covered with a white plaque.[33] Diagnosis is by culture of *Candida albicans* from the lesions or by identifying yeast hyphae in PAS-stained biopsies.[8] The yeast *Cryptococcus neoformans* can also cause oral lesions. Proliferative crater-like nonhealing lesions are characteristic.[34]

Therapeutic decision-making

Proliferative lesions on the oral mucosa or gingiva should always be biopsied because they are very difficult to diagnose based on clinical appearance. Diagnosis of some oral proliferative lesions is based on incisional biopsy, histopathological examination, culture and sometimes antigen detection (e.g., *Cryptococcus*). A specimen of appropriate size can be obtained with biopsy punch or other suitable instrument.

Treatment for fungal infections includes elimination of the underlying cause, if identified, local rinsing with an antifungal agent such as nystatin, and systemic antifungal therapy (e.g., ketoconazole 10 mg/kg daily by mouth for 4–6 weeks).[35]

Treatment for *Leishmania* consists of meglumine antimonate, sodium stibogluconate, liposomal amphotericin B, or allopurinol. Because meglumine and sodium stibogluconate are not routinely available, liposomal amphotericin B or allopurinol are the drugs of choice.[36]

Complications

Complications of fungal infections usually arise from failure to respond to antifungal therapy.[36] There have also been reported side effects of the antifungal therapy ranging from nausea, diarrhea and vomiting to hepatotoxicity. Additionally, some fungi, such as *Cryptococcus neoformans*, produce mucopolysaccharide capsules that protect them from host immune defenses. Disseminated infection is a common complication associated with *Cryptococcus neoformans*. The most frequent site of dissemination is the meninges.[36]

Prognosis

Management of cryptococcal infections can be difficult due to the frequency of underlying medical problems. The triazoles (fluconazole and itraconazole) have been effective against *Cryptococcus*, producing far fewer side effects than amphotericin B and flucytosine.[28] Prognosis with leishmaniasis is variable, as most cases tend to recur. Dogs with renal insufficiency and leishmaniasis have a poorer prognosis.[36]

EOSINOPHILIC GRANULOMA COMPLEX IN THE CAT

The eosinophilic granuloma complex in the cat consists of three clinical entities: (1) eosinophilic granuloma; (2) eosinophilic ulcer; and (3) eosinophilic plaque. Recently, eosinophilic dermatitis has been described and some authors have included it with the eosinophilic granuloma complex.[37,38] These lesions have been grouped together because they can occur simultaneously in the same animal, and present many common aspects, such as occasional peripheral blood eosinophilia, an eosinophilic tissue infiltrate, and an association with various allergies. Only those lesions that may manifest in the oral cavity will be considered here.

Clinical presentation

Eosinophilic granuloma

Eosinophilic granuloma is a linear, well-circumscribed, raised lesion, yellowish-pink in color, usually localized to the caudal aspect of the rear limb, and is often bilateral. It may also be seen on the paws, cheek, lip commissure, chin, pinna of the ear and in the oral cavity. Oral lesions can involve the hard palate, the soft palate or the base of the tongue (Fig. 42.3A).[39–42] When oral lesions are present, dysphagia or ptyalism are usually seen. Large lesions may interfere with prehension and swallowing of food, and in very severe cases they may even compromise breathing.

Eosinophilic granuloma has not been found to have a breed predilection in cats, but it is more commonly found in young animals (2–6

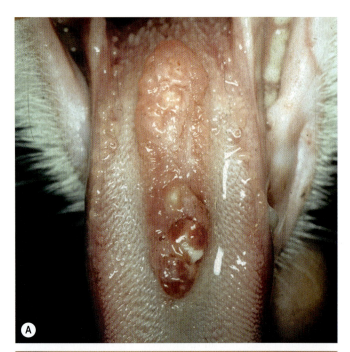

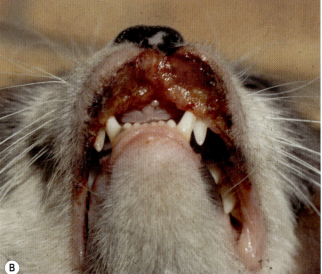

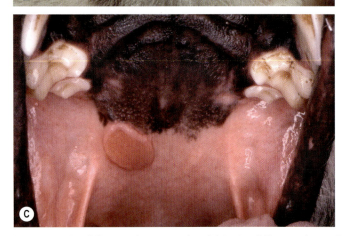

Fig. 42.3 Eosinophilic granuloma complex: (**A**) Eosinophilic granuloma of the tongue in a cat; (**B**) Severe eosinophilic ulcers of the upper lips in a cat; (**C**) Focal eosinophilic stomatitis in a cavalier King Charles spaniel.

years), with a twofold higher incidence in females.[41-43] It has been associated with insect bite allergies (e.g., flea and mosquito bites), food allergy, atopy, immunosuppression, and bacterial and viral (calicivirus) infections.[39,43-48] The etiology of oral eosinophilic granuloma is rarely determined and is often considered idiopathic.[45]

The histology of eosinophilic granuloma resembles a foreign body reaction, appearing as granulomatous inflammation with eosinophilic infiltrates surrounding collagen fibers. Recent reports have revealed that the collagen is not lysed or altered, but rather is coated with the contents of eosinophils.[49,50] These lesions may resolve spontaneously or persist for a prolonged period. Eosinophilic granuloma may be an isolated lesion or manifest as part of the eosinophilic granuloma complex, associated with eosinophilic plaques or deep ulceration (so-called *rodent ulcers*).[45]

Eosinophilic ulcer

An eosinophilic ulcer is typically a well-circumscribed lesion, with raised edges and necrosis of the superficial layers, most frequently located on the upper lip (Fig. 42.3B). It can also occur anywhere on the skin or within the oral cavity. It starts as an erosive and exudative lesion, which may evolve into a major ulcer with swelling of the surrounding tissues. The lesions vary in size, depending on their chronicity, and are usually not painful.[45] The eosinophilic ulcer has been found in cats of all ages and breeds, but with a higher incidence in middle-aged cats and in females.[43] It may be present as part of the eosinophilic granuloma complex, or occur as a single lesion. The etiology of the eosinophilic ulcer may be traumatic, as seen in cases where the lower canines contact the upper lip with a secondary bacterial infection and fibrosis. A number of eosinophilic ulcers may be secondary to flea allergy.[51]

The histological features of the eosinophilic ulcer are often nonspecific. The predominant cell type can vary from a neutrophilic to an eosinophilic infiltrate, and bacterial colonization is common. The transformation of a chronic eosinophilic ulcer into a squamous cell carcinoma has been reported, although this is a rare occurrence.[39]

The differential diagnoses for oral eosinophilic lesions include gingivostomatitis, squamous cell carcinoma, other oral tumor types, food allergy and atopy. Biopsy is useful to exclude the possibility of a malignancy.

Therapeutic decision-making

Medical treatment

To rule out food allergy and atopy, a restricted-ingredient diet can be used and skin testing performed. Thorough control of ectoparasites is essential. If there is no response to dietary change, or if there is evidence of secondary infection, then antibiotics (amoxicillin/clavulanate at the dosage of 20 mg/kg or cephalexin at 20–30 mg/kg BID) is a therapeutic option. Prolonged (4–6 weeks) treatment may be required before a response is seen.[41,42] In those cases where a skin test has identified allergens that could potentially be responsible for the lesions, it is mandatory to control and if possible eliminate exposure to them, performing desensitization when possible.[36,39,41,42] This may be very difficult if not impossible to achieve.

For the many patients refractory to these measures and cases where an underlying etiology could not be identified, corticosteroid treatment is indicated. Prednisolone (1–2 mg/kg BID, gradually reducing the dosage and progressing to alternate-day treatment when a response is seen) or subcutaneous injections of methylprednisolone acetate (20–40 mg/cat every 2 weeks for up to three doses) are usually effective. Therapy should be continued until the lesion or at least the signs completely disappear.[45] Corticosteroids may have profound side effects (adrenocortical suppression, polyphagia, polydipsia, polyuria,

obesity and diabetes mellitus) so it is best to use the minimum effective dose and avoid unnecessary prolonged or repeated treatment. Treatment with megestrol acetate is also effective but it is not recommended because of a high risk of side effects including diabetes mellitus, mammary tumors and uterine problems and should only be used when other options have failed or cannot be used.[52]

Other therapeutic options that have been suggested include ascorbic acid, gold salts, interferon, chlorambucil, cyclosporine and fatty acids, as well as intralesional administration of corticosteroids.[36,53]

Surgical treatment

Before performing any kind of surgery it is recommended to biopsy the lesion to confirm the diagnosis of an eosinophilic lesion and eliminate other differential diagnoses. Conventional surgical excision is indicated for very proliferative lesions that interfere with breathing or swallowing. Severe hemorrhage should be expected. This can be minimized by use of electrosurgery, but caution is needed to avoid thermal injuries to the adjacent tissues. Cautious use of CO_2 laser tissue ablation will also minimize hemorrhage and is anecdotally reported to give good results (see Ch. 8).[54] In the late 1970s and early 1980s some authors obtained good results using cryotherapy, with little or no hemorrhage.[55-57]

Postoperative care and assessment

Postoperative pain control is fundamental to help get cats eating as soon as possible. In some cases it may be necessary to provide postoperative alimentary support via a nasogastric tube. These cases should be hospitalized until they can eat unaided (see Ch. 5).

Complications

Wound dehiscence is a possibility, particularly if the soft palate is involved. Dehiscence is likely if there is excessive tension on the wound margins, when electrosurgery has been overused or if infection is present. Provision of easily swallowed food and daily use of an antiseptic mouth rinse (e.g., 0.12% chlorhexidine gluconate solution) for the first few days is helpful. The other main postoperative complications are hemorrhage, which is usually minor and easy to control, and local recurrence of the disease. Cases should be followed long term to monitor for recurrence, particularly when the etiology has not been determined.

Prognosis

If the etiology has been determined and eliminated, recurrence is unlikely following appropriate medical or surgical therapy; however, idiopathic eosinophilic lesions tend to recur and require ongoing, sometimes lifelong, treatment. Concurrent diseases, particularly those that contraindicate the use of corticosteroids, worsen the prognosis.

ORAL EOSINOPHILIC GRANULOMA COMPLEX IN THE DOG

Oral eosinophilic granuloma in Siberian huskies

The oral eosinophilic granuloma lesions observed in this syndrome are usually found on the tongue: the lateral margins and the frenulum are involved, with raised, firm, yellow–pink lesions that may be ulcerated.[58,59] They can also be seen on the palatal mucosa. Patients with the lingual lesions are commonly presented for halitosis and oral discomfort, whereas the palatal mucosal lesions typically do not cause clinical signs.[8] The histopathological findings are similar to those seen in the feline eosinophilic granuloma complex, with granulomatous inflammation rich in eosinophils. The complete blood count reveals a peripheral eosinophilia in 80% of patients.[8] The eosinophilic granuloma is reported in young animals (1–7 years of age), and is most common in Siberian huskies. In this breed it is believed to be an hereditary or familial condition.[58,59] Recommended treatment is the same as for cats, i.e., corticosteroids or surgical excision. There may be recurrence.[58,59]

Eosinophilic stomatitis in Cavalier King Charles spaniels

Cavalier King Charles spaniels and other dogs with ulcerative eosinophilic stomatitis are typically presented for dysphagia, paroxysmal coughing or anorexia.[60] Oral findings include mucosal ulceration, plaque formation and granulomatous lesions, although the latter to a lesser extent than with the abovementioned eosinophilic granuloma lesions. Both entities are consistent with the spectrum of lesions found with eosinophilic granuloma complex in the cat (Fig. 42.3C). In very severe cases oronasal fistula formation may occur.[61] The etiology of the lesions is unknown, although a familial predisposition is often evident, both in Cavalier King Charles spaniels as well as other affected breeds.[60–63] Peripheral eosinophilia is occasionally seen.[64] A genetic predisposition to eosinophilic syndromes in general may exist, both in Cavalier King Charles spaniels as well as other breeds.[64] Fine needle aspiration or exfoliative cytology may be performed instead of an incisional biopsy due to friability of the tissues, although histopathology is required for a definitive diagnosis. Care should be taken when performing an incisional biopsy of a lesion on the soft palate, as an oronasal fistula may result from a nonhealing biopsy site. Corticosteroids have been variably effective, although spontaneous regression may occur.[60,62,63] Due to the variability in the response to treatment, prognosis remains guarded.[63]

CHRONIC GINGIVOSTOMATITIS IN THE CAT

An in-depth discussion of the etiology, pathophysiology and medical aspects of chronic gingivostomatitis in cats is beyond the scope of this text. Only the aspects that are relevant to case selection for surgical treatment options of this condition are reviewed.

Clinical presentation

Feline chronic gingivostomatitis (FCGS), also called feline lymphocytic-plasmacytic stomatitis, is manifested by chronic inflammation of the gingiva and oral mucosa. No causative agent for this disease has yet been identified. Clinically, patients are presented with varying degrees of inflammation at the gingiva (gingivitis), alveolar and buccal mucosa (mucositis), the area lateral to the palatoglossal folds (often incorrectly referred to as 'faucitis'), tongue (glossitis), palate (palatitis) or any combination thereof.[65] The lesions are often symmetrical. It is more common that the soft tissues in the premolar–molar area are affected than the tissues surrounding the incisor and canine teeth (Fig. 42.4).

Affected cats are presented with dysphagia, ptyalism and anorexia. Physical examination reveals a painful, inflamed mouth and variable lymphadenopathy.

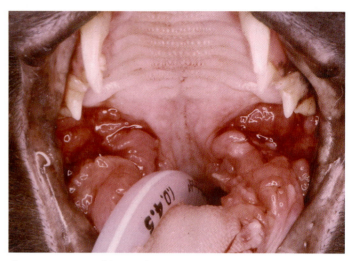

Fig. 42.4 Severe proliferative lesions in a cat with chronic gingivostomatitis.

Preoperative concerns

A systematic approach should be followed in order to identify concurrent disease processes. Routine laboratory work, including a complete blood count, biochemical profile and urinalysis, must be performed to rule out oral manifestations of systemic illness (e.g., renal failure and diabetes mellitus). Elevated serum gamma-immunoglobulins are commonly seen with feline chronic gingivostomatitis.

The FIV/FeLV status of any cat presenting for FCGS must be assessed. The incidence of FeLV infection in cats with FCGS is relatively low (reportedly 0–28%).[66] FIV-positive cats are commonly affected by oral disease (50–80%).[67] However, neither FIV nor FeLV infections are considered causative agents of FCGS. Viral testing (PCR) for feline calicivirus (FCV) and feline herpesvirus type 1 (FHV-1) are also good tests to perform, although the results may be more academic than diagnostic.[68] In one study it was found that most FCGS patients are FCV and FHV positive, although this does not necessarily indicate a causative relationship.[68]

In certain geographic locations many cats affected by FCGS test positive for *Bartonella henselae*.[69] Subsequent treatment of *Bartonella*-positive cats does not seem to improve the outcome of FCGS treatment, and it is unlikely that *Bartonella* plays a major causative role.

A detailed oral examination and full-mouth radiographs are indicated to diagnose concomitant periodontal disease and odontoclastic resorption lesions. Root fragments are also commonly found in cats affected by FCGS, and are thought to play an important role in perpetuating the disease if left in place (see Ch. 15).[70]

An incisional biopsy is routinely obtained. Histopathological findings typically include a diffuse, dense, mixed lymphocytic and plasmacytic infiltrate in the mucosa and submucosa. In some cases the infiltrate is predominately plasmacytic, while a variable amount of neutrophils may be present.[71] Superficial ulceration is also common. The main reason for obtaining a biopsy, however, is to exclude the presence of squamous cell carcinoma, which may present as an ulcerative lesion rather than a typical exophytic tumor. Conversely, FCGS may result in proliferative lesions that are clinically indistinguishable from squamous cell carcinoma, other tumor types such as fibrosarcoma, or non-neoplastic lesions such as eosinophilic granuloma.

Therapeutic decision-making

The findings of the comprehensive preoperative evaluation and the previous treatment history largely determine the choice of treatment.

Initial treatment

Periodontally compromised teeth and teeth affected by resorption should be extracted. The goals of subsequent conservative medical therapy are: (1) oral hygiene to control plaque; (2) antibiotics and/or oral antiseptic rinses to treat secondary bacterial infection; and (3) antiinflammatory drugs to diminish the inflammatory response. Since the secondary bacterial pathogens are believed to be anaerobic,[72] metronidazole is prescribed in conjunction with amoxicillin–clavulanic acid for 2 weeks; clindamycin is a suitable alternative for the latter. Daily brushing and chlorhexidine gluconate rinses should be performed. Prednisone may be administered per os at an antiinflammatory dosage of 0.5–1 mg/kg/day.

A variety of other medical treatment options have been described or have anecdotally been reported.[69] Oral administration of bovine lactoferrin has been shown to improve intractable stomatitis in one experiment, although the study included only seven subjects.[73] Some patients may respond favorably to treatment with piroxicam or cyclosporine.[69]

Treatment of refractory cases

For patients who have not improved following selective extractions and medical management, extraction of all premolar and molar teeth is recommended. The removal of each tooth and its entire root is crucial for this therapy to be beneficial (see Ch. 15). Eighty percent of cats improve shortly after extractions. Of the remaining 20% of cats not responding to extraction of the premolars and molars, half will respond to extraction of the canines and incisors.[74]

The use of CO_2 laser ablation in the management of FCGS is controversial (see Ch. 8). The rational for this technique is that repeated ablation of the inflamed tissue may result in the formation of less-inflamed scar tissue. It is unclear, at this stage, to what extent this occurs and therefore what the success rate is. The incidence of complications, such as postoperative swelling, is unknown. The CO_2 laser may be most useful for the excision of severe, proliferative lesions, which are occasionally found in the areas lateral to the palatoglossal folds.

Postoperative care and assessment

See Chapter 15 for a more detailed discussion of postoperative care. It is essential to ensure adequate nutritional intake as soon as possible, but in some cases it is necessary to provide postoperative alimentary support via a nasogastric tube or an esophagostomy tube (see Chs 4 and 5). These patients should be hospitalized until they can eat on their own.

Prognosis

Feline chronic gingivostomatitis is a frustrating condition to treat. Even following full-mouth extractions, some patients, especially those who have already been subjected to many different medical treatments over long periods, fail to respond.

NONTRAUMATIC DISEASES OF THE JAWS

Disease syndromes

Osteomyelitis

Osteomyelitis can be classified by duration, etiology and method of infection.[75] Chronic osteomyelitis usually results from inadequate treatment of acute osteomyelitis or may be an insidious process.[76]

Osteomyelitis may be bacterial, fungal or rarely viral in origin.[75,76] Most bone infections are of bacterial origin, and approximately half of them are monomicrobial.[75,77] *Staphylococcus* spp. are most commonly isolated. Other aerobic bacteria that may be involved include *Streptococcus* spp., *Escherichia coli*, *Pseudomonas* spp., *Proteus* spp. and *Klebsiella* spp.[75,77] Anaerobes isolated from osteomyelitis lesions include many species that are often found in the oral cavity, namely *Actinomyces*, *Clostridium*, *Bacteroides* and *Fusobacterium* spp.[78] Fungal osteomyelitis is often a component of a systemic mycosis.[77,79] The genera that can be involved include *Coccidioides*, *Blastomyces*, *Cryptococcus*, *Histoplasma* and *Aspergillus*, and some of these are endemic in certain geographic regions.[79]

Osteomyelitis of the jaw most commonly occurs as a complication of trauma and fracture repair (see Ch. 34). Other sources of infection include extension of soft tissue infection, including periodontal disease and periapical disease, and hematogenous spread. A low-grade osteomyelitis causing swelling of the mandible is commonly observed in cats, and is associated with dental disease and retained root tips.[80] This is occasionally also seen in the dog (Fig. 42.5A). Fungal osteomyelitis most commonly occurs as a result of hematogenous spread of the causative organism, which gains entrance to the body by inhalation or through the gastrointestinal tract.

There is no apparent breed disposition for bacterial osteomyelitis, with the possible exception of the foxhound; a series of five related animals with severe osteomyelitis was documented in this breed.[81] Blastomycosis occurs more commonly in coonhounds, pointers and Weimaraners, while a variety of breeds, including the pointer, have been identified to be more at risk for coccidioidomycosis.[79] Cats are more susceptible to histoplasmosis and cryptococcosis than dogs.[79] Osteomyelitis can occur with any of the aforementioned systemic mycoses; involvement of the jaw (Fig. 42.5B) would appear to be rare, although the actual incidence is unknown.[79,82]

Osteomyelitis presents as a firm, warm and painful swelling of the part of the jaw involved. Draining tracts may be present. Animals with fungal osteomyelitis often have signs of systemic disease, which can range from non-specific signs like inappetence, weight loss, lymphadenopathy and fever, to respiratory, ocular, cardiac and nervous symptoms if those systems are involved.[76,79]

Complete blood count and biochemical profile may be near normal or reflect the chronic infection and inflammation present. A very comprehensive examination, including abdominal ultrasound and thoracic radiographs, is indicated if systemic mycosis is suspected.[76,79]

The radiological signs of chronic osteomyelitis of the jaw include new bone production, lysis and remodeling.[75] The periosteal new bone proliferation varies from smooth, lamellated or spiculated.[77,83] Endosteal or periosteal scalloping of the cortex, or a moth-eaten pattern of bone destruction is often evident. The presence of one or more sequestra is typical for osteomyelitis.[77,83]

An incisional biopsy followed by histopathological evaluation and aerobic and anaerobic microbiological culture is recommended to determine the exact nature of the lesion.[76] Specimens for bacterial and fungal culture must be collected and transported appropriately.[77]

The principles of treatment of chronic osteomyelitis of bacterial origin include surgical debridement, sequestrectomy, lavage and administration of appropriate antimicrobial drugs based on culture and sensitivity.[75–77] Open drainage and cancellous bone grafting may be indicated in selected cases.[77] Osteomyelitis associated with dental disease is usually treated by extraction of diseased teeth and root fragments, if present; this is combined with curettage of the affected bone and followed by a therapeutic course of a suitable antibiotic (see Ch. 3). The treatment for mycotic osteomyelitis is long-term antifungal therapy with a suitable agent, such as itraconazole; some animals may require lifelong treatment.[76,77]

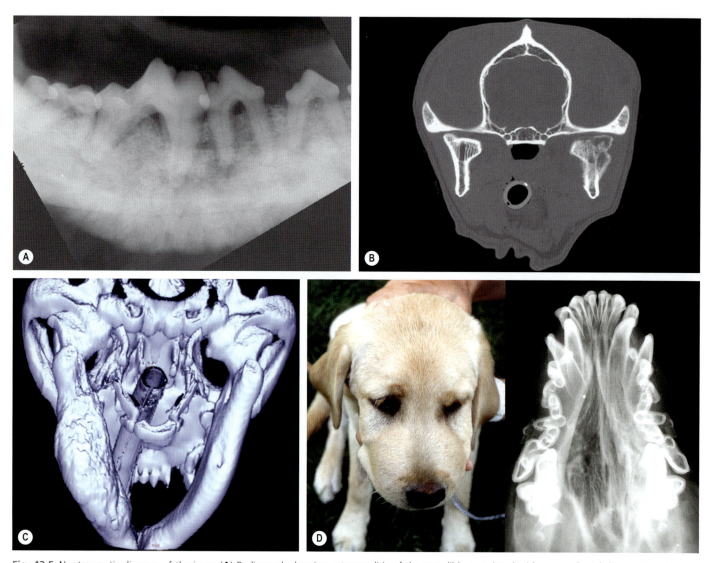

Fig. 42.5 Nontraumatic diseases of the jaws: (**A**) Radiograph showing osteomyelitis of the mandible associated with severe dental disease in a dog; (**B**) Computed tomography image showing fungal osteomyelitis of the right condylar process in a dog, who had a similar lesion in the left tibia; (**C**) Tridimensional reconstruction (caudoventral–craniodorsal view) following computed tomography showing craniomandibular osteopathy affecting the left mandible in a 7-month-old English bulldog; (**D**) Clinical appearance (*left*) and skull radiograph (*right*) of an 8-month-old dog with renal secondary hyperparathyroidism. *(From Self-Assessment Colour Review of Veterinary Dentistry, edited by Frank Verstraete. Manson Publishing Ltd, London, 1999.)*

Craniomandibular osteopathy

Craniomandibular osteopathy (CMO) is an uncommon, noninflammatory, non-neoplastic proliferative bone disease that occurs in dogs of 3–6 months of age. It has been reported most often in West Highland white terriers and Scottish terriers, but also sporadically in a wide variety of other breeds.[84–87] The disease is inherited as an autosomal recessive trait in West Highland white terriers.[88] Affected dogs are typically presented for pain on opening the mouth and inappetence. Other signs include intermittent pyrexia, depression, and palpably enlarged mandibles.[87] The mandibles and tympanic bullae are most commonly affected.[89]

The diagnosis of CMO is based on the characteristic radiographic findings and confirmed by means of histopathological examination of a biopsy. On conventional radiographs or computed tomography, dense osseous proliferations are seen arising from the affected periosteal surfaces (Fig. 42.5C).[87] The histopathological findings include resorption of lamellar bone and replacement with exuberant, coarsely woven, poorly mineralized bony trabeculae, interspersed with fibrous tissue.[87] There are no consistent changes in the complete blood count, biochemical profile and urinalysis, although the alkaline phosphatase may be elevated.[90]

The disease is usually self-limiting, with bone growth ceasing or even regressing at skeletal maturity.[87] Treatment is symptomatic and includes steroidal and nonsteroidal antiinflammatory drugs. Nutritional support is indicated in severe cases.

The prognosis depends of the degree of bony proliferation at the temporomandibular joints, the angular processes and the tympanic bullae, which can limit the range of motion of the jaws.[87]

Idiopathic calvarial hyperostosis

Idiopathic calvarial hyperostosis is a non-neoplastic proliferative bone disease with clinical and histopathological characteristics similar to CMO.[91,92] It may affect the frontal, temporal and occipital bones and has to date only been described in young bull mastiffs. The disease becomes symptomatic around 6 months of age and most cases are self-limiting, with bone growth ceasing and regressing at skeletal maturity.[92,93]

Hyperparathyroidism

Hyperparathyroidism can be primary due to a functional adenoma, or secondary to chronic renal insufficiency or nutritional deficiency.[89,94] Secondary hyperparathyroidism results in resorption of calcium from bone as the body attempts to maintain the calcium homeostasis. Nutritional secondary hyperparathyroidism can occur as a result of diets with a low calcium-to-phosphorous ratio, such as all meat or organs, which contain adequate phosphorous but insufficient calcium.[94,95] This leads to a transient hypocalcemia, which stimulates the secretion of parathyroid hormone (PTH). In renal secondary hyperparathyroidism the reabsorption of phosphate is impaired, which results in hyperphosphatemia. This in turn leads to a lower blood calcium concentration, which stimulates parathyroid gland activity.[89] The effects of PTH on bone include osteoclastic bone resorption and osteocyte-mediated release of calcium and phosphorous.[95] The osteoclasts are activated by osteoclast-activating factors released by the osteoblasts in response to PTH.[95] Concurrent with secondary hyperparathyroidism, the synthesis of 1,25-dihydroxyvitamin D in the kidney is also decreased due to the loss of functional nephrons.[89,95] This leads to a decrease in intestinal calcium absorption and impaired mineralization of osteoid. The combined effect of renal secondary hyperparathyroidism and the decreased 1,25-dihydroxyvitamin D is often referred to as *renal osteodystrophy*.[89,96,97]

The resultant bony changes are most likely to become clinically evident in growing dogs but rarely in cats.[89,98,99] The first bone affected is the mandible, followed by the maxilla, then the other bones of the skull, and finally the long bones. Before the rest of the skeleton is affected, the bones of the jaws may be severely demineralized, and become swollen and malleable. This is evident clinically and is commonly referred to as *rubber jaw* (Fig. 42.5D). The occlusion can be grossly distorted and exfoliation of teeth may occur. Histologically, bone resorption and replacement with fibrous tissue is seen, which is often referred to as *osteitis fibrosa cystica*. In addition, osteomalacia, or poorly mineralized osteoid, may be seen.[100]

The radiological findings are often pathognomonic of the disease. The first radiographic sign is loss of the lamina dura, followed by loss of density of mandibular trabecular and cortical bone (Fig. 42.5D).

Teeth may appear almost unsupported by bone.[89] In the cat, decreased density and thin cortices are seen in the long bones and vertebrae.[89]

Treatment depends on the cause of the hyperparathyroidism. For nutritional secondary hyperparathyroidism the diet should be corrected, in which case remineralization of the bones usually occurs. Treatment of the renal form is based on the medical management of chronic renal failure. The skeletal lesions tend to be more severe with the renal form and therapy may be unrewarding.

Acromegaly

Acromegaly is a chronic endocrine disorder caused by excessive growth hormone (GH) secretion.[101-103] The underlying pathophysiology and clinical presentation of the disease are very different in the dog compared to the cat.

In the dog, acromegaly is very rare.[101] The disease mainly occurs in middle-aged female dogs treated with progestagens or spontaneously during metestrus.[101,103] The excess GH is secreted by foci of hyperplastic ductular epithelium of the mammary gland. In cats, the most common cause of acromegaly is GH-secreting tumors of the pituitary gland, similar to what is seen in human patients.[102] The disease is uncommon and mainly affects elderly male cats. Acromegaly is associated with insulin-resistant diabetes mellitus, especially in the cat. The diagnosis is made by measuring GH concentrations in plasma. Pituitary tumors can be visualized using computed tomography or magnetic resonance imaging.[103]

Acromegaly is associated with enlargement of one or more organs.[102,103] Of importance in maxillofacial surgery is the soft tissue swelling of the face and tongue. The head has a heavy appearance and skin folds may be present. A relative mandibular prognathism and wide spacing of the incisors are often evident.[101-103] Hyperostosis of the skull and periosteal reaction on the mandible has been noted in cats.[102] Soft tissue swelling in the pharyngeal region may give rise to respiratory stridor.[103] The physical changes in cats tend to be less pronounced than in dogs.[103]

The diagnosis of acromegaly is based on clinical findings, plasma GH-concentration, and diagnostic imaging. Biopsy of the maxillofacial soft tissues and bone is not indicated.

Acromegaly in the dog is treated by withdrawal of exogenous progestagens and/or ovariohysterectomy.[103] Irradiation is currently the treatment of choice in cats.[103] The maxillofacial soft tissue features return to normal following treatment; bony changes are permanent but do not require treatment.[103]

REFERENCES

1. Regezi JA, Sciubba JJ, Jordan RC. Oral pathology – clinical pathologic correlations. 4th ed. Philadelphia, PA: WB Saunders Co; 2003.
2. Anonymous. Mosby's dental dictionary. St. Louis, MO: Mosby; 2004.
3. Carranza FA, Hogan EL. Gingival enlargement. In: Newman MG, Takei HH, Carranza FA, editors. Clinical periodontology. 9th ed. Philadelphia, PA: WB Saunders Co; 2002. p. 279–96.
4. Dongari-Bagtzoglou A. Drug-associated gingival enlargement. J Periodontol 2004;75:1424–31.
5. Mavrogiannis M, Ellis JS, Thomason JM, et al. The management of drug-induced

gingival overgrowth. J Clin Periodontol 2006;33:434–9.
6. Lewis JR, Reiter AM. Management of generalized gingival enlargement in a dog – case report and literature review. J Vet Dent 2005;22:160–9.
7. Verstraete FJM, Ligthelm AJ, Weber A. The histological nature of epulides in dogs. J Comp Pathol 1992;106:169–82.
8. Burrows CF, Miller WH, Harvey CE. Oral medicine. In: Harvey CE, editor. Veterinary Dentistry. 1st ed. Philadelphia, PA: WB Saunders Co; 1985. p. 34–58.
9. Kfir Y, Buchner A, Hansen LS. Reactive lesions of the gingiva. A

clinicopathological study of 741 cases. J Periodontol 1980;51:655–61.
10. Burstone MS, Bond E, Litt R. Familial gingival hypertrophy in the dog (boxer breed). Arch Pathol 1952;54:208–12.
11. Hassell TM, Page RC. The major metabolite of phenytoin (Dilantin) induces gingival overgrowth in cats. J Periodontal Res 1978;13:280–2.
12. Kamali F, Ball DE, McLaughlin WS, et al. Phenytoin metabolism to 5-(4-hydroxyphenyl)-5-phenylhydantoin (HPPH) in man, cat and rat in vitro and in vivo, and susceptibility to phenytoin-induced gingival overgrowth. J Periodontal Res 1999;34:145–53.

the three incisors, canine, and first and second premolar teeth. *Bilateral rostral mandibulectomy* (removal of the rostral parts of both mandibles following osteotomy between the second and third premolars) is more commonly performed. If necessary, the osteotomy can be performed as far caudally as between the fourth premolar and first molar teeth.[27] In a *segmental mandibulectomy* part of the body of the mandible is excised, typically including the caudal premolar and one or more molar teeth. A *caudal mandibulectomy* involves excision of the ramus of the mandible, including the condylar and coronoid processes.[28] Although the term *hemimandibulectomy* is often used in the veterinary literature to denote the complete excision of one of the two mandibles, the term *total* or *unilateral mandibulectomy* is more appropriate.

SURGICAL TREATMENT OBJECTIVES

Once the histopathologic nature and clinical stage of the tumor have been determined, a decision must be made with regard to surgical treatment. The type and extent of surgical procedure is based on clinical and radiographic findings, and the propensity of the specific tumor type for local invasion and metastasis.[29] There are four potential goals of oral oncologic surgery: (1) surgery to cure, (2) surgery for debulking, (3) surgery for local control and (4) surgery for palliation. The therapeutic goal of a *curative* surgical procedure is to remove the entire lesion and leave no cells that could proliferate and cause recurrence of the lesion.[30] Surgical excision is considered curative for benign, locally aggressive tumors such as acanthomatous ameloblastoma. It is also possible to achieve cure of malignant tumors (such as squamous cell carcinomas in dogs) if metastasis has not already occurred at the time of the procedure. Debulking, which leaves macroscopic tumor behind, may be performed prior to radiation therapy for large tumors which cannot be completely excised. However, adjuvant treatment is generally less effective when macroscopically visible tumor remains than when residual neoplasia is microscopic.[8] Surgery for local control is typically the goal for patients with malignant oral tumors such as melanoma, where the potential for early metastasis is high and where adjunctive therapy may be performed following surgical excision of the primary tumor. However, some oral cancers cannot be eliminated by any treatment modality. In these cases, surgery for palliation may be undertaken to temporarily relieve pain, improve function and increase quality of life.[29]

TREATMENT PLANNING

Once the surgical objective has been determined, an appropriate treatment plan can be formulated. Whenever possible, the decision-making process should include a team consisting of a veterinary dentist, surgeon, medical oncologist and radiation oncologist[14] in addition to the primary care veterinarian. The client should be informed of the various treatment options and their associated expectations with regard to duration and expense of treatment, prognosis, possible complications, and postoperative appearance and function. Postoperative and follow-up photographs of previous patients should be provided to clients to give them a realistic expectation of their own pet's postoperative appearance.[8]

Treatment planning must include the following:

- appropriate anesthesia and analgesia,
- adequate surgical margins,
- patient positioning for optimum visibility,
- prevention of damage to adjacent teeth; if damage occurs, address appropriately,

- preservation of local blood supply: atraumatic surgical technique; minimal use of electrocautery,
- tension-free closure,
- anticipation and prevention of complications: hemorrhage, infection, dehiscence, dysfunction.

ANESTHESIA AND ANALGESIA

Anesthesia and pain management are discussed in detail in Chapter 4. A multimodal approach to anesthesia and analgesia is indicated for oral oncologic surgery. The perioperative use of opioids,[31–35] nonsteroidal antiinflammatory agents,[36] ketamine infusions,[37–40] local or regional anesthesia[41–43] and/or alpha-2 adrenergic agonists,[33,44,45] in combination with inhaled anesthetics, should be considered for patients undergoing maxillectomy or mandibulectomy.

SURGICAL EXCISION

Four types of excision have been described (Fig. 43.1):[8,29,46,47]

- *Intracapsular excision:* A 'debulking' procedure that leaves behind macroscopically visible tumor. Local recurrence will happen unless surgery is followed by radiation therapy. This type of excision is acceptable for well-differentiated, benign tumors such as odontomas.[14] Debulking is also occasionally performed as palliative therapy for tumors which are too large to be completely excised and where radiation therapy is not elected (Fig. 43.2).
- *Marginal excision:* Excision immediately outside the pseudocapsule of the tumor, within the reactive zone (which consists mostly of inflammatory cells). Some neoplastic cells may remain visible microscopically. This type of excision may be appropriate for a well-differentiated benign tumor such as peripheral odontogenic fibroma (Fig. 43.3).[14] If marginal excision is performed on a malignant tumor, recurrence is likely without adjuvant therapy.

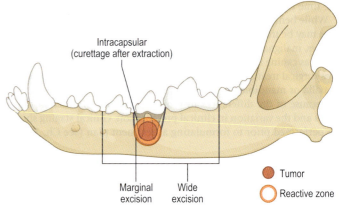

Fig. 43.1 Diagrammatic representation of surgical resection margins. Intracapsular excision may be appropriate for benign, well-differentiated lesions such as odontoma. Marginal excision, immediately outside the pseudocapsule of the tumor, may be appropriate for a well-differentiated benign tumor such as peripheral odontogenic fibroma.[14] Segmental mandibulectomy is an example of wide excision, which involves removal of the tumor, its pseudocapsule, and the reactive zone, with complete margins of normal tissue on all aspects.

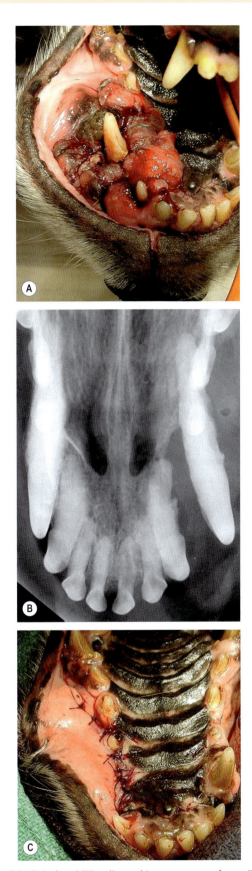

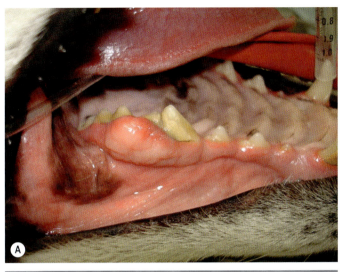

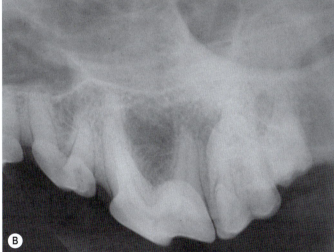

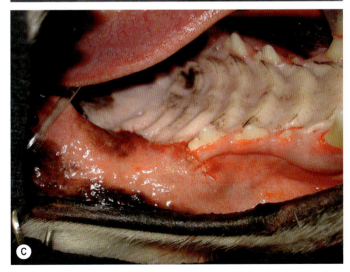

Fig. 43.2 (**A**) Clinical and (**B**) radiographic appearance of a malignant melanoma in a 14-year-old dog. (**C**) Debulking (intracapsular excision) was performed for palliative treatment. The patient is positioned in dorsal recumbency.

Fig. 43.3 (**A**) Clinical and (**B**) radiographic appearance of a peripheral odontogenic fibroma at the left maxillary fourth premolar tooth of an 8-year-old dog. (**C**) En bloc resection (marginal excision) was performed to achieve surgical cure. The patient is positioned in dorsal recumbency.

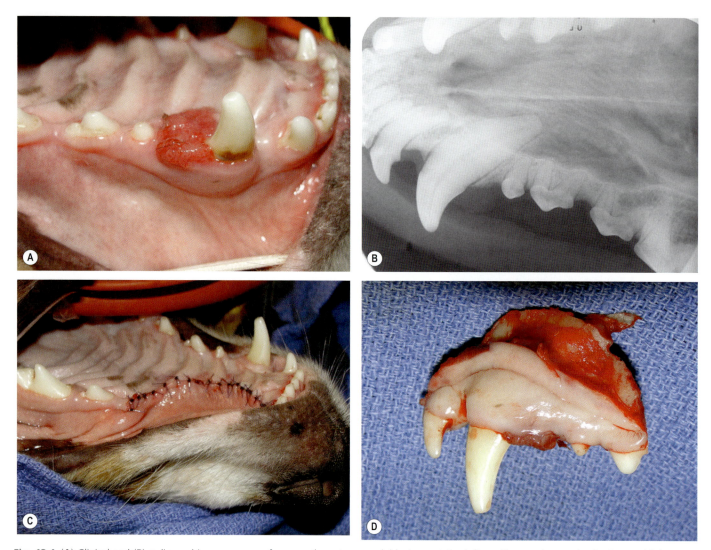

Fig. 43.4 (**A**) Clinical and (**B**) radiographic appearance of an acanthomatous ameloblastoma at the left maxillary canine tooth of a 3-year-old dog. (**C**) Unilateral rostral maxillectomy (wide excision) was performed to achieve surgical cure. The patient is positioned in dorsal recumbency. (**D**) The excised section of maxilla, containing the third incisor, canine, first and second premolar teeth.

- *Wide excision*: Removal of the tumor, its pseudocapsule, and the reactive zone, with complete margins of normal tissue on all aspects. In general, 10 mm of normal tissue is recommended for most malignant tumors.[8,14,48] However, some aggressively infiltrative tumor types, such as fibrosarcoma, may require much wider margins to achieve surgical cure.[48] Partial mandibulectomy or partial maxillectomy (Fig. 43.4) are examples of wide excision. Local recurrence is unexpected.
- *Radical excision:* Removal of the entire anatomical structure or compartment containing the tumor. It is questionable whether a total unilateral mandibulectomy meets the definition of a radical excision or whether it is a very wide excision. This approach is indicated for malignant oral tumors with extensive infiltration, such as fibrosarcoma, or involving a major part of the jaw.[14] Local recurrence is unexpected.

Attention to detail in surgical technique is of great importance in oncologic surgery and the management of oral tumors.[44,45] An oral tumor should be considered an 'infective nidus' of neoplastic cells, all of which may exfoliate into the surgical field and give rise to local recurrence, or enter the circulation and cause distant metastasis. During surgery, an oral tumor should therefore be covered using sterile swabs and handled as little as possible; if necessary, stay sutures may be placed in normal marginal tissue to facilitate manipulation. Other important measures include tying off blood vessels as early as possible in the procedure and electrocoagulating any accidentally exposed tumor surfaces. Once the tumor is excised, a second set of instruments and drapes should be used for the reconstructive stage of the procedure.

Following surgical excision, the margins of the excised tissue should be examined for the presence of neoplastic cells.[14,49] Although sutures may be used to identify the borders of the specimen, using different dyes (Davidson Marking System, Bradley Products Inc., Bloomington, MN) to mark the edges of the specimen enables the pathologist to more accurately identify and orient the sample.[14]

PATIENT POSITIONING

Lateral recumbency is preferred by most veterinarians for mandibulectomy and maxillectomy procedures.[48] Although lateral recumbency offers good exposure of the buccal surfaces of the uppermost teeth and jaws, it only provides fair visualization of the palate and lingual surfaces of the opposite quadrants. Therefore, dorsal recumbency is recommended for maxillectomy.[14,48,50] For mandibulectomy procedures, the authors prefer sternal recumbency, with the head elevated and the maxillas suspended between IV poles or secured to an anesthesia screen.[14,27] The main hazard of dorsal and sternal recumbency is fluid aspiration. The use of a cuffed endotracheal tube and pharyngeal pack is necessary to prevent aspiration. In addition, having continuous suction available is very helpful. In dorsal recumbency, the neck should be fully extended and the head end of the table slightly lowered. To further improve visibility, use of surgical telescopes and a head lamp is beneficial, particularly for surgeries involving the caudal mandible or maxilla.

MANAGEMENT OF ADJACENT TEETH

Although maintaining teeth is secondary to achieving adequate surgical margins and tension-free closure, it is important to consider adjacent teeth when planning the osteotomy. The excised tissue bloc should preferably include intact alveoli as tumors may infiltrate down the periodontal ligament space.[28] If teeth are transected during osteotomy, the remaining roots must be extracted. Osteotomy in a narrow interdental space may injure a tooth that was not planned to be included in the ostectomy. In these cases, it is preferable to widen the surgical margin and transect or extract the adjacent tooth than to compromise the margin in order to avoid injuring the tooth. For example, when performing rostral mandibulectomy, the second premolar tooth should be included in the section to be removed, because performing the osteotomy rostral to the second premolar tooth would transect the root of the canine tooth.

When performing an incisivectomy, great care should be taken not to damage the canine teeth when performing the osteotomy on the distal line angle of the third incisors.[28]

For segmental or caudal mandibulectomies, the blood supply to the teeth in the remaining rostral fragment is transected. This results in devitalization of the rostral teeth, which may require endodontic treatment.[28]

PRESERVATION OF LOCAL BLOOD SUPPLY

Knowledge of surgical anatomy is essential when planning a mandibulectomy or maxillectomy procedure. While major vessels may necessarily be ligated and transected as part of the surgical procedure, it is important to identify and preserve vessels supplying the mucosal flap and skin. For example, when performing a rostral mandibulectomy, it is usually possible to locate the branches of the mental artery as they exit the middle mental foramen at the level of the second premolar; these vessels can be preserved and included as part of the flap used to cover the remaining mandibular bone. Similarly, branches of the infraorbital artery may be preserved when creating a vestibular mucosal–submucosal flap for closure following partial maxillectomy. Specific techniques for maxillectomy and mandibulectomy are described in Chapters 45 and 46, respectively. Although transection of small vessels leads to persistent, diffuse hemorrhage once the mucosa has been incised, the use of electrocautery should be avoided, as it is associated with delayed wound healing and an increased risk of wound dehiscence.[48,51,52] Similarly, although the use of CO_2 lasers for oral mucosal incisions has been described,[53] research suggests that mucosal healing of incisions made with CO_2 lasers is delayed when compared with incisions made with steel blades.[54-56]

TENSION-FREE CLOSURE

The defect resulting from removal of a portion of the mandible or maxilla must be reconstructed. This is typically achieved by means of mucosal and submucosal flaps from the adjacent soft tissues; although techniques for mandibular reconstruction (using a free ulnar autograft, a microvascular coccygeal autograft, a split-rib graft, and the use of a buttress plate and biodegradable mesh filled with cancellous bone) have been described,[57-60] they are not routinely performed.

The tissue from which the vestibular flap originates will depend on the location and extent of the tumor to be resected; detailed surgical techniques for maxillectomy and mandibulectomy are described in Chapters 45 and 46, respectively. The flap must be undermined extensively to enable it to be brought into apposition with the hard palate mucoperiosteum (in the case of maxillectomy) or the sublingual mucosa (in the case of mandibulectomy) without tension.[48] If excision of the tumor precludes closure of the defect with a vestibular mucosal–submucosal flap, a myocutaneous free flap can be transferred to the site with microvascular techniques,[48] which are discussed in Chapter 9.

ANTICIPATION AND PREVENTION OF COMPLICATIONS

Hemorrhage

Hemorrhage is the primary intraoperative complication encountered during mandibulectomy or maxillectomy.[14] Blood typing and cross-matching are indicated, especially before a maxillectomy.[61] Because severe hemorrhage results when one of the main arteries (the inferior alveolar artery during a mandibulectomy and the infraorbital, sphenopalatine and major palatine arteries during a maxillectomy) is transected prior to ligation, every attempt should be made to identify and ligate the arteries prior to transection. A mandibulectomy technique has been described which employs an osteotomy bur (Lindemann bur, Hu-Friedy Mfg. Inc., Chicago, IL) on an oral surgery handpiece (INTRAsurge 300, KaVo America Corp., Lake Zurich, IL) to transect the ventral third of the mandible and make a shallow incision in the bone on the buccal and lingual aspects of the mandible over the mandibular canal without damaging the neurovascular bundle. Following the osteotomy, the mandible is separated, revealing the intact inferior alveolar blood vessels, which are then double-ligated and transected without hemorrhage.[14]

During a maxillectomy, if the margin of excision extends beyond the major palatine artery, that artery should be identified and ligated immediately to reduce hemorrhage.[48] Diffuse bleeding may occur following trauma to the turbinates during a maxillectomy, and can be a significant source of hemorrhage. Application of pressure, identification and ligation of blood vessels, and placement of absorbable hemostatic agents are all useful methods of controlling hemorrhage.[14] The focal use of electrocoagulation may also be employed. Both the surgeon and the anesthetist should be adequately prepared and skilled to handle extensive blood loss. Preoperative, bilateral temporary carotid artery ligation has been described[62] but is rarely indicated.

Postoperatively, hemorrhage may occur if a ligature becomes undone, or if hemostatic agents become dislodged as blood pressure rises. Hospitalization is indicated to allow careful monitoring for hemorrhage during the first 12 hours after surgery.

Infection

Due to the excellent blood supply of the oral soft tissues, wound healing in the oral cavity is typically rapid and uncomplicated, and infectious complications are uncommon. However, delayed wound healing and a higher incidence of wound infection should be anticipated in the presence of immunosuppressive systemic illness, following long-term administration of corticosteroids, in animals undergoing chemotherapy, or if the surgical site has previously been irradiated.[14]

Ideally, the teeth will have been scaled and polished during the anesthetic episode for clinical staging, diagnostic imaging and biopsy.[62] This provides a cleaner surgical field and less inflamed gingival tissues at the time of the maxillectomy or mandibulectomy.[14]

Most oral oncologic surgical procedures involve 'clean-contaminated' surgical wounds, and intraoperative antibiotic prophylaxis is warranted.[63] Ampicillin, amoxicillin-clavulanic acid, certain cephalosporins, and clindamycin are appropriate choices.[64–68] The use of antibiotics is discussed in detail in Chapter 3.

Surgical technique plays an important role in preventing infectious complications. In addition to employing aseptic technique, the surgeon must be careful not to traumatize the oral soft tissues, including the wound edges as well as more deeply situated tissues. Electrocoagulation should be used judiciously.[69] Irrigation must be used during osteotomy, ostectomy and osteoplasty to prevent thermal necrosis of bone.[28]

Dehiscence

Wound dehiscence is a relatively common complication following maxillectomy, with a reported incidence of 7–33%; the majority of cases which dehisced were caudal maxillectomies.[10,70,71] As previously mentioned, tension-free closure of the vestibular mucosal–submucosal flaps is essential to proper technique, and will largely prevent dehiscence.[48,50] Overzealous use of electrocoagulation may also result in dehiscence.[69]

Although uncommon, wound dehiscence following mandibulectomy may occur at the rostral end of the mandible, especially at the alveolar margin, resulting in bone exposure.[27,48] Small areas of dehiscence may heal by second intention while larger areas may have to be debrided and closed surgically.[28] Dehiscence of the commissurorrhaphy performed concomitantly with unilateral total mandibulectomy may also occur, and is repaired by delayed primary closure.[28]

Because wound dehiscence may occur as a result of tumor recurrence, biopsy of the dehisced wound edges is indicated if surgical repair is performed on a dehisced area.[50]

Postoperative dysfunction

Following mandibulectomy in the dog, it is common for the tongue to hang out laterally (unilateral rostral mandibulectomy or total mandibulectomy) or ventrally (bilateral rostral mandibulectomy). The patient's ability to prehend food may be affected, and drooling may be significant; performing a commissurorrhaphy will help to keep the tongue in the mouth and reduce drooling following total unilateral mandibulectomy.[28] Drooling following a bilateral rostral mandibulectomy can be reduced by carefully reconstructing the lower lip in a raised position.[27] If a bilateral rostral mandibulectomy is performed farther caudally than the second premolar tooth, the patient may require assisted feeding for a short time after surgery in order for the tongue to return to normal function.[48,50]

Segmental, caudal or total unilateral mandibulectomy will generally result in significant postoperative malocclusion. Typically, the intact mandible and the rostral part of the operated mandible, if present, drift toward the side of the resection. If both mandibular canine teeth are still present, they will traumatize the hard palate.[61] Crown reduction and endodontic treatment of the exposed pulp, or extraction of the mandibular canine tooth or teeth, is indicated to resolve and prevent further ulceration.[61] Alternatively, an 'elastic training device' using orthodontic buttons and bands to maintain normal occlusion has been described.[72] Malocclusion can be particularly severe in cats, and temporary maxillomandibular fixation using interdental bonding has been suggested to prevent this complication.[27]

Although bilateral rostral maxillectomy in the dog results in considerable deformity, caused by drooping of the nose, this does not seem to affect breathing through the nostrils.[50] Following maxillectomy, some mandibular teeth can occlude with the vestibular flap and cause mild and transient ulceration;[61] in addition, the ability to pick up objects and retrieve toys and sticks may be impaired, particularly after bilateral rostral maxillectomy.[19]

When premolar and molar teeth are removed as part of a maxillectomy or mandibulectomy, the natural cleaning action of mastication is prevented, resulting in rapid accumulation of plaque and calculus on the teeth of the opposing quadrant. Frequent routine periodontal treatment is therefore indicated.[61]

Cats are much more likely than dogs to display significant morbidity following major oral surgery, with 98% of cats experiencing one or more of the following symptoms in the first 4 weeks following mandibulectomy: tongue protrusion, malocclusion, dehiscence, drooling, pain, and difficulty eating or grooming.[73] More than three-fourths of cats for whom long-term follow-up was available displayed one or more of the above symptoms for the duration of their lives, and nearly half (18 of 38 cats with available follow-up beyond 4 weeks postoperatively) developed local tumor recurrence, in spite of adjuvant therapy in several cases.[73]

Client satisfaction following mandibulectomy and maxillectomy in dogs has been reported to be 85%, and was proportional to the postoperative survival time.[74] A similar percentage of clients with cats who had undergone mandibulectomy reported that they would choose the same course of action given the same circumstances, despite the fact that 76% of the cats who survived had adverse effects for the rest of their lives.[73]

REFERENCES

1. Withrow SJ. Cancer of the oral cavity. In: Withrow SJ, MacEwen EG, editors. Small animal clinical oncology. 3rd ed. Philadelphia, PA: W.B. Saunders; 2001. p. 305–18.
2. Stebbins KE, Morse CC, Goldschmidt MH. Feline oral neoplasia: a ten-year survey. Vet Pathol 1989;26:121–8.
3. Todoroff RJ, Brodey RS. Oral and pharyngeal neoplasia in the dog: a retrospective survey of 361 cases. J Am Vet Med Assoc 1979;175:567–71.
4. Brodey RS. A clinical and pathologic study of 130 neoplasms of the mouth and pharynx in the dog. Am J Vet Res 1960; 21:787–812.
5. Brodey RS. The biological behaviour of canine oral and pharyngeal neoplasms. J Small Anim Pract 1970;11:45–53.
6. Harvey CE, Emily PP. Oral neoplasms. In: Harvey CE, Emily PP, editors. Small animal dentistry. St. Louis, MO: Mosby – Year Book; 1993. p. 297–311.

7. Harvey HJ. Cryosurgery of oral tumors in dogs and cats. Vet Clin North Am Small Anim Pract 1980;10:821–30.

8. Berg J. Surgical therapy. In: Slatter DG, editor. Textbook of small animal surgery. 3rd ed. Philadelphia, PA: Saunders; 2003. p. 2324–8.

9. Schwarz PD, Withrow SJ, Curtis CR, et al. Mandibular resection as a treatment for oral cancer in 81 dogs. J Am Anim Hosp Assoc 1991;27:601–10.

10. Schwarz PD, Withrow SJ, Curtis CR, et al. Partial maxillary resection as a treatment for oral cancer in 61 dogs. J Am Anim Hosp Assoc 1991;27:617–24.

11. Kosovsky JK, Matthiesen DT, Manfra Marretta S, et al. Results of partial mandibulectomy for the treatment of oral tumors in 142 dogs. Vet Surg 1991; 20:397–401.

12. Salisbury SK, Lantz GC. Long-term results of partial mandibulectomy for treatment of oral tumors in 30 dogs. J Am Anim Hosp Assoc 1988;24:285–94.

13. Salisbury SK, Richardson DC, Lantz GC. Partial maxillectomy and premaxillectomy in the treatment of oral neoplasia in the dog and cat. Vet Surg 1986;15:16–26.

14. Verstraete FJ. Mandibulectomy and maxillectomy. Vet Clin North Am Small Anim Pract 2005;35:1009–39.

15. Ellis III E. Surgical management of oral pathologic lesions. In: Hupp JR, Ellis III E, Tucker MR, editors. Contemporary oral and maxillofacial surgery. 5th ed. St. Louis, MO: Mosby; 2008. p. 449–68.

16. O'Mara RE. Skeletal scanning in neoplastic disease. Cancer 1976;37:480–6.

17. Seguin B. Tumors of the mandible, maxilla and calvarium. In: Slatter DG, editor. Textbook of small animal surgery. 3rd ed. Philadelphia, PA: Saunders; 2003. p. 2488–502.

18. Anonymous. Nomina anatomica veterinaria. 5th ed. Hannover, Columbia, Gent and Sapporo: Editorial Committee, World Association of Veterinary Anatomists; 2005.

19. Lascelles BD, Henderson RA, Seguin B, et al. Bilateral rostral maxillectomy and nasal planectomy for large rostral maxillofacial neoplasms in six dogs and one cat. J Am Anim Hosp Assoc 2004;40: 137–46.

20. Kirpensteijn J, Withrow SJ, Straw RC. Combined resection of the nasal planum and premaxilla in three dogs. Vet Surg 1994;23:341–6.

21. O'Brien MG, Withrow SJ, Straw RC, et al. Total and partial orbitectomy for the treatment of periorbital tumors in 24 dogs and 6 cats: a retrospective study. Vet Surg 1996;25:471–9.

22. Brown JS, Kalavrezos N, D'Souza J, et al. Factors that influence the method of mandibular resection in the management of oral squamous cell carcinoma. Br J Oral Maxillofac Surg 2002;40:275–84.

23. Arzi B, Verstraete FJ. Mandibular rim excision in seven dogs. Vet Surg 2010;39: 226–31.

24. Peled M, Machtei EE, Rachmiel A. Osseous reconstruction using a membrane barrier following marginal mandibulectomy: an animal pilot study. J Periodontol 2002; 73:1451–6.

25. Walker KS, Reiter AM, Lewis JR. Step-by-step: marginal mandibulectomy in the dog. J Vet Dent 2009;26:194–8.

26. Reynolds D, Fransson B, Preston C. Crescentic osteotomy for resection of oral tumours in four dogs. Vet Comp Orthop Traumatol 2009;22:412–6.

27. Dernell WS, Schwarz PD, Withrow SJ. Mandibulectomy. In: Bojrab MJ, editor. Current techniques in small animal surgery. 4th ed. Baltimore, MD: Williams & Wilkins; 1998. p. 132–42.

28. Verstraete FJ. Mandibulectomy and maxillectomy. Vet Clin North Am Small Anim Pract 2005;35:1009–39.

29. Gilson SD, Stone EA. Principles of oncologic surgery. Compend Cont Educ Pract Vet 1990;12:827–38.

30. Ellis III E. Surgical management of oral pathologic lesions. In: Peterson LJ, Ellis III E, Hupp JR, editors. Contemporary oral and maxillofacial surgery. 4th ed. St. Louis, MO: Mosby; 2003. p. 479–502.

31. Buback JL, Boothe HW, Carroll GL, et al. Comparison of three methods for relief of pain after ear canal ablation in dogs. Vet Surg 1996;25:380–5.

32. Hofmeister EH, Egger CM. Transdermal fentanyl patches in small animals. J Am Anim Hosp Assoc 2004;40:468–78.

33. Itamoto K, Hikasa Y, Sakonjyu I, et al. Anaesthetic and cardiopulmonary effects of balanced anaesthesia with medetomidine-midazolam and butorphanol in dogs. J Vet Med A Physiol Pathol Clin Med 2000;47:411–20.

34. Wilson DV. Advantages and guidelines for using opioid agonists for induction of anesthesia. Vet Clin North Am Small Anim Pract 1992;22:269–72.

35. Ilkiw JE. Balanced anesthetic techniques in dogs and cats. Clin Tech Small Anim Pract 1999;14:27–37.

36. Lascelles BD, McFarland JM, Swann H. Guidelines for safe and effective use of NSAIDs in dogs. Vet Ther 2005;6:237–51.

37. Boscan P, Pypendop BH, Solano AM, et al. Cardiovascular and respiratory effects of ketamine infusions in isoflurane-anesthetized dogs before and during noxious stimulation. Am J Vet Res 2005;66:2122–9.

38. Pascoe PJ, Ilkiw JE, Craig C, et al. The effects of ketamine on the minimum alveolar concentration of isoflurane in cats. Vet Anaesth Analg 2007;34:31–9.

39. Pypendop BH, Solano A, Boscan P, et al. Characteristics of the relationship between plasma ketamine concentration and its effect on the minimum alveolar concentration of isoflurane in dogs. Vet Anaesth Analg 2007;34:209–12.

40. Solano AM, Pypendop BH, Boscan PL, et al. Effect of intravenous administration of ketamine on the minimum alveolar concentration of isoflurane in anesthetized dogs. Am J Vet Res 2006;67:21–5.

41. Beckman B, Legendre L. Regional nerve blocks for oral surgery in companion animals. Compend Cont Educ Pract Vet 2002;24:439–44.

42. Lantz GC. Regional anesthesia for dentistry and oral surgery. J Vet Dent 2003;20:181–6.

43. Woodward TM. Pain management and regional anesthesia for the dental patient. Top Companion Anim Med 2008;23: 106–14.

44. Benson GJ, Grubb TL, Neff-Davis C, et al. Perioperative stress response in the dog: effect of pre-emptive administration of medetomidine. Vet Surg 2000;29:85–91.

45. Vaisanen M, Raekallio M, Kuusela E, et al. Evaluation of the perioperative stress response in dogs administered medetomidine or acepromazine as part of the preanesthetic medication. Am J Vet Res 2002;63:969–75.

46. Soderstrom MJ, Gilson SD. Principles of surgical oncology. Vet Clin North Am Small Anim Pract 1995;25:97–110.

47. Enneking WF. Surgical procedures. In: Enneking WF, editor. Musculoskeletal tumor surgery. 1st ed. New York: Churchill Livingstone; 1983. p. 89–122.

48. Salisbury SK. Maxillectomy and mandibulectomy. In: Slatter DH, editor. Textbook of small animal surgery. 3rd ed. Philadelphia, PA: W.B. Saunders; 2003. p. 561–72.

49. Mann FA, Pace LW. Marking margins of tumorectomies and excisional biopsies to facilitate histological assessment of excision completeness. Semin Vet Med Surg (Small Anim) 1993;8:279–83.

50. Dernell WS, Schwarz PD, Withrow SJ. Maxillectomy and premaxillectomy. In: Bojrab MJ, editor. Current techniques in small animal surgery. 4th ed. Baltimore, MD: Williams & Wilkins; 1998. p. 124–32.

51. Liboon J, Funkhouser W, Terris DJ. A comparison of mucosal incisions made by scalpel, CO2 laser, electrocautery, and constant-voltage electrocautery. Otolaryngol Head Neck Surg 1997; 116:379–85.

52. Kahnberg KE, Thilander H. Healing of experimental excisional wounds in the rat palate. II. Histological study of electrosurgical wounds. Swed Dent J 1984;8:49–56.

53. Taney KG, Smith MM. Surgical extraction of impacted teeth in a dog. J Vet Dent 2006;23:168–77.

54. Sinha UK, Gallagher LA. Effects of steel scalpel, ultrasonic scalpel, CO2 laser, and monopolar and bipolar electrosurgery on

wound healing in guinea pig oral mucosa. Laryngoscope 2003;113:228–36.

55. Mison MB, Steficek B, Lavagnino M, et al. Comparison of the effects of the CO2 surgical laser and conventional surgical techniques on healing and wound tensile strength of skin flaps in the dog. Vet Surg 2003;32:153–60.

56. Hendrick DA, Meyers A. Wound healing after laser surgery. Otolaryngol Clin North Am 1995;28:969–86.

57. Boudrieau RJ, Mitchell SL, Seeherman H. Mandibular reconstruction of a partial hemimandibulectomy in a dog with severe malocclusion. Vet Surg 2004;33:119–30.

58. Strong EB, Rubinstein B, Pahlavan N, et al. Mandibular reconstruction with an alloplastic bone tray in dogs. Otolaryngol Head Neck Surg 2003;129:417–26.

59. Bracker KE, Trout NJ. Use of a free cortical ulnar autograft following en bloc resection of a mandibular tumor. J Am Anim Hosp Assoc 2000;36:76–9.

60. Yeh L-S, Hou S-M. Repair of a mandibular defect with a free vascularized coccygeal vertebra transfer in a dog. Vet Surg 1994; 23:281–5.

61. Salisbury SK. Aggressive cancer surgery and aftercare. In: Morrison WB, editor. Cancer in dogs and cats – medical and surgical management. 2nd ed. Jackson, WY: Teton NewMedia; 2002. p. 249–301.

62. Hedlund CS. Surgery of the oral cavity and oropharynx. In: Fossum TW, editor. Small animal surgery. 2nd ed. St. Louis, MO: Mosby; 2002. p. 274–306.

63. Peterson LJ. Principles of surgical and antimicrobial infection management. In: Topazian RG, Goldberg MH, Hupp JR, editors. Oral and maxillofacial infections. 4th ed. Philadelphia, PA: W.B. Saunders; 2002. p. 99–111.

64. Callender DL. Antibiotic prophylaxis in head and neck oncologic surgery: the role of Gram-negative coverage. Int J Antimicrob Agents 1999;12(Suppl 1):S21–7.

65. Johnson JT, Kachman K, Wagner RL, et al. Comparison of ampicillin/sulbactam versus clindamycin in the prevention of infection in patients undergoing head and neck surgery. Head Neck 1997;19:367–71.

66. Harvey CE, Thornsberry C, Miller BR, et al. Antimicrobial susceptibility of subgingival bacterial flora in cats with gingivitis. J Vet Dent 1995;12:157–60.

67. Harvey CE, Thornsberry C, Miller BR, et al. Antimicrobial susceptibility of subgingival bacterial flora in dogs with gingivitis. J Vet Dent 1995;12:151–5.

68. Mueller SC, Henkel KO, Neumann J, et al. Perioperative antibiotic prophylaxis in maxillofacial surgery: penetration of clindamycin into various tissues. J Craniomaxillofac Surg 1999;27: 172–6.

69. Salisbury SK, Thacker HL, Pantzer EE, et al. Partial maxillectomy in the dog. Comparison of suture material and closure techniques. Vet Surg 1985; 14:265–76.

70. Harvey CE. Oral surgery. Radical resection of maxillary and mandibular lesions. Vet Clin North Am Small Anim Pract 1986;16:983–93.

71. Wallace J, Matthiesen DT, Patnaik AK. Hemimaxillectomy for the treatment of oral tumors in 69 dogs. Vet Surg 1992; 21:337–41.

72. Bar-Am Y, Verstraete FJ. Elastic training for the prevention of mandibular drift following mandibulectomy in dogs: 18 cases (2005–2008). Vet Surg 2010;39: 574–80.

73. Northrup NC, Selting KA, Rassnick KM, et al. Outcomes of cats with oral tumors treated with mandibulectomy: 42 cases. J Am Anim Hosp Assoc 2006;42:350–60.

74. Fox LE, Geoghegan SL, Davis LH, et al. Owner satisfaction with partial mandibulectomy or maxillectomy for treatment of oral tumors in 27 dogs. J Am Anim Hosp Assoc 1997;33:25–31.

Chapter 44

Surgical treatment of tongue, lip and cheek tumors

Bernard Séguin

DEFINITIONS[1,2]

Cheeks (buccae): the cheeks form the caudal portion of the lateral margins of the vestibular cavity. Dogs possess small cheeks because of the large mouth opening. They are the lateral wall of the vestibule caudal to the commissures of the lips on either side, continuous with the lips.

Lips (labia oris): the lips are the fleshy margins of the opening of the mouth. The upper lip (*labium superius*) is associated with the maxilla and the lower lip (*labium inferius*) is associated with the mandible. The lips form the rostral and lateral margins of the vestibule of the mouth. The upper and lower lips meet at the angles of the mouth (*angulus oris*), forming the commissures of the lips.

Mouth (os): the mouth in its restrictive definition is limited to the opening between the lips. In a broader sense it designates the entire oral cavity, in which are located the tongue and the teeth. The oral cavity proper (*cavum oris proprium*) is bounded dorsally by the hard palate and the rostral part of the soft palate, laterally and rostrally by the dental arches and teeth, and ventrally by the tongue and the reflected mucosa under the tongue. The vestibule of the mouth (*vestibulum oris*) is the space external to the teeth, gingiva and alveolar mucosa, and internal to lips and cheeks.

Tongue (lingua): the tongue is mostly a large muscle (*m. lingualis proprius*) located on the floor of the oral cavity proper. It aids in prehension, chewing and swallowing and is the location of the papillae and the taste buds (*caliculi gustatorii*).

SURGICAL ANATOMY

Tongue[2]

The intricate movement of the tongue is made possible by extrinsic and intrinsic muscles. The extrinsic muscles are the styloglossus, hyoglossus, and genioglossus. The intrinsic muscle (*m. lingualis proprius*) contains superficial and deep longitudinal, perpendicular, and transverse fibers. The lingual mucosa is thick and heavily keratinized on the dorsal surface of the tongue and on the ventral surface becomes thinner and unkeratinized. Ventrally, it also forms an unpaired, median mucosal fold, the lingual frenulum. The frenulum attaches the body of the tongue to the floor of the oral cavity.

The blood supply to the tongue is primarily through the paired lingual arteries, which are one of the largest branches of the external carotid arteries. The lingual arteries are closer to the ventral surface and midline. There are several anastomoses between the left and right lingual arteries found at the level of the root, body and tip of the tongue. The lingual veins are in close proximity to their respective lingual arteries.

The tongue is innervated by the lingual nerve, a branch of the trigeminal (V), the chorda tympani, a branch of the facial (VII), the glossopharyngeal (IX), and the hypoglossal (XII) nerves. The only nerve responsible for the motor function of the tongue is the hypoglossal nerve. It runs parallel to the lingual artery. All nerves play a role in the sensory function of the tongue such as tactile, pain, thermal, taste, or proprioception.

Lips and cheeks

The lips and cheeks consist of three basic layers: the external layer is the integument, the middle layer consists of muscles and fibroelastic tissue, and the internal layer is the mucosa. The blood supply is provided by the inferior and superior labial arteries bringing blood to the lower and upper lip, respectively. Both are branches of the facial artery, arising from the external carotid. The inferior labial artery anastomoses with the caudal mental and the sublingual arteries. The superior labial artery forms anastomoses with the lateral inferior palpebral, malar, lateral nasal and masseter arteries. These anastomoses ensure a significant collateral blood supply to the lips.

The lips and cheeks are innervated by the trigeminal and facial nerves. Severing branches of the facial nerve when attempting a tumor excision can lead to droopy lips and drooling, especially in dogs with more pendulous lips. Because the lips do not play a role in the prehension of food in dogs and cats, severing these nerves at the level of the lips or cheeks minimally affects quality of life.

The parotid duct opens into the vestibular area, at the caudal margin of the maxillary fourth premolar tooth. In some instances, it

DOI: 10.1016/B978-0-7020-4618-6.00044-0

is necessary to excise this area during tumor removal. The duct can be ligated and the salivary gland will atrophy, or the duct can be preserved and transposed. However, preservation of the duct should not be attempted if it could compromise the completeness of the tumor removal.

Lymphatic drainage[3]

There are three lymph centers in the head, namely, the lymphocentrum parotideum, lymphocentrum mandibulare and lymphocentrum retropharyngeum. Lymphatic drainage of the tongue, cheek and lips is mainly to the lymphocentrums mandibulare and retropharyngeum. Therefore the mandibular nodes, tonsils and retropharyngeal nodes are of clinical interest. Lymph vessels of the head and neck can cross over the midline and therefore nodes on both sides of the head and neck should be evaluated even in the presence of a unilateral lesion. The efferent lymph vessels of the lymphocentrums of the head are part of the afferent vessels of the lymphocentrum cervicale. Therefore the superficial cervical (clinically known as prescapular) lymph nodes should also be evaluated when a neoplasm of the head is present.

THERAPEUTIC DECISION-MAKING

The amount of tissue to be excised depends on the size of the tumor and its histologic type. Therefore performing a biopsy in order to find out the type of tumor is imperative before attempting definitive excision. As a general rule, benign tumors can be removed by performing a marginal excision, whereas malignant tumors require a wide excision (see Ch. 43). When planning the excision, the primary goal is to achieve a complete excision of the tumor (i.e., 'clean' margins). Once the amount of tissue to be removed in order to achieve a complete excision has been determined, the remaining function needs to be anticipated in light of the reconstructive options. If function is projected to be greatly comprised and to severely affect quality of life, then a different therapeutic option must be sought. Adjuvant or neoadjuvant radiation therapy or chemotherapy may be necessary and therefore a multidisciplinary approach must always be kept in mind (see Ch. 43).

Tongue tumors

The tongue plays a much more important role in the prehension of food and water in the cat than in the dog. The tongue is also important for grooming in cats, which is an important function for the quality of life of a cat. Therefore dogs are better at adapting following a partial glossectomy. Malignant tumors that are located on the rostral half of the tongue can be removed by full-thickness partial glossectomy. Tumors located in the caudal aspect of the tongue can be excised if they are superficial, especially if in the dorsal aspect. It has been shown that dogs tolerate 40–60% of their tongue being excised.[4] Based on a limited number of cases, it appears that dogs can tolerate 75–100% amputation of their tongue while achieving an acceptable functional outcome and be able to adapt to their disability.[4,5] However, such extensive glossectomy may not always reliably achieve the same prognosis. The cat may only be able to tolerate 50% of its tongue being excised.[6]

Benign tumors, such as granular cell myoblastoma, can be removed with conservative and close margins, i.e., by marginal excision. Malignant tumors require a full-thickness glossectomy, which will be a wedge, transverse or longitudinal glossectomy. Smaller tumors located near the lateral edge of the tongue a few centimeters away from the

tip can be removed with a wedge glossectomy. If the lingual artery is sacrificed, it is possible for the ipsilateral rostral aspect of the tongue to survive because of the existing anastomoses between the paired lingual arteries. If the surgery leaves a significant portion of the rostral aspect of the tongue and the lingual artery was sacrificed, it may be safer to perform a longitudinal glossectomy as the anastomoses may not be sufficient to maintain the viability of the ipsilateral rostral aspect of the tongue. A longitudinal glossectomy is also indicated for larger tumors that are limited to one side of the tongue. If the tumor invades both sides of the tongue or comes too close to the midline, such that both lingual arteries would be sacrificed during tumor excision, a transverse glossectomy is recommended.

Lip and cheek tumors[7]

Following tumor excision, the next priority is restoration of function. For the lips and cheeks, this mainly involves preventing drooling and leakage of oral contents. Cosmesis largely depends on the restoration of a smooth lip margin. Selection of the most appropriate method of closure is based on size and location of the defect, the inherent tissue elasticity of the species, breed, and particular individual patient, and the tissues available in the vicinity that can be used in the reconstruction to close the defect. It has been stated that, as a general rule, approximately half of the upper lip (from the philtrum to the commissure) can be removed and the defect closed primarily without resorting to more advanced reconstruction techniques.[8] The cosmetic appearance of the pet can be an important factor in the decision-making for some clients. Providing information to the clients about the prognosis following tumor excision, including the expected quality of life and cosmetic appearance, is crucial. This will lead to greater client satisfaction regarding their decision. Most reconstruction techniques will create some rostral displacement of the commissure of the lips on the ipsilateral side of the tumor resection: the larger the defect, the more noticeable the displacement. The buccal rotation, the labial buccal reconstruction with inverse tubed skin, and the upper or lower labial pedicle rotation flap techniques create the most significant rostral displacement of the commissure.

Malignant tumors require a full-thickness excision of the lip or cheek in order to insure a complete excision at the deep margin. As a general rule, the simplest technique of excision and lip/cheek reconstruction should always be employed. However, since complete excision is one of the primary goals, the larger the tumor, the larger the defect will be and therefore the more complex and involved the technique for reconstruction will be.

As a general rule, techniques for the upper lip and lower lip are similar. Smaller tumors can be removed by performing a wedge resection. Larger tumors are removed by performing a rectangular resection. The defect can be closed in a 'Y' fashion or, for larger defects, it can be closed by performing a full-thickness labial advancement technique. The lower lip is easier to advance compared with the upper lip, with the mucosa/submucosa being the most significant restricting layers. For tumors that are at the most rostral aspect of the lower lips, i.e., at the level of the incisor teeth, a bilateral labial advancement technique can be performed to close the defect on the rostral midline. For larger defects of the upper or lower lip, a labial pedicle rotation flap technique can be performed. Large defects of the upper lip can be reconstructed with a buccal rotation technique. Excision of the entire upper lip is possible with reconstruction using a buccolabial pedicle flap. Very large defects of the upper lip or cheek, with or without upper lip and/or lower lip involvement, can be reconstructed by using skin flaps. Small gaps in the mucosal surface can heal by second intention. Large mucosal defects are most likely to create scarring, contraction and distortion of the lips if left to heal by second intention. Therefore the skin flap can be used as a substitute for the oral mucosal lining. Alternatively, an experimental technique has been described where the mucosa from under the tongue is grafted under a proposed skin flap, which will eventually be transferred as a free microvascular skin graft to the cheek/lip area to be reconstructed.[9] The time period between the grafting of the oral mucosa to the underside of a skin flap to the transfer of the skin graft to the facial area can be 2–3 weeks. By that time, the underside of the skin flap will be partially lined with oral mucosa, which will enable reconstruction of large cheek and labial defects.[9]

Dogs with more pendulous upper lips with a tumor that is situated at the dorsal aspect of the lip can be treated with an upper lip pull-down technique. It is important to assure that adequate tissue margins are available before attempting this technique of tumor excision and lip reconstruction. Dogs with malignant tumors extending closer to the alveolar mucosa and gingiva may require a full-thickness lip excision combined with a partial maxillectomy or mandibulectomy.

SURGICAL TECHNIQUES – GLOSSECTOMY

Stay sutures can be placed slightly away from the proposed incision site before the incision is performed. These stay sutures will help to manipulate the tongue with minimal use of tissue forceps and hence decrease the trauma to the tongue. Because the tongue is very well vascularized, copious bleeding is usually present during surgery of the tongue. Hemostasis can be achieved by ligation of larger vessels, pressure or judicious use of electrocoagulation. Through-and-through horizontal mattress sutures can be placed a few millimeters away from the incision to help control hemorrhage. Temporary occlusion of the carotid arteries can be performed before attempting glossectomy in order to minimize blood loss; however, this is rarely required and blood loss can usually be controlled without having to resort to carotid occlusion. The edges of the incised tongue can be sutured using simple continuous or simple interrupted patterns with fine monofilament absorbable suture.

Marginal excision

A fusiform incision is made around the tumor into the tongue and the tumor is excised by partial-thickness glossectomy. The defect in the tongue is closed with simple interrupted or simple continuous suture pattern by apposition of the lingual mucosa.

Wedge glossectomy (Fig. 44.1)

A full-thickness wedge-shape incision is performed around the tumor. The defect can be closed by apposing the ventral mucosa to the dorsal mucosa therefore closing it longitudinally, which will cause a narrowing of the tongue, or it can be closed transversely by suturing the dorsal mucosa together and the ventral mucosa together, which will cause a deviation of the tip of the tongue to the side of the resection.

Transverse glossectomy (Fig. 44.2)

A full-thickness incision is made transversely across the tongue caudal to the tumor. The defect is closed by apposing the dorsal mucosa with the ventral mucosa. Depending on the shape of the tumor, it may be possible to create a V-shaped incision with the apex of the 'V' directly caudally on midline. This defect is closed by apposing the dorsal mucosa on either side together and the ventral mucosa as well.

Longitudinal glossectomy (Fig. 44.3)

A full-thickness longitudinal incision is made along the midline from the tip of the tongue to the caudal extent of the tumor. The incision is then brought to the lateral edge of the tongue providing an adequate margin of normal tissue. The defect is closed by apposing the ventral and dorsal mucosal layers together along the length of the incision.

SURGICAL TECHNIQUES – EXCISION OF LIP AND CHEEK TUMORS AND RECONSTRUCTION[7]

Techniques for the upper lip and cheek

Wedge excision (Fig. 44.4 and 26.3)

A wedge excision is performed from the lip with the tip away from the labial margin. The defect is closed by apposing the edges starting with the lip margins to ensure proper alignment. A two-layer closure is performed by suturing the mucosa first and then the skin.

Rectangular excision and Y-closure (Fig. 44.5)

The tumor is removed by performing a rectangular incision around it, removing the labial margin as well. The defect is closed by apposing the labial margins accurately first. Then the rest of the defect is sutured in a 'Y' fashion with a two-layer closure (mucosa and skin).

Full-thickness labial advancement technique (Fig. 44.6)

After removing the tumor with a rectangular incision, the remaining lip caudal to the defect is mobilized by performing a full-thickness incision at the dorsal aspect of the lip, parallel to the dental arcade. The length of the mobilizing incision depends on the size of the defect needing repair. The flap should stretch over the defect without excessive tension. The labial margins are accurately apposed and the edges of mucosa are reapposed to reconstruct the vestibule. The skin is closed as a second layer. Tension sutures can be used in areas of moderate tension.

Buccal rotation flap (Fig. 44.7)

The tumor is removed with a rectangular incision. The lip margin caudal to the rectangular defect is removed for a length equal to the height of the rectangle (i.e., dorsoventral dimension). The caudoventral corner of the rectangle is brought into the rostrodorsal corner. A two-layer closure is performed by suturing the mucosal edges together and then the skin edges.

Lower labial pedicle rotation flap[8] (Fig. 44.8)

The tumor is excised with a wedge or rectangular resection. Approximately 80% to 90% of the lip margin (from philtrum to commissure) can be excised. A full-thickness lower lip flap is created by making an incision parallel to the lip margin and 30–40 mm away from it. The incision begins at the caudal aspect of the upper lip defect and runs several centimeters cranially (long enough to be able to appose it with the rostral edge of the upper lip defect). The flap is rotated after releasing the restrictive soft tissues from the mandible such that the caudal edge of the flap meets the rostral edge of the upper lip defect. The margin of the lower lip flap becomes the margin of the upper lip

433

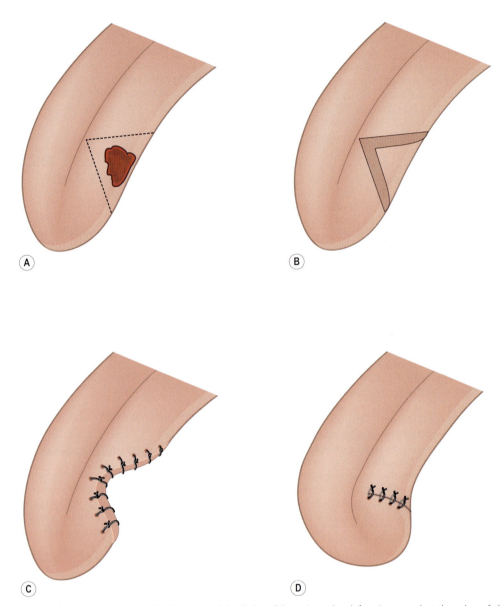

Fig. 44.1 Wedge glossectomy. (**A**) Proposed wedge incision around the lesion. (**B**) A triangular defect is created at the edge of the tongue. (**C**) The incision can be closed by suturing the dorsal mucosa with the ventral mucosa. (**D**) Alternatively, the incision can be closed by suturing the two edges of the ventral mucosa together and the same with the dorsal mucosa.

where the defect was. The buccal mucosa is sutured. Small gaps can be left open to allow wider opening of the jaws. The skin is closed in an inverted 'Y' fashion over the defect.

Buccolabial pedicle flap (Fig. 44.9)

The tumor is excised where the entire upper lip is removed in the process. With this technique to reconstruct the upper lip, the lower labial pedicle rotation flap technique is modified by extending the labial flap into the cheek, thereby elongating the flap and allowing larger defects of the upper lip to be reconstructed. In order to close the lip defect, the flap created from the cheek and lower lip is full thickness such that the deep aspect of the flap is covered with buccal mucosa. An incision is made from the caudal aspect of the defect at the level of the junction between the labial mucosa and gingiva, and runs caudally to the level of the most caudal aspect of the vestibule. The height (the ventrodorsal dimension) of the flap is made to be of

equal dimension as the height of the resected lip. A ventral incision is made from the caudal incision of the buccal flap extending to the ventral aspect of the lower lip to about half of the length of the lower lip. This creates a buccolabial flap with the pedicle being at the rostral aspect of the flap, ventral to the lower lip. The caudal aspect of the flap in its orthotopic position is rotated rostrally to join the rostral aspect of the upper lip defect. Restrictive soft tissues are released from the mandible to relieve tension on the flap. The incised mucosa of the flap is sutured to the edges of the mucosa of the defect with an absorbable suture material. By apposing the cut edges of mucosa, the buccal cavity is reconstructed. The edges of the skin are apposed where the caudal aspect of the flap (in its orthotopic position) meets with the rostral and dorsal aspects of the upper lip defect, and the ventral border of the flap (in its orthotopic position) meets with the dorso-caudal aspect of the defect. The skin edges are sutured with an absorbable suture material for the subcuticular layer and with nonabsorbable sutures for the dermis. Because the most rostral aspect of the new lip

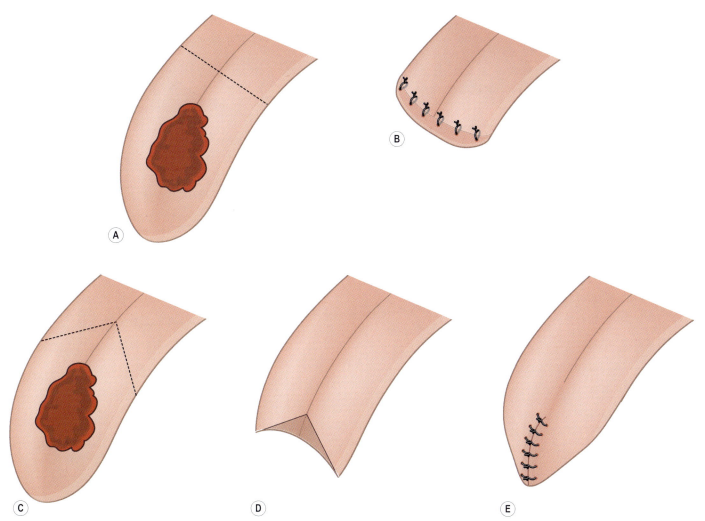

Fig. 44.2 Transverse glossectomy. (**A**) Proposed transverse incision of the tongue, caudal to the lesion. (**B**) The incision is closed by suturing the ventral and dorsal mucosae together. (**C**) Alternatively, the incision is made into a 'V' with the tip of the 'V' being caudal. (**D**) This results in a triangular defect at the rostral aspect of the tongue. (**E**) The incision is closed by suturing the ventral mucosa together and the same with the dorsal mucosa, creating a longitudinal suture line.

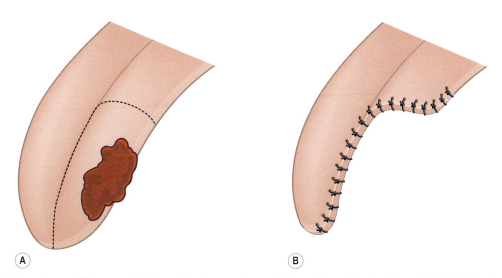

Fig. 44.3 Longitudinal glossectomy. (**A**) Proposed incision of the tongue along midline and caudal to the lesion. (**B**) The incision is closed by suturing the ventral mucosa and dorsal mucosa together.

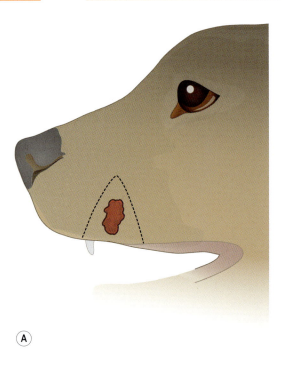

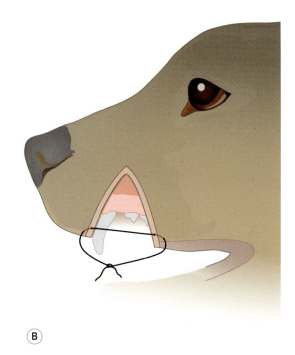

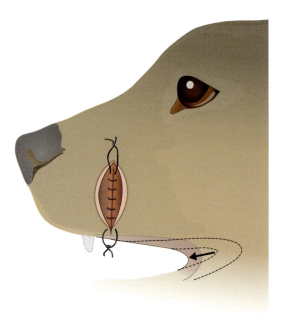

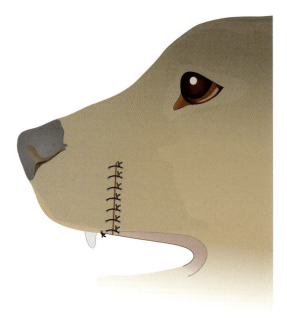

Fig. 44.4 Wedge excision of lip. (**A**) Proposed full-thickness wedge incision around lesion with tip away from lip margin. (**B**) The defect is closed by apposing the lip margin first to ensure proper alignment. (**C**) A two-layer closure is performed by suturing the mucosa first. (**D**) The second layer is closed by suturing the skin. The commissure of the lips will move rostrally (*arrow*). *(From Atlas of Small Animal Wound Management and Reconstructive Surgery, 3rd Edition, by M. Pavletic, 2010. Reproduced with permission of John Wiley & Sons, Inc.)*

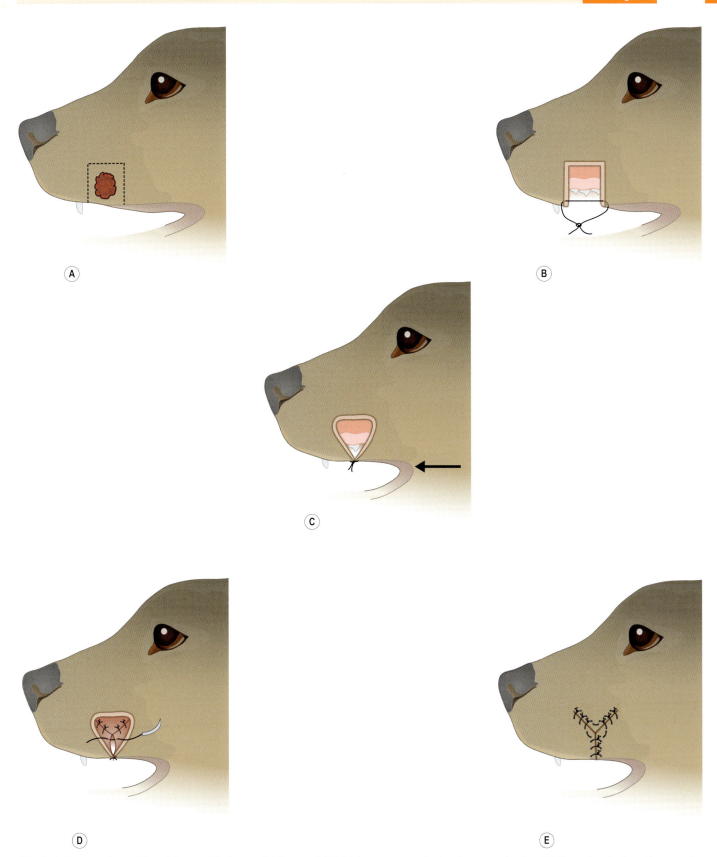

Fig. 44.5 Rectangular excision of lip and 'Y' closure. (**A**) Proposed full-thickness rectangular incision around lesion. (**B**) The defect is closed by apposing the lip margin first to ensure proper alignment. (**C**) The commissure of the lips will move rostrally (*arrow*). (**D**) A two-layer closure is performed in a 'Y' fashion, starting with the mucosa. (**E**) The second layer is closed by suturing the skin. *(From Atlas of Small Animal Wound Management and Reconstructive Surgery, 3rd Edition, by M. Pavletic, 2010. Reproduced with permission of John Wiley & Sons, Inc.)*

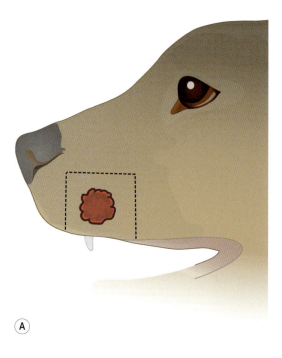

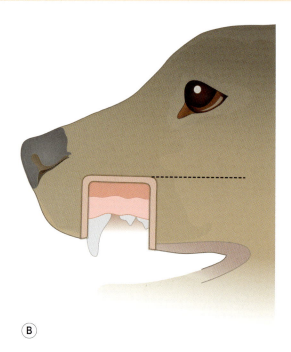

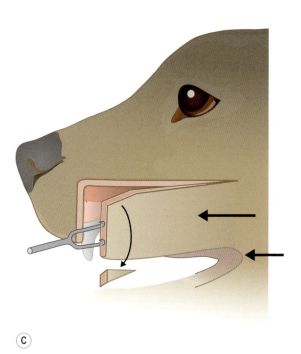

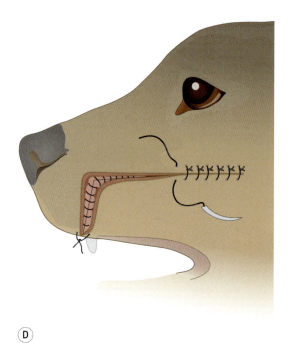

Fig. 44.6 Rectangular excision and full-thickness labial advancement technique. (**A**) Proposed full-thickness rectangular incision around lesion. (**B**) A full-thickness incision is performed at the level of the dorsal extent of the excision, the incision being parallel to the dental quadrant or lip margin. The length of the incision will depend on the size of the defect. (**C**) The labial flap is advanced rostrally, which will also cause rostral advancement of the commissure of the lips (*bottom arrow*). A triangular full-thickness piece of the flap can be removed from the caudorostral aspect of the flap to assure that the lip margin will be leveled to account for the difference in height in the lip. (**D**) The labial flap is sutured to the rostral lip in a two-layer fashion, starting at the lip margin and suturing the mucosa first. *(From Atlas of Small Animal Wound Management and Reconstructive Surgery, 3rd Edition, by M. Pavletic, 2010. Reproduced with permission of John Wiley & Sons, Inc.)*

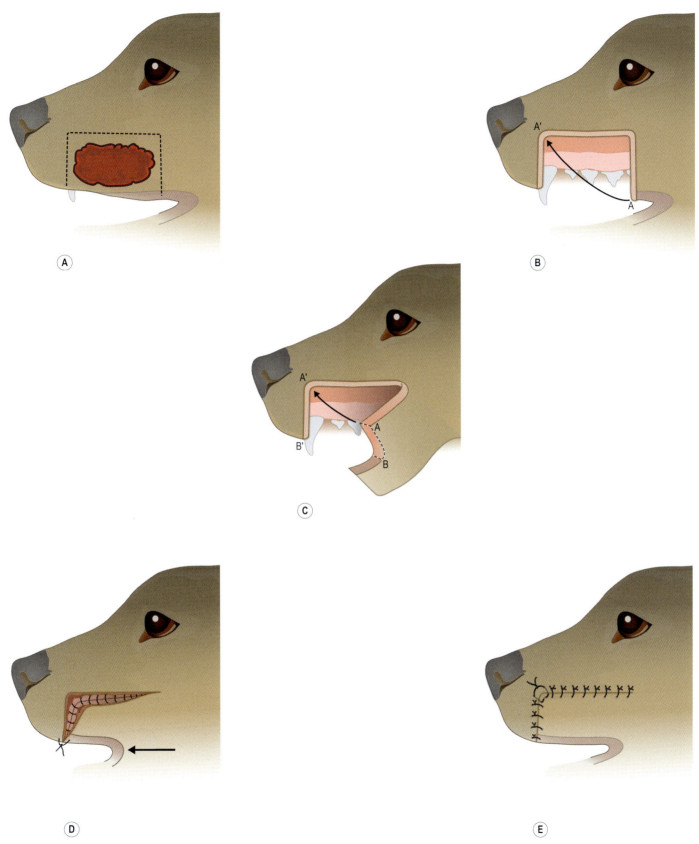

Fig. 44.7 Buccal rotation flap. (**A**) Proposed full-thickness rectangular incision around the lesion. (**B**) The caudoventral corner of the defect (A) will be apposed to the rostrodorsal corner of the defect (A'). (**C**) A segment of the lip margin is removed equal to the height of the defect in the lip. (**D**) The defect is closed in a two-layer fashion by apposing the caudal lip margin (B) to the rostral lip margin (B') and then suturing the mucosa. This causes the commissure of the lips to move rostrally (*arrow*). (**E**) The skin is sutured. Tension sutures can be used in areas of moderate tension. *(From Atlas of Small Animal Wound Management and Reconstructive Surgery, 3rd Edition, by M. Pavletic, 2010. Reproduced with permission of John Wiley & Sons, Inc.)*

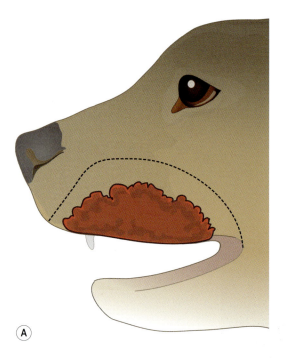

(A)

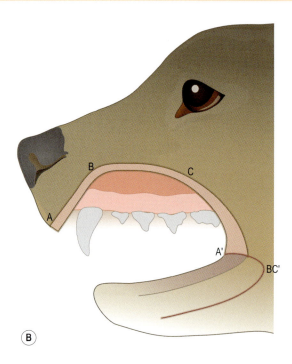

(B)

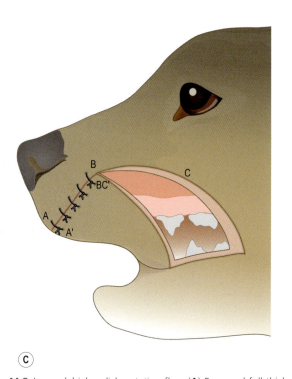

(C)

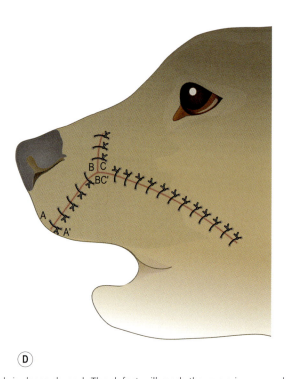

(D)

Fig. 44.8 Lower labial pedicle rotation flap. (**A**) Proposed full-thickness incision, which is dome-shaped. The defect will reach the commissure caudally. (**B**) A full-thickness labial flap is created with the lower lip. A first incision is made at the commissure, perpendicular to the lower lip margin. The length is equal to the height of the lower lip. A second incision is made parallel to the dental quadrant or lip margin starting at the first incision and running rostrally. The incision is long enough that it is possible to appose the flap to the rostral edge of the upper lip defect. (**C**) The labial flap is rotated and the lip margins are apposed (A' to A) The width of the flap is sutured to the rostrodorsal aspect of the defect (BC' to B). (**D**) A point along the dorsal border of the defect caudal to the transposed flap (C) is apposed to the flap without excessive tension (C to BC'). A two-layer closure is performed. Because suturing the buccal mucosa completely can greatly reduce mandibular range of motion, a defect in the mucosa can remain and allowed to heal by second intention. The skin is sutured in a 'Y' fashion. This technique creates a significant rostral transposition of the opening of the mouth on the side of the surgery.

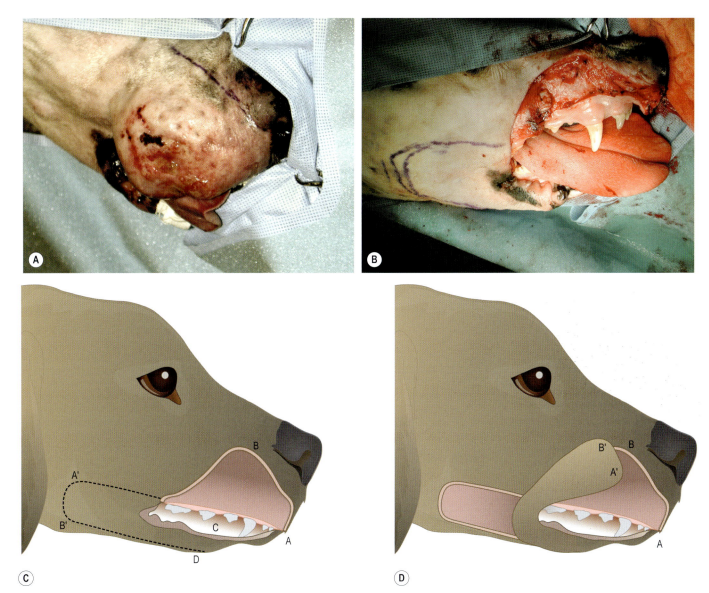

Fig. 44.9 Buccolabial pedicle flap. (**A**) A mast cell tumor is present on the right-upper lip before surgical excision. The dog is in left lateral recumbency and the nose is to the right of the figure. (**B**) The tumor has been excised where the entire upper lip was removed in the process. The limits of the proposed flap are demarcated with a surgical skin marker. (**C**) An incision is made from the caudal aspect of the defect at the level of the junction between the labial mucosa and gingiva, and runs caudally to the level of the most caudal aspect of the vestibulum. The height (the ventrodorsal dimension) of the flap is made to be of equal dimension as the height of the resected lip. A ventral incision is made from the caudal incision of the buccal flap extending to the ventral aspect of the lower lip to about half of the length of the lower lip. This creates a buccolabial flap with the pedicle being at the rostral aspect of the flap, ventral to the lower lip. The base of the flap is between points C and D. In transferring the flap into the defect, point A' will meet point A and point B' will meet with point B. (**D**) The caudal aspect of the flap in its orthotopic position is rotated rostrally to join the rostral aspect of the upper lip defect such that point A' will meet point A and point B' will meet with point B. Restrictive soft tissues are released from the mandible to relieve tension on the flap.

does not have a normal lip margin at the mucocutaneous junction, the skin is sutured to the buccal mucosa of the flap. The defect in the cheek (created by the transfer of the flap) is closed by simply apposing the ventral and dorsal edges together in three layers (mucosa, subcuticular, and dermis).

Upper labial pull-down technique (Fig. 44.10)

A full-thickness fusiform incision is created around the tumor, preserving the lip margin. The long axis of the defect is parallel to the lip margin. The labial mucosa is sutured to the oral mucosa. The skin

defect is closed. This technique can be combined with a maxillectomy if the tumor is very close to the alveolar mucosa and gingiva.

Transposition skin flap (Fig. 44.11)

The tumor is excised, creating a defect in the upper lip. A transposition skin flap is created caudal to the defect, ventral to the ear. Skin will be used to replace oral mucosa. The flap should be about twice as wide as the lip excised, since half of the flap is required to replace the mucosal defect The flap is inverted rostrally to cover the defect such that the skin is inside the mouth. What was the dorsal border of the

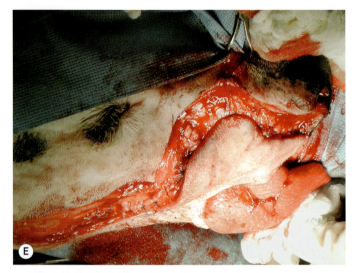

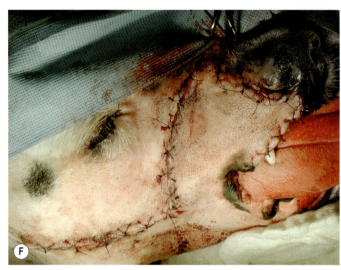

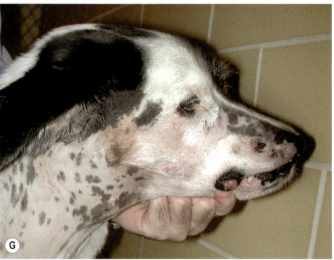

Fig. 44.9, cont'd. (**E**) The incised mucosa of the flap is sutured to the edges of the mucosa of the defect with an absorbable suture material. By apposing the cut edges of mucosa, the buccal cavity is reconstructed. The defect in the cheek is also closed by apposing the ventral and dorsal edges of the mucosa. (**F**) The edges of the skin are apposed in the same fashion. Because the most rostral aspect of the new lip does not have a normal lip margin at the mucocutaneous junction, the skin is sutured to the buccal mucosa of the flap. (**G**) Photograph of the dog 43 days after surgery. The flap is viable and has healed into its heterotopic position. The tip of the maxillary canine tooth remains uncovered.

skin flap is sutured to the oral mucosa. The flap is then folded onto itself and what was the ventral border of the flap as it was created is now sutured to the skin at the dorsal edge of the upper lip defect. The skin defect from the flap bed is also closed.

Techniques for the lower lip

The techniques described for the upper lip are also applicable for the lower lip. The full-thickness labial advancement technique and upper labial pedicle rotation flap techniques are reviewed with specific attention to the application to the lower lip.

Full-thickness labial advancement technique (Fig. 44.12)

After removing the tumor with a rectangular incision, the remaining lip caudal to the defect is mobilized by performing a full-thickness incision at the ventral aspect of the lip, parallel to the dental quadrant. The length of the mobilizing incision depends on the size of the defect needing repair. The flap should stretch over the defect without excessive tension. The labial margins are accurately apposed and the edges of mucosa are reapposed to reconstruct the vestibule. Care must be

taken to recreate the interdental attachment between lip and the oral mucosa at the level of the space between the canine tooth and the first premolar tooth in order to prevent drooping of the lower lip. The skin is closed as a second layer. Tension sutures can be used in areas of moderate tension.

Upper labial pedicle rotation flap (Fig. 44.13)

The tumor is excised with a wedge or rectangular resection. Approximately 80% to 90% of the lip margin (from rostral midline to commissure) can be excised. A full-thickness upper lip flap is created by making an incision parallel to the lip margin for a distance equal to the height of the lower lip. The incision begins at the caudal aspect of the lower lip defect and runs several centimeters cranially (long enough to be able to appose it with the rostral edge of the lower lip defect). The flap is rotated after releasing the restrictive soft tissues from the maxilla such that the caudal edge of the flap meets the rostral edge of the lower lip defect. The margin of the upper lip flap becomes the margin of the lower lip where the defect was. The buccal mucosa is sutured. Small gaps can be left open to allow wider opening of the jaws. The skin is closed in an inverted 'Y' fashion over the defect.

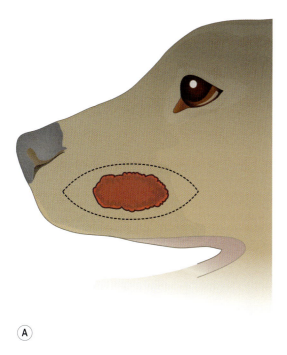

(A)

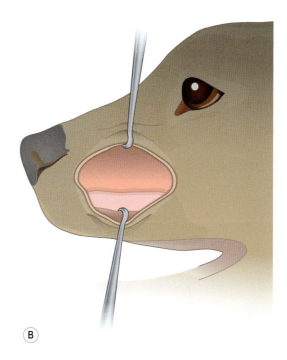

(B)

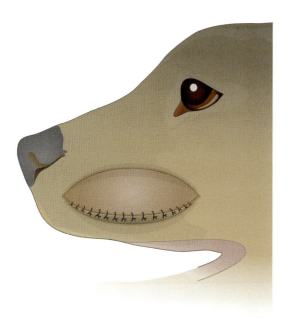

(C)

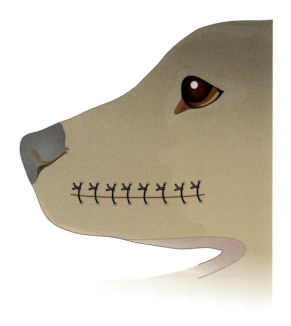

(D)

Fig. 44.10 Upper labial pull-down technique. (**A**) Proposed full-thickness fusiform incision around the lesion, preserving the lip margin. The long axis of the incision is parallel to the lip margin. (**B**) It is possible to also remove part of the maxilla to ensure an adequately deep margin when the tumor invades or buttresses against the maxilla. (**C**) A two-layer closure is performed by suturing the labial mucosa to the oral mucosa. (**D**) The closure is completed by suturing the skin. *(From Atlas of Small Animal Wound Management and Reconstructive Surgery, 3rd Edition, by M. Pavletic, 2010. Reproduced with permission of John Wiley & Sons, Inc.)*

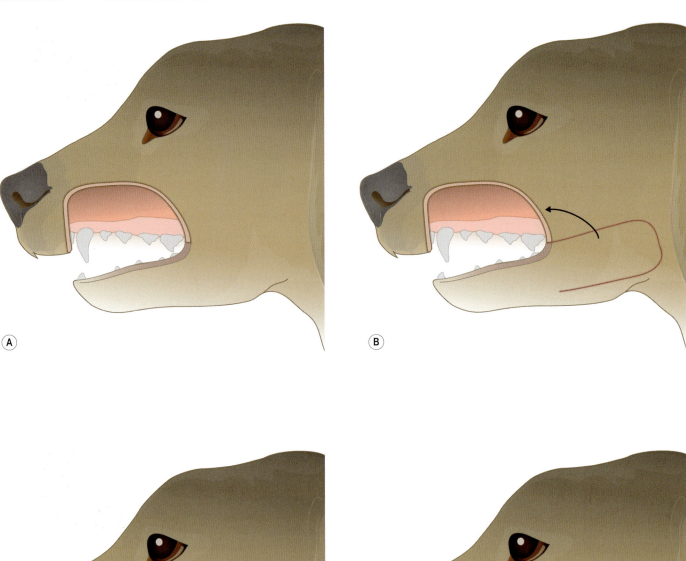

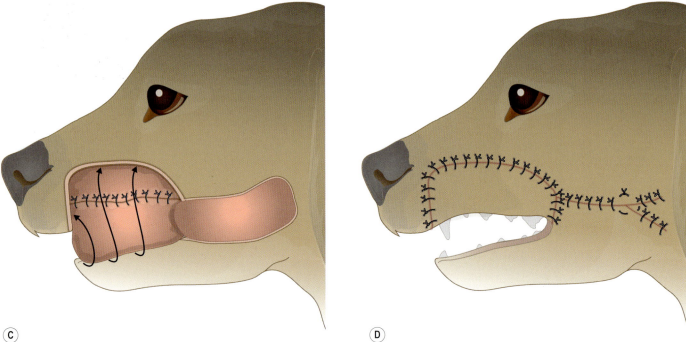

Fig. 44.11 Transposition skin flap. (**A**) Proposed full-thickness incision around lesion, removing most of the upper lip. (**B**) A single pedicle skin flap is created caudal to the defect and ventral to the ear. The base of the flap is at its rostral aspect and is aligned with the buccal–labial border. The width of the flap is twice the height of the defect since the flap will be folded in half. (**C**) The flap is folded onto its base rostrally and its dorsal border is sutured to the oral mucosa. The flap is then folded along its long axis such that its ventral border will be sutured to the skin border of the defect dorsally. (**D**) The remaining borders of the flap are sutured to the skin borders of the defect and the donor site of the flap is also sutured. *(From Atlas of Small Animal Wound Management and Reconstructive Surgery, 3rd Edition, by M. Pavletic, 2010. Reproduced with permission of John Wiley & Sons, Inc.)*

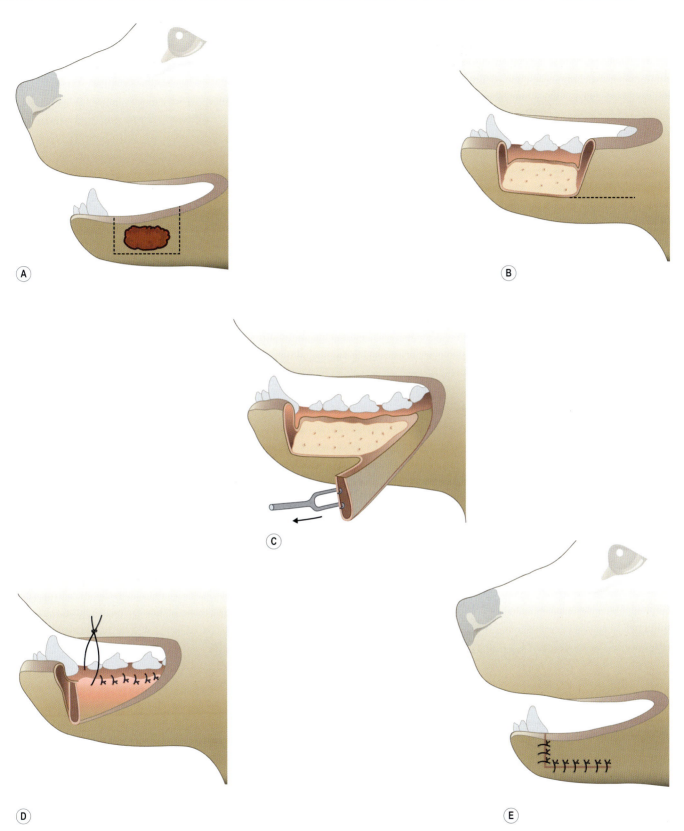

Fig. 44.12 Full-thickness labial advancement technique. (**A**) Proposed full-thickness rectangular incision around the lesion. (**B**) A full-thickness incision is performed at the level of the ventral extent of the excision, the incision being parallel to the dental quadrant or lip margin. The length of the incision will depend on the size of the defect. (**C**) Rostral traction on the lower lip helps to determine the length of the incision required. (**D**) A two-layer closure is performed by first suturing the labial mucosa to the buccal mucosa. Sutures are placed to recreate the labial frenulum located between the mandibular canine and first premolar teeth. (**E**) The closure is completed by suturing the skin. *(From Atlas of Small Animal Wound Management and Reconstructive Surgery, 3rd Edition, by M. Pavletic, 2010. Reproduced with permission of John Wiley & Sons, Inc.)*

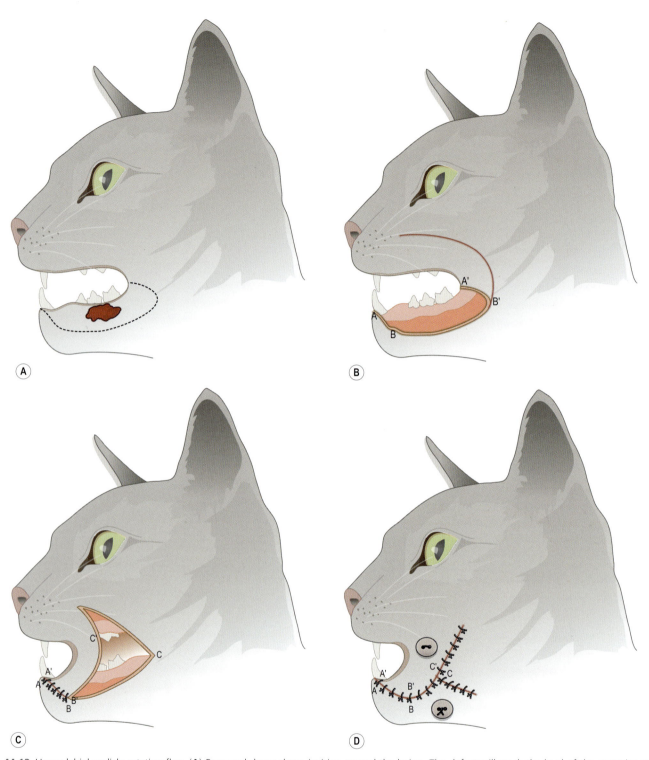

Fig. 44.13 Upper labial pedicle rotation flap. (**A**) Proposed dome-shape incision around the lesion. The defect will reach the level of the commissure caudally. (**B**) A full-thickness labial flap is created with the upper lip. A first incision is made at the commissure, perpendicular to the lower lip margin. The length is equal to the height of the lower lip. A second incision is made parallel to the teeth or lip margin starting at the first incision and running rostrally. The incision is long enough that it is possible to appose the flap to the rostral edge of the lower lip defect. (**C**) The labial flap is rotated and the lip margins are apposed (A' to A) The width of the flap is sutured to the rostroventral aspect of the defect (B' to B). (**D**) The point at the caudoventral aspect of the defect (C) is apposed to the caudal aspect of the flap without excessive tension (C to C'). A two-layer closure is performed. Because suturing the buccal mucosa completely can greatly reduce mandibular range of motion, a defect in the mucosa can remain and be allowed to heal by second intention. The skin is sutured in a 'Y' fashion. This technique creates a significant rostral transposition of the opening of the mouth on the side of the surgery. Buttons can be placed dorsal and ventral to the suture line to relieve some of the tension and help prevent dehiscence by wide opening of the mouth.

Techniques for the lower lip, upper lip and cheek reconstruction

Following excision of a tumor that creates a defect in the cheek, lower lip and upper lip, such large defects usually will require a skin flap for reconstruction.

Labial buccal reconstruction with inverse tubed skin flap[7] (Fig. 44.14)

A full-thickness wide excision of a tumor has been performed. The upper and lower lips are apposed at the rostral end of their respective defect. A transposition flap is created in the skin adjacent to the defect. A portion of the flap is partially tubed in inverse fashion at the base of the flap such that the skin is lining the inside of the tube. The flap is reflected rostrally such that the skin becomes intraoral. The skin edges are sutured to the edges of the gingival mucosa. The skin dorsal and ventral to the defect is advanced over the flap and sutured. The skin adjacent to the defect created from the transposition flap is also advanced and sutured. A narrow opening is left over the short tubed segment. This tubed segment can be excised when healing is complete and neovascularization to the flap is adequate, i.e., 4 to 6 weeks postoperatively.

Free microvascular skin flap grafted with oral mucosa[9]

This technique has been used experimentally in dogs and may prove to be very valuable in certain instances in clinical settings. The objective of the technique is to be able to reconstruct very large full-thickness lip and cheek defects by being able to provide both a mucosal and skin replacement. It is a staged procedure where the first step is to elevate a skin flap such as the medial saphenous cutaneous free flap, which is based on the saphenous artery and medial saphenous vein. Mucosa from the ventral surface of the tongue is harvested by injecting saline under the mucosa, which will help elevate it. Two or more pieces of full-thickness mucosa (20×20 mm in size) are excised. The pieces of mucosa are trimmed into smaller pieces (10×20 mm) and the lingual mucosal grafts are sutured to the undersurface of the skin flap. A skin expander or a sheet of silicone can be used to separate the graft from the subcutaneous tissue. The skin flap in sutured back into its orthotopic position. The skin expander can be used to try to expand the skin and mucosal grafts. Fourteen to 21 days later, the skin flap is harvested with its new oral mucosa lining on the undersurface, with preservation of its vascular pedicle. The vessels are transected and the skin/mucosal graft is transferred to the cheek and/or lip defect. Microvascular surgery is performed for anastomosis of the vascular pedicle of the graft with the superficial temporal artery and rostral auricular vein or the infraorbital artery and superior labial vein. The graft is then sutured into the defect with a two- or three-layer closure and the donor bed is also closed primarily. One of the disadvantages of this procedure, other than requiring microvascular surgery, is the fact that it is a staged procedure and therefore requires careful planning in time between the removal of the tumor, harvesting and seeding of the oral mucosa, and transfer of the skin graft to reconstruct the lip/cheek defect.

COMPLICATIONS

Complications following glossectomy

Complications are infrequent and may include hemorrhage, dehiscence, necrosis of part of the tongue and inability to eat or drink. Slow hemorrhage in the early postoperative period will usually resolve without any intervention, whereas significant hemorrhage usually requires heavy sedation or anesthesia and applying pressure for 5 minutes. If the hemorrhage persists, the sutures need to be removed and the source of bleeding identified so that it can be ligated or electrocoagulated. Dehiscence rarely requires intervention. Small defects will heal by second intention. Larger defects may need resuturing. Necrosis of the rostral border of the tongue occurs when the blood supply has been compromised too much. In two dogs, debridement and resuturing was not necessary.[4] If the necrosis leads to anorexia or other systemic signs, surgical intervention would become necessary. Inability to eat or drink in the early postoperative period is probably the most common complication following glossectomy. Intravenous fluid therapy can be used to manage patients that are dehydrated, and a feeding tube (esophagostomy or gastrostomy tube) can be placed in order to feed the patient (see Ch. 5). The feeding tube can be placed under the same anesthesia as the glossectomy in patients that are more likely to have problems in the postoperative period, such as cats or dogs that undergo a large excision (i.e., 50% or more). It can take up to 4 weeks for dogs to be able to eat and drink unassisted following major glossectomy (removal of >75% of the tongue).[5] In one study, one dog suffered a complication following a 100% glossectomy, which was ptyalism.[5]

Complications following excision of lip and cheek tumors and reconstruction

The most common complication is dehiscence. Because most procedures lead to the rostral displacement of the labial commissure, this in turn leads to a decrease in how wide the mouth can be opened. When the animal is eating, opening the jaws can put too much tension on the incision line and cause dehiscence. To prevent dehiscence, tension sutures can be used. Some surgical techniques used to repair a large defect in the upper lip can lead to unilateral deviation of the nasal planum (e.g., full-thickness labial advancement technique) when there is enough tension on the rostral suture line from elastic retraction of the flap. This deviation usually subsides over the next 2 to 3 weeks following surgery. Infection is uncommon in spite of performing surgery in a contaminated site probably due to the rich vascular supply to the area. If the chosen technique left a large mucosal defect, the lip can undergo excessive contraction, which can lead to drooling and leakage of food when eating. The same outcome can occur if the chosen techniques failed to restore adequate lip function.

PROGNOSIS

Prognosis following glossectomy

The prognosis for tongue tumors will vary with the site, type and grade of tumor.[6] Tumors in the rostral tongue have a better prognosis for any of the following reasons: earlier detection since it is more likely to be seen by the client; the rostral tongue may have less abundant lymphatic and vascular channels as opposed to the caudal tongue; rostral lesions are easier to excise with wide margins.[6] Dogs with squamous cell carcinoma have a 1-year survival of approximately 50%.[4,6] In one study, no dog with complete resection of the squamous cell carcinoma had local recurrence.[4] The overall metastatic rate in this study was 37.5%. Histologic grade appears to be a prognostic factor for survival for dogs with lingual squamous cell carcinoma.[4] For malignant melanoma of the tongue in dogs, the median survival was not reached in one case series and was over 551 days.[10] Granular cell myoblastoma of the tongue is a highly curable cancer. The prognosis for other tumor types is unknown due to the lack of information.[11]

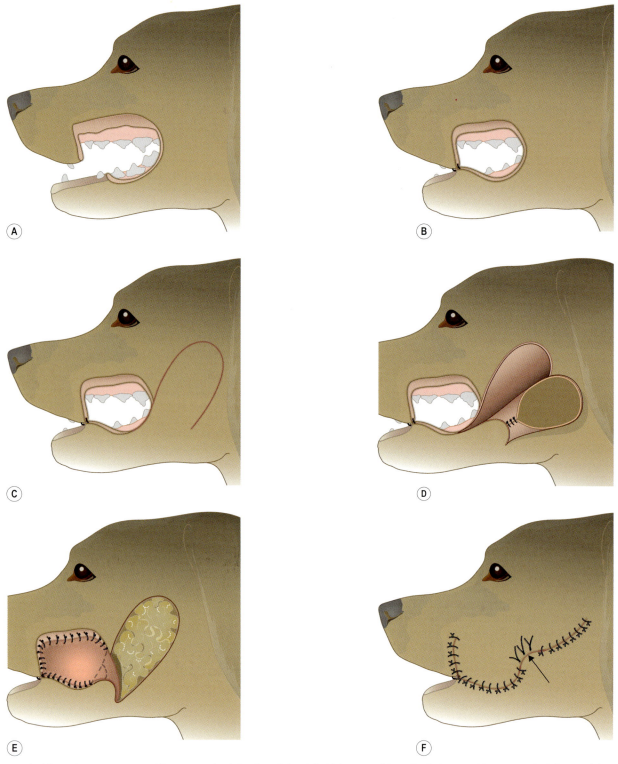

Fig. 44.14 Labial buccal reconstruction with inverse tubed skin flap. (**A**) A full-thickness excision of a lesion requiring removal of the caudal portions of the upper and lower lips and part of the cheek. (**B**) The lower and upper lip margins are apposed. (**C**) A transposition skin flap is created with its base being rostral. The flap is long enough to reach the rostral aspect of the defect and wide enough to reach the dorsal and ventral borders of the defect. (**D**) The rostral part of the flap is tubed. The length of the portion tubed is that part of the flap that will be reflected onto itself so that the skin distal to the tube can replace the buccal mucosal defect. (**E**) The flap is reflected rostrally and the skin edges are sutured to the mucosal edges in a simple interrupted pattern. (**F**) The skin is advanced over the transposition flap, inverse tube segment and donor bed. There will be a narrow opening of the skin-lined tube (*arrow*). *(From Atlas of Small Animal Wound Management and Reconstructive Surgery, 3rd Edition, by M. Pavletic, 2010. Reproduced with permission of John Wiley & Sons, Inc.)*

Long-term control of tongue tumors in cats is rarely reported with 1-year survival rate for tongue squamous cell carcinoma less than 25%.[11]

Prognosis following excision of lip and cheek tumors and reconstruction

The three most important prognostic factors are histologic type of the tumor (including grade if applicable), status of the surgical margins (i.e., complete versus incomplete excision), and stage.

Tumors that are incompletely excised have a higher likelihood of local recurrence, and malignant tumors and tumors that have metastasized carry a worse prognosis. Little information exists regarding outcome and survival following excision of lip and cheek tumors specifically.

REFERENCES

1. Evans HE. The digestive apparatus and abdomen. In: Evans HE, editor. Miller's anatomy of the dog. 3rd ed. Philadelphia, PA: WB Saunders Co; 1993. p. 385–95.

2. Chibuzo GA. The tongue. In: Evans HE, editor. Miller's anatomy of the dog. 3rd ed. Philadelphia, PA: WB Saunders Co; 1993. p. 396–414.

3. Bezuidenhout AJ. The lymphatic system. In: Evans HE, editor. Miller's anatomy of the dog. 3rd ed. Philadelphia, PA: WB Saunders Co; 1993. p. 717–57.

4. Carpenter LG, Withrow SJ, Powers BE, et al. Squamous cell carcinoma of the tongue in 10 dogs. J Am Anim Hosp Assoc 1993;29:17–24.

5. Dvorak LD, Beaver DP, Ellison GW, et al. Major glossectomy in dogs: a case series and proposed classification system. J Am Anim Hosp Assoc 2004;40:331–7.

6. Withrow SJ. Tumors of the gastrointestinal system; A. cancer of the oral cavity. In: Withrow SJ, MacEwen EG, editors. Small animal clinical oncology. 3rd ed. Philadelphia, PA: WB Saunders Co; 2001. p. 305–18.

7. Pavletic MM. Facial reconstruction. In: Pavletic MM, editor. Atlas of small animal reconstructive surgery. 2nd ed. Philadelphia, PA: WB Saunders Co; 1999. p. 297–329.

8. Smeak DD. Lower labial pedicle rotation flap for reconstruction of large upper lip defects in two dogs. J Am Anim Hosp Assoc 1992;28: 565–9.

9. Miyawaki T, Degner D, Jackson IT, et al. Easy tissue expansion of prelaminated mucosa-lined flaps for cheek reconstruction in a canine model. Plast Reconstr Surg 2002;109: 1978–85.

10. Kudnig ST, Ehrhart N, Withrow SJ et al. Survival analysis of oral melanoma in dogs. Vet Cancer Soc Proc 23:39, 2003.

11. Liptak JM, Withrow SJ. Oral tumors. In: Withrow SJ, Vail DM, editors. Withrow and MacEwen's small animal clinical oncology. 4th ed. Philadelphia, PA: Elsevier – Saunders; 2007. p. 455–75.

Chapter | 45 |

Maxillectomy techniques

Gary C. Lantz

DEFINITIONS

Partial maxillectomy techniques involve removal of various segments of the incisive, nasal, maxilla, palatine, vomer, lacrimal and zygomatic bones with adjacent neoplastic and normal soft tissues and teeth. The term *premaxillectomy* is often used in the veterinary literature to denote an excision confined to the incisive bone. However, the term *premaxilla* is not accepted veterinary anatomical nomenclature;[1] the term *incisivectomy* is therefore more appropriate. The term *hemimaxillectomy* is equally confusing and incorrect if used to describe the surgical excision of one maxilla. Removing most of one maxillary bone (typically combined with the excision of all or parts of the incisive and palatine bones) is a complete or total, unilateral *maxillectomy*. The term *hemimaxillectomy* could be used to denote the excision of half of one maxillary bone, but the term *partial maxillectomy* is more appropriately used for this. An *orbitectomy* involves removal of portions of bones that comprise the orbit including the maxilla, palatine, zygomatic, lacrimal and frontal bones.[2]

Closure of the resulting oronasal surgical defects is accomplished using vestibular (i.e., alveolar and buccal) mucosal–submucosal flaps that may be combined with palatal mucoperiosteal flaps. An en-bloc resection is resection 'as a whole,'[3] in this case referring to removal of the neoplasm and all soft and hard tissues within the boundaries of the predetermined surgical margins. An oronasal fistula is an abnormal opening (here, surgically created) connecting the oral cavity with the nasal cavity or maxillary recess.[4] In the dog, the maxillary recess extends approximately from the level of the distal root of the third premolar to the second molar teeth.[5] Alveolar juga are the smooth topographical elevations on the maxilla overlying maxillary tooth roots. Juga of the canine and fourth premolar teeth are the most prominent and easily palpated.[5]

INDICATIONS

Partial maxillectomy techniques are most commonly indicated for excision of malignant and benign oral neoplasms. They are also warranted as salvage procedures for oronasal fistula repair secondary to periodontal disease, treatment of severely comminuted maxillary fractures and repair of traumatic palatal defects that cannot be closed using palatal soft tissue flaps.

BACKGROUND

Partial maxillectomy for the treatment of oral neoplasms was introduced by Withrow et al.[6] Clinical investigation for treatment of neoplastic[7-15] and non-neoplastic[16] oral conditions, wound healing[17] and review publications[18-27] have followed, documenting healing and clinical treatment results.[28]

PREOPERATIVE CONCERNS

Diagnosis

Whether an oral mass is the primary complaint or an incidental finding during physical examination, an early diagnosis should be aggressively pursued. The biologic behavior and clinical staging using TNM (tumor, node, metastasis) classification of patients with oral tumors has been described (see Ch. 38).[24,29] The initial database must include a complete physical examination including the oropharyngeal region and histopathologic diagnosis of a biopsy of the mass. The biopsy site is planned so it can be excised during the maxillectomy surgery. Skull radiographs are obtained. Lack of radiographic evidence of bone involvement does not rule out malignancy.[30] Periosteal or bony invasion is assumed with any oral mass that is fixed to bone on palpation. Radiographs may help determine invasion along tooth roots in the periodontal ligament spaces. For most maxillary tumors, computed tomography or magnetic resonance imaging is indicated to determine the feasibility of surgery and to aid preoperative planning. Advanced imaging can help determine if the infraorbital canal or periodontal ligament spaces have been invaded.

Client communications

When clinical staging is completed, treatment options reviewed with the client, and surgery elected, several topics should be discussed with the client. These include: (1) intent of surgery (local cure or palliation)

© 2012 Elsevier Ltd
DOI: 10.1016/B978-0-7020-4618-6.00045-2

and prognosis; (2) operative concerns (blood loss, anesthesia risk); (3) postoperative appearance and oral function; and (4) recommended follow-up evaluation and treatment. Postoperative appearance of the patient is a concern for most clients. A photograph album including preoperative and postoperative photographs of patients that have had various types of maxillectomy aids this aspect of client communications.

Preoperative management

Antibiotics

A prophylactic course of antibiotics is administered intravenously in most patients. The first injection is administered at the time of anesthetic induction and repeated as needed (see Ch. 3). A therapeutic course is used in debilitated or immunosuppressed or immunocompromised patients. Commonly used intravenous antibiotics are first-generation cephalosporins, ampicillin and clindamycin. Oral formulations of these drugs or amoxicillin-clavulanic acid are used to complete a therapeutic course if indicated.

Oral cavity disinfection

Depending on overall oral health, preoperative periodontal treatment may be needed. Elective oral surgery should not be performed in a patient with heavy dental calculus or extensive, active periodontal disease. In the event of severe oral infection secondary to periodontal disease, general oral health is addressed initially and maxillectomy performed in 7 to 10 days when the infection is controlled and the oral tissues are less inflamed. Rapid growth of the neoplasm may preclude delay in surgery.

Surgical preparation of the oral cavity prior to maxillectomy is routine (see Ch. 6).

Anesthetic considerations

As with any major surgery, a preoperative minimal database should consist of physical examination, complete blood count, serum biochemistry profile and urinalysis. Coagulation parameters are screened by means of the mucosal bleeding test.[31] Further tests for coagulopathies are indicated if the mucosal bleeding test results are abnormal or if the patient has a history of bleeding tendency. The presence of von Willebrand's disease should be evaluated in Doberman pinschers. More extensive resections have greater blood loss potential. Blood cross-matching is routinely performed. Blood products and colloidal fluids should be available in the event of severe blood loss. Placement of two intravenous and one arterial catheter is recommended.

Preemptive analgesia

A multimodality approach to analgesia administered before the onset of surgery is most effective.[32] Typically, the patient receives an opioid and a nonsteroidal antiinflammatory drug prior to induction of general anesthesia and intubation. Regional blocks are routinely used, except if the tumor is located in the immediate vicinity of the nerve to be blocked. The surgeon should be familiar with regional anesthesia techniques administered at the infraorbital and major palatine foramina (see Ch. 4). Bilateral blocks may be needed, depending upon the proposed excision.

Patient positioning

For the majority of patients, positioning in dorsal recumbency allows good visualization of the surgical field (see Ch. 6). The head is secured into position with a vacuum-charged surgical positioning system (Vac-Pac, Olympic Medical, Seattle, WA). A mouth gag is positioned away from the surgery site to keep the mouth open. The endotracheal tube is secured to the lower jaw and the tongue retracted from the surgery site. Alternatively, a pharyngotomy intubation can be performed (see Ch. 57). The table is slightly tilted to lower the head and provide gravity-dependent drainage for irrigation fluid and blood. Visualization of the surgery site in patients with larger masses extending more dorsolateral on the maxilla can be improved by tilting and rotating the head to allow adequate access to the palate and dorsolateral surface of the maxilla.

After positioning, a layer of water-repellant gauze sponge packing (Exodontia Sponges, Henry Schein, Port Washington, NY) is placed in the pharynx around the endotracheal tube then covered with a layer of absorbent gauze.

SURGICAL ANATOMY[5]

The major and minor palatine, sphenopalatine and infraorbital arteries originate from the maxillary artery. The malar artery originates from the infraorbital artery. The facial artery originates from the external carotid artery (Fig. 45.1). The greater palatine foramen is located at a level approximately equal to the distal surface of the maxillary fourth premolar tooth and midway between the palate midline and dental arch. The major palatine artery, vein and nerve exit this foramen, and course along the length of the palate in the palatine sulcus. The palatine sulcus is located halfway between the midline and dental arch, making it relatively easy to find and ligate the major palatine vessels. The artery enters the nasal cavity through the palatine fissure as the rostral septal branch of the nasal septum. At the level of the palatine fissure an arterial branch originates from the major palatine artery and courses on the palate through the interdental space between the canine and third incisor teeth to terminate on the lateral aspect of the incisive bone. This artery may be transected during incisivectomy ('premaxillectomy') techniques. The sphenopalatine artery terminates in many branches supplying the nasal cavity, septum and conchae. The infraorbital artery exits the infraorbital foramen and divides into the lateral nasal and dorsal nasal arteries which supply the soft tissues of the muzzle. The lateral nasal artery anastomoses with the superior labial branch of the facial artery. These arteries provide the blood supply to the vestibular mucosal–submucosal flaps commonly used to close maxillectomy defects. Terminal branches of the malar artery may be encountered during partial orbitectomy.

The major nerves encountered are the dorsal buccal branch of the facial nerve and the infraorbital nerve (Fig. 45.2). The dorsal buccal nerve provides motor innervation for the muscles of the upper lip. This nerve is normally not injured during maxillectomy and motor control of the muscles is maintained. The infraorbital nerve originates from the maxillary division of the trigeminal nerve and provides sensory innervation to the nose, upper lip, nasal mucosa and maxillary teeth. Transection of this nerve during maxillectomy creates sensory loss that is not clinically relevant. The branches of both nerves are visible during the reflection of a vestibular mucosal–submucosal flap for maxillectomy defect closure.

THERAPEUTIC DECISION-MAKING

Types of osseous excisions

The general types of partial maxillectomy techniques are shown in Figure 45.3. The extent of any excision is determined by the oral physical examination and diagnostic imaging findings, the

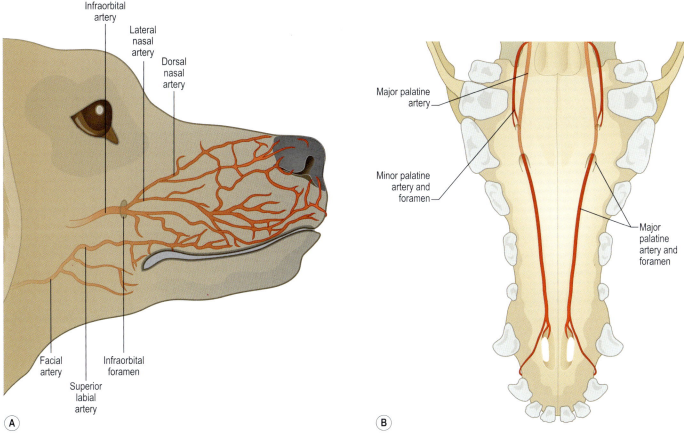

Fig. 45.1 Blood supply to the upper jaw: (**A**) Lateral aspect. (**B**) Palatal aspect.

histopathological diagnosis, the recommended surgical margins, the intent of the surgery and the tissue available for defect closure.

SURGICAL TECHNIQUE

General surgical principles

Surgical plan[23–26,33]

The surgical plan for a maxillectomy procedure includes the following important points: (1) plan for adequate surgical margins; (2) plan for complete mucosal closure; (3) perform atraumatic surgery and preserve local blood supply; (4) employ minimal use of electrosurgery; (5) harvest large mucosal flaps to avoid suture line tension; (6) use double-layer closure if possible; and (7) support suture lines with grossly healthy bone if possible.

Surgical margins

Surgical margins are indicated by the biological behavior of the neoplasm as determined from the preoperative histopathological diagnosis, radiographic findings of bone involvement and oral physical examination findings (see Ch. 43). The preoperative histopathological diagnosis is essential for definitive surgical planning. In general, a minimum of 10-mm margins should be obtained for all benign and malignant neoplasms except fibrosarcoma, where a minimum margin of 20 mm is recommended due to the higher local recurrence rate.[23–26] These recommendations have not been correlated with clinical

outcome. Wider margins can be obtained for malignant neoplasms if a tension-free oral mucosal reconstruction can be obtained. The surgical margins are measured and marked around the circumference of the mass using a sterile surgical marker before starting the surgery. If the neoplasm is found to penetrate cortical bone and enter the nasal cavity, the adjacent turbinates are excised.

Postoperative radiographs of the excised specimen or surgery site are made to document adequate gross surgical margins. The entire specimen is sent for histopathological examination to confirm the diagnosis and to assess the bone and soft tissue margins for neoplastic cells. Finding neoplastic cells on the excision margin implies incomplete removal of local microscopic disease and the need to consider adjunct radiation or chemotherapy.[25]

Surgical incision

The incision is made along the measured and marked surgical margins. The initial incision is a light scoring of the mucosa to produce a minimally bleeding incision line. Once the margins of the proposed resection are verified the incision is taken to bone. Once incised, the alveolar mucosal margins may retract and result in some distortion of proposed margins. The described incision method maintains accurate surgical margins. In the regions of larger vessels and nerves, the dissection is continued to identify, ligate and transect the vessels and transect the nerves. Hemorrhage is controlled by ligation, pressure and minimal focal use of electrocoagulation.[23–26]

A concurrent rostral–caudal oriented skin incision in the dorsal midline or dorsolateral muzzle may aid dissection of more dorsally extended masses.[34] A segment of skin may need to be excised to obtain adequate surgical margins.[25] This is achieved using a rostral–caudal

453

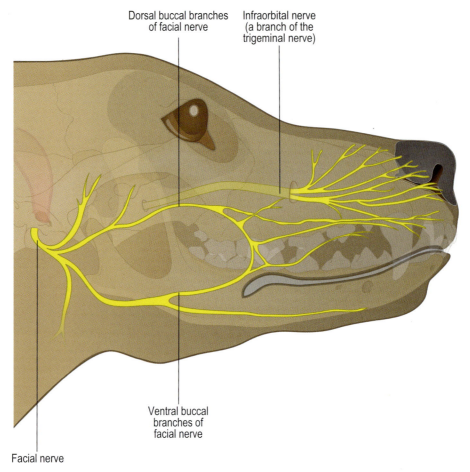

Dorsal buccal branches of facial nerve

Infraorbital nerve (a branch of the trigeminal nerve)

Ventral buccal branches of facial nerve

Facial nerve

Fig. 45.2 Some of the superficial branches of the facial and trigeminal nerves.

oriented fusiform excision and linear closure. Rostral–caudal orientation generally parallels the course of most neurovascular structures and reduces iatrogenic injury potential to these structures. Concurrent lip wedge resection may be needed to obtain tumor-free surgical margins.

Management of adjacent teeth

Maintaining teeth is secondary to achieving adequate surgical margins and tension-free closure of the surgical defect. Ostectomy performed at a narrow interdental space may result in injury requiring extraction of a tooth adjacent to the ostectomy site if inadvertent severe periodontal or endodontal injury (root canal exposure) occurred during ostectomy. Ostectomy at the level of a wider interdental space may not result in similar tooth injury. Therefore, to minimize tooth loss, the ostectomy margins are planned to transect a tooth at the margin level (Fig. 45.4). This may require margin extension, which is acceptable. Margins should never be compromised to save teeth. Once the en-bloc tissue mass is excised, the remnant of the transected tooth is extracted. The adjacent teeth and periodontal structures are not injured, leaving a margin of attached and free gingiva adjacent to the ostectomy. The alveolar bone covering the roots of adjacent teeth must remain intact. Careful attention is needed, with additional bone removal around adjacent teeth, as it may be very difficult to visually differentiate bone from dentin. Removal of this alveolar bone results in chronic root exposure to the nasal cavity and will result in periodontal disease, probable endodontic involvement and abscess formation. Inadvertent root exposure requires extraction of the involved tooth.

The apex of each maxillary canine tooth is located dorsal to the maxillary second premolar tooth. Therefore, rostral resections to ensure complete removal of the alveolus of the canine tooth include the first and second premolar teeth.

Ostectomy and osteoplasty

The soft tissues are subperiosteally elevated away from the ostectomy site. The ostectomy is performed as determined by the premeasured surgical margins. The resection is planned so that all root structures and preferably all intact alveoli of teeth within the surgical margins are part of the en-bloc excision.

Any remaining tooth root fragments from transected teeth at the resection periphery are extracted after the en-bloc tissue segment is removed.

Ostectomy may be performed with a thin osteotome and mallet. The instruments are used with gentle technique to slowly advance the depth of bone cut. Aggressive use may result in fractures of remaining bone and injury to nasal cavity and periocular tissues and the eyeball. Increased resistance will be found when tooth roots are encountered and may require extraction of the tooth or deviation of the ostectomy course to include the entire tooth.

Power equipment that cuts bone with saw blades or burs offers the most efficient ostectomy method. The most control is gained when using a surgical handpiece and bone-cutting burs. Ostectomy margins can be cut with rounder borders that facilitate flap closure as opposed to the straight cuts and sharp angles that result when using a saw blade. Carbide steel bone-cutting burs may leave a roughened edge. Medium-grit diamond tapered cylinder burs produce a smooth cut.

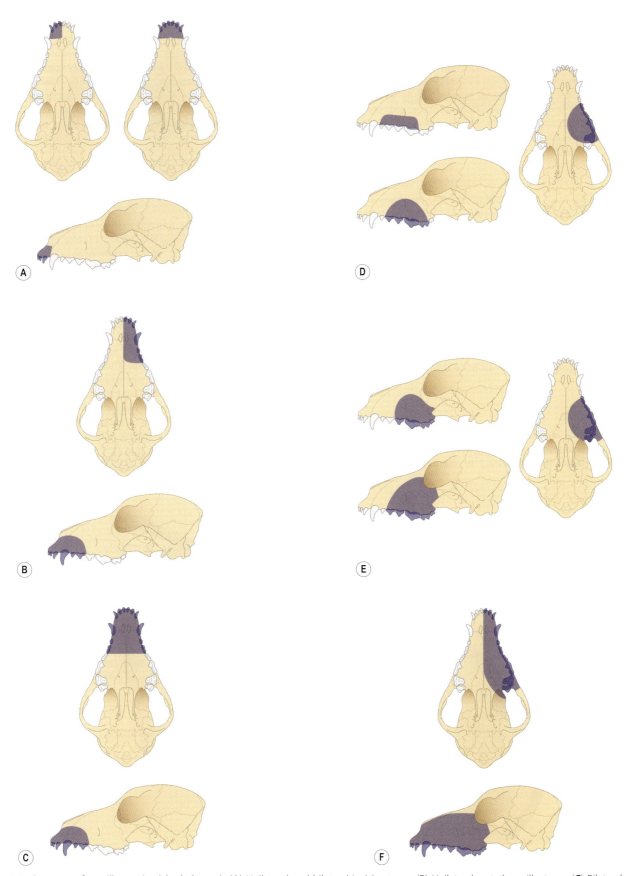

Fig. 45.3 Major types of maxillectomies (*shaded areas*). (**A**) Unilateral and bilateral incisivectomy. (**B**) Unilateral rostral maxillectomy. (**C**) Bilateral rostral maxillectomy. (**D**) Central or segmental maxillectomy. (**E**) Caudal maxillectomy. (**F**) Unilateral (complete) maxillectomy.

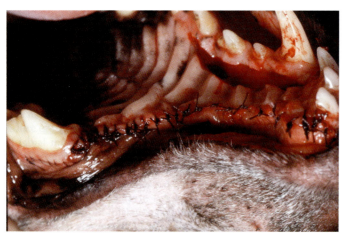

Fig. 45.11 Reconstruction using vestibular mucosal–submucosal, palatal mucoperiosteal and alveolar mucosa–periosteal transposition flaps after en-bloc resection of a large ameloblastoma. The combination of flaps eliminated suture line tension and reduced the concave deformity of the lip.

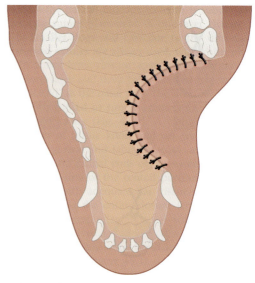

Fig. 45.13 Closure of a large central maxillectomy defect using a vestibular mucosal–submucosal flap. A concave deformity of the face will result.

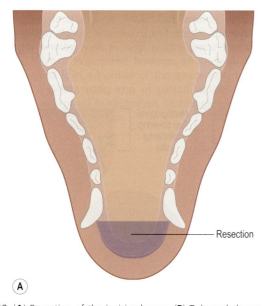

Resection

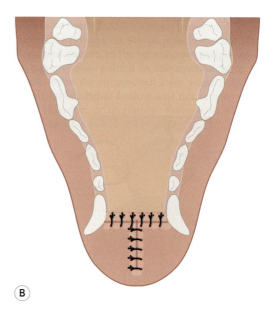

(A) (B)

Fig. 45.12 (A) Resection of the incisive bones. (B) T-shaped closure.

CENTRAL AND CAUDAL MAXILLECTOMY

Central and caudal maxillectomies create a temporary communication between the oral cavity and nasal cavity. Transection of the major palatine artery, vein and nerve is often required. Careful transection of the palatal mucoperiosteum allows ligation and transection of the vessels at the rostral and caudal extent of the resection. It may be necessary to extend the excision beyond the midline, depending on the size of the tumor; if so, the ability to close the defect will depend on the width of the maxilla and amount of remaining labial mucosa. Excision of larger masses with appropriate surgical margins will leave less labial tissue for closure of the defect. There is often enough labial mucosa to extend to the midline and sometimes beyond the midline; however, this must be evaluated for each patient (Fig. 45.13).

Another closure option for large maxillary defects is bilateral buccal mucosal–submucosal flaps. A buccal mucosal–submucosal labial flap is harvested from adjacent to the maxillectomy site as described. On the opposite side of the maxilla, the rostral–caudal length of the second flap is determined. A sulcular incision is made on the buccal and palatal side of the teeth at the level of this flap. Buccal diverging vertical releasing incisions are made through the attached gingiva into the alveolar and buccal mucosa. Care is taken to not transect neurovascular structures emerging from the infraorbital foramen. The vestibular flap and palatal mucoperiosteum margins are subperiosteally elevated, the teeth extracted, and the alveolar margin height is slightly reduced with an osteoplasty bur. Any remaining palatal mucoperiosteum lying between the maxillectomy surgical defect and the second flap is excised or denuded of epithelium with a bur. The free gingiva, including the sulcular epithelium, is excised from the second flap; this

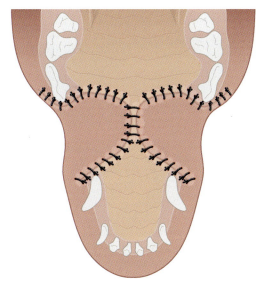

Fig. 45.14 Closure of a large maxillectomy defect using bilateral vestibular mucosal–submucosal flaps. Creating the flap on the opposite side requires extraction of teeth, reduction in the alveolar bone height and diverging vertical releasing incisions. A bilateral concave deformity of the face may result.

flap now consists of attached gingiva, alveolar mucosa and buccal mucosa–submucosa and periosteum. It is lengthened as needed to meet the original buccal mucosal–submucosal flap from the maxillectomy site for a tension-free closure. Lengthening is accomplished by extension of the vertical releasing incisions and/or release of the periosteum at the flap base. The defect is closed as described (Fig. 45.14).

Orbitectomy[2]

Caudal maxillectomy techniques may require removal of portions of bones that comprise the orbit. Removal of the ventral orbital margin (inferior partial orbitectomy) is most commonly performed for resection of caudal maxillary neoplasia. Surgery involves excision of the rostral zygomatic arch and caudal maxilla and, possibly, lacrimal and palatine bones. Resection of larger more dorsally located tumors require intraoral and dorsal cutaneous incisions to allow access to the tumor circumference.[34] Partial inferior orbitectomy will not result in displacement of the eyeball as all supporting periorbital soft tissues remain intact. The defect is closed by suturing a vestibular mucosa–submucosa flap to palatal mucoperiosteum, and, possibly, to soft palate. More extensive tumor involvement may require resection of the coronoid process of the mandible with associated muscles of mastication. Enucleation is considered if the eye, its neurovascular supply or large portion of an eyelid is infiltrated with neoplasia or lies within the desired surgical margins.

When performing a caudal maxillary resection including partial inferior orbitectomy one may be unable to completely cut all the bone surrounding the tumor. Bone at the level of the rostromedial aspect of the pterygopalatine fossa and the caudomedial wall of the infraorbital canal (portions of palatine and maxilla bones) cannot be accessed to cut with a bur or saw. In this situation, all bone cuts are made and this remaining inaccessible area is fractured by lateral displacement of the tumor/bone segment. This now isolated tumor/segment is gently manipulated rostrally, the maxillary artery is ligated and divided, and the maxillary nerve is divided as they enter the infraorbital canal. Any visible branches of superior alveolar nerves are divided as they enter accessory canals in the caudal maxilla.

Additional technical considerations

Some partial maxillectomy techniques may require the ostectomy to cross the infraorbital canal or removal of the entire infraorbital canal. The level of the canal may be identified by one of several landmarks including: (1) palpating the lateral bone rim of the infraorbital foramen which is found dorsal to the distal root of the maxillary third premolar tooth; (2) palpating the alveolar jugum of the maxillary fourth premolar tooth, the dorsal extent of which lies ventrolateral or lateral to the canal; and (3) by visually tracing the infraorbital neurovascular structures caudally to the level of the foramen. The canal is opened by ostectomy of the buccal bone plate. The artery and vein are ligated and transected and the nerve transected. The resection ostectomy may proceed without risk of inadvertently severing these vessels, resulting in profuse hemorrhage. Removal of the entire infraorbital canal, if needed as part of an inferior partial orbitectomy, is accomplished as described above. Based on clinical experience, sacrifice of the infraorbital artery does not jeopardize vestibular mucosal–submucosal flap vitality. Assumedly, the blood supply from the superior labial branch of the facial artery and the lateral nasal artery from the contralateral infraorbital artery is sufficient to maintain the flap.

For caudal maxillectomy, the parotid and zygomatic salivary papillae are identified and preserved. If the papillae are included within the excision margins, the salivary ducts are identified and ligated.

The nasolacrimal duct is transected in various maxillectomy techniques. Epiphora generally does not result. Although not specifically studied, the proximal transected end of the duct apparently heals and forms a new ostium for continued tear drainage into the nasal cavity. Healing may occur similarly to various salvage procedures for nasolacrimal duct disruption.[35,36] Stent placement is not required. Surgical trauma to the lacrimal bone and disruption of the lacrimal sac may result in epiphora.

POSTOPERATIVE CARE AND ASSESSMENT

Extubation

Immediately after completion of the surgery, all debris including tissue fragments and blood clots is removed from the oral cavity. Suction is applied to the pharyngeal area around the gauze packing. The gauze packing is removed and the oropharyngeal area closely inspected to ensure removal of all debris and fluid. The patient is then extubated.

Pain management

Depending on the magnitude of the surgery, most pain is evident in the first 24 to 72 hours postoperatively (see Ch. 4). Signs suggestive of continued pain include tachycardia, hypertension, salivation, pale mucous membranes and dilated pupils. Vocalization may occur related to pain, anxiety or fear. The spectrum of behavior can range from lethargy to restlessness, agitation or delirium. Additional analgesic intervention is needed in the presence of these signs. Concurrent tranquilization will calm the delirious patient. Opioid administration is continued in the first 1 to 3 days postoperatively by intermittent injection or, more effectively, by continuous-rate infusion. Residual discomfort (less intense pain related to resolving inflammation) will last longer and is managed with nonsteroidal antiinflammatory drugs. Clinical behavior including increasing activity level, eating, drinking and grooming suggest adequate pain management and patient comfort.

Nutritional support

Multielectrolyte intravenous fluids are continued until normal eating and drinking occur as analgesic medications are being reduced and patients become more alert. Oral water is offered at 24 hours postoperatively. Soft food is then offered. Most patients with mild to moderate maxillectomies will drink and eat at this time provided higher levels of opioid administration, which may sedate the patient, are no longer needed. Patients that have more extensive surgery may require a longer course of opioids and may not voluntarily eat or drink for 2 to 3 days. Placement of an enteral feeding tube is rarely needed but is recommended as a method of reducing suture line stresses when closure of large defects using bilateral vestibular mucosal–submucosal flaps is performed. Placement of a feeding tube is also considered in the debilitated patient (see Ch. 5).

Postoperative patient appearance[23,26]

Swelling of the surgery site is usually resolved by 3 to 7 days postoperatively. Cosmetic appearance is generally good and depends on the extent of excision. Smaller excisions or larger excisions leaving abundant vestibular mucosa–submucosa for flap harvesting result in unnoticeable or minimal cosmetic abnormalities (Fig. 45.15). Bilateral incisivectomy results in some drooping of the nose and possible caudal retraction of the rostral lip margin. Unilateral incisivectomy may result in slight facial concavity and lip margin elevation. Concurrent lip wedge resection may result in additional lip margin deformity (Fig. 45.16). Unilateral rostral maxillectomy including the canine tooth creates a more pronounced concavity with lip elevation (Fig. 45.17) and possible ipsilateral mandibular canine tooth protrusion lateral to the upper lip (Fig. 45.18). Extensive bilateral rostral maxillectomies create relative mandibular prognathism and nose droop (Fig. 45.19). More extensive central and caudal maxillectomies may result in facial concavity with elevation of the lip margin (Fig. 45.20).

Homecare and follow-up

Most patients are sent home after 2 to 4 days postoperatively. A soft food diet and removal of chew toys is recommended for 2 to 3 weeks. The client is shown how to administer any oral medications so as not to disrupt the suture line. Medications may be concealed in soft food. If oral manipulation is needed, the manipulation is performed away from the surgery site. The surgery site is examined in 2 weeks and any skin sutures removed. The surgery site is reexamined at 1 month postoperatively and any residual oral sutures removed at this time. Most oral sutures are absorbed or extruded in approximately 3 weeks. A complete physical examination, including the surgical site, is performed at 3-month intervals for 1 year. In the case of malignant neoplasms, three-view thoracic radiographs are obtained at these examinations.

COMPLICATIONS

Intraoperative complications

Hemorrhage is the major intraoperative complication. Extensive blood loss may occur from premature transection of the major palatine and infraorbital arteries. Temporary carotid artery ligation before starting the maxillectomy has been described to aid in the control of

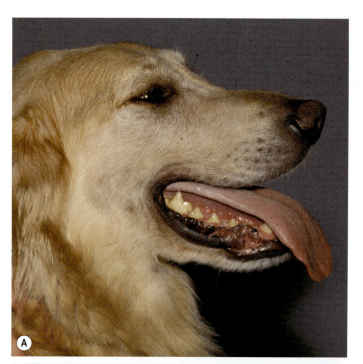

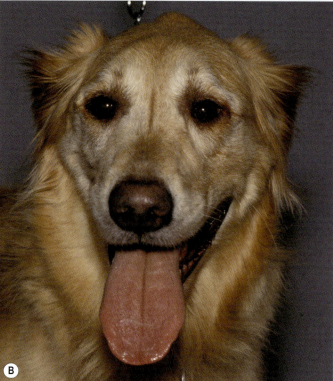

Fig. 45.15 (**A**) Lateral and (**B**) frontal view of a dog that underwent a right central maxillectomy. Abundant tissue for creation of a large vestibular mucosal–submucosal flap was available, which resulted in excellent cosmetic results.

hemorrhage but is rarely needed.[37] Hemorrhage is controlled as it is encountered by pressure, ligation or focal use of electrocoagulation. If necessary, thrombin-soaked gelatin sponges are placed in the nasal cavity and left for 10 to 15 minutes. In the event of persistent nasal cavity hemorrhage, which is unusual, gauze packing is left in the nasal cavity and removed in approximately 24 hours.[22] In the event

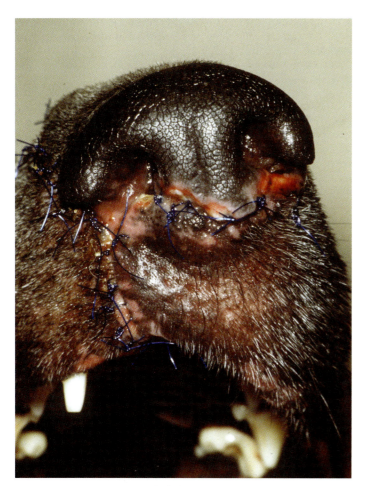

Fig. 45.16 Incisivectomy with wide lip wedge resection. Bilateral full-thickness advancement flaps were used for closure of the lip margin.

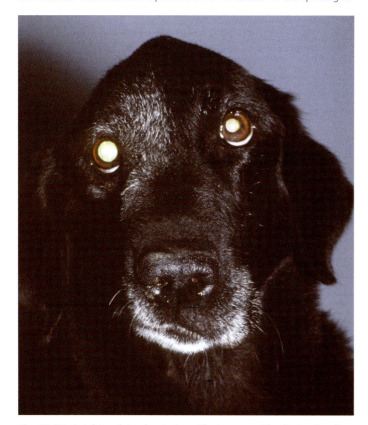

Fig. 45.17 A right unilateral rostral maxillectomy resulting in lip elevation.

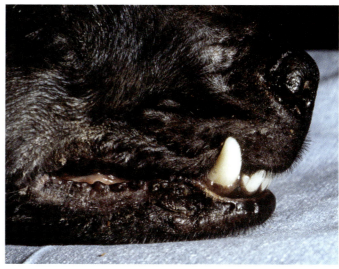

Fig. 45.18 Mandibular canine tooth protrusion and concavity of the face after unilateral rostral–central maxillectomy.

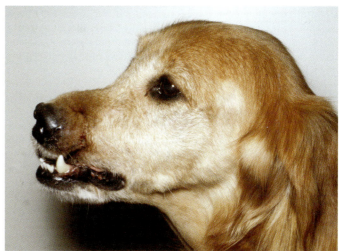

Fig. 45.19 Extensive bilateral rostral maxillectomy created relative mandibular prognathism. The nose droop was corrected by suturing the nose to the rostral aspect of the maxillas.

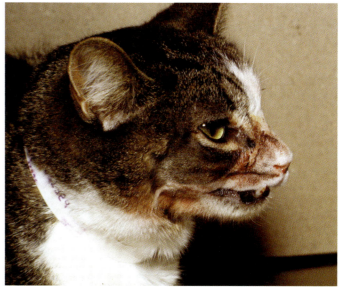

Fig. 45.20 Concavity of the face after extensive unilateral rostral–central maxillectomy.

of brisk hemorrhage, it is essential that the surgeon keep track of the approximate amount of blood loss in gauze sponges and the suction unit; if such occurs, the physiologic responses of the patient such as tachycardia and reduced blood pressure indicate the need for volume replacement.

Postoperative complications

Bilateral surgery may result in temporary occlusion of one or both nasal passages. The patient may experience anxiety in the early postoperative period due, in part, to inability to breathe through the nose. Tranquilization combined with adequate analgesia will eliminate the anxiety and allow open-mouth breathing. Sneezing and a small amount of serosanguineous nasal discharge may be present for several days. More radical excision and removal of all turbinates from one side of the nasal cavity may result in permanent serous nasal discharge.[26]

Superficial ulceration of the vestibular mucosal–submucosal flap may occur secondary to contact with mandibular teeth. This is generally not a chronic problem, as keratinization of these contact areas increases over time and ulceration ceases in a few weeks.

The ipsilateral mandibular canine tooth may protrude intermittently or continuously to the lateral surface of the upper lip. This is usually a cosmetic problem but occasionally causes ulceration of the labial mucosa and/or skin. If indicated, the tooth protrusion is corrected by crown height reduction and partial coronal pulpectomy, direct pulp capping and restoration.[38,39]

Dehiscence is often a result of technical error, with extrinsic tension on the wound edges being the most important cause.[25] Occurrence is minimized by following the principles of oral surgery. Inadequate suture placement (small bite depth, wide spacing), suture line tension, excessive use of electrosurgery and marginal necrosis of the flap contribute to dehiscence. Dehiscence most commonly occurs within the first few days but may occur later. Repair of a dehiscence that results in an oronasal fistula is usually deferred for 2 to 4 weeks. This delay allows for resolution of flap inflammation and reestablishment of the blood supply of the flap. The fistula is treated by debridement of soft tissue and bone margins and mobilization of adequate mucosal tissues for a tension-free closure. A two-layer closure is preferred. Excised tissues are sent for histopathological evaluation to rule out local tumor recurrence as the cause for wound healing failure.

Dehiscence of an incisivectomy which exposes the ventral lateral nasal cartilages usually does not need repair and heals by second intention.

Periodontal abscessation of a tooth adjacent to the surgery site may develop as a result of chronic root exposure to the nasal cavity, with resulting periodontal and possible endodontic disease. This is caused by removal of alveolar bone during the partial maxillectomy. Diagnostic findings may include intraoral swelling at or adjacent to the surgery site, a parulis (an elevated mucosal nodule at the site of an intraoral sinus tract draining a chronic abscess), a periapical radiolucency in the involved area, and oral sensitivity that may improve when treated with antibiotics. Tooth extraction, debridement, and antibiotics based on culture and sensitivity results resolve this complication. Tissues are submitted for histopathologic examination to rule out local neoplasm recurrence as a contributing factor.

Local tumor recurrence is common with certain tumor types. Suspicious areas noted during recheck examination must be biopsied to differentiate neoplasm recurrence from suture reaction and scar tissue.

PROGNOSIS

The overall prognosis for maxillectomy techniques regarding oral function, operative and postoperative complications, postoperative appearance and client satisfaction is good to excellent.[15,18-26] This seems directly related to the surgeon's experience with appropriate patient selection, technical performance of the surgery, and preoperative owner communications to set realistic expectations. Less positive results may occur in patients with more aggressive disease and more radical surgery. One study reported an overall 85% client satisfaction with maxillectomy and mandibulectomy procedures. The satisfaction level correlated with the postoperative survival time of the patient.[15]

Local recurrence rates, survival times and biologic behavior of benign and malignant oral tumors reported in various clinical studies have been reviewed (see also Ch. 40).[25-29] Fibrosarcoma has the highest local recurrence rate (46%) followed by melanoma (25%), osteosarcoma (25%), squamous cell carcinoma (15%) and benign neoplasms (0–4%).[25,29] Early recognition, accurate diagnosis and aggressive, planned resection are essential for optimal results.

REFERENCES

1. Anonymous. Nomina anatomica veterinaria. 5th ed. Hannover, Columbia, Gent and Sapporo: World Association of Veterinary Anatomists; 2005.
2. O'Brien MG, Withrow SJ, Straw RC, et al. Total and partial orbitectomy for the treatment of periorbital tumors in 24 dogs and 6 cats: a retrospective study. Vet Surg 1996;25:471–9.
3. Venes D. Taber's Cyclopedic medical dictionary. Philadelphia, PA: FA Davis; 2001. p. 694.
4. Zwemer T. Mosby's dental dictionary. St. Louis, MO: Mosby Inc.; 1998. p. 353, 366.
5. Evans HE. The digestive apparatus and abdomen. In: Evans HE, editor. Miller's anatomy of the dog. 3rd ed. Philadelphia, PA: WB Saunders Co; 1993. p. 385–462.
6. Withrow SJ, Nelson AW, Manley PA, et al. Premaxillectomy in the dog. J Amer Anim Hosp Assoc 1985;21:49–55.
7. White RAS, Gorman NT, Watkins SB, et al. The surgical management of bone-involved oral tumours in the dog. J Small Anim Pract 1985;26:693–708.
8. Emms SG, Harvey CE. Preliminary results of maxillectomy in the dog and cat. J Small Anim Pract 1986;27:291–306.
9. Salisbury SK, Richardson DC, Lantz GC. Partial maxillectomy and premaxillectomy in the treatment of oral neoplasia in the dog and cat. Vet Surg 1986;15:16–26.
10. White RAS, Gorman NT. Wide local excision of acanthomatous epulides in the dog. Vet Surg 1989;18:12–14.
11. Schwarz PD, Withrow SJ, Curtis CR, et al. Partial maxillary resection as a treatment for oral cancer in 61 dogs. J Amer Anim Hosp Assoc 1991;27:617–24.
12. White RAS. Mandibulectomy and maxillectomy in the dog: long term survival in 100 cases. J Small Anim Pract 1991:32:69–74.
13. Wallace J, Matthiesen DT, Patnaik AK. Hemimaxillectomy for the treatment of oral tumors in 69 dogs. Vet Surg 1992; 21:337–41.
14. Kirpensteijn J, Withrow SJ, Straw RC. Combined resection of the nasal planum and premaxilla in three dogs. Vet Surg 1994;23:341–6.
15. Fox LE, Geoghegan SL, Davis LH, et al. Owner satisfaction with partial mandibulectomy or maxillectomy for treatment of oral tumors in 27 dogs. J Amer Anim Hosp Assoc 1997;33:25–31.

16. Salisbury SK, Richardson RC. Partial maxillectomy for oronasal fistula repair in the dog. J Amer Anim Hosp Assoc 1986;22:185–92.

17. Salisbury SK, Thacker HL, Pantzer EE, et al. Partial maxillectomy in the dog comparison of suture materials and closure techniques. Vet Surg 1985;14:265–76.

18. Harvey CE. Oral surgery, radical resection of maxillary and mandibular lesions. Vet Clin North Amer 1986;16:983–93.

19. Harvey CE, Emily PP. Small animal dentistry. St. Louis, MO: Mosby Inc.; 1993. p. 312–77.

20. Birchard S, Carothers M. Aggressive surgery in the management of oral neoplasia. Vet Clin North Amer Small Anim Pract 1990;20:1117–40.

21. Matthiesen DT, Marretta SM. Results and complications associated with partial mandibulectomy and maxillectomy techniques. Probl Vet Med 1990;2:248–75.

22. Salisbury SK. Problems and complications associated with maxillectomy, mandibulectomy, and oronasal fistula repair. Probl Vet Med 1991;3:153–69.

23. Salisbury SK. Maxillectomy and mandibulectomy. In: Slatter DH, editor. Textbook of small animal surgery. 3rd ed. Philadelphia, PA: WB Saunders Co; 2003. p. 561–72.

24. Hedlund C. Surgery of the digestive system, surgery of the oral cavity and oropharynx. In: Fossum TW, editor. Small animal surgery. 3rd ed. St. Louis, MO: Mosby; 2007. p. 339–47.

25. Dernell WS, Schwarz PD, Withrow SJ. Maxillectomy and premaxillectomy. In: Bojrab MJ, editor. Current techniques in small animal surgery. 4th ed. Philadelphia, PA: Williams and Wilkins; 1998. p. 124–32.

26. Salisbury SK. Aggressive cancer surgery and aftercare. In: Morrison WB, editor. Cancer in dogs and cats: medical and surgical management. Philadelphia, PA: Williams and Wilkins; 1998. p. 265–321.

27. Verstraete FJM. Mandibulectomy and maxillectomy. Vet Clin North Am Small Anim Pract 2005;35:1009–39.

28. Lascelles BD, Henderson RA, Seguin B, et al. Bilateral rostral maxillectomy and nasal planectomy for large rostral maxillofacial neoplasms in six dogs and one cat. J Am Anim Hosp Assoc 2004; 40:137–46.

29. Liptak JM, Withrow SJ. Cancer of the gastrointestinal tract, oral tumors. In: Withrow SJ, Vail DM, editors. Small animal clinical oncology. 4th ed. Philadelphia, PA: WB Saunders; 2007. p. 455–75.

30. Anderson JG, Revenaugh AF. Canine oral neoplasia. In: DeForge DH, Colmery BH, editors. An atlas of veterinary dental radiology. Ames, IA: Iowa State University Press; 2000. p. 87–104.

31. Marks SL. The buccal mucosal bleeding time. J Am Anim Hosp Assoc 2000;36:289–90.

32. Woolf CJ, Chong MS. Preemptive analgesia-treating postoperative pain by preventing the establishment of central sensitization. Anesth Analg 1993;77:362–79.

33. Hupp JR. Principles of surgery. In: Peterson LJ, Ellis III E, Hupp JR, et al, editors. Contemporary oral and maxillofacial surgery. 4th ed. St. Louis, MO: Mosby; 2003. p. 42–8.

34. Lascelles BD, Thomson MJ, Dernell WS, et al. Combined dorsolateral and intraoral approach for the resection of tumors of the maxilla in the dog. J Am Anim Hosp Assoc 2003;39:294–305.

35. van der Woerdt A, Wilkie DA, Gilger BC, et al. Surgical treatment of dacryocystitis caused by cystic dilatation of the nasolacrimal system in three dogs. J Am Vet Med Assoc 1997;211:445–7.

36. Gelatt KN, Gelatt JP. Small animal ophthalmic surgery: practical techniques for the veterinarian. Oxford, UK: Butterworth Heinemann; 2001. p. 125–41.

37. Hedlund CS, Tangner CH, Elkins AD, et al. Temporary bilateral carotid artery occlusion during surgical exploration of the nasal cavity of the dog. Vet Surg 1983;12:83–5.

38. Niemiec BA. Assessment of vital pulp therapy for nine complicated crown fractures and fifty-four crown reductions in dogs and cats. J Vet Dent 2001;18:122–6.

39. Niemiec BA, Mulligan TW. Vital pulp therapy. J Vet Dent 2001;18:154–6.

Chapter 46

Mandibulectomy techniques

Gary C. Lantz

DEFINITIONS

Mandibulectomy techniques involve removal of various segments of a mandible, one entire mandible, or one mandible with a rostral portion of the other mandible, with adjacent neoplastic and soft tissues. Closure of the surgical defects is accomplished using buccal mucosal–submucosal and alveolar mucosal flaps. A *rim excision*, with reference to mandibulectomy, is defined as a partial segmental excision leaving the ventral border of the mandible intact.[1] The term *hemimandibulectomy* is often used in the veterinary literature to denote the complete excision of one of the two mandibles. The term *total mandibulectomy* is more appropriate. The term *hemimandibulectomy* should only be used to denote the excision of half of one mandible, but the term *partial mandibulectomy*, with a reference to which part (rostral, central or caudal) is more appropriately used for this. Similarly, when referring to the excision of one entire mandible and half of the other mandible, the term *one-and-one-half mandibulectomy* is preferred over *three-quarter mandibulectomy*.

INDICATIONS

Mandibulectomy techniques are most commonly indicated for excision of malignant and benign oral neoplasms. They are also used as salvage procedures for mandibular fractures that are severely comminuted or complicated by missing bone fragments or severe periodontitis (see Ch. 34).[2,3]

BACKGROUND

Partial mandibulectomy techniques for the treatment of oral neoplasms were introduced by Withrow and Holmberg.[4] Clinical investigation for treatment of neoplastic[5–16] and non-neoplastic oral conditions[2,3] and review publications[16–25] have followed, documenting clinical results.

PREOPERATIVE CONCERNS

Diagnosis

The histopathologic diagnosis of an oral mass must be aggressively pursued and the patient 'staged' using the TNM (tumor, node, metastasis) classification.[22,23] Further details are found in Chapters 38 and 45. Especially relevant to mandibulectomy techniques is to assess how far apically tumors originating on the gingiva have infiltrated. This will largely determine whether a surgically aggressive or more conservative approach is indicated. It is also very important to determine whether and to what extent the root of the tongue is involved; computed tomography with soft tissue contrast enhancement or nuclear magnetic resonance imaging are especially useful in this respect. Computed tomography is also helpful in determining the extent of bone and mandibular canal involvement.

Client communication

Topics to discuss with the client include intent of surgery (local cure or palliation) and prognosis, operative concerns (blood loss, anesthesia risk), postoperative appearance and oral function, and recommended follow-up. A photograph album including preoperative and postoperative photographs of patients that have had various types of partial mandibulectomy aids this aspect of client communication.

THERAPEUTIC DECISION-MAKING

Types of osseous excisions

The most common types of mandibulectomy are shown in Figure 46.1. The extent of any excision is determined by the oral physical examination and diagnostic imaging findings, the histopathological diagnosis, the recommended surgical margins, intent of the surgery and the tissue available for closure of the defect.

© 2012 Elsevier Ltd
DOI: 10.1016/B978-0-7020-4618-6.00046-4

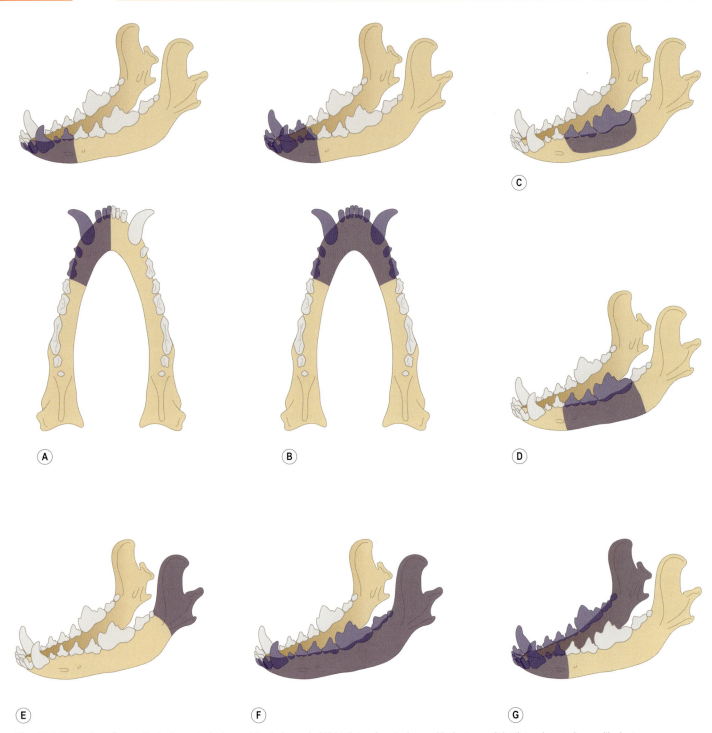

Fig. 46.1 Examples of mandibulectomy techniques (*shaded areas*). (**A**) Unilateral rostral mandibulectomy. (**B**) Bilateral rostral mandibulectomy. (**C**) Central or segmental mandibulectomy with preservation of the mandibular canal and ventral margin ('rim excision'). (**D**) Central or segmental mandibulectomy (full thickness). (**E**) Caudal mandibulectomy. (**F**) Total mandibulectomy. (**G**) One-and-a-half mandibulectomy.

Preoperative management

The reader is referred to Chapter 45 and other chapters for anesthetic considerations, preemptive analgesia, antibiotics and oral cavity disinfection.

Patient positioning

Dorsal and lateral recumbency

The head is secured into position with a vacuum-charged surgical positioning system (Vac-Pac, Olympic Medical, Seattle, WA). This device allows the head to be held in any position. A mouth gag is positioned away from the surgery site to keep the mouth open. The endotracheal tube is secured to the muzzle and the tongue retracted from the surgery site and packed off with gauze sponges. For bilateral rostral mandibulectomy, the patient is placed in dorsal recumbency, with the neck flexed to allow access to both oral and cutaneous surfaces of the rostral mandibles. For unilateral rostral or central mandibulectomy, the patient is placed in lateral or dorsal recumbency with the head rotated to facilitate visualization of the surgical field. The head is held parallel with the table top or the rostral end of the muzzle and lower jaw slightly elevated to improve site access. The neck is extended when the patient is in lateral recumbency. For caudal and total mandibulectomy, the patient is placed in lateral recumbency with the neck extended and the rostral end of the muzzle and lower jaw elevated so the surgeon can look into the open mouth.

After positioning, a layer of water-repellant gauze (Exodontia Sponges, Henry Schein, Melville, NY) packing is placed in the pharynx around the endotracheal tube then covered with a layer of absorbent gauze.

Sternal recumbency

Sternal recumbency, with the head elevated and the maxilla suspended, is an alternative method of positioning for mandibulectomy procedures. The maxilla is suspended by perforating the maxillary canine teeth through a long strip of adhesive tape. The ends of the tape are then extended and wrapped high around IV poles placed on either side of the patient's head. The mandible should be level with or slightly lower than the surface of the surgery table.

Sternal recumbency offers excellent visualization of the mandible and oral cavity. In this position, all mandibulectomy procedures can be performed using an intraoral approach.

The main hazard of sternal recumbency is fluid aspiration. The use of a cuffed endotracheal tube and pharyngeal pack is necessary to prevent aspiration. Having continuous suction available is very helpful.

SURGICAL ANATOMY[26–28]

The inferior alveolar artery originates from the maxillary artery. It enters the mandibular foramen, and traverses the mandibular canal with numerous arterioles branching to the bone and teeth. There are no direct vascular anastomoses across the fibrocartilaginous mandibular symphysis; however, small extraosseous arterioles span the symphysis in the submucosal tissue. Blood supply to the cortical bone at the symphysis is from endosteal and periosteal surfaces. This extraosseous supply may be important to the viability of a rostral mandibular segment after interruption of the inferior alveolar artery secondary to a caudal or central mandibulectomy. The inferior alveolar artery terminates in the caudal, middle and rostral mental arteries.

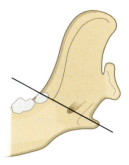

Fig. 46.2 Lingual aspect of mandibular ramus. The mandibular foramen is located in the middle of and immediately ventral to an imaginary line between the palpable landmarks of the angular process and the distal aspect of the mandibular third molar tooth.

The mandibular canal mainly contains the inferior alveolar artery, vein and nerve, and some loose connective tissue and fat. The nerve is dorsolateral, the artery is in the central area and vein ventromedial. Bone convexities from the apical alveolar bone of the mandibular teeth border the lingual or dorsal lingual aspect of the canal. The mandibular canal terminates at the mental foramina.

The mandibular foramen is located on the medial aspect of the mandible. It is immediately below and centered on a line from the tip of the angular process to the distal aspect of the third molar tooth in the dog (Fig. 46.2) and the first molar tooth in the cat. Palpation of these landmarks during caudal mandibulectomy aids in dissection of the inferior alveolar artery and nerve as they enter the foramen. The middle mental foramen in the dog is at the level of the rostral root of the second premolar tooth, immediately distal to the apex of the canine tooth and approximately midway between the alveolar margin and ventral bone margin (Fig. 46.3A). In the cat, this foramen is located at the level of the apex of the canine tooth. The caudal mental foramen is at the level of the third premolar tooth and approximately midway between the alveolar margin and ventral margin in the dog and cat. The rostral mental foramen is generally at the level of the second incisor tooth and a short distance ventral to the alveolar margin. Multiple small foramina may be present.

The apex of the large curved root of the mandibular canine tooth in the dog extends as far as the apex of the distal root of the second premolar tooth. Therefore, bone resection to remove the canine tooth alveolus would also result in removal of the first and second premolar teeth. In the cat, the apex of the canine tooth is immediately rostral to the mesial root of the third premolar tooth. Complete removal of the bone segment encasing the canine tooth root may also require removal of the third premolar tooth and surrounding bone.

The inferior labial artery originates from the facial artery and supplies the soft tissue of the lower lip. The sublingual artery also originates from the facial artery and courses along the medial aspect of the mandible. The ventral buccal branch of the facial nerve provides motor innervation to the muscles of the lip. The mandibular branch of the trigeminal nerve provides motor innervation to the muscles of mastication and sensory innervation to the lower lips, rostral two-thirds of the tongue, mandibular teeth (as the inferior alveolar nerve) and buccal cavity. The muscles of mastication insert on the ramus of the mandible and some lingual and hyoid muscles insert on the body of the mandible (Fig. 46.3B).

The mandibular and sublingual salivary ducts are visible through the thin oral mucosa and course lateral to the tongue frenulum to end in the sublingual caruncle located just rostrolateral to the rostral margin of the frenulum.

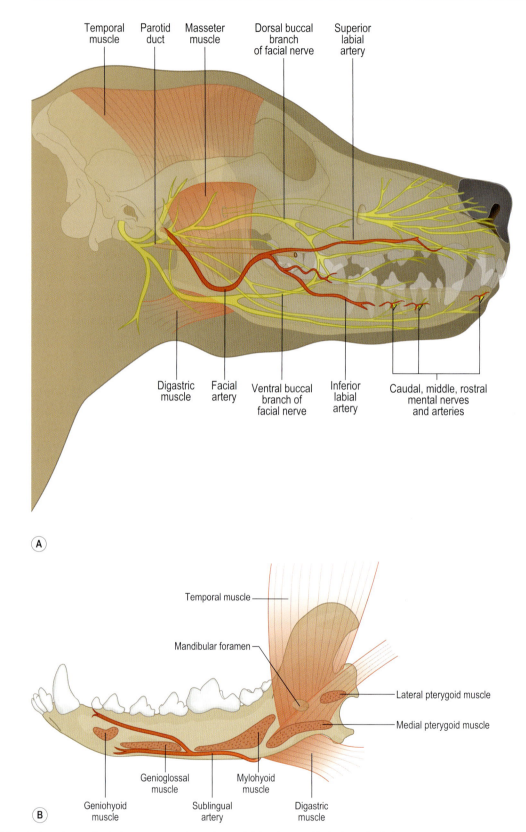

Fig. 46.3 (A, B) Surgical anatomy of arteries, nerves and muscles pertaining to mandibulectomy techniques.

SURGICAL TECHNIQUE

General surgical principles[21–23]

Surgical plan

The surgical plan for a mandibulectomy procedure includes the following important points: (1) plan for adequate surgical margins; (2) plan for complete mucosal closure; (3) perform atraumatic surgery and preserve local blood supply; (4) employ minimal use of electrosurgery; (5) harvest large mucosal flaps to avoid suture line tension; (6) use double-layer closure if possible; and (7) support suture lines with grossly healthy bone if possible.

Surgical margins

Surgical margins are indicated by the biological behavior of the neoplasm as determined by the preoperative histopathological diagnosis, and diagnostic imaging and oral physical examination findings (see Ch. 43). The preoperative histopathological diagnosis is essential for definitive surgical planning. In general, a minimum of 10-mm margin should be obtained for all benign and malignant neoplasms except fibrosarcoma where a minimum margin of 20 mm is recommended due to the higher local recurrence rate.[21–23] These recommendations have not been correlated with clinical outcome. Wider margins are obtained for malignant neoplasms if a tension-free oral mucosal reconstruction can be obtained. The surgical margins are measured and marked around the circumference of the mass using a sterile surgical marker before starting the surgery. It is important to remember that the periodontal ligament spaces and mandibular canal may facilitate neoplastic cell infiltration. Therefore, if the canine tooth is included in the measured surgical margins, the ostectomy is usually performed between the second and third premolar teeth (in the dog) to ensure complete removal of the canine tooth alveolus. Invasion of the mandibular canal by a malignancy requires total mandibulectomy.

Postoperative radiographs of the excised specimen or surgery site are made to document adequate gross surgical margins. The entire specimen is sent for histopathological examination to confirm the diagnosis and to assess the bone and soft tissue margins for neoplastic cells. Finding neoplastic cells on the excision margin implies incomplete removal of local microscopic disease and the need to consider adjunct radiation or chemotherapy.

Surgical incision

The incision is made along the measured and marked surgical margins. The initial incision is a light scoring of the mucosa to produce a minimally bleeding incision line. Once the margins of the proposed excision are verified the incision is taken to bone. Once incised, the alveolar mucosal margins may retract and result in some distortion of the proposed margins. The described incision method maintains accurate surgical margins. In the regions of foramina, the dissection is continued to identify, ligate and transect the vessels and transect the nerves. Hemorrhage is controlled by ligation, pressure and minimal focal use of electrocoagulation. Depending on surgical margins, muscles attaching to the mandible are subperiosteally elevated or transected.

Concurrent lip wedge excision may be needed to obtain adequate surgical margins. This is true for large neoplasms along the body of the mandible and when a bilateral rostral mandibulectomy is performed. Wedge excision is also performed during the latter procedure to remove excess skin. Lip excision compromises blood supply to the remaining rostral lip segment; however, viability is maintained by submucosal arterial branches.

Management of adjacent teeth

Maintaining teeth is secondary to achieving adequate surgical margins and tension-free closure. Ostectomy performed at a narrow interdental space may result in injury requiring extraction of a tooth adjacent to the ostectomy site if inadvertent severe periodontal or endodontic injury (root canal exposure) occurred during ostectomy. Ostectomy at the level of a wider interdental space may not result in similar tooth injury. Therefore, to minimize tooth loss, the ostectomy margins are planned to transect a tooth at the margin level (Fig. 46.4). This may require margin extension, which is acceptable. Margins should never be compromised to save teeth. Once the en-bloc tissue mass is excised, the remnant of the transected tooth is extracted. The adjacent teeth and periodontal structures are not injured, leaving a margin of attached and free gingiva adjacent to the ostectomy.

Ostectomy and osteoplasty

Ostectomy often removes a full-thickness (dorsoventral) segment of the mandible. However, in the case of smaller neoplasms, adequate surgical margins may be achieved by partial-thickness excision or *rim*

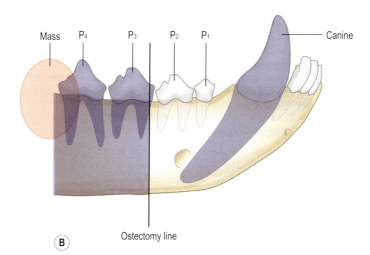

Fig. 46.4 Ostectomy lines for (**A**) rostral mandibulectomy, and (**B**) caudal mandibulectomy in relation to adjacent teeth. Transecting a tooth at the time of excision will not injure adjacent teeth; the remaining tooth fragment is removed after the en-bloc excision is completed. The specific level of ostectomy is dependent upon measured surgical margins.

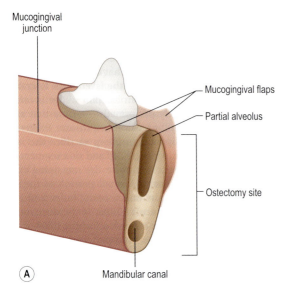

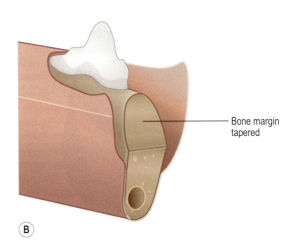

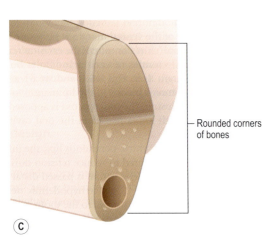

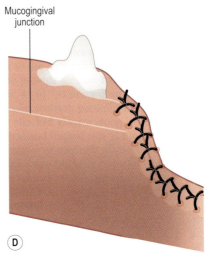

Fig. 46.6 Tapering the alveolar bone margin to reduce suture line tension. The adjacent tooth was transected during ostectomy; the root remnant has been extracted leaving a partial alveolus. (**A**) Alveolar margin and sulcular incisions are made and the attached gingiva and proximal alveolar mucosa are subperiosteally elevated. (**B**) The alveolar margin bone is tapered approximately 30–60 degrees. (**C**) Osteoplasty is performed by rounding the bony edges. (**D**) The attached gingiva and alveolar mucosa is closed over the surgical defect.

as needed. Mucosal incisions are made along the measured surgical margins. However, it is often unnecessary to incise the cheek to achieve surgical margins and have good site exposure, especially when dorso-lateral or sternal positioning is used. Using the intraoral approach, a mucosal incision is made over the rostral edge of the ramus then extended in a buccal and lingual direction around the mandibular body along surgical margins. After dissection of the caudal part of the mandibular body and ostectomy, dissection along the ramus is performed. The insertions of the muscles of mastication are subperiosteally elevated or the muscle body transected, depending on surgical margins. If needed, the masseter is excised as part of the en-bloc excision. The digastric and pterygoid muscles are elevated or transected, as determined by surgical margins. The mandibular foramen is located and the inferior alveolar artery is ligated and transected close to the

foramen to avoid injury to the maxillary artery. The inferior alveolar nerve is also transected as close as possible to the foramen, in order to avoid damage to the lingual nerve. The temporalis muscle insertions on the medial and lateral aspects of the ramus and coronoid process are elevated or transected, as determined by the surgical margins. The temporomandibular joint is located by palpation during manipulation of the caudal mandibular en-bloc segment. The capsule is incised on the medial aspect. As the mandible is manipulated to aid visualization, adjacent soft tissues are gently 'wiped' off the capsule and the capsule incision extended laterally. The rostral and caudal aspects of the capsule are incised in this manner and the lateral ligament is incised last. It is essential that dissection and joint capsule incision occur immediately adjacent to the condylar process to avoid injury to adjacent vessels and nerves. The tortuous course and close

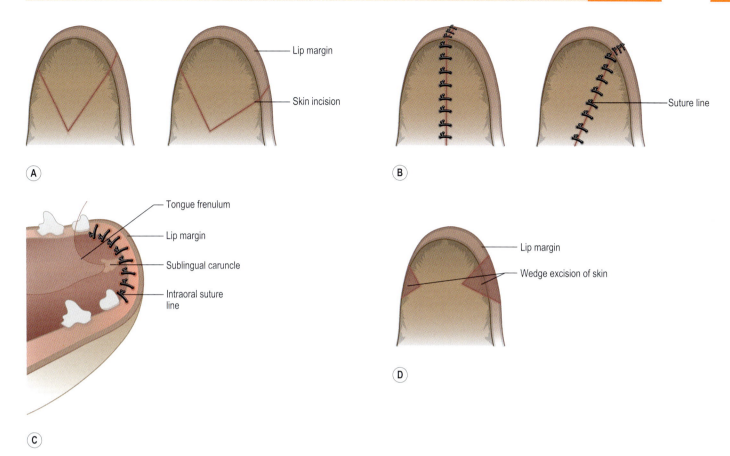

Fig. 46.7 Bilateral rostral mandibulectomy. The patient is in dorsal recumbency. (**A**) The wedge incision (either symmetrical, left, or asymmetrical, right) incorporates the surgical margins and estimated excess skin and lip for closure. (**B**, **C**) Closure results in a linear skin suture line and a transverse oral mucosal suture line. (**D**) Alternative skin and lip closure with bilateral removal of full-thickness labial tissue.

proximity of the maxillary artery on the ventromedial aspect of the joint, and its local branches, make them vulnerable to inadvertent transection. Once the joint is disarticulated, any remaining soft tissue attachments are cut. A local anesthetic 'splash' block may be applied to the surgery site. Placement of local hemostatic agents (see Ch. 7) may be needed to help control bleeding from transected muscles. Oral mucosal tissues are opposed using simple interrupted sutures. Closure is routine.

Unilateral (total) mandibulectomy

Penetration of the mandibular canal implies potential spread of neoplasm along the length of the mandible, indicating the need for total mandibulectomy. This procedure can be performed with the patient in lateral recumbency using an incision of the cheek. This may facilitate the caudal dissection, especially in some large patients and in patients with more caudally located masses necessitating excision of the masseter muscle, and transection rather than subperiosteal elevation of other muscles. The procedure can be performed intraorally with the patient in sternal recumbency. The intraoral incision is started as described for caudal mandibulectomy and continued along the predetermined surgical margins. The mandibular symphysis is split using a thin osteotome and mallet and the body and ramus dissected free of all tissue attachments, as described above for the various partial mandibulectomy techniques. If necessary for surgical margins, the tongue frenulum can be removed without altering tongue function. Soft tissue excision may extend toward the opposite mandible.

However, this excision margin is limited by the need for primary mucosal closure. Extensive removal of sublingual muscle may result in impairment of tongue function. The mandible is excised intact.

The commissure is moved rostrally to minimize drooling and help prevent tongue protrusion. Commissurorrhaphy is performed by excision of the lip margin followed by a three-layer closure. The new commissure is approximately at the level of the mandibular second premolar tooth. A full-thickness horizontal mattress suture may be placed to span between the upper and lower lip immediately rostral to the new commissure. This suture is tied over buttons or suture bolsters. Its purpose is to restrain mouth opening to keep tension off the commissure suture line and promote normal healing.

Stabilization of mandibular segments

To date, reconstruction following mandibulectomy is infrequently performed.[30] An ulnar autograft combined with rigid internal fixation was used to bridge a central mandibulectomy site for benign neoplasm excision, with good results.[31] This technique has the potential to eliminate mandibular instability and malocclusion and improve cosmetic results for central mandibulectomies. Stabilization of the remaining lower jaw after bilateral rostral mandibulectomy has been attempted using orthopedic pins,[32] screws,[4,7] and screws and bone graft.[33] The screws and pins are placed before the excision is performed. Mandibular instability is avoided and prehension is similar to that of patients not having any stabilization technique performed.

A microvascular bone autograft using coccygeal vertebrae has been reported for fracture reconstruction of a central mandibular defect in a dog.[34] Microvascular transfer of bone autografts is the preferred method of mandibular reconstruction in humans and may be of benefit to selected small animal patients.[35]

POSTOPERATIVE CARE AND ASSESSMENT

Most aspects of postoperative care, including pain management and nutritional support, are similar to those described for maxillectomy (see Ch. 45).

Postoperative patient appearance[21–23]

Swelling of the surgical site is usually resolved by 3 to 7 days postoperatively. Cosmetic appearances are generally good and depend on the extent of excision. Smaller excisions result in unnoticeable or minimal cosmetic abnormalities. Regrowth of hair will conceal many surgically created facial asymmetries. Unilateral rostral mandibulectomy without canine tooth removal results in no obvious abnormality. When the canine tooth is removed, the tongue hangs out from that side when panting. Bilateral rostral mandibulectomy results in relative mandibular brachygnathism and the most noticeable uncosmetic appearance (Fig. 46.8). The tongue protrudes from the mouth during panting. Drooling may occur. Central mandibulectomy results in a mild facial concavity. Caudal and complete mandibulectomy result in facial concavity and tongue protrusion from the side of surgery during panting (Fig. 46.9). Malocclusion occurs as the remaining mandible shifts toward the operated side.

Homecare and follow-up

Most patients are sent home in 2 to 3 days postoperatively. A soft food diet and removal of chew toys is recommended for 2 to 3 weeks. The client is shown how to administer any oral medications so as not to disrupt the suture line. Medications are concealed in soft food snacks. If oral manipulation is needed, the manipulation is performed away from the surgical site. The surgical site is examined in 2 weeks and any skin sutures removed. The surgical site is reexamined at 1 month postoperatively and any residual oral sutures removed at this time. Most oral sutures are extruded in approximately 2 to 3 weeks. A complete physical examination, including the surgical site, is performed at 3-month intervals for 1 year. In case of malignant neoplasms, three-view thoracic radiographs are obtained at these examinations.

COMPLICATIONS[19–23]

Intraoperative complications

Hemorrhage is the major intraoperative complication. It is managed as it is encountered by ligation, pressure or focal use of electrocoagulation. The risk for excessive bleeding is the highest during ostectomy and during dissection of the caudal mandible. Blood loss during ostectomy is minimized by cutting the bone of the ventral mandible last and isolating and ligating the inferior alveolar artery. In the event of inadvertent transection of the artery, rapid completion of the ostectomy is done and the vessel retrieved and ligated. If the artery retracts into the canal and cannot be retrieved, the mandibular canal is packed with a suitable hemostatic agent (see Ch. 7). Careful dissection for disarticulation of the temporomandibular joint is required to avoid vascular injury and profuse hemorrhage.

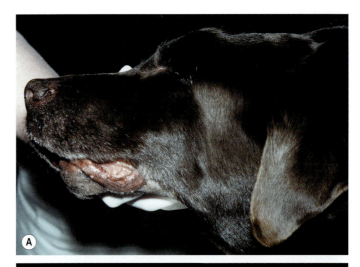

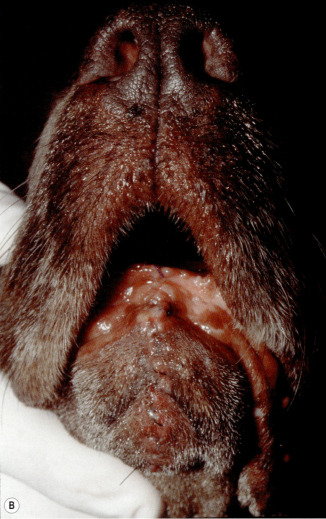

Fig. 46.8 (**A**) Lateral and (**B**) ventrodorsal view of a patient after bilateral rostral mandibulectomy.

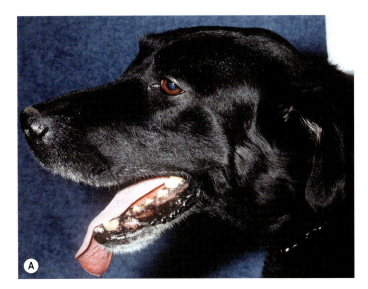

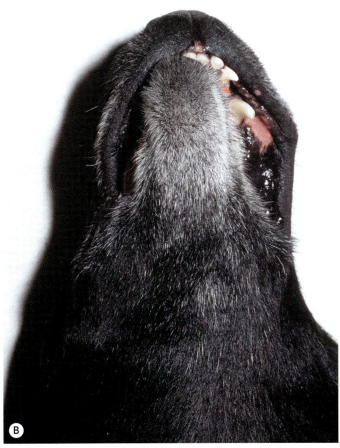

Fig. 46.9 (**A**) Lateral and (**B**) ventrodorsal view of a patient after a total mandibulectomy of the right mandible. Lateral tongue protrusion during panting and mandibular drift to the right side are visible.

Dehiscence

Dehiscence of the commissurorrhaphy may occur and is repaired by delayed primary closure. A small dehiscence over the ostectomy site exposing bone will usually heal by second intention. A larger dehiscence requires debridement and resuturing.

Functional complications

Malocclusion

The contralateral mandible is initially unstable and drifts toward the midline. Elastic training using orthodontic buttons and power chain between the buccal aspect of the maxillary fourth premolar tooth and the lingual aspect of the mandibular canine tooth is a simple method for prevention of mandibular drift but requires good client compliance.[36] Abnormal contact with the remaining mandibular canine tooth may result in palatal or upper lip ulceration. Crown reduction and partial coronal pulpectomy, or extraction of the mandibular canine tooth, is needed to resolve the palatal ulceration.[37] The remaining mandible may occasionally drift away from the midline. When this happens the mandibular and maxillary teeth meet end on. Clicking is briefly audible until the mandible drifts medially. The unstable mandibular movement is reduced 4–6 weeks after surgery; however, occlusion may remain abnormal. Long-term follow-up of clinical cases does not suggest abnormal temporomandibular joint clinical effects. After experimental unilateral rostral mandibulectomy, temporomandibular degenerative joint disease occurred and did not impair the dogs at 3 and 6 months postoperatively.[38]

Prehension

Most patients prehend and drink normally after partial mandibulectomy. Patients with more extensive excisions practice eating and adapt after a short period of time. Some dogs spill a large amount of food around the food-bowl during this period. Food with a consistency similar to ground meat or soaked kibble seems the easiest to prehend. Hand-feeding may be permanently necessary with some patients after a one-and-one-half mandibulectomy. These patients usually adapt to drinking by a combination of lapping and sucking water.

Drooling

Drooling occurs with bilateral rostral mandibulectomies and total mandibulectomies. Drooling often decreases over time. If the new lip margin is immediately rostral to the sublingual caruncles when closing a bilateral rostral mandibulectomy, the mandibular and sublingual salivary ducts may be ligated to reduce drooling potential. Moving the commissure rostrally during closure of a total mandibulectomy usually prevents drooling.

Tongue protrusion

Lateral tongue protrusion occurs when a mandibular canine tooth is absent, as in a unilateral rostral mandibulectomy or total mandibulectomy. Ventral tongue protrusion occurs following a bilateral rostral mandibulectomy. The protrusion is most evident when panting. Dessication of the tongue rarely occurs.

Ranula

A ranula may result from surgical trauma to the salivary duct or papilla or postoperative swelling that temporarily impairs flow of saliva from the sublingual caruncle. This condition may occur at 1 to 2 days postoperatively and usually resolves by 5 to 7 days. Treatment is not needed.

Dental calculus

The ipsilateral maxillary fourth premolar tooth and molar teeth may accumulate dental calculus more rapidly, as compared to the contralateral side, in patients with central, caudal and total mandibulectomies. There is an apparent compromise of normal oral cleansing,

Chapter 47

Clinical behavior and management of odontogenic cysts

Thomas P. Chamberlain & Frank J.M. Verstraete

INTRODUCTION

Odontogenic cysts (OC) are epithelium-lined structures that appear in the tooth-bearing areas of both jaws and are considered uncommon in domestic animals.[1,2] OC reported in dogs and cats include dentigerous cysts, periapical cysts and odontogenic keratocysts.[1,3–13] In humans, the majority of cystic jaw lesions are discovered incidentally on screening studies.[14] Much diagnostic confusion exists between the study of veterinary and human OC because unified terminology and classification schemes do not exist.[1] OC arise within islands of remnants of odontogenic epithelium (dental lamina, rests of Malassez) located in the periodontal ligament stroma.[1] Cystic lesions often have multilayered walls of epithelium that resemble ameloblastic epithelium in some areas.[1] Different OC have variable clinical and biological behaviors.[15–17] Adequate treatment planning requires accurate histopathologic diagnosis by pathologists with training in odontogenic tumor and cyst pathology.[15–17] Any epithelial tumor may become cystic as central degeneration of neoplastic epithelium occurs and the converse is true in that malignant transformation of OC lining has also been reported.[1] In humans, histological evidence as well as immunohistochemical markers of cellular proliferation indicate that the architecture of some OC may actually be neoplastic versus truly cystic.[15–17] Genetic factors are thought to play a major role in the etiology of human OC; however, cytomegalovirus has been detected as a common inhabitant of both inflammatory and noninflammatory human OC.[18,19] Histopathology is the main modality for definitive diagnosis of OC, as immunochemistry and molecular diagnostic techniques are not yet clinically used.[20]

DENTIGEROUS CYST

Pathophysiology

Although they are the second most common type of odontogenic cyst in humans, dentigerous cysts (DC) are infrequent in dogs and cats.[8–12,21,22] A recent study indicated that DC are the most prevalent odontogenic cyst in dogs.[23] By definition, DC are associated with unerupted normal or malformed teeth, and arise from proliferation of tissue remnants of the enamel organ or reduced enamel epithelium.[21,22,24] The pathogenesis is uncertain; however, trauma is thought to be the main etiologic factor.[9] In humans, there is increasing evidence that genetic mechanisms are involved in cyst genesis.[24] As for other odontogenic cysts, DC expansion occurs by common pathways involving passive osmotic fluid accumulation, proliferation of epithelial cells, and release of mediators of osteoclastic bone resorption.[25,26]

Clinical features

Dentigerous cysts should be a primary consideration for any oral swelling in an edentulous area of either jaw.[22] Age of initial diagnosis ranges between 6 months and 10 years; however, the highest frequency of DC is discovered between 2 and 3 years of age.[23] Although DC are identified in a variety of breeds, the brachycephalic breeds are overrepresented.[23] The mandibular first premolars are the most commonly affected teeth in dogs; however, DC associated with unerupted maxillary and mandibular canine teeth are also observed.[23] As for humans, the most common location for canine DC is in the mandible.[23] In the early stages of cyst formation, patients are generally asymptomatic. As the cyst enlarges, the mucosa overlying the cyst may appear slightly blue or purple (Fig. 47.1A). Asymmetry with tooth displacement, severe resorption of adjacent teeth and pain are possible sequela of progressive cyst enlargement.[9,11,12] Fluid-filled osseous cyst walls may be palpable.[10] DC can become large lesions and expand the cortical bone of the maxilla or mandible.[17] In humans, cystic growth rate is estimated to be 2–14 mm per year.[27,28] Malignant transformation of the epithelial lining cells to primary osseous carcinoma and ameloblastoma has been reported in humans but appears to be extremely rare.[11,13,22] Because DC are often discovered as incidental findings, the significance of frequent oral examinations and the routine use of full-mouth intraoral radiographs should be emphasized.[23]

DOI: 10.1016/B978-0-7020-4618-6.00047-6

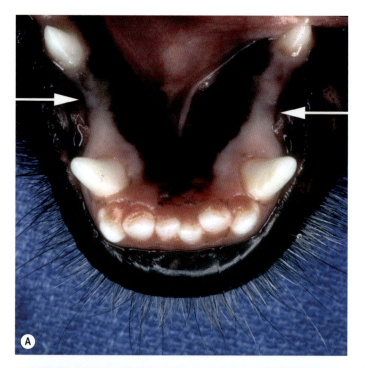

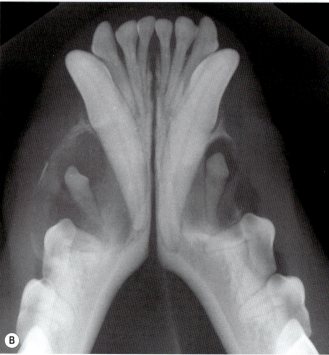

Fig. 47.1 (**A**) Clinical and (**B**) radiographic appearance of bilateral dentigerous cysts associated with unerupted mandibular first premolars. Note the bluish appearance of the mucosa overlying the cyst cavities (**A** arrows). (From Self-Assessment Colour Review of Veterinary Dentistry, edited by Frank Verstraete. Manson Publishing Ltd, London, 1999.)

The radiologic features of DC are considered nearly pathognomonic (Fig. 47.1B).[10] The crown of the unerupted tooth will be enclosed by a radiolucent halo of variable size attached to the cemento-enamel junction.[9,10,12,22] Although generally structureless, a thin, well-defined, radiopaque margin of cortical bone (well circumscribed) may be visible surrounding all or part of the radiolucent cyst.[9,10,12,14,22] Cysts

may be unilocular or occasionally multilocular, and the unerupted tooth may be displaced.[21] Resorption of adjacent teeth may also be noted.[21] The cyst wall is composed of a thin layer of connective tissue and nonkeratinized stratified squamous epithelium of 2–6 cell layers thick and resembles reduced enamel epithelium.[21] Occasionally, secondary inflammatory cell infiltrates and epithelial hyperplasia may be observed.[21]

Management

Treatment involves a surgical approach using a mucogingival–periosteal flap to accomplish removal of the unerupted tooth, complete enucleation of the cyst wall, curettage, osteoplasty and bone grafting if bone defects are extensive.[22] Prior to primary surgical closure, careful evaluation of the surgical site is mandatory, and submission of the entire cyst wall for thorough histopathologic examination and definitive diagnosis is necessary.[22] Incomplete removal of cystic epithelium may result in recurrence of the dentigerous cyst and/or neoplastic transformation.[21,22] Bone grafting may be required if the size of the dentigerous cyst compromises the integrity of the jaw. Because these lesions are often asymptomatic for long periods of time, patients may easily be lost to follow-up.[15] Follow-up should continue for 2 years or until there is complete reossification of the cyst cavity.[15]

PERIAPICAL CYST

Pathophysiology

Although the periapical (PC) or radicular cyst is the most common OC diagnosed in humans, they have been infrequently reported in dogs and cats.[4–7,21] PC are strictly inflammatory cysts associated with a pre-existing periapical granuloma of a nonvital tooth.[18,20,25] Periapical granulomas are the most common finding associated with failed endodontic treatment in humans.[25] Infected root canal content is the source of bacterial endotoxins and necrotic debris that stimulate a chronic inflammatory response in the periapical area.[29] PC are believed to develop from endotoxin and immune stimulation of small odontogenic residues (epithelial rests of Malassez) within periapical tissues.[18,25,29] The 'true' periapical cyst is completely enclosed by epithelium and attached by a cord of epithelium to the root apex, whereas the 'pocket' periapical cyst has a cavity confluent with the root canal.[30] Cyst formation may represent formation of a physical barrier that confines necrotic pulp contents to the root canal, thus preventing spread into the surrounding bone and other tissues.[29,31] Once remnant epithelial cells begin proliferating, there are several theories as to how apical cyst formation actually occurs, and this may be genetically programmed.[29] At the center of the developing mass, cells eventually become necrotic. As the result of accumulating protein concentrations, osmotic pressure rises, and fluid ingress occurs as cavitation and passive cyst expansion occurs.[4,25,31] As the result of cellular degeneration, many proinflammatory cytokines, growth factors and inflammatory mediators accumulate, promoting osteoclastic bone resorption and cyst expansion.[25,26,32]

Clinical features

A nonvital tooth is a prerequisite to PC formation, though many nonvital teeth are initially asymptomatic.[25] In dogs, few necrotic and/or infected teeth are associated with clinical symptoms recognizable by pet owners.[33] The only evidence of pulp necrosis may be intrinsic tooth staining.[33] In humans, most PC are asymptomatic and discovered during routine dental radiographic examinations as round to ovoid, well-circumscribed, unilocular periapical lucencies that are contiguous with the lamina dura of the involved tooth.[14,25] Depending upon the stage at diagnosis, some cysts in dogs may demonstrate relatively wide areas of radioluceny (Fig. 47.2A).[4,5] Radiographically, a PC cannot be distinguished from a granuloma.[14,25] With longstanding PC, resorption of the affected tooth as well as adjacent teeth may occur (Fig. 47.2B).[4,14] With periapical granulomas, resorption of the affected tooth may be seen; however, resorption of adjacent teeth would be unexpected.[25] Although some types of ultrasound and computed tomography scans have demonstrated ability to differentiate between periapical granulomas and cysts, the gold standard for definitive identification of a periapical cyst versus a granuloma is histopathologic assessment through serial sections of lesions removed in their entirety.[25,31,34,35]

Periapical cysts are lined by nonkeratinized stratified squamous epithelium of variable thickness, and the underlying supportive connective tissue may be focally or diffusely infiltrated with a population of mixed inflammatory cells.[25,36] Plasma cell infiltrates, multinucleated foreign body-type giant cells and dystrophic mineralization may also be observed.[25]

Management

As for all teeth with nonvital pulp, management by tooth extraction with curettage of the periapical region or an endodontic procedure should be performed.[25] If endodontic treatment is elected, initial treatment of inflammatory periapical lesions should be with conservative, nonsurgical measures.[31] In apical pocket cysts, intracanal toxins can be eliminated by nonsurgical endodontic procedures, and these lesions may completely resolve.[25,26,31,34,35] Proliferation of periapical tissues will be inhibited by the removal of bacterial endotoxins, proinflammatory cytokines, inflammatory mediators and cellular growth factors.[25,31] Further degradation of the periapical lesion may be augmented by resumption of normal apoptotic mechanisms of epithelial cell death.[36,37] Although root canal treatment may remove endotoxins from canals associated with true PC, remaining cystic epithelium (*residual cysts*) still contains inflammatory mediators capable of sustaining or enlarging the cyst.[29–31] True PC must be treated by apicoectomy or extraction, because irritants cannot be removed nonsurgically.[38,39] Because many diseased teeth are asymptomatic to the owners for long periods of time, and significant complications of cyst expansion may occur, treatment follow-up should last until the complete ossification of the cyst cavity has occurred, i.e., at least 2 years (Fig 47.2C).[15,25] Failure to remove all of the epithelial cyst lining at the time of tooth extraction and periapical curettage may result in renewed epithelial proliferation and development of a *residual cyst* (cyst recurrence).[14,29] Any medication that can prevent release of inflammatory mediators and/or proinflammatory cytokines might be able to inhibit proliferation of epithelial cell rests in apical periodontitis, so administration of nonsteroidal

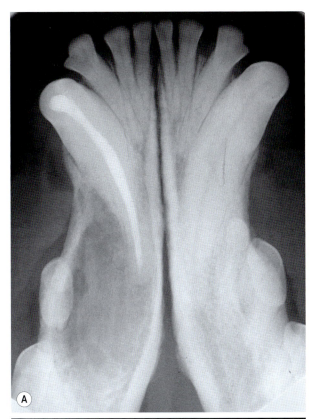

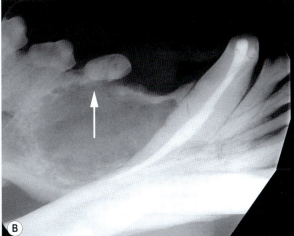

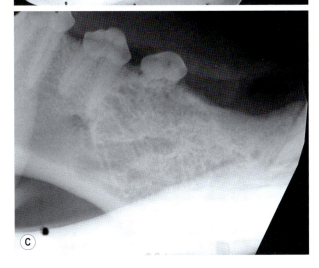

Fig. 47.2 (**A**) Occlusal and (**B**) lateral views of the left mandibular canine tooth. Note the resorption of the roots of the second premolar tooth (*arrow*). This 9-year-old dog was presented for evaluation of a gingival mass at the right mandibular canine tooth, and the clients had no recollection of root canal treatment having been performed on the left mandibular canine tooth. Extraction was performed, and no bone graft was placed at the client's request. Histopathology confirmed the clinical diagnosis of periapical cyst. (**C**) Six months later, the dog was returned for a follow-up radiograph, which verified complete filling of the cyst cavity with new bone. (*From: Lommer MJ. Diagnostic imaging in veterinary dental practice. Periapical cyst. J Am Vet Med Assoc. 2007;230:997–9.*)

antiinflammatory drugs may have beneficial effects in addition to postoperative analgesia.[31]

ODONTOGENIC KERATOCYST-LIKE LESION (OKC-LIKE) – KERATOCYSTIC ODONTOGENIC TUMOR

Pathophysiology

Although commonly encountered in humans, OKC are rare in dogs and other domestic animals.[1,3,20,21] A recent study of odontogenic cysts in dogs identified nine cysts that had histopathologic features that were suggestive of, but not diagnostic- of, the human OKC.[23] These were identified as the second most common type of canine cyst encountered and the term 'OKC-like lesion' or 'canine odontogenic parakeratinized cyst' was proposed.[23] The odontogenic keratocyst (OKC) is classified as a developmental cyst originating from dental lamina remnants in the maxilla or mandible.[21,22] OKC are characterized by aggressive and destructive behavior with a marked propensity to recur.[21] Because they often appear as ordinary cysts, they may be underdiagnosed and undertreated, leading to unnecessary recurrences.[40] Increasing evidence supports the theory that OKC development may be genetically programmed.[24] In humans, the presence of the cytomegalovirus is a common feature of OKC walls; however, the relationship to cyst pathogenesis is unknown.[19] Studies of PC and OKC indicate that cyst expansion and bone resorption are mediated by the common mechanisms of passive osmosis and cellular production of cytokines.[16] Markers of biologic proliferation indicate that the OKC should be considered as an aggressive odontogenic tumor rather than merely a benign cyst, hence the recent suggested name change to keratocystic odontogenic tumor.[36,41]

Clinical features

Patients may be asymptomatic up to the point where facial distortion (Fig. 47.3A), drainage, pain, difficulties with prehension, mastication and/or other complications become obvious as a result of cyst expansion. OKC in humans may occur in any position of either jaw and multiple cysts may be present.[20,21] In dogs, the maxilla is the most frequently affected jaw, there is no specific age for presentation, and miniature schnauzers were the most commonly represented breed.[23] OKC are not associated with unerupted teeth. Upon surgical exploration, a fluid-filled, cystic cavity is identified below the gingiva and mucosa (Fig. 47.3B). Radiographically, OKC may present as a well-circumscribed unilocular or multilocular radiolucency with smooth or scalloped margins (Fig. 47.3C).[14,21,27] Although displacement of adjacent teeth may occur, only rarely is there root resorption.[28]

Histopathologic assessment remains the mainstay for diagnosis of human OKC.[20,21] The microscopic feature of parakeratotic keratinization of the cyst lining is highly characteristic.[1,3,16,20,21] The cyst lining is composed of a thin connective tissue periphery supporting a stratified squamous layer of 6–10-cell thickness.[16,20,21] The basal layer consists of well-developed, palisaded, cuboidal or columnar cells with a higher mitotic index and intensely stained nuclei.[16,20,21] Budding of the basal layer and daughter, microcyst formation may be encountered.[20,21] The luminal surface cells are parakeratinized, refractile and form a corrugated rim.[20,21] The lumen may contain variable amounts of desquamated keratin.[27] If secondary inflammation occurs, an inflammatory cell infiltrate and hyperplasia may ensue, disrupting the characteristic appearance.[20] Therefore, submitting large areas or the entirety of the cyst for histopathologic assessment is important.[20]

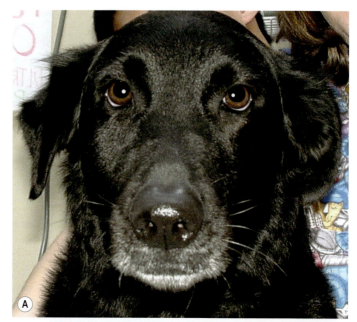

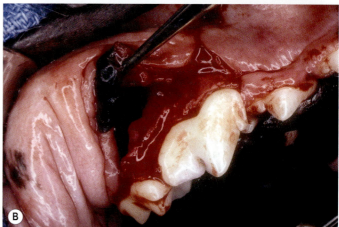

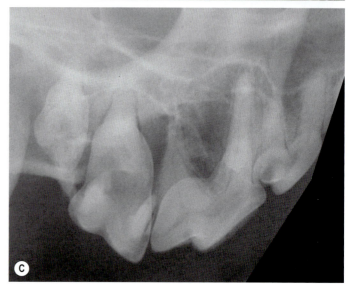

Fig. 47.3 (A) Clinical, **(B)** intraoperative, and **(C)** radiographic appearance of an odontogenic keratocyst-like lesion adjacent to the right maxillary fourth premolar and first and second molar teeth in a dog.

The canine OKC-like cysts differ in that they lack the basal cell hyperchromasia and palisading typical of the human OKC form.[23]

Management

In the human literature, treatment of the OKC remains controversial as there is no consensus on what is appropriate.[42] Treatment goals are focused on prevention of recurrence and minimizing surgical morbidity.[42] Post-treatment recurrence rates are high and have been reported to be 6–62%.[28] Friability and thinness of the cyst wall contribute to incomplete surgical removal as the most common reason for the high rate of recurrence.[3,42,43] Conservative management includes simple enucleation (with or without curettage), marsupialization or decompression.[27,28,42–44] Conservative management is an alternative when extensive surgery may be unacceptable.[28] Treatment of OKC with enucleation alone is associated with the highest rate of recurrence.[28,43]

Decompression and marsupialization have the advantage of preserving vital structures. These procedures may reduce the size of the lesion; however, a second procedure can be expected to completely remove the cyst.[45] The preferred definitive treatment by one human oral surgeon is decompression/marsupialization to decrease the size of the lesion, followed by definitive surgery (aggressive curettage) and liquid nitrogen cryotherapy.[45,46] Conservative approaches may not be the best management choice if patient follow-up is a concern. Aggressive treatment includes surgical peripheral ostectomy or resection.[43] Peripheral ostectomy is associated with the highest morbidity; however, significantly reduced rates of recurrence are noted.[28,43] In summary, aggressive surgical removal of OKC may be justified when the high recurrence rate is considered; however, in select patients (especially in large OKC), conservative management to promote cyst shrinkage, followed by later resection or other adjunctive therapy, may be advantageous.[21] To evaluate for completeness of excision and treatment success, long-term clinical and radiographic follow-up is mandatory.[21,27,28,43,45,47] In the study involving nine OKC-like lesions, treatment was identical to that performed for dentigerous cysts; however, in the long-term follow-up period, recurrence was not observed.[23]

REFERENCES

1. Poulet FM, Valentine BA, Summers BA. A survey of epithelial odontogenic tumors and cysts in dogs and cats. Vet Pathol 1992;29:369–80.

2. Gardner DG. An orderly approach to the study of odontogenic tumours in animals. J Comp Pathol 1992;107:427–38.

3. Nicoll SA, Sylvestre AM, Remedios AM. Odontogenic keratocyst in a dog. J Am Anim Hosp Assoc 1994;30:286–9.

4. Lommer MJ. Diagnostic imaging in veterinary dental practice. Periapical cyst. J Am Vet Med Assoc 2007;230:997–9.

5. Beckman BW. Radicular cyst of the premaxilla in a dog. J Vet Dent 2003;20:213–17.

6. French SL, Anthony JM. Surgical removal of a radicular odontogenic cyst in a four-year-old Dalmatian dog. J Vet Dent 1996;13:149–51.

7. Doran I, Pearson G, Barr F, et al. Extensive bilateral odontogenic cysts in the mandible of a dog. Vet Pathol 2008; 45:58–60.

8. Gardner DG. Dentigerous cysts in animals. Oral Surg Oral Med Oral Pathol 1993;75: 348–52.

9. Manfra Marretta S, Patnaik AK, Schloss AJ, et al. An iatrogenic dentigerous cyst in a dog. J Vet Dent 1989;6:11–13.

10. Lobprise HB, Wiggs RB. Dentigerous cyst in a dog. J Vet Dent 1992;9:13–15.

11. Kramek BA, O'Brien TD, Smith FO. Diagnosis and removal of a dentigerous cyst complicated by ameloblastic fibro-odontoma in a dog. J Vet Dent 1996;13:9–11.

12. Gioso MA, Carvalho VG. Maxillary dentigerous cyst in a cat. J Vet Dent 2003;20:28–30.

13. Anderson JG, Harvey CE. Odontogenic cysts. J Vet Dent 1993;10:5–9.

14. DelBalso AM. An approach to the diagnostic imaging of jaw lesions, dental implants, and the temporomandibular joint. Radiol Clin North Am 1998;36: 855–90, vi.

15. Meningaud JP, Oprean N, Pitak-Arnnop P, et al. Odontogenic cysts: a clinical study of 695 cases. J Oral Sci 2006;48:59–62.

16. Thosaporn W, Iamaroon A, Pongsiriwet S, et al. A comparative study of epithelial cell proliferation between the odontogenic keratocyst, orthokeratinized odontogenic cyst, dentigerous cyst, and ameloblastoma. Oral Dis 2004;10:22–6.

17. Toida M. So-called calcifying odontogenic cyst: review and discussion on the terminology and classification. J Oral Pathol Med 1998;27:49–52.

18. Shear M. The aggressive nature of the odontogenic keratocyst: is it a benign cystic neoplasm? Part 2. Proliferation and genetic studies. Oral Oncol 2002;38:323–31.

19. Andric M, Milasin J, Jovanovic T, et al. Human cytomegalovirus is present in odontogenic cysts. Oral Microbiol Immunol 2007;22:347–51.

20. Regezi JA. Odontogenic cysts, odontogenic tumors, fibroosseous, and giant cell lesions of the jaws. Mod Pathol 2002; 15:331–41.

21. Regezi JA, Sciubba JJ, Jordan RC. Cysts of the jaws and neck. In: Regezi JA, Sciubba JJ, Jordan RC, eds. Oral pathology: clinical pathologic correlations. 5th ed. St. Louis, MO: Saunders Elsevier; 2008. p. 237–60.

22. Verstraete FJM. Self-assessment color review of veterinary dentistry. 1st ed. Ames, IA: Iowa State University Press; 1999.

23. Verstraete FJ, Zin BP, Kass PH, et al. Clinical signs and histologic findings in dogs with odontogenic cysts: 41 cases (1995–2010). J Am Vet Med Assoc 2011;239:1470–6.

24. Stenman G, Magnusson B, Lennartsson B, et al. In vitro growth characteristics of human odontogenic keratocysts and dentigerous cysts. J Oral Pathol 1986; 15:143–5.

25. Nobuhara WK, del Rio CE. Incidence of periradicular pathoses in endodontic treatment failures. J Endod 1993;19: 315–18.

26. Meghji S, Qureshi W, Henderson B, et al. The role of endotoxin and cytokines in the pathogenesis of odontogenic cysts. Arch Oral Biol 1996;41:523–31.

27. Maurette PE, Jorge J, de MM. Conservative treatment protocol of odontogenic keratocyst: a preliminary study. J Oral Maxillofac Surg 2006;64:379–83.

28. Bsoul SA, Paquette M, Terezhalmy GT, et al. Odontogenic keratocyst. Quintessence Int 2002;33:400–1.

29. Muglali M, Komerik N, Bulut E, et al. Cytokine and chemokine levels in radicular and residual cyst fluids. J Oral Pathol Med 2008;37:185–9.

30. Nair PNR, Pajarola G, Schroeder HE. Types and incidence of human periapical lesions obtained with extracted teeth. Oral Surg Oral Med Oral Pathol Oral Radiol Endod 1996;81:93–102.

31. Lin LM, Huang GT, Rosenberg PA. Proliferation of epithelial cell rests, formation of apical cysts, and regression of apical cysts after periapical wound healing. J Endod 2007;33:908–16.

32. Hayashi M, Ohshima T, Ohshima M, et al. Profiling of radicular cyst and odontogenic keratocyst cytokine production suggests common growth mechanisms. J Endod 2008;34:14–21.

33. Hale FA. Localized intrinsic staining of teeth due to pulpitis and pulp necrosis in dogs. J Vet Dent 2001;18:14–20.

34. Walton DR. Periapical biopsy? Oral Surg Oral Med Oral Pathol Oral Radiol Endod 2000;89:533–4.

35. Spatafore CM, Griffin Jr JA, Keyes GG, et al. Periapical biopsy report: an analysis of over a 10-year period. J Endod 1990;16:239–41.

36. Majno G, Joris I. Apoptosis, oncosis, and necrosis. An overview of cell death. Am J Pathol 1995;146:3–15.

37. Saikumar P, Dong Z, Mikhailov V, et al. Apoptosis: definition, mechanisms, and relevance to disease. Am J Med 1999;107:489–506.

38. Nair PN. New perspectives on radicular cysts: do they heal? Int Endod J 1998;31:155–60.

39. Lin LM, Gaengler P, Langeland K. Periradicular curettage. Int Endod J 1996;29:220–7.

40. Chapelle KA, Stoelinga PJ, de Wilde PC, et al. Rational approach to diagnosis and treatment of ameloblastomas and odontogenic keratocysts. Br J Oral Maxillofac Surg 2004;42:381–90.

41. Barnes L, Eveson JW, Reichart P, et al. World Health Organization classification of tumours – pathology and genetics of head and neck tumours. Lyon, France: IARC Press; 2005.

42. Voorsmit RA, Stoelinga PJ, van Haelst UJ. The management of keratocysts. J Maxillofac Surg 1981;9:228–36.

43. Morgan TA, Burton CC, Qian F. A retrospective review of treatment of the odontogenic keratocyst. J Oral Maxillofac Surg 2005;63:635–9.

44. Blanchard SB. Odontogenic keratocysts: review of the literature and report of a case. J Periodontol 1997;68:306–11.

45. Pogrel MA. Treatment of keratocysts: the case for decompression and marsupialization. J Oral Maxillofac Surg 2005;63:1667–73.

46. Schmidt BL, Pogrel MA. The use of enucleation and liquid nitrogen cryotherapy in the management of odontogenic keratocysts. J Oral Maxillofac Surg 2001;59:720–5.

47. Blanas N, Freund B, Schwartz M, et al. Systematic review of the treatment and prognosis of the odontogenic keratocyst. Oral Surg Oral Med Oral Pathol Oral Radiol Endod 2000;90:553–8.

Chapter 48

Advanced maxillofacial reconstruction techniques

Mark M. Smith

DEFINITION

Axial-pattern flap: a pedicle flap of skin and subcutaneous tissue that incorporates a direct cutaneous artery and vein into its base.

THERAPEUTIC DECISION-MAKING

Animals with no radiographic signs of distant metastasis should be considered for aggressive therapy. The concept of complete local excision of all visible tumor followed by, or concurrent with, chemotherapy or radiation therapy for treatment of presumed micrometastasis has achieved marked acceptance in human oncologic therapy and is being applied in veterinary medicine.[1–4] Surgery is integral to this multimodality treatment plan, especially for large, aggressive neoplasms.[5–8] Resective surgery plus radiation and/or chemotherapy are usually well tolerated by dogs and cats, leaving conservative management for debilitated and geriatric patients.[9]

The goal of surgery for oral neoplasms in small animals is generally curative resection or palliation.[10] The ideal surgical procedure is one that offers the greatest possibility of cure, restores or maintains function, and has an acceptable cosmetic result. Extended dissection from the primary site may improve the incidence of free margins related to surgical resection of direct metastatic pathways, especially for neoplasms of the floor of the mouth. The cranial cervical area may be approached in conjunction with reconstructive surgery. Direct observation of regional lymph nodes allows assessment of gross transcapsular spread of the tumor, which may warrant wider margins for adhered lymph nodes.[11,12]

Cutaneous maxillofacial defects can also result from trauma, complications of radiation therapy or failure of another reconstructive surgical technique.[13,14] Second-intention wound management of such cutaneous defects is usually not possible based on the inherent mobility of functional areas of the head and an unacceptable cosmetic appearance of the wound during the management period. Further, the result of second-intention healing may contribute to impaired function of the eyelids, nares or mouth.[15] Surgical techniques have been developed for cutaneous maxillofacial reconstruction which obviate the need to utilize second-intention healing. These surgical treatment methods include subdermal plexus flaps or random-pattern flaps, the labial advancement flap, and the buccal rotation technique (see Chs 26 and 44).[16,17]

Axial-pattern flaps have been developed in dogs and cats to augment the treatment options for wounds with large skin defects.[16] Axial-pattern flaps have enhanced perfusion compared with subdermal plexus flaps because the former incorporates a direct cutaneous artery and vein at the flap base.[16] This enhanced vascular supply allows formation and transfer of a relatively large area of skin in a single-staged procedure to aid cutaneous reconstruction.[17] Identification and development of an axial-pattern flap for cutaneous maxillofacial reconstruction is of particular importance based on the aforementioned limitations of second-intention healing in this region.

The superficial temporal artery (STA) and caudal auricular artery (CAA) axial-pattern flaps provide tissue with direct cutaneous blood supply for maxillofacial reconstruction.

SURGICAL ANATOMY AND SURGICAL TECHNIQUES

Caudal auricular axial-pattern flap

Anatomical studies have shown that branches of the CAA provide blood supply to the cranial aspect of the cervical skin in dogs and cats.[18,19] The sternocleoidomastoid branches supply skin, platysma and subcutaneous fat, and eventually anastomose with the superficial cervical artery. These vessels emerge from deeper tissues in the area between the lateral aspect of the wing of the atlas and the vertical ear canal.[20]

Guidelines for flap location were based on these studies (Fig. 48.1). A palpable depression between the lateral aspect of the wing of the atlas and the vertical ear canal is the cranial border of the flap. The flap base is centered over the lateral aspect of the wing of the atlas. The flap is positioned in the center of the neck within ventral and dorsal lines paralleling the measured flap base width and the same width of measurement centered on the spine of the

© 2012 Elsevier Ltd
DOI: 10.1016/B978-0-7020-4618-6.00048-8

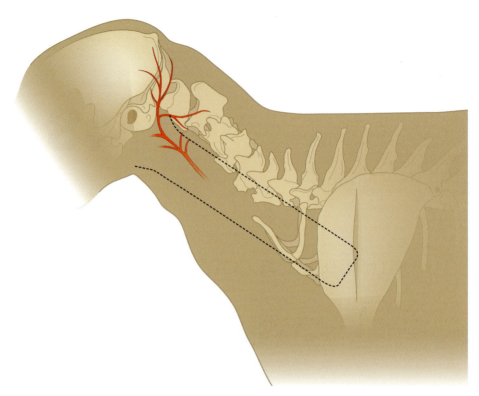

Fig. 48.1 Illustration showing location of the caudal auricular axial-pattern flap (*broken lines*) and the sternocleoidomastoid branch of the caudal auricular artery in relation to the wing of the atlas and the scapula.

scapula. Flap dimensions are based on the feasibility of primary wound closure of the donor site and required length to transfer the distal flap to the facial area. Flap length may vary and does not necessarily extend to the spine of the scapula. The surgical plane of dissection is between the cervical neck fascia and the subcutaneous fat since direct cutaneous arteries are located in the subcutaneous tissues.

Superficial temporal axial-pattern flap

Branches of the STA provide blood supply to the skin and frontal muscle in the temporal region in dogs and cats.[21–23] The STA originates at the base of the zygomatic arch in a subcutaneous position, and extends rostrally along the zygomatic arch with small branches extending to the skin of the temporal region and the frontalis muscle.

The landmarks for the base of the STA flap are the caudal aspect of the zygomatic arch caudally and the lateral orbital rim rostrally (Fig. 48.2). Flap width is limited by the eye rostrally and the ear caudally, and is therefore equivalent to the length of the zygomatic arch. The skin is incised and the thin frontal muscle identified superficial to the fascia of the temporal muscle. The flap is carefully elevated, deep to the frontal muscle, toward the flap base. A small superficial branch of the rostral auricular nerve plexus may be present at the cranial border of the flap over the ipsilateral eye adjacent to the flap base. Incision of this branch and the surrounding subcutaneous tissue enhances flap rotation. Flap length may vary and does not necessarily extend to the contralateral zygomatic arch. In fact, flap length approximating 75% of the distance from one zygomatic arch to the other is associated with reliable complete flap survival.

Transection of the small superficial branch of the rostral auricular nerve plexus does not result in functional deficits of the eyelids.

Wound dehiscence occurs at areas of flap necrosis. Redundant tissue over the eye due to rotation of flap tissue centrally, and mild tension over the contralateral eye may occur secondary to primary closure of the donor site. However, in clinical cases, there were no associated clinical problems related to these transient abnormalities.

Application and surgical closure

The CAA and STA axial-pattern flaps have been developed and transferred immediately to allow extensive reconstruction as a component of definitive surgery. This characteristic is particularly useful in facial reconstruction following radical resection or extensive trauma, because the transferred flap provides full-thickness skin that is durable in an area of movement (Figs 48.3 and 48.4).

Flaps should be handled with care, and the base of the flap including the vascular pedicle should not be dissected or excessively manipulated, in order to avoid potential direct or indirect (vasospasm) vascular trauma that might negatively impact flap viability. Peripheral continuous or simple interrupted sutures are used to appose skin. Subcutaneous or tacking sutures to decrease dead space are not recommended since they may occlude direct cutaneous vascular supply. Passive or active drainage systems may be used to prevent seroma formation. They should be placed beneath the flap, exiting through a separate site caudoventral to the flap base, in a position not expected to influence circulation to the flap. A Stent bandage may be used to cover the drain exit site.

The donor site is closed in two layers including a subcutaneous–subcuticular pattern with tacking 'bites' in the muscular fascia aimed at decreasing dead space. Any wound tension associated with donor site closure should be directed away from the flap, especially the flap base where the direct cutaneous vasculature is located.

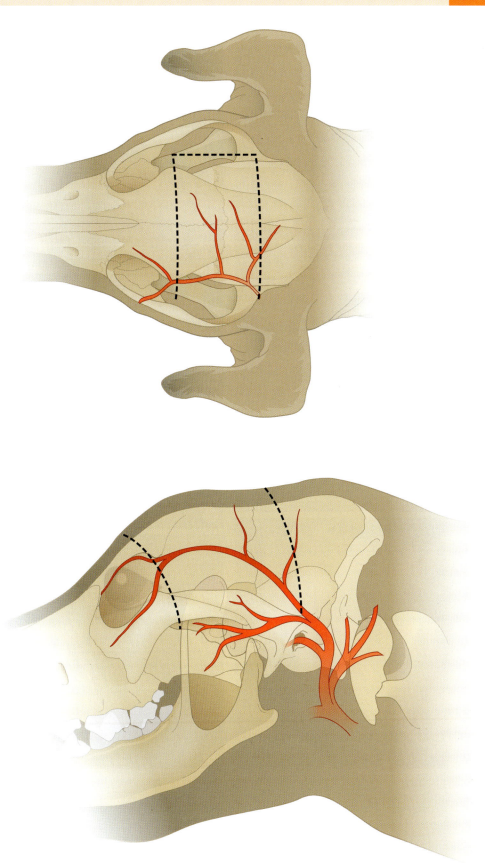

Fig. 48.2 Illustration showing the location of the superficial temporal axial pattern flap (*broken lines*) and the cutaneous branch of the superficial temporal artery in relation to the zygomatic arch and orbital rim.

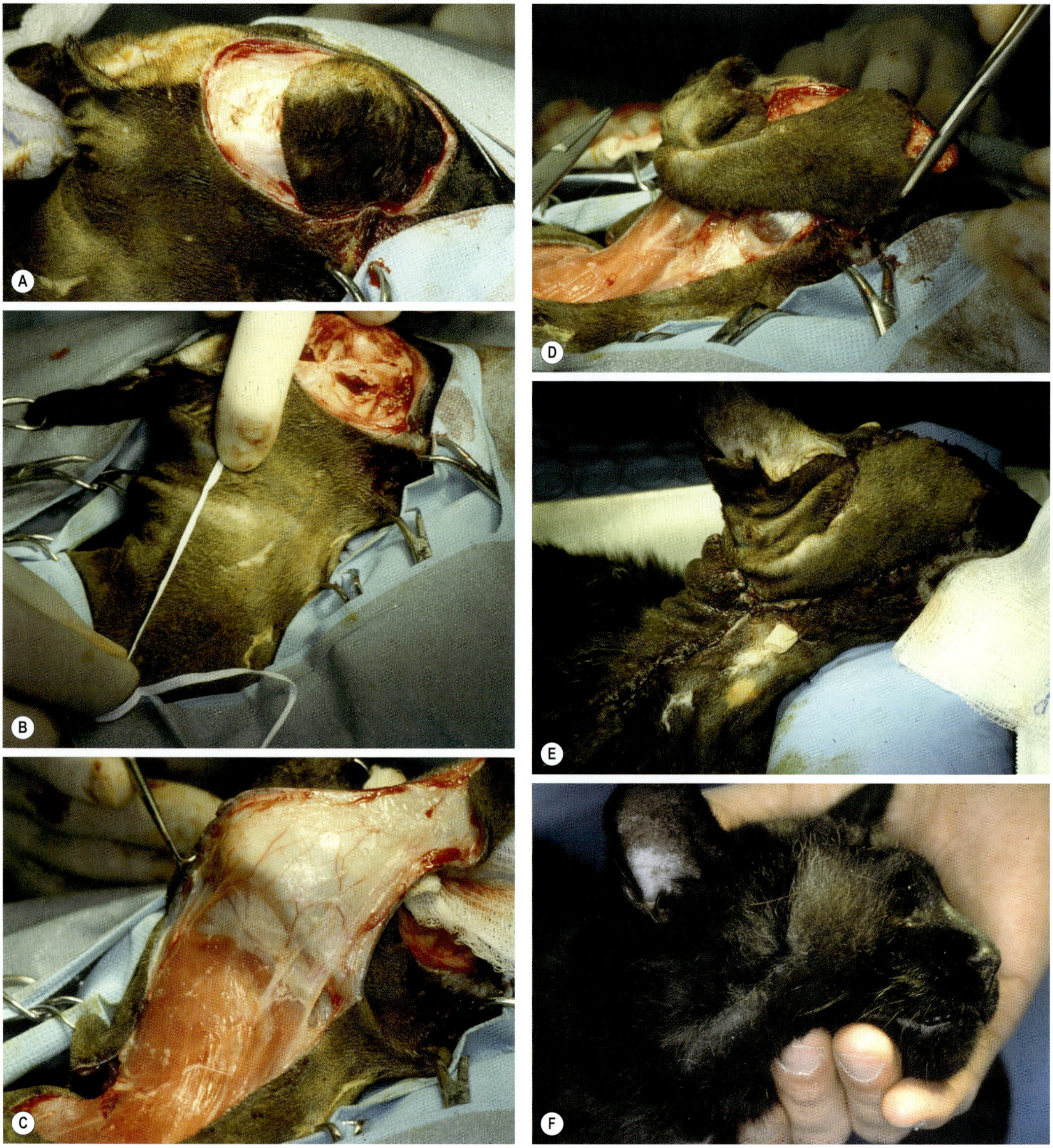

Fig. 48.3 En bloc resection and partial orbitectomy for fibrosarcoma in a 12-year-old cat: (**A**) Wide surgical margins are included with the lesion. (**B**) The length of the caudal auricular axial-pattern flap (CAA) is measured using umbilical tape. (**C**) The flap is elevated, revealing the direct cutaneous vascular supply. (**D**, **E**) A bridge incision communicates the donor and recipient sites followed by CAA apposition and donor site wound closure. (**F**) The 6-week postoperative examination indicates complete flap survival with cosmesis similar to enucleation.

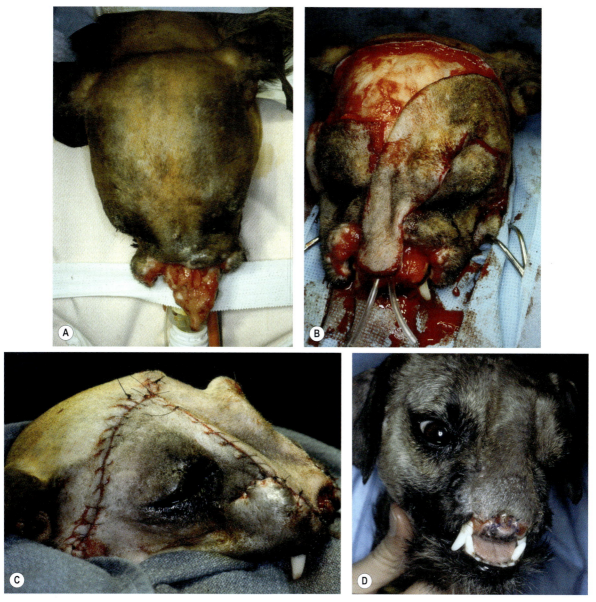

Fig. 48.4 (**A**) Preoperative photograph showing the dorsal view of a 1-year-old Border terrier following maxillofacial trauma. (**B**) The superficial temporal axial pattern flap (STA) is elevated. (**C**) The flap is sutured to the defect providing full-thickness skin to cover the wound. (**D**) Follow-up photograph.

Other techniques

Rectus abdominis myoperitoneal flap

The rectus abdominis myoperitoneal flap has been used for oral reconstruction in the dog.[24] Muscle flaps promote rapid revascularization of the wound. Wounds are resistant to infection, based on the muscle flap's ability to effectively deliver antimicrobials, antibodies, and cellular components of the immune system. Disadvantages of using muscle flaps in the oral cavity include contraction, an inability to lubricate, and delayed reepithelialization by the oral squamous lining leading to scarring and restricted motion. Self-mutilation of the flap is also possible, necessitating the recommendation of interdental bonding during the healing period.[24] The rectus abdominis myoperitoneal flap is an alternative for oral reconstruction and requires microvascular methods for application.

Skin grafts

Full- or partial-thickness skin grafts have application for cutaneous defects of the maxillofacial area. Skin grafts are difficult to manage in this location because of the mobility of the area and the requirement for a bandage to promote graft stability and revascularization.[25] A tie-down bandage or closed-suction bandage may facilitate wound stability, leading to a successful outcome (Fig. 48.5).

Angularis oris axial-pattern flap

The angularis oris axial-pattern flap has recently been described in dogs for repair of defects in the hard and soft palate to the distal margin of the canine tooth. The flap includes a surface of buccal mucosa, is well vascularized, and has been shown to be quite robust and highly mobile.[26]

491

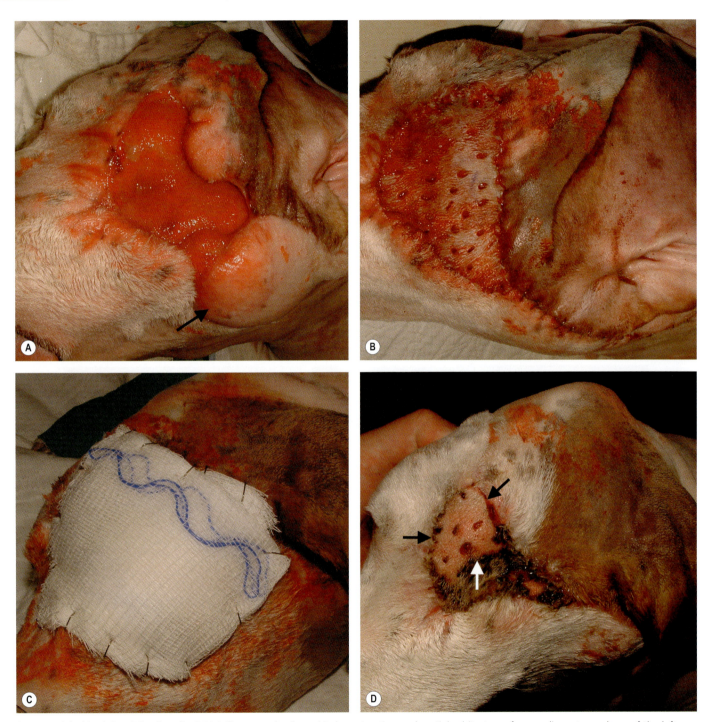

Fig. 48.5 (**A**) Skin defect following distal CAA flap necrosis after orbital exenteration and partial orbitectomy for a malignant neoplasm of the left ocular region. Note the area of granulation tissue and the distal aspect of the remaining CAA flap (*arrow*). (**B**) A free skin graft was applied to the area. (**C**) A Stent bandage was applied. (**D**) Approximately 60–70% of the skin graft was viable (*arrows*) 14 days following surgery. (*Photographs courtesy of Dr. M. King.*)

Bone reconstruction

The surgical goal of maintaining function may be achieved without bone reconstruction. Bone reconstruction is usually a low priority when considering methodology for reconstruction following resection of parts of the mandible or maxilla. This surgical philosophy is influenced by a number of factors. A good to excellent clinical result may be obtained using only soft tissue reconstructive techniques (see Chs 45 and 46).[27] Patients undergoing extensive maxillectomies have a propensity to eat and drink normally following appropriate healing, which maintains the remaining oral and nasal cavities without oronasal communication. Bone reconstruction may improve cosmesis; however, corticocancellous autografts or allografts require rigid fixation and a prolonged revascularization phase. Grafts of this type would be prone to infection and sequestrum formation, based on their placement in a contaminated environment.[28] Successful application of bone grafts would serve a functional purpose if used as a platform for the installation and incorporation of dental implants. A free vascularized tibial bone graft has been used in a mandibular body defect in an experimental canine model. This graft, which required microvascular technique, went on to bony union more readily than a cortical tibial autograft.[29]

Although reconstruction may be achieved in humans using distraction osteogenesis and dental implants,[30] the cost of these procedures may prohibit their use in veterinary medicine.

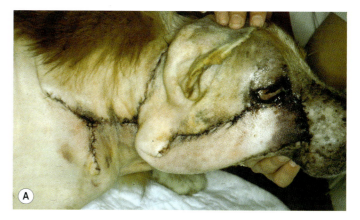

POSTOPERATIVE CARE AND ASSESSMENT

Immediate postoperative care

Skin cleansing of wound drainage and dressing changes are performed daily. Drains are removed by 48 hours postoperatively, or when there is minimal drainage. An Elizabethan collar may be indicated to prevent self-mutilation.

Assessment – viability of axial-pattern flaps

The most detrimental complication associated with the use of axial-pattern flaps for wound reconstruction is devitalization of the flap apex, or end. Because of the nature of axial-pattern flap utilization, partial-flap necrosis occurs at an area where the flap is most important. This is particularly problematic in oral and maxillofacial reconstruction where second-intention healing following flap necrosis and wound dehiscence is not a viable management option.

Clinical signs of flap necrosis include a demarcated discolored (black/purple) area, palpably decreased temperature of the discolored area, decreased hair growth in the devitalized area, and wound dehiscence with drainage of a serosanguineous or purulent fluid if there is concurrent infection. The clinician should be deliberate when deciding when to revise the flap. Early intervention may result in even more tension applied to the flap and continued flap necrosis. It is advisable to wait 4–7 days until flap viability is ascertained and the risk of further devitalization is minimal. Another advantage of

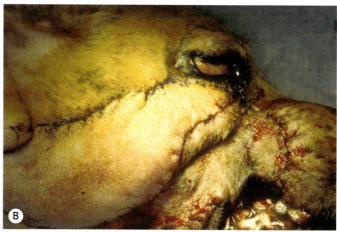

Fig. 48.6 (**A**) Postoperative photograph showing skin discoloration demarcating viable and nonviable skin in a caudal auricular axial-pattern flap (CAA) used for maxillofacial reconstruction of a traumatic facial defect. (**B**) The CAA flap revision is performed by elevation and resection of the devitalized area followed by primary wound closure.

deliberate management is the improved blood flow to the base of the flap at the time when flap revision is performed (Fig. 48.6). Generally, the revision of a devitalized flap is successful, taking advantage of the increased blood flow and redundant skin present at the base of the flap.

REFERENCES

1. Owen LN. TNM classification of tumours in domestic animals. Geneva: World Health Organization; 1980.
2. Forastiere AA. Management of advanced stage squamous cell carcinoma of the head and neck. Am J Med Sci 1986;291:405–15.
3. Lo TC, Salzman FA, Swartz MR. Radiotherapy for cancer of the head and neck. Otolaryngol Clin North Am 1985;18:521–31.
4. Hammer AS, Couto CG. Adjuvant chemotherapy for sarcomas and carcinomas. Vet Clin North Am Small Anim Pract 1990;20:1015–36.
5. Page RL, Thrall DE. Clinical indications and applications of radiotherapy and hyperthermia in veterinary oncology. Vet Clin North Am Small Anim Pract 1990;20:1075–92.
6. Bradney IW, Hobson HP, Stromberg PC. Rostral mandibulectomy combined with intermandibular bone graft in treatment of oral neoplasia. J Am Anim Hosp Assoc 1987;23:611–15.
7. Salisbury SK, Lantz GC. Long-term results of partial mandibulectomy for treatment of oral tumors in 30 dogs. J Am Anim Hosp Assoc 1988;24:285–94.
8. White RAS. Mandibulectomy and maxillectomy in the dog: long term survival in 100 cases. J Small Anim Pract 1991;32:69–74.
9. Fox LE, Geoghegan SL, Davis LH, et al. Owner satisfaction with partial mandibulectomy or maxillectomy for treatment of oral tumors in 27 dogs. J Am Anim Hosp Assoc 1997;33:25–31.
10. White RAS: Mandibulectomy and maxillectomy in the dog: results of 75 cases. Vet Surg 1987;16:105.
11. Close LG, Brown PM, Vuitch MF, et al. Microvascular invasion and survival in cancer of the oral cavity and oropharynx. Arch Otolaryngol Head Neck Surg 1989;115:1304–9.

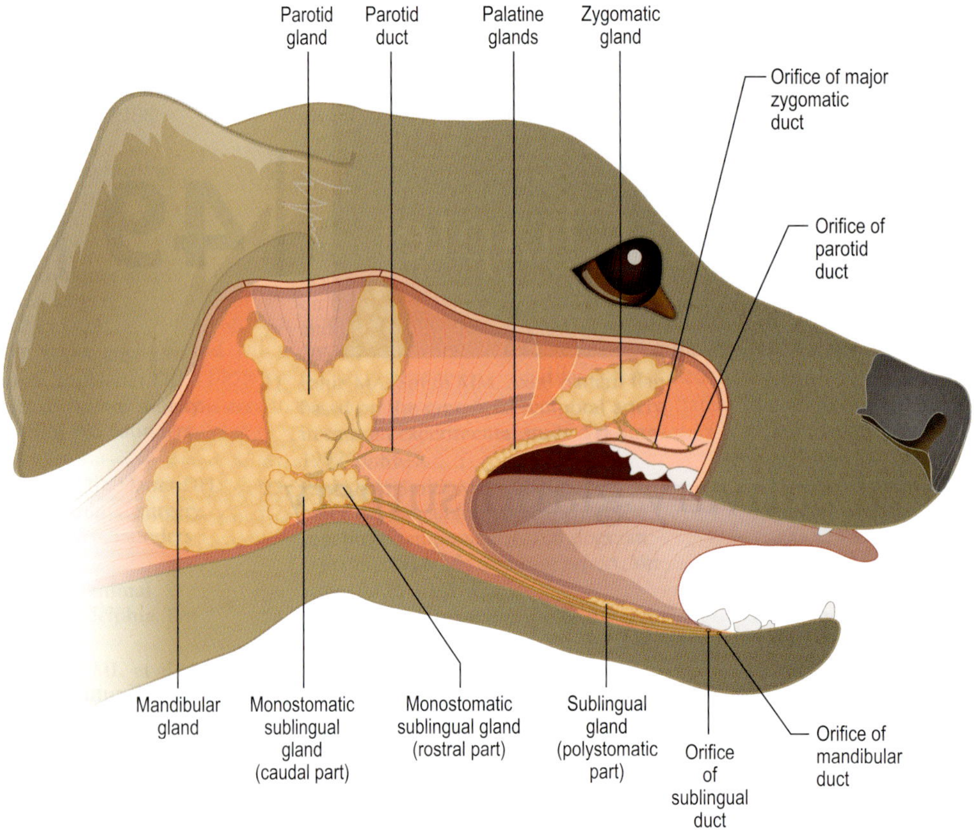

Fig. 49.1 Topographical anatomy of the major salivary glands in the dog.

under the mucosa of the mouth. These lobules empty into the main sublingual duct through four to six smaller ducts. The main sublingual duct runs with the mandibular duct between the styloglossus muscle medially and the mylohyoid muscle laterally in a rostromedial direction towards a small sublingual caruncle, lateral to the frenulum. The ducts have one common or separate openings (in which case the mandibular opening is the most rostral one). The polystomatic sublingual gland consists of 6–12 separate lobules that empty directly into the oral cavity instead of emptying into the sublingual duct. The lobules lie submucosally on both sides of the body of the tongue, rostral to the lingual branch of the mandibular nerve. Blood supply of the monostomatic sublingual gland is from the glandular branch of the facial artery. The sublingual artery (a branch of the lingual artery) supplies the polystomatic sublingual gland.

Molar glands in the cat

The buccal molar gland in the cat is located between the orbicularis oris muscle and the mucous membrane of the lower lip at the angle of the mouth.[4] It empties into the buccal cavity through several small ducts. The lingual molar gland lies in the membranous molar pad just lingual to the mandibular first molar tooth. The gland has multiple small openings into the oral cavity.[5]

Other salivary glands

A small buccal lymph node is found in just under 10% of dogs and is located dorsal to the zygomatic muscle and rostral to the masseter muscle in the region where the superior labial vein drains into the facial vein.[6] Other salivary glands are located in the submucosa and muscles of the tongue (lingual glands), the submucosa of the buccal cavity (minor buccal glands), the submucosa of the lips (labial glands) and the submucosa of the ventral side of the soft palate (palatine glands).[7]

EXAMINATION TECHNIQUES

Diagnostic imaging

Plain radiographs may be diagnostic if a radiopaque foreign body or a salivary calculus is present.[8] Contrast radiography (sialography) is performed under general anesthesia and may be helpful to locate salivary duct tears causing mucocele, to determine which glands should be removed surgically.[9] An iodine-based water-soluble dye (Télébrix 350, Laboratoire Guerbet, France) in a dosage of 1 mL/kg body weight is injected after cannulation of the duct with a 25- or 26-gauge catheter. For cannulation of the parotid duct, the mucosa caudal to the parotid papilla is grasped and pulled rostromedially to straighten the distal portion of the duct. The sublingual duct can only be cannulated when a separate opening is present just caudal to the larger opening of the mandibular duct on the sublingual caruncle.

Computed tomography (CT) and magnetic resonance imaging (MRI) may be useful in the investigation of the extent of salivary gland tumors to determine the feasibility of surgical resection (Fig. 49.2A). Ultrasound is helpful in the differentiation of cystic lesions from inflammation or tumors, and as guidance during biopsy procedures.

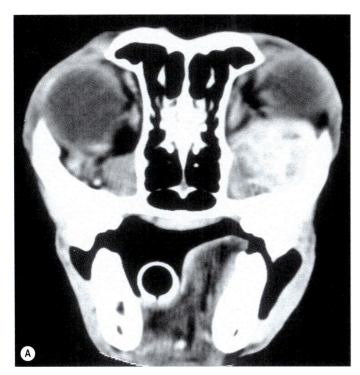

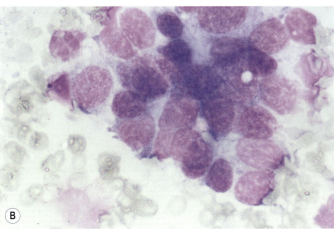

Fig. 49.2 (**A**) CT image of an adenocarcinoma of the zygomatic salivary gland with craniolateral displacement of the eye in an 11-year-old dog. *(Courtesy of Dr. S.A.E.B. Boroffka, Utrecht University.)* (**B**) Fine needle aspirate demonstrating the neoplastic cells (May-Grünwald-Giemsa stain; 1000×). *(Courtesy of Dr. E. Teske, Utrecht University.)*

Salivary gland biopsy

Diseased salivary glands can be biopsied to determine the presence or absence of saliva, inflammation or neoplastic cells (Fig. 49.2B). Indications for obtaining a biopsy include enlarged, painful or cystic salivary glands.[10-13] Fine needle aspiration (FNA) biopsies are minimally invasive and generally do not require local or general anesthesia. Ultrasound may be helpful to obtain a representative sample of the abnormality. Saliva or cell types of the FNA biopsy can be identified by cytologic examination. Histologic characteristics and invasive growth can only be examined in larger tissue samples obtained by Tru-Cut, punch or surgical (incisional) biopsy (Tru-Cut biopsy needle, Travenol Laboratories, Inc., Deerfield, IL; Baker Cummons punch biopsy, Key Pharmaceuticals, Inc., Miami, FL). Local or general

anesthesia is required. With a Tru-Cut biopsy, a piece of tissue 1–2 mm in width and 10–15 mm long is obtained with a 14–18-gauge needle. A closed or open (after incision of the skin) method is used. Punch biopsies will provide a composite of normal and abnormal tissue but are limited in depth. Incisional biopsies are used when less-invasive techniques are not diagnostic. After incising the skin, the gland is localized. The capsule, if present, is incised. Unless there is an obvious lesion visible, a lobule of salivary gland tissue is isolated and its duct ligated prior to excision. The surrounding salivary tissue should be handled atraumatically to prevent extravasation of saliva. Care should be taken in removing the biopsy tract during curative resection of malignancies.

SURGICAL DISEASES OF THE SALIVARY GLANDS

Salivary gland and duct injury

Most injuries of the salivary glands and ducts are caused by sharp or blunt trauma to the head or by surgery, and may eventually result in salivary mucocele (see Ch. 50) or salivary fistula. Bite wounds or trauma that is caused by stick penetration injury may result in infected mucoceles that are difficult to differentiate from ordinary abscesses. Injuries resulting in stenosis or blockage of a salivary duct will not cause visible long-term complications.[14]

Microsurgical reconstruction of a lacerated duct may be performed with or without stenting. In an experimental study on salivary duct surgery in the dog it was concluded that a massive scarring process postoperatively interferes with uncomplicated healing. Long-term stenting (14 days or more) was found to increase the success rate of salivary duct surgery.[15]

Salivary fistula

Salivary fistula of the parotid gland may be caused by severing of the parotid duct. The saliva accumulates in the subcutaneous tissues, forming a mucocele, or it finds a new way out through a nonphysiologic opening in the skin, resulting in a permanent fistula.[14] If primary anastomosis or oral reimplantation of the duct is not feasible, ligation of the parotid duct 'upstream' is the most easy way to solve the problem.[14,15] The rupture can be localized by sialography.[9] The 'upstream' part of the duct is cannulated with a 00 tear-duct cannula (Shepard tear duct cannula, Eickemeyer, Hamburg, Germany) or a monofilament nylon suture. The duct is exposed through a lateral skin incision between the buccal nerves on the masseter muscle. The duct is undermined, the cannula or suture is withdrawn and the duct is double-ligated with monofilament nonresorbable suture material.[14]

Sialoliths

Sialoliths are calcifications found in salivary glands or ducts (Fig. 49.3).[8,12,16-18] In the dog, they typically occur in the parotid duct and are occasionally caused by an ascending foreign body.[19] Sialoliths may also form within the walls of longstanding mucoceles and in inactive salivary glands.[18,19] Obstruction of a duct may cause a painful swelling of the gland and eventual rupture of the duct.[8] Sialoliths do not cause salivary mucoceles. The diagnosis can be made by plain radiographs or sialography. A sialolith within a duct is removed by incising the duct over the stone through the oral mucosa. By flushing the duct, small remnants of the obstruction are removed. The incision is not sutured.[20]

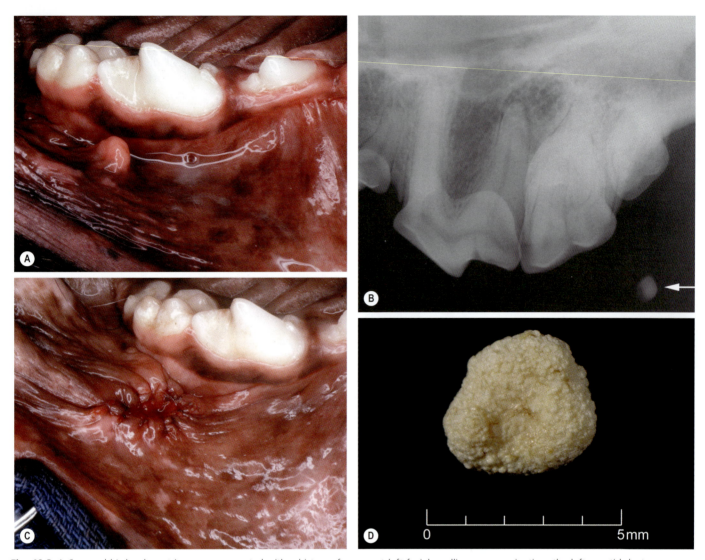

Fig. 49.3 A 6-year-old Labrador retriever was presented with a history of recurrent left facial swelling; on examination, the left parotid duct was palpably enlarged. (**A**) A hyperplastic left parotid papilla, caused by a sialolith lodged at the papilla. (The dog is in dorsal recumbency.) (**B**) Radiograph showing the sialolith (*arrow*). (**C**) Following excision of the hyperplastic papilla and removal of the sialolith, a sialodochostomy was performed. (**D**) Sialolith following removal. *(Courtesy of Dr. F.J.M. Verstraete, University of California, Davis.)*

Salivary gland neoplasia

Salivary gland tumors are rare in the dog and cat, with a reported incidence of 0.17%.[10] Adenocarcinomas of the larger salivary glands as well as carcinomas originating from the salivary tissues in the superficial submucosa of the oral cavity have been described.[11,12,21] Occasionally, malignant tumors of nonsalivary tissue origin occur within the salivary glands.[22,23] The presenting complaint in most cases is a mass being noted by the client, sometimes with halitosis and dysphagia. Tumors of the zygomatic gland may result in exophthalmos.[13] Metastases of malignant salivary neoplasia to lymph nodes, lung, liver, pancreas, heart, adrenal glands, diaphragm, body wall and bone have been reported.[10,21,24-26] Benign tumors of the salivary glands are very rare in dogs and cats; lipomas and adenomas have been reported.[10,27] The prognosis of malignant salivary neoplasia, in general, is poor, but with early diagnosis and aggressive treatment of the disease with radical surgery and radiation, survival times of over 1 year are achievable in some patients.[13,28] Surgical excision of a salivary gland malignancy should always include the biopsy of the draining lymph nodes (parotid, mandibular and retropharyngeal lymph nodes).

Surgical excision of the mandibular gland

Surgical excision of the mandibular gland is performed through a skin incision caudal to the mandible, avoiding the maxillary and linguofacial veins (see Ch. 50). After incising the platysma muscle, the fibrous tissue of the mandibular gland capsule is identified. Unlike during excision of this gland for the treatment of mucocele, the capsule preferably is not opened if the gland contains malignant neoplasia. Dissection is continued in a rostral direction, where a ligature is placed on normal sublingual gland tissue before removing the neoplastic mandibular gland.

Surgical excision of the parotid gland

Surgical excision of a parotid gland with malignant neoplasia is a surgical challenge because of the diffuse nature of the gland and the presence of the facial nerve. The parotidoauricularis muscle is separated from its vertical ear canal attachment and retracted. The caudal auricular vein is ligated and divided. The parotid gland is dissected beginning at its dorsocaudal angle. Small vessels are ligated or electrocoagulated. Ventrally, the parotid gland is separated from the mandibular salivary gland and the vertical ear canal. The facial nerve, located at the beginning of the horizontal ear canal, is avoided during dissection.

Surgical excision of the zygomatic gland

Surgical excision of the zygomatic gland can be performed using a lateral or a dorsal approach.[29-31] The lateral approach is more commonly used. For the lateral approach the skin over the dorsal rim of the zygomatic arch is incised. The palpebral fascia, retractor anguli oculi lateralis muscle, and orbital ligament are incised at the periosteum and reflected dorsally. The dorsal rim of the zygomatic arch is removed with bone rongeurs. The zygomatic gland can be removed by gentle blunt dissection. The zygomatic branch of the buccal artery is ligated.

The dorsal approach is performed through a skin incision over the frontal bone margin of the periorbita. After incising the palpebral fascia at its bone attachment, the orbital ligament can be divided if additional exposure is needed. The tissues are reflected ventrally and the affected gland and periorbital fat are removed by gentle blunt dissection. The lateral superior palpebral artery can be ligated. Temporary dysfunction of the upper eyelid after surgery can be managed with artificial tears.

Salivary gland necrosis

Salivary gland necrosis in dogs causes severe pain on swallowing and palpation, nausea, vomiting and anorexia. The disease, which mainly affects the mandibular salivary gland, has been described under several different names, namely sialadenitis, salivary gland infarction, salivary gland necrosis and necrotizing sialometaplasia.[32-36] Ischemic necrosis of the glandular tissues, inflammation, and regenerative hyperplasia of the ductal epithelium are described in most cases. Different etiologic agents have been proposed as the cause of this disease: viral infections, fungi, cervical trauma, limbic epilepsy and lesions of the esophagus.[12,32-34,37,38] Surgical excision of the affected salivary glands alone does not resolve the clinical signs in most cases.[34,35] Some patients responded well to adjuvant therapy with anticonvulsants.[32,34,36,39] In dogs that were treated successfully for esophageal lesions caused by *Spirocerca lupi*, the salivary signs disappeared.[38]

COMPLICATIONS

Postoperative complications after surgery of the salivary glands or ducts may include dysfunction caused by laceration of nerves, mucocele, seroma and infection. Mucoceles are treated by the complete resection of the affected gland or by marsupialization (see Ch. 50). Persistent seromas may require drainage. Infection is treated with drainage and antibiotics. Complications are prevented if close attention is paid to the anatomy and aseptic technique. The use of a surgical magnifying loupe is recommended.

REFERENCES

1. Evans HE. Miller's anatomy of the dog. 3rd ed. Philadelphia, PA: WB Saunders; 1993. p. 415–19.
2. Carlson GW. The salivary glands. Embryology, anatomy, and surgical applications. Surg Clin North Am 2000; 80:261–73.
3. Evans HE. Miller's anatomy of the dog. 3rd ed. Philadelphia, PA: WB Saunders; 1993. p. 724.
4. Done, SH, Goody PC, Evans SA, et al. The cat. In: Done, SH, Goody PC, Evans SA, et al, editors. Color atlas of veterinary anatomy, vol. 3. London: Mosby; 2001. 10.4.
5. Okuda A, Inouc E, Asari M. The membranous bulge lingual to the mandibular molar tooth of a cat contains a small salivary gland. J Vet Dent 1996; 13:61–4.
6. Casteleyn CR, van der Steen M, Declercq J, et al. The buccal lymph node (lymphonodus buccalis) in dogs: Occurrence, anatomical location, histological characteristics and clinical implications. Vet J 2008;175:379–83.
7. Banks WJ. Applied veterinary histology. 2nd ed. Baltimore, MD: Williams & Wilkins, 1986.

8. Jeffreys DA, Stasiw A, Dennis R. Parotid sialolithiasis in a dog. J Small Anim Pract 1996;37:296–7.
9. Harvey CE. Sialography in the dog. J Am Vet Rad Soc 1969;10:18–27.
10. Carberry CA, Flanders JA, Harvey HJ, et al. Salivary gland tumors in dogs and cats: a literature and case review. J Am Anim Hosp Assoc 1988;24:561–7.
11. Carpenter JL, Bernstein M. Malignant mixed (pleomorphic) mandibular salivary gland tumors in a cat. J Am Anim Hosp Assoc 1991;27:581–3.
12. Spangler WL, Culbertson MR. Salivary gland disease in dogs and cats: 245 cases (1985–1988). J Am Vet Med Assoc 1991; 198:465–9.
13. Hammer A, Getzy D, Ogilvie G et al. Salivary gland neoplasia in the dog and cat: survival times and prognostic factors. J Am Anim Hosp Assoc 2001;37: 478–82.
14. Harvey CE: Parotid salivary duct rupture and fistula in the dog and cat. J Small Anim Pract 1977;18:163–8.
15. Dumpis, J, Feldmane L. Experimental microsurgery of salivary ducts in dogs. J Craniomaxillofac Surg 2001;29: 56–62.

16. Mulkey OC, Knecht CD. Parotid salivary gland cyst and calculus in a dog. J Am Vet Med Assoc 1971;159: 1774.
17. Chastain CB. What is your diagnosis? J Am Vet Med Assoc 1974;164:415.
18. Teunissen GHB, Teunissen-Strik AL. Speichelzyste mit Calculi-ahnlichen Knotchen in der Zystenwand und der mandibularen Speicheldruse [Ptyalocele with calculi-like granules in the cyst wall and the mandibular salivary gland]. Kleintierpraxis 1986;31:343–4, 346.
19. Triantafyllou A, Harrison JD, Garrett JR, et al. Increase of microliths in inactive salivary glands of cat. Arch Oral Biol 1992;37:663–6.
20. Harvey CE. Oral cavity. The tongue, lips cheeks, pharynx, and salivary glands. In: Slatter DH, editor. Textbook of small animal surgery. 2nd ed. Philadelphia, PA: WB Saunders; 1993. p. 510–20.
21. Karbe E, Schiefer B. Primary salivary gland tumors in carnivores. Can Vet J 1967;8: 212–15.
22. Carberry CA, Flanders JA, Anderson WI, et al. Mast cell tumor in the mandibular salivary gland in a dog. Cornell Vet 1987; 77:362–6.

23. Thomsen BV, Myers RK. Extraskeletal osteosarcoma of the mandibulary salivary gland in a dog. Vet Pathol 1999;36:71–3.

24. Koestner A, Buerger I. Primary neoplasms of the salivary glands in animals compared to similar tumors in man. Pathol Vet 1965;2:201–26.

25. Liu SK, Harvey HJ. Metastatic bone neoplasms in the dog. In: Bojrab MJ, editor. Pathophysiology in small animal surgery. Philadelphia, PA: WB Saunders; 1981. p. 712–15.

26. Bright JM, Bright RM, Mays MC. Parotid carcinoma with multiple endocrinopathies in a dog. Compend Cont Educ Pract Vet 1983;5:728–34.

27. Brown PJ, Lucke VM, Sozmen M, et al. Lipomatous infiltration of the canine salivary gland. J Small Anim Pract 1997; 38:234–6.

28. Evans SM, Thrall DE. Postoperative orthovoltage radiation therapy of parotid salivary gland adenocarcinoma in three dogs. J Am Vet Med Assoc 1983;182: 993–4.

29. Knecht CD. Treatment of diseases of the zygomatic salivary gland. J Am Anim Hosp Assoc 1970;6:13–19.

30. Smith MM. Surgery of the canine salivary system. Compend Cont Educ Pract Vet 1985;7:457–64.

31. Brown NO. Salivary gland diseases. Diagnosis, treatment, and associated problems. Probl Vet Med 1989;1: 281–94.

32. Kelly DF, Lucke VW, Denny HR, et al. Histology of salivary gland infarction in the dog. Vet Pathol 1979;16:438–3.

33. Harvey CE. Oral, dental, pharyngeal, and salivary gland disorders. In: Ettinger SJ, Feldman EC, editors. Textbook of veterinary internal medicine. 3rd ed. Philadelphia, PA: WB Saunders; 1989. p. 1203–54.

34. Mawby DI, Bauer MS, Loyd-Bauer PM, et al. Vasculitis and necrosis of the mandibular salivary glands and chronic vomiting in a dog. Can Vet J 1991;32:562–4.

35. Cooke MM, Guilford WG. Salivary gland necrosis in a wire-haired fox terrier. N Z Vet J 1992;40:69–72.

36. Brooks DG, Hottinger HA, Dunstan RW. Canine necrotizing sialometaplasia: a case report and review of the literature. J Am Anim Hosp Assoc 1995;31:21–5.

37. Kelly DF, Lucke VM, Lane JG, et al. Salivary gland necrosis in dogs. Vet Rec 1979;104:268.

38. Schroeder H, Berry WL. Salivary gland necrosis in dogs: a retrospective study of 19 cases. J Small Anim Pract 1998;39:121–5.

39. Chapman BL, Malik R. Phenobarbitone-responsive hypersialism in two dogs. J Small Anim Pract 1992;33:549–52.

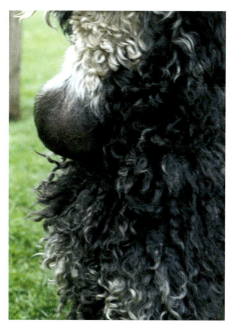

Fig. 50.4 Longstanding cervical sialocele with hair loss and thinning of overlying skin in an Old English sheepdog.

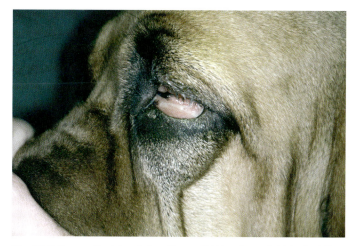

Fig. 50.5 Zygomatic sialocele in a 6-year-old bloodhound. Note that the eye is displaced dorsally by the lesion that has expanded in the floor of the orbit.

overlying skin (Fig. 50.4). Nevertheless, spontaneous ulceration of the skin or rupture of the sialocele wall is highly improbable. It is also unusual for overt trauma (such as an oropharyngeal injury due to stick penetration) to rupture the sublingual or mandibular duct and to provoke the formation of a sialocele, although one published case series included five dogs with a reliable history of pharyngeal stick penetration in the period immediately preceding development of a sialocele.[8] The distension of a ranula may produce an obvious deviation of the tongue, and the patient may find it difficult to close the mouth because the teeth tend to occlude onto the sialocele. A common feature of sialoceles arising in the pharyngeal position is that they provoke dyspnea, as the expanding lesions tend to obstruct the airway.[9] This was the case in all eight dogs presented with a sialocele in this location in the author's series.[8] On superficial inspection, lesions at this site might resemble a tonsillar mass.

Less frequently, sialoceles arise through leakage of saliva from the ducts of the parotid or zygomatic glands,[10–13] and trauma to the duct system is most commonly responsible. Trauma to the parotid duct or inflammatory reactions adjacent to it may cause stenosis, and initially there will be a palpable distension over the cheek region where the duct dilates. However, there will be a tendency for the glandular tissue to atrophy as pressure increases within the distension, except in the presence of low-grade infection which stimulates the continued production of saliva. The parotid duct lies relatively superficially as it passes over the face of the masseter muscle and is more vulnerable to rupture by an incisive wound than the other major ducts; under these conditions a fistula will develop, with a discharge of saliva directly to the skin surface. Rarely, a sialocele develops from the zygomatic gland to cause orbital swelling or proptosis (Fig. 50.5), and this must be differentiated from a retrobulbar abscess or orbital tumor: a fluctuant swelling may be present beneath the oral mucosa caudal to the last molar tooth. Ultrasonography of the orbit will help to make a definitive diagnosis of zygomatic sialocele. Obstructions in the small glandular aggregations in the mouth may give rise to blister-like cystic lesions, particularly around the soft palate (Fig. 50.6).

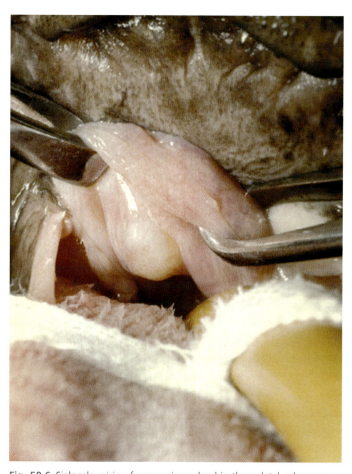

Fig. 50.6 Sialocele arising from a minor gland in the palatal submucosa in a French bulldog presenting with dyspnea.

Sialoceles in cats almost invariably form by leakage of saliva from a ductule of the sublingual gland, causing a sublingual sialocele.[8] However, there has been a single report of a lesion at the pharyngeal site causing obstructive dyspnea,[14] and another case report in which a sialocele from the zygomatic gland arose in the ventral region of the orbit.[15]

PREOPERATIVE ASSESSMENT

Diagnosis of sialocele

The diagnosis of cervical and sublingual sialoceles generally presents no difficulties. The lesions consist of thin-walled, painless, fluctuant swellings. Also, cervical sialoceles can be differentiated from abscesses because the skin overlying a sialocele is never adherent to the underlying lesion unless there has been previous surgical interference. Aspiration of the contents of the sialocele confirms the diagnosis (Fig. 50.7). The stagnant saliva in a sialocele is thick and tenacious; it is difficult to draw through an 18-gauge needle and will form strings when expressed from a syringe. Sometimes it is bloodstained, but so is the pus which might gather in an abscess in this area in the dog. However, pus, while tacky, cannot be described as tenacious. In referral practice, diagnosis by examination of the aspirated fluid can be confused if there has been recent drainage of the sialocele, in which case the vacated space may fill temporarily with serum. The side of origin of a unilateral sialocele in the cervical site is usually obvious in the early stages, but as sialoceles at this site become more pendulous, there is a tendency to migrate towards the ventral midline. Unless the client's

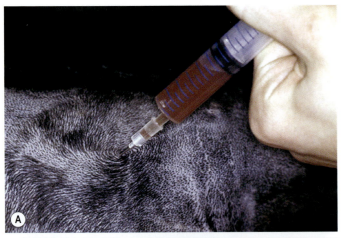

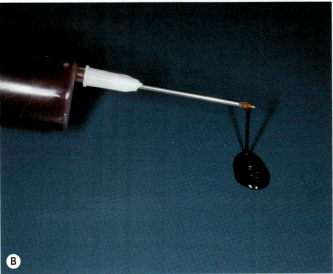

Fig. 50.7 (**A**) Aspiration of the contents of a cervical sialocele. Note that the stagnant saliva is bloodstained. (**B**) Aspirated saliva is viscous.

memory is dependable, it can be difficult to decide which side is involved. Thus, the major diagnostic challenge with sialoceles can be to determine from which side a cervical sialocele has arisen. If this is difficult in the normal standing position, the dilemma may be clarified by placing the patient in dorsal recumbency, after which the swelling should gravitate more towards the side of origin. Sialography (the radiographic study of the salivary glands following the introduction of contrast medium through the duct papillae) may appear to offer the definitive diagnostic technique.[1,4] However, cannulation of the papillae can be very time-consuming and frustrating, making this an unsuitable procedure for general practice. The ventral surgical approach to treatment described below affords a simpler means to resolve the dilemma.

Saliva is saturated by calcium hydroxyapatite and calcium salts, which may precipitate within a salivary duct to form sialoliths. Occlusion of a salivary duct by sialolith(s) is one of the proposed causes of sialoceles. However, histologic studies have suggested that sialoliths are not implicated in the majority of sialoceles.[16] On the other hand, stagnant saliva within a sialocele often contains tapioca-like particles of semi-mineralized aggregates of calcium salts. The discovery of such particles at surgery reinforces the diagnosis of sialocele.

THERAPEUTIC DECISION-MAKING

Objectives of surgery

The primary purpose of this section is to describe two methods to extirpate the sublingual and mandibular glands, one using the traditional lateral surgical approach and the other using the ventral approach, and to comment upon their relative merits and detractions. In a series of 166 dogs with sialocele referred for surgical correction, the lateral route was used for 120 operations and the ventral technique was employed 60 times.[8] The apparent disparity in addition arises because there were 10 bilateral cases (6.25%) and in four instances where there was recurrence after excision of the glands by the lateral approach, secondary surgery by the ventral method was used. Cats are far less frequently subject to sialocele formation: over the same time period, only seven feline cases were presented, all of which arose at the sublingual site and were treated successfully, four by the lateral route and three ventrally.

In referral practice it is likely that many patients will already have been subjected to one or more of a variety of techniques attempting to resolve the sialoceles. Drainage, as opposed to diagnostic aspiration of saliva, is the most likely. However, persistence of a sialocele after attempted extirpation of the mandibular and sublingual glands is not an uncommon finding, particularly when the lateral approach to surgery has been employed. Not all such failures can be attributed to the shortcomings of the lateral technique because some clinicians may be confused in the identification of the salivary glands. Instances have been documented where a complete glandular chain was found on each side after the salivary glands were purported to have been excised. Possibly the local lymph nodes had been removed in error.[8]

SURGICAL ANATOMY

General anatomy

The anatomy of the salivary glands is presented in detail in Chapter 49 and is simply summarized here. In the dog and cat there are four pairs of major salivary glands: the parotid, zygomatic, mandibular and sublingual. In addition to the major glands, salivary tissue is generously distributed in the oral and pharyngeal submucosa. The major section of the sublingual gland, the caudal (monostomatic) portion, shares a common capsule with the mandibular gland and (as the name suggests) drains by a single duct to the sublingual caruncle. Rarely, the distal segment of this duct is united with the mandibular gland duct.[4] A number of small tributary ducts lead from the lobules of the sublingual gland into the monostomatic duct.

Topographical anatomy

The mandibular gland forms a palpable spherical mass adjacent to the angle of the mandible, in the fork where the linguofacial branch joins the jugular vein. It lies within a tough fibrous capsule which extends rostromedially to envelope the mandibular duct and the sublingual glandular chain and duct. The mandibular gland receives its blood supply through the glandular branch of the facial artery, which enters the capsule at the rostromedial aspect, close to the exit point of the mandibular duct. The mandibular duct, together with the sublingual glandular chain and duct, travels rostrally between the medial pterygoid and digastricus muscles, effectively passing through a tunnel over the dorsal surface of the latter. On leaving the tunnel, the chain passes between the styloglossus and mylohyoid muscles and eventually comes to lie beneath the oral mucosa at the lateral aspect of the tongue. Whichever method of surgical excision is used, communication with the sialocele should be identified during the surgery so that the stagnant saliva within can be drained without creating a separate incision. In rare cases, a sialocele may have become very pendulous, resulting in stretching of the overlying skin to a point where a cosmetic procedure is required to excise the redundant skin. This is more conveniently performed when the ventral approach is used, as it simply entails creating an bi-elliptical rather than a linear incision.

SURGICAL TECHNIQUES

Lateral approach to excision of mandibular and sublingual glands[17]

The patient is positioned in lateral recumbency with the affected side uppermost (Fig. 50.8A). The neck is extended over a roll placed behind the underside ear. An incision is made over the mandibular gland, lying in the division between the jugular and linguofacial veins (Fig. 50.8B–D). After clearing the overlying fat and connective tissue, the tough capsule of the mandibular gland is incised in order to shell out the gland within (Fig. 50.8E, F). The dissection continues between the medial pterygoid and digastricus muscles, with gentle tension applied to the glandular chain (Fig. 50.8G, H). Amputation of the chain is made as far rostrally as access between these two muscles will permit (Fig. 50.8I). The surgery concludes with routine closure of the overlying soft tissues and skin.

Ventral approach to excision of mandibular and sublingual glands[8,18]

The patient is positioned in dorsal recumbency with the neck extended over a sandbag. A longitudinal incision is made medial to the ramus of the mandible, and extended caudally beyond the level of the angular process where the mandibular gland is palpable (Fig. 50.9A, B). A midline incision is used in cases when it is unclear from which side the sialocele has arisen. When the sialocele is in the cervical location, the ventral approach usually necessitates passage

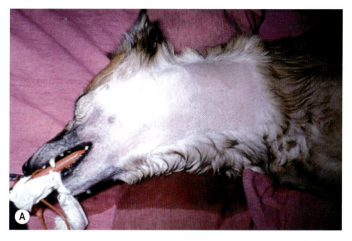

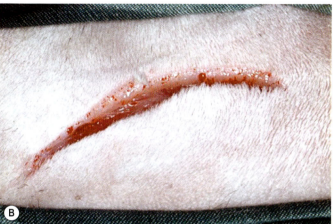

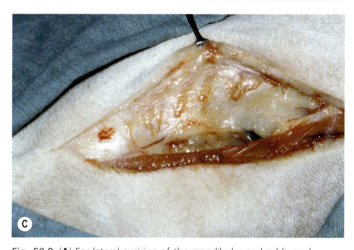

Fig. 50.8 (**A**) For lateral excision of the mandibular and sublingual salivary glands, the patient is positioned in lateral recumbency with the head extended over a sandbag or roll. (**B**) The skin incision is made directly over the mandibular gland. (**C**) The underlying panniculus muscle is divided. *Continued*

through the sialocele itself. This should be regarded as a help and not a hindrance, particularly with midline sialoceles, because tracts will be seen leading from the cyst to the diseased salivary tissue, thereby confirming the side and level of origin (Fig. 50.9C). The dissection is continued through the subcutaneous tissues caudally, and the mandibular gland is identified deep to the bifurcation of the external

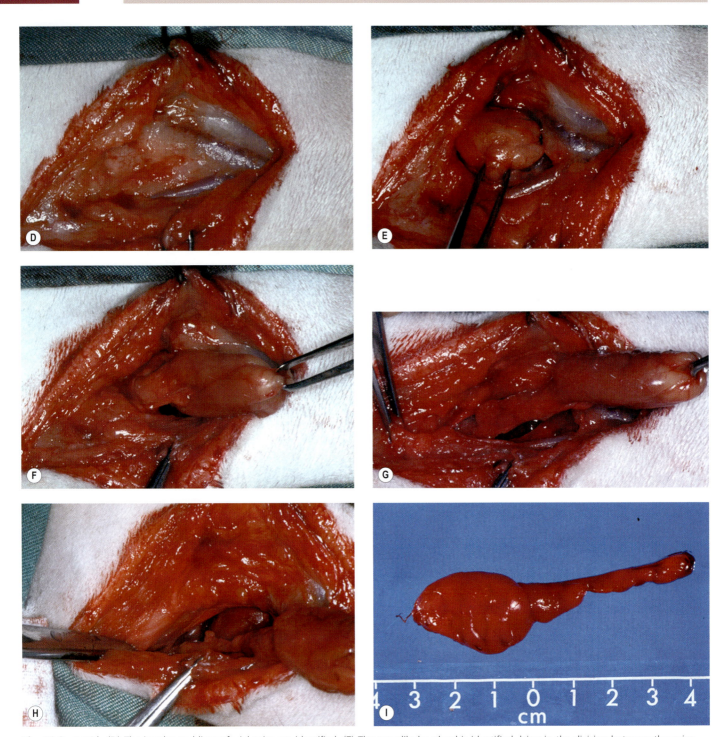

Fig. 50.8, cont'd. (**D**) The jugular and linguofacial veins are identified. (**E**) The mandibular gland is identified, lying in the division between the veins. (**F**) The mandibular gland is freed from its capsule and drawn laterally. (**G, H**) The chain of the sublingual gland if freed as it passes between the medial pterygoid and digastricus muscles. It is at this stage that the contents of the sialocele may well up into the incision. (**I**) Mandibular and sublingual glandular chain after amputation.

jugular vein (Fig. 50.9D). The arterial and venous blood supply enters the capsule from the rostromedial aspect; these vessels should be identified and ligated. The glandular tissue is dissected free from its capsule and the caudal lobules of the sublingual chain are also freed. When this route is used, the dissection rostrally is inhibited by the presence of the digastricus muscle, which crosses the path of the

glandular chain (Fig. 50.9E). Thus, at this point, attention is transferred to the rostral portion of the sublingual chain. The line of dissection passes through the tissues between the tongue and the body of the mandible by splitting between the mylohyoid and styloglossal muscles longitudinally. At this level, the sublingual chain is located together with the mandibular duct as it passes dorsal to the digastricus

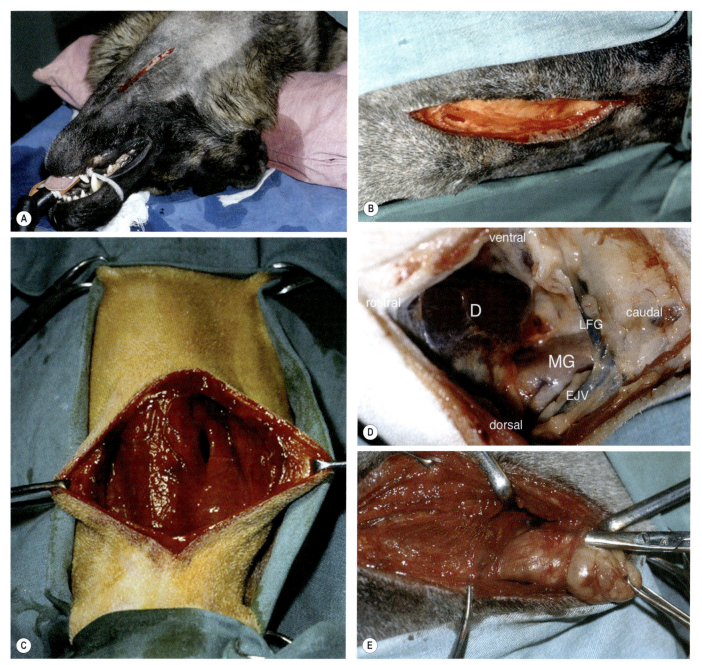

Fig. 50.9 (**A**, **B**) For ventral excision of the mandibular and sublingual salivary glands, the dog or cat is positioned in dorsal recumbency with the neck extended. The surgical drapes have been removed to show patient positioning. The skin incision is made medial to the mandible on the affected side or at the midline if the side of origin of the sialocele is uncertain or bilateral. The incision extends caudally to the level of the mandibular gland. (**C**) When the sialocele is incised, a tract can be seen leading to the glandular tissue on the afflicted side. (**D**) Cadaver dissection showing relationship of mandibular gland (MG) to the external jugular vein (EJV), linguofacial vein (LFG) and digastricus muscle (D). The right side is exposed and the dog is in dorsal recumbency. (**E**) The mandibular gland is separated from its capsule.

muscle. In cases where previous excision of the glandular chain has been inadequately performed, the stump of residual glandular tissue can be found here. The introduction of a finger or retractor beneath the belly of the digastricus from the caudal aspect helps to free the glandular chain and creates a tunnel through which the glandular tissue can be passed to the rostral portion of the surgical field (Fig.

50.9F, G). The complete chain is then amputated cranial to the most rostral glandular lobule. Structures to identify and preserve during the dissection include the hypoglossal and lingual nerves and the lingual artery. A Penrose drain may be used to prevent seroma formation in the dead space created by the surgery. Otherwise, closure of the incision is routine.

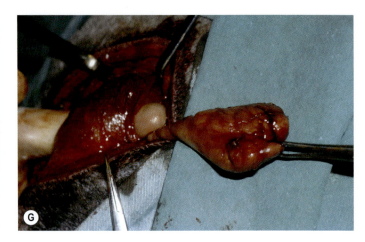

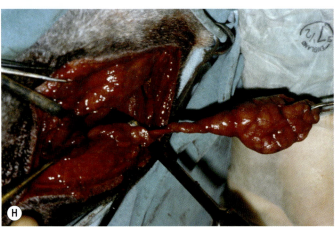

Fig. 50.9, cont'd. (**F**) The sublingual glandular chain passes dorsal to the digastricus muscle. (**G**) Blunt dissection with a finger creates a tunnel dorsal to the digastricus muscle through which the chain of glands can be passed. (**H**) The full length of the glandular chain has been freed and lies medial to the digastricus muscle immediately before amputation.

Advantages and disadvantages of lateral versus ventral approaches for sialoadenectomy: results of two techniques to excise the mandibular and sublingual salivary glands

Although the lateral approach to ablation of the mandibular and sublingual salivary glands is traditionally advocated, the technique has two shortcomings, either or both of which may lead to failure and persistence of the sialocele. The triangular space formed by the linguofacial and jugular veins, combined with the caudal border of the mandible, limits access as the dissection proceeds between the medial pterygoid and digastricus muscles. Thus, residual glandular tissue from the more rostral lobules of the sublingual gland is invariably left behind. If one of these should be the source of the salivary leakage, the sialocele will persist. Alternatively, if the contralateral chain (inaccessible by the lateral approach) is the source of the salivary leakage, the sialocele will persist.

Box 50.2 illustrates the results from one study where sialoceles persisted in a substantial number of dogs when the lateral approach to glandular excision had been attempted before referral. These failures were attributed to one of three causes: (1) the surgery had been performed on the incorrect side, (2) the rostral part of the glandular chain had not been excised on the correct side, and (3) poor anatomical appreciation of the region had led to failure to identify the mandibular gland and the entire glandular chain remained in situ.[8]

Box 50.3 reproduces the results reported in 120 operations when the lateral method was used. Cases with follow-up intervals of less

Box 50.2 **Treatments used in 166 dogs with sialoceles before referral**[8]	
Previous surgery	Number
No previous surgery	77
Drainage of sialocele (excludes diagnostic centesis)	65
Excision of sialocele	17
Marsupialization	6
Excision of mandibular and sublingual salivary glands:	21
Once	18
Twice	2
Three times	1

than 2 months were not included, and the longest period over which data were available was 12.5 years. Although the results were generally favorable, recurrence or persistence of the sialocele was recorded in six cases. Two of these were euthanized without a request for further treatment, but the other four were subjected to secondary surgery by the ventral route. In each case, it was established that residual rostral lobules of the sublingual gland were responsible.

The major detraction of the ventral technique is that it is more tedious to perform than the lateral method. The ventral approach to the surgery has two advantages over the lateral technique: (1) it allows exposure and excision of the entire sublingual chain and, (2) it permits the flexibility to remove the glandular chain on either or both sides through a single incision. The ventral approach provides the only

Box 50.3 Results of surgery to excise mandibular and sublingual glands[8]

Lateral approach: 120 operations

Lost to follow-up	36
Operations with follow-up: 2–185 months	84
Recurred/persisted (including 2 euthanasia)	6 (7%)
Resolved, no complication	75 (89%)
Resolved after delayed healing	3 (4%)
Total resolved	**78 (92%)**

Box 50.4 Results of surgery to excise mandibular and sublingual glands[8]

Ventral approach: 60 operations

Lost to follow-up	6
Operations with follow-up: 2–122 months	54
Recurred/persisted	0
Resolved, no complication	50 (93%)
Resolved after delayed healing	4 (7%)
Total resolved	**54 (100%)**

effective option when lateral surgery has already failed, as was the case with 25 of the operations reported. However, in 35 cases of sialocele it was used as the primary surgical technique. The technique was also used uneventfully in three cats.

The results of 60 operations to extirpate the mandibular and sublingual glands by the ventral approach are presented in Box 50.4. There was no record of recurrence or persistence of a sialocele after glandular excision by this method. One dog required a second interference 6 hours after the initial surgery to control hemorrhage from a branch of the lingual artery, and four dogs showed partial wound dehiscence with delayed healing by second intention.

The results of a second study of 41 cases of canine sialocele treated by excision of the salivary glands using the ventral route have been similar: none of the 31 dogs available for follow-up showed recurrence of the sialocele and seven sustained transient wound complications.[18]

In light of the evidence reviewed above, excision of the mandibular and sublingual glands by the ventral approach should be the primary treatment of choice for sialoceles in the dog. It is also recommended that this be the preferred option to treat the disorder whenever it arises in cats.

Intraoral marsupialization of a ranula

Marsupialization consist of the partial excision of the wall of a ranula followed by coaption of the lingual mucosa to the lining of the sialocele to form a 'pseudofistula', allowing saliva filling the sialocele to drain into the oral cavity.[7] The technique has not been subjected to statistical scrutiny and is probably only of historical interest, having its origins at a time when it was still believed that the lining contributed to the contents of the sialocele. Nevertheless, some success has been reported, especially when nonabsorbable sutures have been used to appose the inflammatory lining of the sialocele to the oral mucosa. However, the recurrence rate with marsupialization is such that removal of the salivary glandular chain offers a greater likelihood of a successful outcome (see also Box 50.2).[7,8]

Zygomatic sialoadenectomy

The indications for the removal of the zygomatic salivary gland are very rare and include traumatic rupture, sialocele and neoplasia. Upon clinical presentation of a patient with proptosis (especially when the globe is displaced dorsally), diagnosis may be made by ultrasonography and fine needle aspiration. If ultrasonography confirms a fluid-filled structure and saliva is identified upon aspiration, the diagnosis of zygomatic sialocele is confirmed, while soft tissue echogenicity and a cellular aspirate is more suggestive of neoplasia and is an indication for histopathologic analysis. In addition, oral inspection may reveal a swelling caudal to the maxillary molar teeth which will fluctuate in the case of a sialocele but will be firmer in the case of a neoplastic disorder.

The zygomatic salivary gland lies in the floor of the orbit and is protected by the overlying arch of the zygoma which restricts surgical access. The author's preferred method for zygomatic sialoadenectomy is to remove the ventral half of the zygomatic arch after dissecting between the aponeurosis of the masseter muscle and the periosteum (Fig. 50.10A–C). The gland is generally obscured by orbital fat, which is cleared before the gland is withdrawn by gentle traction (Fig. 50.10D). The incision is closed by sutures placed between the periosteum and the masseteric fascia, followed by closure of the subcutis and skin in a routine fashion. The advantage of this technique is cosmetic in that it preserves the facial outline. More generous exposure can be achieved by a full-thickness zygomatic osteotomy.[12,13]

POSTOPERATIVE CARE, ASSESSMENT AND COMPLICATIONS

Excision of the mandibular and sublingual salivary glands

Mandibular and sublingual sialoadenectomy should be regarded as sterile surgical procedures that do not enter the upper alimentary or respiratory tracts. Thus, normal rigorous aseptic techniques are adopted during preparation for surgery, and prophylactic antibiotic therapy is not required. There are no reports in the literature of a dog or cat which developed deep suppuration after sialoadenectomy, and the author's experience supports this. Short-term incisional dehiscence may result from self-trauma by the patient, but this is sufficiently uncommon that the routine use of a protective plastic collar is not necessary.

In the immediate postoperative period, careful observation is necessary to monitor for tense swelling at the surgical site. Such swelling might arise if hemorrhage from the nutrient vessels of the mandibular salivary gland has not been controlled, or if the lingual artery has been inadvertently damaged, during surgery. The proximity of the upper respiratory tract renders the patient at risk to asphyxiation if such a swelling is not recognized and the cause addressed promptly.

The dead space previously occupied by the fluid contents of the sialocele is likely to fill with serum even after the Penrose drain has been withdrawn, but the resultant seroma should never become tense or painful. Clients should be advised that some filling at the site is inevitable, and that this does not indicate that the surgery has been unsuccessful. The seroma will normally have regressed by the time the skin sutures are removed 10–14 days postoperatively. Longer-term swelling (weeks or months after a lateral approach to sialoadenectomy) suggests that the sublingual gland has been incompletely excised.

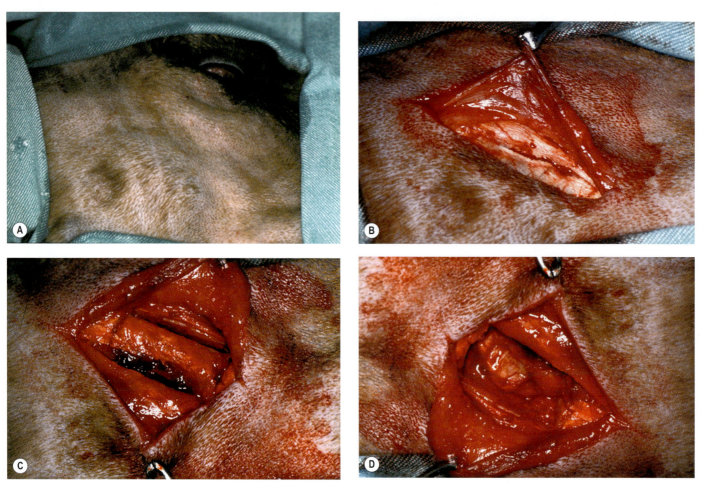

Fig. 50.10 (A) The area ventral to the zygomatic arch has been prepared for surgery. (B) The zygomatic arch is exposed at its ventral margin where the aponeurosis of the masseter muscle attaches. (C) The ventral section of the zygomatic arch is resected to leave the dorsal arch intact. (D) The infraorbital fat has been cleared to expose the underlying salivary gland, which is removed by gentle traction.

REFERENCES

1. Glen JB. Salivary cysts in the dog: identification of sublingual duct defects by sialography. Vet Rec 1966;78:488–92.

2. Spreull JS, Head KW. Cervical salivary cysts in the dog. J Small Anim Pract 1967;8:17–35.

3. Harvey CE. Canine salivary mucocoele. J Am Anim Hosp Assoc 1969;5:155–64.

4. Glen JB. Canine salivary mucocoeles. Results of sialographic examination and surgical treatment of fifty cases. J Small Anim Pract 1972;13:515–26.

5. DeYoung DW, Kealy JK, Kluge JP. Attempts to produce salivary cysts in the dog. Am J Vet Res 1978;39:185–6.

6. Knecht CD, Phares J. Characterization of dogs with salivary cyst. J Am Vet Med Assoc 1971;158:612–13.

7. Bellenger CR, Simpson DJ. Canine sialocele – 60 clinical cases. J Small Anim Pract 1992;33:376–80.

8. Lane JG. Surgical options in the treatment of salivary mucocoeles. Proceedings of 19th Congress of World Small Animal Veterinary Association 1994; 568–72.

9. Weber WJ, Hobson HP, Wilson SR. Pharyngeal mucoceles in dogs. Vet Surg 1986;15:5–8.

10. Mulkey OC, Knecht CD. Parotid salivary gland cyst and calculus in a dog. J Am Vet Med Assoc 1971;159:1774.

11. Termote S. Parotid salivary duct mucocoele and sialolithiasis following parotid duct transposition. J Small Anim Pract 2003;44:21–3.

12. Schmidt GM, Betts CW. Zygomatic salivary mucoceles in the dog. J Am Vet Med Assoc 1978;172:940–2.

13. Bartoe JT, Brightman AH, Davidson HJ. Modified lateral orbitotomy for vision-sparing excision of a zygomatic mucocele in a dog. Vet Ophthalmol 2007;10:127–31.

14. Feinman JM. Pharyngeal mucocele and respiratory distress in a cat. J Am Vet Med Assoc 1990;197:1179–80.

15. Speakman AJ, Baines SJ, Williams JM, et al. Zygomatic salivary cyst with mucocele formation in a cat. J Small Anim Pract 1997;38:468–70.

16. Spangler WL, Culbertson MR. Salivary gland disease in dogs and cats: 245 cases (1985–1988). J Am Vet Med Assoc 1991; 198:465–9.

17. Kealy JK. Salivary cyst in the dog. Vet Rec 1964;119–20.

18. Ritter MJ, von Pfeil DJ, Stanley BJ, et al. Mandibular and sublingual sialocoeles in the dog: a retrospective evaluation of 41 cases, using the ventral approach for treatment. N Z Vet J 2006; 54:333–7.

Chapter | 51 |

Cheiloplasty

Daniel D. Smeak

LIP FOLD RESECTION

Dogs with infections involving the lips are typically presented for treatment of their severe halitosis or facial pruritus. Skin fold intertrigo is a frictional dermatitis that occurs in areas where two skin surfaces are intimately apposed.[1] If moisture, sebum, glandular secretions and excretions such as tears, saliva and urine are present, these areas provide an environment that favors skin maceration and bacterial overgrowth.[1] Although bacteria play a central role in the pathogenesis of fold dermatitis, they rarely invade tissues, so its designation as a fold pyoderma is technically inaccurate.[1] The surface bacteria act on trapped secretions and sebum and produce breakdown products, which are irritating and odoriferous.[1] Lip fold intertrigo is found caudal to the mandibular canine teeth where the lower lips are contacted by the tips of the maxillary canine teeth (Fig. 51.1). Lip fold resection eliminates these folds so there is no further accumulation of food and saliva to trigger infection.[2]

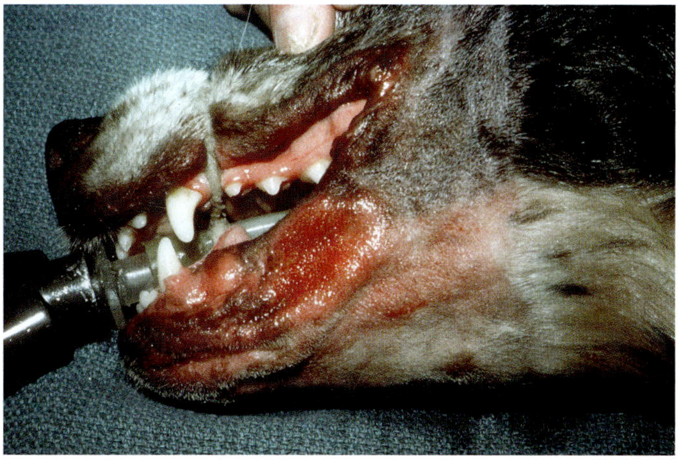

Clinical characteristics

The affected area is usually red, glistening and ulcerated and, unless the condition is severe, the lesion is confined to a sharply demarcated area within the recesses of the folds. There may be a film of purulent exudate and debris covering the area. On physical examination, the problem is often not obvious until the fold is stretched, revealing the affected area. This condition is most common in dogs with large, pendulous upper lips and prominent lower lip lateral folds such as St. Bernards, schnauzers and brachycephalic breeds, but spaniels and setters appear to be particularly predisposed. Food, hair and saliva collect in these folds, causing inflammation and fetid odors. Since the condition is due to a conformational problem, the course of the disease is chronic and usually only temporarily improved by medical therapy.

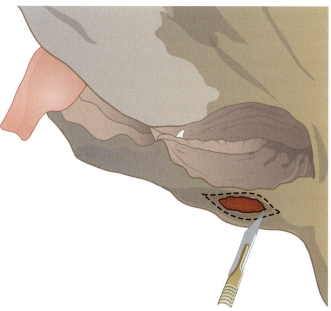

Fig. 51.1 Severe lip fold pyoderma in a dog.

Fig. 51.2 The lip fold is excised with a fusiform incision around its margin (*dashed line*).

© 2012 Elsevier Ltd
DOI: 10.1016/B978-0-7020-4618-6.00051-8

Associated conditions

Lip fold pyoderma should be differentiated from other conditions that cause halitosis and/or facial dermatitis such as dental disease, canine acne, juvenile pyoderma, contact or food allergic dermatitis and other immune-related diseases that cause ulceration of the mucocutaneous areas. If the condition is not limited to the lateral folds, or the lip conformation is not considered abnormal, surgical treatment should not be considered and other dermatological problems should be investigated.

Preoperative considerations

Attempt to improve the local tissue condition before surgery by swabbing the folds daily with 2% acetic/2% boric acid solution wipes (MalAcetic Wet Wipe/Dry Bath, Dermapet, Potomac, MD) or shampoo. Use of topical 2% mupirocin (Bactoderm, Beecham Laboratories, Bristol, TN) or silver sulfadiazine, and systemic antibiotics such as clavulanic acid/amoxicillin may be helpful if there is staphylococcal colonization of the folds. Administer a single intravenous dose of a cephalosporin antibiotic just before surgery.

Surgical technique

Place the patient in dorsal recumbency to allow access to both lip folds. Prepare the region for aseptic surgery. Create a fusiform incision, parallel to the body of the mandible, around the affected area to include a rim of normal skin (Fig. 51.2). Elevate the underlying subcutaneous tissue attachments to the outlined skin segment without invading the inner buccal mucosa. Control hemorrhage, and close the subcutaneous tissue and skin routinely.

Postoperative considerations

Use an Elizabethan collar or bucket to prevent self-inflicted trauma. Continue the medical therapy described above and keep the area clean and dry until suture removal. Healing is complete and permanent following elimination of the fold with surgical excision.[2]

ANTI-DROOL CHEILOPLASTY

Anti-drool cheiloplasty (ADC) is an elective surgical procedure in which the lower lip is permanently attached in a dorsally suspended position to the upper lip.[3]

Purpose and indications

The suspended lower lip reduces the loss of food and saliva from the lateral vestibules of the oral cavity. Indications for ADC include congenital overabundance and eversion of the caudal lower lip, frequently seen in large- and giant-breed dogs such as the St. Bernard and Newfoundland, and acquired loss of lip motor function from trauma or nerve damage.[3] Most clients seek this procedure because they are tired of cleaning the mess left after their dog eats or drinks.

Preoperative considerations

Withhold food from patients for 12 hours before surgery. No prophylactic antibiotics are required. Be sure the endotracheal tube cuff is positioned in the trachea and properly inflated to prevent aspiration of blood during the procedure. Irrigate food and saliva from the oral cavity with water prior to aseptic preparation of the lip. Place the dog in lateral recumbency and prepare the regional skin with povidone-iodine scrub and daub the buccal mucosa with povidone-iodine solution. Avoid chlorhexidine antiseptics in or around the face because unintentional ocular contact will result in severe chemosis and conjunctivitis. Place the patient in lateral recumbency; stabilize the head and drape the lip region without altering the normal relaxed lip position or the ability to fully open the mouth during the procedure.

Surgical technique

Grasp the irregular lower lip mucocutaneous margin about 20–30 mm rostral to the commissure with an Allis tissue forceps, and elevate the lip dorsally until it is taut when an assistant is asked to fully open the dog's mouth (Fig. 51.3). Mark this spot on the upper lip skin (cheek) with a surgical pen or lightly scratch the skin with a scalpel blade. In most patients this mark roughly corresponds to the level of the distal root of the upper fourth premolar tooth. Start a horizontal cheek incision (parallel to the palate), 25–30 mm long, from a point intersecting the marked lip area and an imaginary line drawn from the medial canthus of the eye to the commissure of the lips (Fig. 51.4). Align

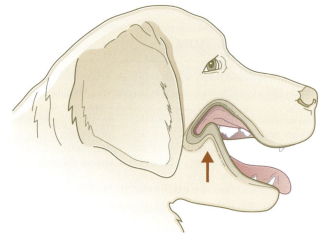

Fig. 51.3 Grasp the lower lip, 20–30 mm rostral to the commissure, and elevate it until the lip is taut when the mouth is fully opened. This will mark the dorsal extent of the horizontal cheek incision.

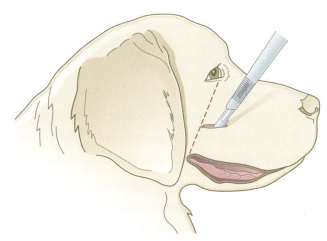

Fig. 51.4 Completed full-thickness horizontal cheek incision. The caudal aspect of the incision intersects a line drawn from the medial canthus to the commissure (dotted line).

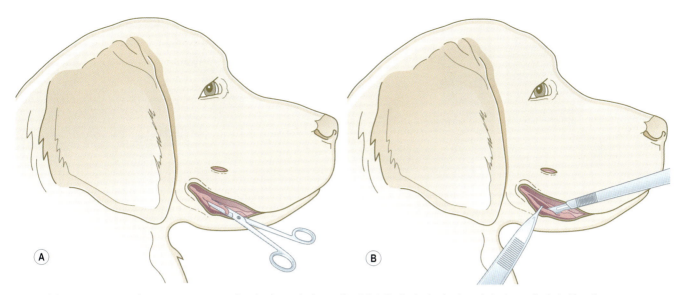

Fig. 51.5 (**A**) Excise a 25-mm-long mucocutaneous border from the lower lip. (**B**) Split the incised edge of the lower lip in half to form separate cutaneous and mucosal flaps.

dissection through deeper cheek tissue directly under the original skin incision, but avoid the superior labial vein coursing just rostrodorsal to this incision. Continue dissection until the buccal mucosa is incised along the limits of the original skin incision, and control hemorrhage before proceeding. Resect a 2-mm mucocutaneous margin of the lower lip with Mayo scissors beginning 20 mm from the commissure and extend the cut rostrally for 25 mm (Fig. 51.5A). Split the cut edge of the lip longitudinally with a scalpel blade to a depth of 7.5–10 mm to create a mucosal and a cutaneous flap (Fig. 51.5B). Pull the flaps through the cheek incision with stay sutures placed at the rostral and caudal aspects of the lower lip incision.

The key goal of the suture pattern described in this procedure is to appose as much raw tissue surface as possible between the cheek incision and lower lip flaps.[3] The mattress pattern must hold the lower lip flaps in eversion within the cheek incision to create a robust and permanent lip adhesion. Appose the everted edges of the lip and cheek with two to three equally spaced and preplaced horizontal mattress sutures using 2–0 or 0 monofilament nonabsorbable suture material. Insert the needle split-thickness through the cheek about 1 cm from the incision. With the flaps everted and elevated from the cheek incision, advance the needle through the raw surface of the facing flap, through the base of the lower lip, out through the opposite flap, and through the cheek skin, again split-thickness. Reverse the needle direction and drive the needle through the lower lip in mirror image to the first needle pass (Fig. 51.6). Tighten each suture just enough to appose the incised edges of the lip and cheek. Moderate swelling occurs after the procedure and this may cause excess intrinsic suture tension, so avoid cinching these mattress sutures too tightly. Check the buccal aspect of the cheek incision to assure the sutures were correctly placed and lower lip flaps are everted within the upper cheek (Fig. 51.7) When skin is not well apposed, close the cheek incision with simple interrupted 3–0 or 4–0 monofilament nonabsorbable sutures. If bilateral ADCs are planned, undrape and roll the dog, and repeat the procedure on the other side. Bilateral ADCs take approximately 30–45 minutes to complete.

Postoperative considerations

Patients are usually released from the hospital the day following the procedure. Feed dogs their routine diet after surgery. Irrigate the oral

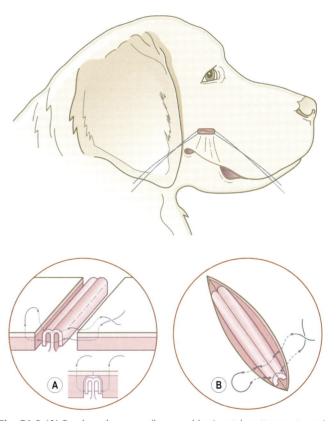

Fig. 51.6 (**A**) Preplace three equally spaced horizontal mattress sutures in the lower lip to cause eversion of the flaps within the cheek incision. (**B**) Close-up of suture pattern.

vestibules after meals with water-filled syringes to remove food debris. Clients should not permit chewable toys or fetching for 2 months after surgery. Fit a short Elizabethan collar on the patient until suture removal to prevent self-mutilation. Remove sutures 3 weeks after surgery.

513

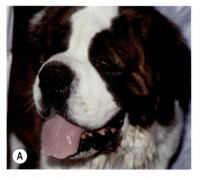 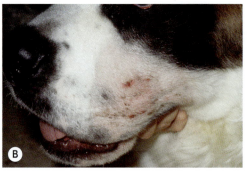 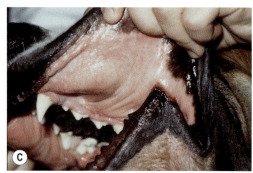

Fig. 51.7 Gross appearance of a patient before and after ADC. (**A**) Preoperative appearance. (**B**) Following suture removal. (**C**) Appearance of buccal surface at suture removal.

Complications and prognosis

Anti-drool cheiloplasty does not appear to cause excessive discomfort after surgery. Dogs are not reluctant to open their mouths the day after surgery and they eat without difficulty. A small indentation or fine incision scar is evident after healing is complete. Excessive tension on the mattress sutures causes suture cutout and abscessation around suture tracks (Fig. 51.8). If this occurs, remove sutures as soon as possible after the mucosal incisions have healed; otherwise, an orocutaneous fistula may occur. Treat the wound open and let it heal by second-intention closure. This procedure is highly successful in reducing drooling associated with congenital lower lip eversion and lip paralysis but it does not totally eliminate drooling. Advise clients that drooling is reduced to a level similar to dogs with normal lip conformation.[3]

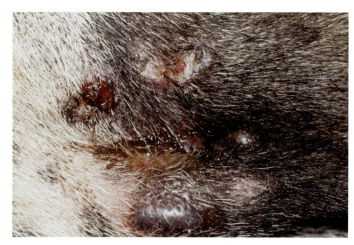

Fig. 51.8 Suture-induced draining cheek wounds at 3 weeks after surgery.

REFERENCES

1. Scott DW, Miller Jr WH, Griffin CE. Environmental skin diseases. In: Scott DW, Miller Jr WH, Griffin CE, editors. Muller & Kirk's small animal dermatology. 5th ed. Philadelphia, PA: WB Saunders; 1995. p. 859–89.

2. Bellah JR. Surgical management of specific skin disorders. In: Slatter DH, editor. Textbook of small animal surgery. 2nd ed. Philadelphia, PA: WB Saunders; 1993. p. 341–4.

3. Smeak DD. Anti-drool cheiloplasty: clinical results in six dogs. J Am Anim Hosp Assoc 1989;25:181–5.

Chapter | 52 |

Inferior labial frenoplasty and tight-lip syndrome

Steven E. Holmstrom

DEFINITIONS

Frenectomy: excision of the frenulum

Frenoplasty: correction of an abnormally attached frenulum by surgically repositioning it

Frenotomy: incision or transection of the frenulum

Inferior labial frenulum (or frenum): a fibroelastic band of tissue attaching the lower lip to the gingiva on the distal aspect of the mandibular canine tooth

Tight-lip syndrome: a condition seen exclusively in Shar-Pei dogs whereby the lower lips curl lingually and over the mandibular incisors, and occasionally the mandibular canine teeth

Vestibule: the space external to the teeth, gingiva, and alveolar mucosa, and internal to lips and cheeks

PREOPERATIVE CONCERNS

Frenoplasty and tight-lip correction are performed to treat patients for an anatomical defect that is likely of genetic origin. If possible, these procedures should be performed on neutered patients to prevent the retention of these traits in the gene pool. The clients should be informed that many organizations have rules against performing corrective surgical procedures on animals intended for breeding or showing.

SURGICAL ANATOMY

A general description of the anatomy of the lips can be found in Chapter 44.

The inferior labial frenulum is a poorly described structure consisting of a fibroelastic band of tissue attaching the lower lip to the gingiva on the distal aspect of the mandibular canine tooth. It contains the neurovascular bundle, including the middle mental nerve

and blood vessels, emerging from the middle mental foramen. The middle mental foramen is located ventral to the mesial root of the second premolar tooth, while the smaller rostral mental foramen and caudal mental foramen can be found ventral to the second incisor and third premolar teeth, respectively. The skin of the chin is tightly attached to the underlying tissues. The structure of the lower lips has not been described in depth. The margin of the lower lip as far caudally as the canine tooth is hairless over a width of approximately 5 mm. Caudal to the canine teeth the hairless zone increases to 10 mm in width, and conical papillae occur.[1] A well-keratinized area is present where the maxillary canine tooth comes in contact with the lower lip when the mouth is in a fully closed position.

The Shar-Pei is a dog breed of Chinese origin.[2] The breed is thought to have been in existence since the Han dynasty, around 200 BC. The literal translation of Shar-Pei is 'sand skin.' Many people develop rashes on their forearms after contact with the Shar-Pei's fur. They have loose skin covering the head and body, small ears and an unusual muzzle shape. The head is covered with profuse wrinkles on the forehead continuing into side wrinkles framing the face. The broad muzzle is one of the distinctive features of the breed. The lips and top of the muzzle are well padded and may cause a slight bulge at the base of the nose.[2]

On the rostral aspect of the lower lip there is normally a space between the lip, and the teeth and gingiva. This space is reduced or missing in affected Shar-Pei dogs.

INFERIOR LABIAL FRENOPLASTY

Clinical presentation

In some dogs, an excessively tight inferior labial frenulum may be present and the resulting abnormally narrow vestibulum entraps food and debris. This results in infection of the periodontium at the disto-buccal surface of the mandibular canine teeth. In addition to periodontal disease, this condition may lead to inflammation and infection of the lower lip (cheilitis) lateral and rostral to the inferior labial frenulum.

© 2012 Elsevier Ltd
DOI: 10.1016/B978-0-7020-4618-6.00052-X

Therapeutic decision-making

There are three indications for frenoplasty. Patients showing dermatological signs of chronic infection and inflammation of the lower lip are initially treated by medical means; if unsuccessful, they may benefit from frenoplasty by exteriorizing the lip out of the moist environment of the oral cavity. Patients with chronic periodontal disease of the distal portion of the mandibular canines may also benefit from frenoplasty, in combination with conventional periodontal treatment and home care. Finally, inferior labial frenoplasty may be performed as an ancillary procedure in the Shar-Pei dog with tight-lip syndrome (see below).

Frenectomy (excision of the frenulum) or simple frenotomy (incision or transection of the frenulum) is rarely if ever indicated.

Surgical technique

The lower lip at the attachment of the frenulum is grasped with thumb forceps and held taut. A scalpel is used to cut the frenulum midway between the lip and gingiva in a sagittal direction. The incision is extended with sharp or blunt dissection into the frenulum to relieve the pull of the muscular attachments. Care is taken not to sever the middle mental nerve and blood vessels. The lip will relax laterally when the attachments have been completely severed and a diamond-shaped cut will be created. The objective of suturing is to prevent the natural adhesion and reattachment of the cut portions of the frenulum. This is accomplished by placing several simple interrupted, absorbable sutures in a transverse direction, bringing the rostral and caudal edges of the incision together, similar to a Heineke-Mikulicz procedure in gastrointestinal surgery.

Postoperative care and assessment

The oral cavity and surgical area should be irrigated twice daily with a 0.05–0.12% chlorhexidine gluconate solution to keep the area clean for 2 weeks.

Complications

Hemorrhage may be caused by the inadvertent transection of the mental artery or vein. Reattachment of the frenulum may occur if the wound is left unsutured. Chronic cheilitis and localized periodontitis affecting the mandibular canine teeth may persist. Wound dehiscence is uncommon and is generally treated conservatively by wound irrigation, allowing the wound to heal by second intention; further surgical revision may be required if this again results in an abnormally tight frenulum.

TIGHT-LIP CORRECTION IN THE SHAR-PEI

Clinical presentation

Because of the reduced space between the lower lip, rostrally, and corresponding teeth and gingiva in affected Shar-Pei dogs, the lower lip can curl up and over the incisors and sometimes the canines (Fig. 52.1). The lip is traumatized, being crushed between the mandibular and maxillary incisors. Further scarring and contracture aggravate this condition. Affected dogs are presented with the mandibular lips tightly pressed against, or covering, the incisor and canine teeth. These teeth may be displaced lingually and predisposed to early periodontal disease. The client may report reluctance to eat, odor or hemorrhage. Skin and oral infections and displaced or rotated teeth are also common.

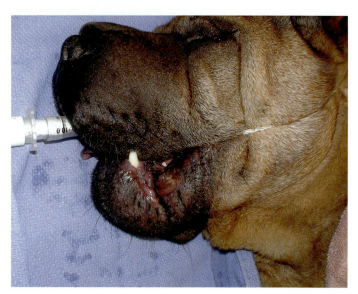

Fig. 52.1 Typical appearance of a tight-lipped Shar-Pei. Note the lower lip is rolled up and over the mandibular incisor teeth. This causes the patient to bite its lip.

Therapeutic decision-making

Surgical repositioning of the retroverted rostral portion of the lip off the incisive edges of the incisors reduces the tension between the lip and teeth, and increases the depth of the vestibule.

The age of the patient is an important consideration. In young animals cheiloplasty is performed to prevent pain and to allow proper growth of the jaw. One technique is to make a releasing incision that separates the lip from its gingival attachment and instruct the client to manipulate the incision daily to prevent the skin from being pulled back to its previous position.[3] An alternative to this would be to place either an oral mucosa graft or Penrose tubing to increase the space in the vestibule.[4–7]

For older patients, where the patient is biting on its lip causing pain and infection, cheiloplasty is also indicated. In addition, two other techniques are available, which may be performed concurrently. One technique involves a ventral mandibular incision, freeing of the attachment of the skin/gingiva to the mandible and suturing the gingiva to the mandible so that the lip is no longer in occlusion with the teeth.[5] In patients with excess skin on the chin or when the two previously described techniques do not work, skin of the chin may be resected.[3]

Antibiotic prophylaxis (see Ch. 3) is generally indicated for these procedures.

Surgical techniques

Cheiloplasty – surgical repositioning of the rostral lower lip

The objective of the cheiloplasty procedure is to increase the amount of vestibule present by separating the lower lip from the chin.

The patient is placed in ventral recumbency with a maxillary support bar (Fig. 52.2A) and the lower lip is retracted to expose the mandibular teeth. The incision can be made on either the mucogingival junction or the mucocutaneous junction (Fig. 52.2B). In either case, the incision should extend from one inferior labial frenulum side to the other (Fig. 52.2C). The soft tissues between the skin and fascia are dissected free (Fig. 52.2D). Once dissected free, the fascia is inverted

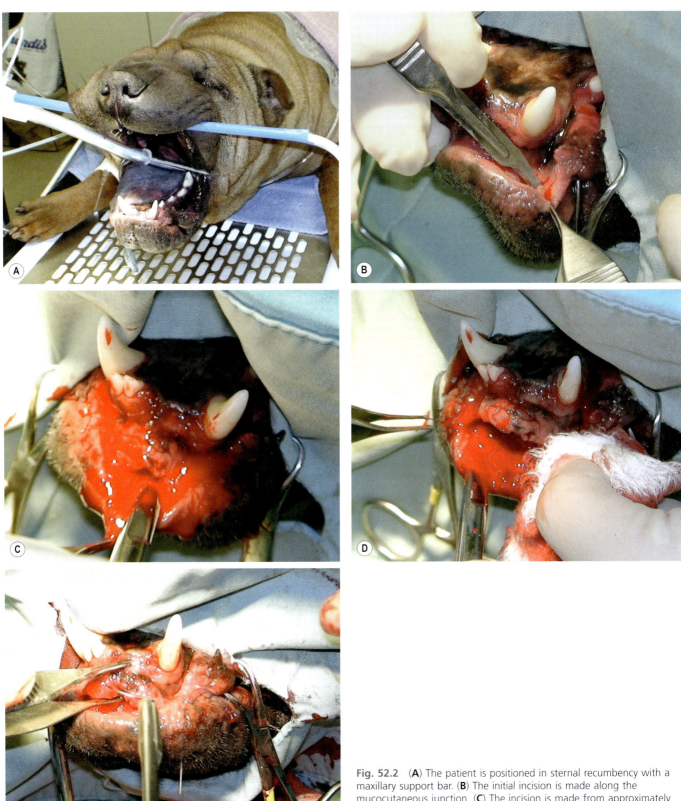

Fig. 52.2 (**A**) The patient is positioned in sternal recumbency with a maxillary support bar. (**B**) The initial incision is made along the mucocutaneous junction. (**C**) The incision is made from approximately one mandibular frenulum to the other. (**D**) Fascia is dissected off the skin and will serve as the graft to enlarge the vestibule. (**E**) The fascia is sutured to the mucous membrane portion of the mucogingival incision.

and sutured to the mucous membrane (Fig. 52.2E). Minor hemorrhage is encountered when the rostral mental arteries are transected. One technique is to keep the surgically created space open by daily manipulation of the tissues to prevent reattachment. This technique requires a great deal of cooperation between the client and patient.

An alternative to intensive home care is to place either a buccal mucosal graft from the cheek or a Penrose drain to physically separate the operated tissue and maintain the deepened lower vestibule.

Sterilized aluminum foil may be used to create a template to use as a guide in outlining the buccal mucosa graft from the cheek. The template should be created 10–20% larger than the anticipated area to fill. Once dissected free, the mucosal graft is sutured to the wound edges of the lip and oral mucosa that was incised away from the lip.

An alternative is to suture a Penrose drain of appropriate size to fill the void instead of the buccal mucosal graft. This is held in place with monofilament sutures until the underlying defect epithelializes. This typically takes 2–3 weeks, hence the need for long-lasting resorbable suture material (e.g., polydioxanone) or nonabsorbable suture material.

Ventral mandibular approach

The objective of this approach is to free up the skin covering the mandible and tack the skin so that the lip is pulled ventrally.

An approximately 20-mm incision is made over the mandibular symphysis in a craniocaudal direction. This allows the insertion of sharp scissors to undermine the skin from the muscle. A suture of 2–0 or 3–0 polydioxanone is passed as far dorsally as possible toward the lip, taking an anchoring bite of subcuticular tissue in order to pull the lip ventrally. The suture is tacked down to the periosteum as far caudally as possible on the mandibular symphysis. The suture is tightened and tied with a reinforced surgeon's knot. Additional sutures, laterally to the right and left, are placed as necessary in order to accomplish the goal of repositioning the skin tissue effectively and cosmetically. The skin is sutured with fine nonabsorbable monofilament suture material.

Skin resection

The objective of this technique is to excise excessive skin from the ventral mandible (chin).

The patient is placed in dorsal recumbency. The chin tissues are pinched to approximate the position of the skin when the tissue is excised. It may be helpful to do this prior to aseptic preparation and to use a permanent marking pen to mark the planned incision. The incision should be symmetrical. A fusiform incision through the skin and subcutaneous tissue is made and the redundant lip tissue is undermined and excised using Metzenbaum scissors. The

subcutaneous tissues are sutured with one to three layers of 3–0 absorbable material in a continuous pattern. Skin closure is routine, using either an intradermal pattern with absorbable suture material, or meticulously placed single-interrupted sutures using fine, nonresorbable material, in order to avoid scar formation.

Postoperative care and assessment

Cheiloplasty

The oral cavity and surgical area should be irrigated twice daily with a 0.05–0.12% chlorhexidine gluconate solution to keep the area clean for 2 weeks. If a Penrose drain is used, it should be removed in 2–3 weeks.

Ventral mandibular approach

The client is advised not to give hard treats, chew toys (soft or hard), or allow oral play for 3 weeks. Recommendations for daily home oral hygiene are routine. The patient is rechecked in 1 week and the skin sutures are removed in 10–14 days.

Skin resection

The patient is rechecked in 1 week and skin sutures are removed in 10–14 days.

Complications

Cheiloplasty

Dehiscence of the suture line or premature removal of the Penrose drain can allow the tissues to join back together in the tight-lip position. An Elizabethan collar may be necessary to prevent self trauma and premature dislodgment of the Penrose drain.

Ventral mandibular approach

Breakdown of suture may occur if a sufficient anchor for the suture is not taken, or if the patient is not restricted from self-destructive oral behavior. Wound infection may also occur if aseptic technique was not used.

Skin resection

Wound infection, and rubbing at the incision with consequent dehiscence of the skin sutures, are two potential complications observed following resection of excessive skin from the ventral mandible. An Elizabethan collar may be required to prevent self-trauma.

REFERENCES

1. Evans HE. Miller's anatomy of the dog. 3rd ed. Philadelphia, PA: WB Saunders Co; 1993. p. 385–7.
2. Anonymous. Chinese Shar-Pei. http://www.akc.org/breeds/recbreeds/sharpei.cfm, accessed December 3, 2003.
3. McCoy DE. Surgical management of the tight lip syndrome in the Shar-Pei dog. J Vet Dent 1997;14:95–6.
4. Wiggs RB, Lobprise HB. Veterinary dentistry principles and practice. Philadelphia, PA: Lippincott-Raven; 1997. p. 248–9.
5. Lobprise HB, Wiggs RW. The veterinarian's companion for common dental procedures. Lakewood, CA: AAHA Press; 2000. p. 89–92.
6. Holmstrom SE, Frost P, Eisner ER. Veterinary dental techniques for the small animal practitioner. 2nd ed. Philadelphia, PA: WB Saunders Co; 1998. p. 167–214.
7. Holmstrom SE, Frost P, Eisner ER. Veterinary dental techniques for the small animal practitioner. 3rd ed. Philadelphia, PA: WB Saunders Co; 2004. p. 282–90.

Chapter | **53** |

Management of maxillofacial osteonecrosis

Sandra Manfra Marretta & Milinda J. Lommer

DEFINITIONS

Bone sequestrum: a piece of necrotic bone that has become separated from vital bone

Osteomyelitis: an inflammatory process of the bone marrow, cortex and possibly the periosteum

Osteonecrosis of the jaw: exposed necrotic bone in the maxillofacial region that fails to heal after 6 to 8 weeks in patients with no history of craniofacial radiation[1]

Osteoradionecrosis: devitalization of bone by cancericidal doses of radiation[2]

PREOPERATIVE CONCERNS

Osteonecrosis is an infrequently diagnosed condition in the maxillofacial region of dogs and cats. Recognition of maxillofacial osteonecrosis includes evaluation of pertinent clinical history and thorough preoperative evaluation of the patient. Animals with osteonecrosis may be presented with a history of fetid breath, severe oral pain, facial swelling, reluctance or inability to eat, severe purulent nasal discharge or exophthalmos.[3,4] Preoperative concerns in animals with maxillofacial osteonecrosis include medical stabilization of the patient prior to surgical intervention and evaluation of underlying conditions that may be contributing to the osteonecrosis.

ETIOPATHOGENESIS

Osteonecrosis may be described as radiation-induced, traumatic or nontraumatic. In humans, nontraumatic osteonecrosis has been associated with corticosteroid usage, alcoholism (and resulting alterations in lipid metabolism), infections, hyperbaric events, storage disorders, marrow-infiltrating diseases, coagulation defects, autoimmune diseases,[5] herpes zoster infection-associated trigeminal neuralgia[6–8] and bisphosphonate administration.[9–11] There are also many idiopathic cases, in which the underlying cause is never identified.

In companion animals, osteonecrosis is most commonly seen following radiation therapy (osteoradionecrosis). While it is generally believed that osteoradionecrosis occurs as a result of vascular compromise,[12] an infectious etiology for osteoradionecrosis has recently been suggested.[13]

In the absence of previous radiation therapy or trauma, it is likely that the pathogenesis of osteonecrosis is multifactorial. Spontaneous, idiopathic osteonecrosis has been reported in cats[14] and is well recognized in the human knee[15–17] and femoral head.[18,19] A genetic basis for predisposition to idiopathic femoral head necrosis, due to genetic polymorphism resulting in decreased nitric oxide production, has been suggested.[20]

The development of nontraumatic osteonecrosis appears to involve vascular compromise, bone and cell death and/or defective bone repair.[5] Recent research suggests regional endothelial cell dysfunction may be the underlying mechanism, uniting the multiple associated risk factors with a single common pathway.[21]

THERAPEUTIC DECISION-MAKING

Therapeutic decision-making in animals with maxillofacial osteonecrosis is, in part, dependent upon the etiology and location of the osteonecrosis. Maxillofacial osteonecrosis can occur in dogs and cats as a complication of maxillofacial injuries, traumatic extraction techniques, chronic infection and radiation therapy for the treatment of oral tumors. Some cases of idiopathic maxillofacial osteonecrosis in dogs may be associated with previously undetected chronic osteomyelitis and bone infarction.[22] The incidence of maxillofacial osteonecrosis has recently increased in humans and has been associated with the administration of high doses of bisphosphonates in cancer patients.[1,9,11,23,24] The potential for an increase in the incidence of maxillofacial osteonecrosis in animals may become a reality as veterinary oncologists utilize these drugs at high doses in the management of animals with cancer.[25] Accurate preoperative assessment and adherence to basic principles in the management of maxillofacial osteonecrosis can help insure a successful outcome in most cases, depending on the initial cause of the maxillofacial osteonecrosis.

© 2012 Elsevier Ltd
DOI: 10.1016/B978-0-7020-4618-6.00053-1

A complete preoperative evaluation of animals with maxillofacial osteonecrosis includes: a complete history, complete general physical examination on the awake patient, a thorough oral examination on the sedated or anesthetized patient, hematologic testing, cytologic examination of the lesion, and radiographic evaluation including thoracic, dental and skull radiographs. Radiographic signs of acute osteomyelitis include decreased density of the involved bone, with scattered regions of radiolucency[26] which may be radiographically indistinguishable from neoplasia. In chronic osteomyelitis, the bone typically appears more radiopaque and sclerotic, and there may be periosteal new bone formation.[24] There is often a fine granular appearance. Areas of necrosis appear even more radiopaque than the surrounding bone, and may exist as sequestra, surrounded by a radiolucent border.[24] Computed tomography and magnetic resonance imaging are superior to conventional radiography in evaluating osteonecrosis[5,24] and should be performed as part of the diagnostic work-up for patients with osteonecrosis whenever possible.

FACTORS TO CONSIDER IN THE SURGICAL MANAGEMENT OF MAXILLOFACIAL OSTEONECROSIS

Factors to be considered in the surgical management of patients with maxillofacial osteonecrosis include underlying contributory factors and location of the maxillofacial osteonecrosis.

Osteonecrosis and bone sequestra occurring as a complication of maxillofacial fractures or traumatic extraction techniques can usually be managed by localization and surgical removal of the bone sequestrum. This is most frequently accomplished by creating a mucoperiosteal flap via an intraoral approach, but occasionally an incision through the skin may be necessary, depending on the proximity of the sequestrum to the surface of the oral mucosa or skin (Fig. 53.1).

Osteonecrosis caused by chronic osteomyelitis can be managed by removal of the bone sequestrum, appropriate bone debridement and long-term appropriate medical therapy. Both bacterial and mycotic organisms may be associated with maxillofacial osteomyelitis and osteonecrosis in dogs and cats. Cytological evaluation of lesions in dogs and cats with maxillofacial osteonecrosis may be particularly helpful in the diagnosis of mycotic infections (Fig. 53.2).

Osteoradionecrosis occurs when maxillofacial osteonecrosis occurs as a complication of radiation therapy in the treatment oral tumors. In these cases, the surgical treatment becomes more complicated since the integrity of the surgical site is compromised. The long-term effects of radiotherapy to the oral mucosa are characterized by a predisposition to breakdown and delayed healing, even after minor insult.[2] Oral surgery in animals with osteoradionecrosis, including repair of oronasal fistulas and surgical extractions, may result in dehiscence of the surgical site and progressive extension of the osteonecrosis in spite of aggressive attempts at surgical and medical management (Fig. 53.3). Minor trauma to previously irradiated oral mucosa may create ulcerations that take weeks or months to heal and may be difficult to differentiate from recurrent malignant disease.[2] The persistence of local neoplasia with associated necrotic bone remains a possibility, as does the potential for distant metastasis. The progressive nature of osteoradionecrosis can be a complicating factor in the management of patients following radiation therapy for maxillofacial tumors. The bone within the radiation beam becomes virtually nonvital from an endarteritis that results in elimination of the fine vasculature within the bone.[2] The turnover rate of any remaining viable bone is slowed to the point of being ineffective in self-repair.[2] The bone of the mandible is denser and has a poorer blood supply than that of the maxilla,

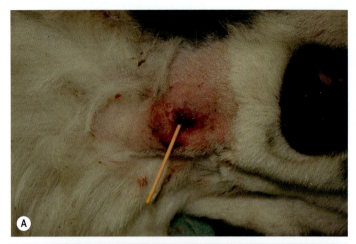

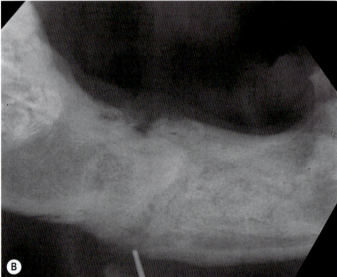

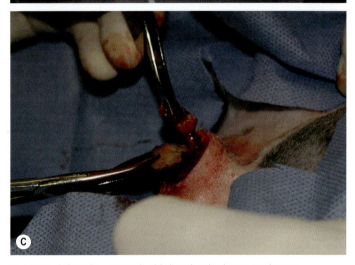

Fig. 53.1 (**A**) In this 6-month-old dog that had sustained severe mandibular trauma from a dog bite at 8 weeks of age, a gutta-percha point has been placed in a cutaneous draining tract at the right caudal mandible. (**B**) Dental radiographs of the right mandible revealed a bone sequestrum ventral to the mandible and adjacent to the gutta-percha point. (**C**) An incision was made around the margins of the cutaneous draining tract and the sequestrum was located and removed.

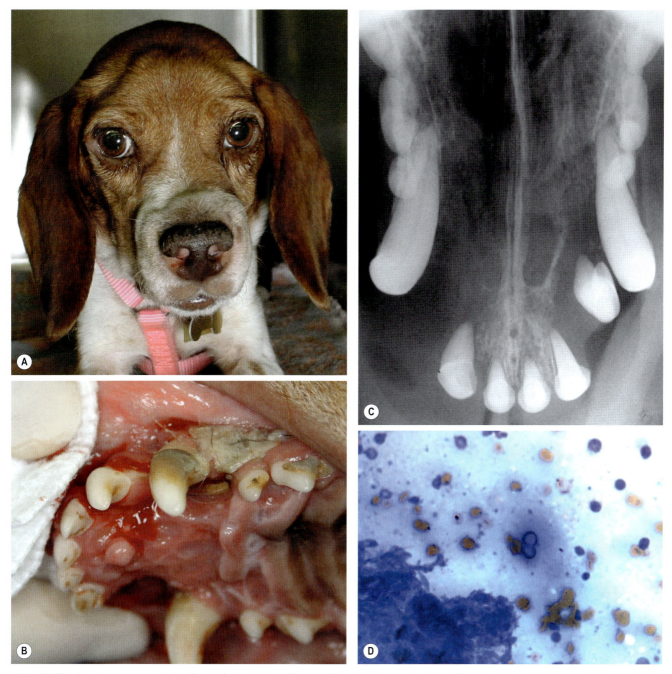

Fig. 53.2 (A) This beagle was presented with painful rostral maxillary swelling of unknown duration. **(B)** Intraoral examination revealed necrotic bone in the region of the canine tooth with loss of normal mucosal integrity. **(C)** Severe rostral maxillary bone lysis was evident on a maxillary occlusal radiograph. **(D)** An impression smear of an incisional biopsy of the abnormal mucosa revealed budding organisms consistent with blastomycosis.

causing the mandible to be the most commonly affected maxillofacial region with nonhealing mucosal ulcerations and osteoradionecrosis.[2]

Idiopathic maxillofacial osteonecrosis (maxillofacial osteonecrosis of unknown etiology) occurs infrequently and has been previously described in dogs (Fig. 53.4).[3,4] A disproportionate number of cocker spaniels have been reported with bone sequestra and osteomyelitis of unknown etiology.[3] Other breeds may also be affected with this condition. The potential for recurrence of osteonecrosis exists, in either the same location or other sites in the mandible or maxilla, in patients previously treated for idiopathic maxillofacial osteonecrosis (Fig. 53.5).

GENERAL PRINCIPLES IN THE SURGICAL MANAGEMENT OF MAXILLOFACIAL OSTEONECROSIS

The general principles of the surgical management of maxillofacial bone sequestra and osteomyelitis have been previously described.[4] The initial step in the surgical management of maxillofacial osteonecrosis is the appropriate surgical approach. The approach typically involves a large mucoperiosteal flap surrounding the area of

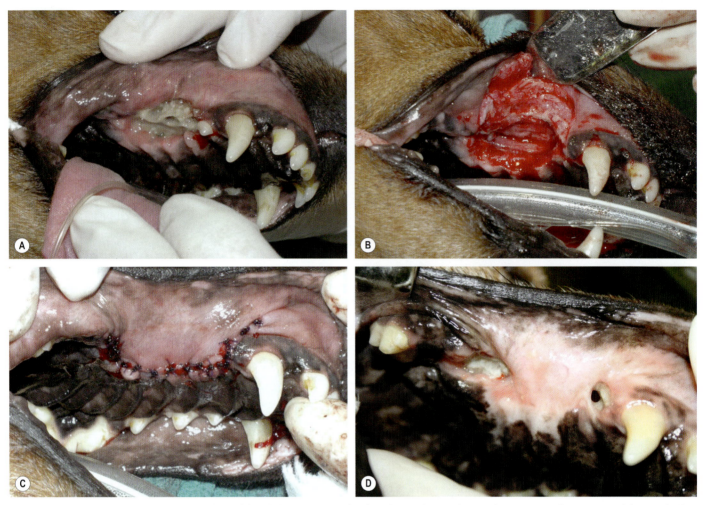

Fig. 53.3 Osteoradionecrosis in an 11-year-old dachshund that was treated with radiation therapy for nasal squamous cell carcinoma. (**A**) Note the loss of oral mucosa and exposed, necrotic bone. (**B**) A large buccal mucoperiosteal flap has been created. (**C**) Following removal of the underlying necrotic bone and the maxillary first premolar tooth, the buccal mucoperiosteal flap was sutured without tension to close the oronasal fistula. (**D**) Two months postoperatively, extension of the osteoradionecrosis and recurrence of oronasal fistulas at the mesial and distal aspects of the previous surgical site were evident.

osteonecrosis. In most cases, either a draining tract (mucosal or cutaneous), cleft in the mucosa or the complete separation of the mucosa from teeth with exposure of underlying necrotic bone is evident. An incision is made around the defect, thereby debriding the edges of the draining tract, cleft or edges of the mucosa separated from the underlying necrotic bone. Any remaining teeth located in the necrotic bone are extracted. The underlying necrotic bone is removed either en bloc (if not attached to the surrounding bone) or with a rongeur until all necrotic bone is removed. Alternatively, a partial mandibulectomy or maxillectomy may be performed to remove all abnormal bone. Debridement is adequate when the remaining bone appears normal and bleeds readily. Intraoperative fungal and aerobic and anaerobic bacterial culture and sensitivity testing is performed. Tissue is submitted for cytologic and histopathologic examination to rule out an underlying neoplasia and to facilitate in the detection of infectious agents. The area is liberally flushed with sterile saline and the mucoperiosteal flap is closed without tension in a simple interrupted pattern with monofilament absorbable suture material. Skin incisions are closed routinely with a nonabsorbable suture material in a simple interrupted pattern.

POSTOPERATIVE CARE AND ASSESSMENT

Broad-spectrum antibiotic therapy, such as amoxicillin-clavulanic acid is initiated until bacterial culture and sensitivity results are available. Antibiotic therapy based on results of bacterial culture and sensitivity testing should be continued for a minimum of 6–8 weeks. Nonsteroidal antiinflammatory medications and other analgesics are also recommended to help manage postoperative swelling and pain.

COMPLICATIONS

Complications associated with the surgical management of maxillofacial osteonecrosis include: local recurrence and progression of the maxillofacial osteonecrosis in spite of aggressive surgical debridement, or the development of osteonecrosis in other areas of the maxilla or mandible. Recurrence of oronasal fistulas from mucoperiosteal flap dehiscence is also a potential complication.

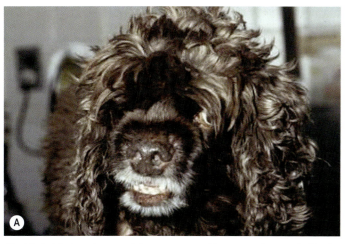
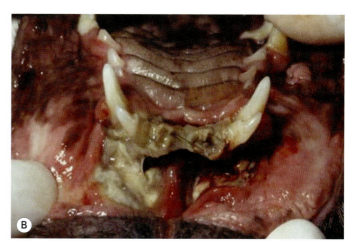

Fig. 53.4 (**A**) A cocker spaniel was presented because of severe halitosis and painful rostral maxillary swelling. (**B**) Note the osteonecrosis present in the region of the missing first and second incisors and the alveolar bone of the third incisors and canine teeth.

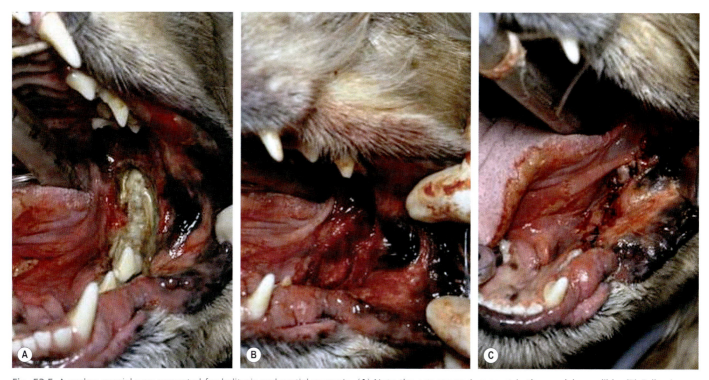

Fig. 53.5 A cocker spaniel was presented for halitosis and partial anorexia. (**A**) Note the osteonecrosis present in the caudal mandible. (**B**) Following thorough curettage of the overlying necrotic bone, healthy, bleeding bone is exposed. (**C**) A mucoperiosteal flap is then created to cover the debrided bone.

When the cause of the maxillofacial osteonecrosis is associated with trauma or traumatic surgical extractions, recurrence is less likely if all bony sequestra are removed during initial debridement. When maxillofacial osteonecrosis occurs as a complication of radiation therapy, the risk of recurrence of local osteonecrosis increases. The development of maxillofacial osteonecrosis at other sites may be a potential complication in dogs presented for idiopathic maxillofacial osteonecrosis.

The incidence of oronasal fistula dehiscence repair following the surgical treatment of maxillofacial osteonecrosis is greatest in animals previously treated with radiation therapy for maxillary or nasal tumors. In these cases, in spite of aggressive debridement of nonvital bone, the disease process often progresses into surrounding bone, resulting in local recurrence. This may be associated with progressive radiation osteonecrosis, local tumor recurrence or both.

PROGNOSIS

The prognosis for animals presented with maxillofacial osteonecrosis largely depends on the initial cause of the osteonecrosis. For cases in which the cause of the maxillofacial osteonecrosis is traumatic, the prognosis is generally excellent following appropriate surgical and medical management. For cancer patients with osteoradionecrosis, the prognosis is generally fair to guarded. The prognosis in animals with idiopathic osteonecrosis is fair to good following appropriate surgical and medical management.

REFERENCES

1. Watts N, Marciani R. Osteonecrosis of the jaw. Southern Medical Journal 2008; 101:160–5.
2. Ellis E. Management of the patient undergoing radiotherapy or chemotherapy. In: Peterson LJ, Ellis E, Hupp JR, et al, editors. Contemporary oral and maxillofacial surgery. 4th ed. St. Louis, MO: Mosby; 2003. p. 405–16.
3. Manfra Marretta S, Brine E, Smith C, et al. Idiopathic mandibular and maxillary osteomyelitis and bone sequestra in cocker spaniels. Proc Vet Dent Forum 1997;119.
4. Manfra Marretta S. Maxillofacial surgery. Vet Clin North Am Small Anim Pract 1998;28:1285–96.
5. Assouline-Dayan Y, Chang C, Greenspan A, et al. Pathogenesis and natural history of osteonecrosis. Semin Arthritis Rheum 2002;32:94–124.
6. Pillai KG, Nayar K, Rawal YB. Spontaneous tooth exfoliation, maxillary osteomyelitis and facial scarring following trigeminal herpes zoster infection. Prim Dent Care 2006;13:114–16.
7. Siwamogsthan P, Kuansuwan C, Reichart P. Herpes zoster in HIV infection with osteonecrosis of the jaw and tooth exfoliation. Oral Dis 2006;12:500–5.
8. Meer S, Coleman H, Altini M, et al. Mandibular osteomyelitis and tooth exfoliation following zoster-CMV co-infection. Oral Surg Oral Med Oral Pathol Oral Radiol Endod 2006;101:70–5.
9. Ruggiero SL, Mehrotra B, Rosenberg TJ, et al. Osteonecrosis of the jaws associated with the use of bisphosphonates: a review of 63 cases. J Oral Maxillofac Surg 2004;62:527–34.

10. Landesberg R, Wilson T, Grbic J. Bisphosphonate-associated osteonecrosis of the jaw: conclusions based on an analysis of case series. Dent Today 2006;25:54–7.
11. Marx R, Sawatari Y, Fortin M, et al. Bisphosphonate-induced exposed bone (osteonecrosis/osteopetrosis) of the jaws: risk factors, recognition, prevention, and treatment. J Oral Maxillofac Surg 2005; 63:1567–75.
12. Peterson LJ. Odontogenic infections. In: Peterson LJ, editor. Contemporary oral and maxillofacial surgery. 3rd ed. St. Louis, MO: Mosby; 1998. p. 426–8.
13. Store G, Olsen I. Scanning and transmission electron microscopy demonstrates bacteria in osteoradionecrosis. Int J Oral Maxillofac Surg 2005;34:777–81.
14. Queen J, Bennet D, Carmichael S, et al. Femoral neck metaphyseal osteopathy in the cat. Vet Rec 1998;142:159–62.
15. Myers T, Cui Q, Kuskowski M, et al. Outcomes of total and unicompartmental arthroplasty for secondary and spontaneous osteonecrosis of the knee. J Bone Joint Surg Am 2006;88:76–82.
16. Kim J, Finger D. Spontaneous osteonecrosis of the knee. J Rheumatol 2006;33:1416.
17. Lotke P, Nelson C, Lonner J. Spontaneous osteonecrosis of the knee: tibial plateaus. Orthop Clin North Am 2004;35:365–70.
18. Specchiulli F, Mele M, Capocasale N, et al. The early diagnosis of idiopathic femoral osteonecrosis. Ital J Orthop Traumatol 1988;14:519–26.

19. Sugano N, Atsumi T, Ohzono K, et al. The 2001 revised criteria for diagnosis, classification, and staging of idiopathic osteonecrosis of the femoral head. J Orthop Sci 2002;7:601–5.
20. Koo K, Lee J, Lee Y, et al. Endothelial nitric oxide synthase gene polymorphisms in patients with nontraumatic femoral head osteonecrosis. J Orthop Res 2006; 24:1722–8.
21. Séguin C, Kassis J, Busque L, et al. Non-traumatic necrosis of bone (osteonecrosis) is associated with endothelial cell activation but not thrombophilia. Rheumatology 2008;47:1151–5.
22. Magremanne M, Vervaet C, Dufrasne L, et al. Avascular mandibular necrosis. Rev Stomatol Chir Maxillofac 2007;108: 539–42.
23. Pogrel MA. Bisphosphonates and bone necrosis. J Oral Maxillofac Surg 2004;62: 391–2.
24. Chiandussi S, Biasotto M, Dore F, et al. Clinical and diagnostic imaging of bisphosphonate-associated osteonecrosis of the jaws. Dentomaxillofac Radiol 2006;35:236–43.
25. Tomlin JL, Sturgeon C, Pead MJ, et al. Use of the bisphosphonate drug alendronate for palliative management of osteosarcoma in two dogs. Vet Rec 2000;147:129–32.
26. Lee L. Inflammatory Lesions of the Jaws. In: White SC, editor. Oral radiology, principles and interpretation. 5th ed. Philadelphia, PA: Mosby; 2004. p. 374–80.

Chapter 54

Management of unerupted teeth

Loïc F.J. Legendre

DEFINITIONS

Embedded tooth: a tooth that is unerupted, usually because of a lack of eruptive force[1]

Extrusion: movement of a tooth in a coronal direction

Impacted tooth: a tooth that is prevented from erupting by some physical barrier in the eruption path, such as crowding from adjacent teeth[1,2]

Operculectomy: excision of the soft tissue overlying an unerupted tooth

Operculum: oral mucosa overlying an unerupted tooth

Pericoronitis: inflammation of the operculum overlying an unerupted tooth or around the crown of a partially erupted tooth

The term unerupted includes both impacted and embedded teeth. An embedded tooth is unerupted usually because of a lack of eruptive force.[1] An impacted tooth is prevented from erupting by some physical barrier in the eruption path, such as crowding from adjacent teeth.[1,2] Impaction is the most common condition.[2] It may lead to root resorption, root dilaceration, pericoronitis, jaw fracture, formation of odontogenic cysts and tumors.[2] A tooth may stop erupting without being blocked by another tooth but rather by a bone shelf and thickened gingiva not being resorbed properly (Fig. 54.1A).[3]

Corrective treatment is divided into three steps: surgical exposure, attachment to tooth, and orthodontic movement to bring tooth into position.[4] Surgical exposure typically entails an operculectomy, the surgical removal of the often thickened oral mucosa overlying an unerupted tooth.[2,5,6] The orthodontic movements required to realign an unerupted tooth may be complex, and orthodontic treatment typically includes extrusion, which means that the tooth is slowly moved in an axial direction out of its alveolus.[4]

SURGICAL ANATOMY

Location of an unerupted tooth

Preoperative planning and choice of surgical approach are based on the location of the unerupted tooth. It is sometimes difficult to ascertain the exact location of the affected tooth, and preoperative radiographs are essential. Two techniques are commonly utilized: the vertical and the horizontal tube shift techniques. These techniques are based on the principle that the movement of an image in relation to a reference object is dependent on the change in angulation of the X-ray beam. With the horizontal shift technique, the X-ray tube is moved mesiodistally on a horizontal plane, moving the affected tooth in the same direction as the tube shift when palatally impacted, and in the opposite direction when labially impacted. With the vertical shift technique, the vertical angulation of the X-ray tube is altered. The tooth located farthest from the X-ray beam will be moved in the direction opposite to the beam (Fig. 54.2). Either technique requires at least two radiographs to determine the exact position of the affected tooth.[3,7,8] Accurate localization is crucial for approaching the tooth with minimal damage to the surrounding structures.

THERAPEUTIC DECISION-MAKING

Treatment options for unerupted teeth include extraction, attempts to allow normal eruption or orthodontic movement of the teeth. The decision as to which option to take depends on several factors. Age is of prime importance. When dealing with deciduous teeth, careful neglect under close observation is indicated only until the adult teeth are due to erupt. Immature impacted teeth will sometime conveniently erupt unaided once the obstruction is removed. This happens very rarely once root formation is complete.[4] Adult impacted teeth should be treated before complications arise.[2] The type of tooth will also affect the decision; a functionally important tooth warrants more effort to save it, and extrusion would then be recommended. Surgical exposure and orthodontic treatment amount to a lengthy, complex procedure that is rarely undertaken in veterinary dentistry. Presence of complicating factors similarly affects the outcome. Reasons for extracting as opposed to moving teeth are: (1) existing lesions or pain from pericoronitis, periodontitis, periapical abscess, cyst or neoplasm, impingement on and external resorption of adjacent teeth, and inflammation; (2) abnormal, dysplastic teeth; (3) aberrant position making it impossible to move the affected tooth; and (4) lack of space for the unerupted tooth to move into.[4] Extraction is contraindicated

DOI: 10.1016/B978-0-7020-4618-6.00054-3

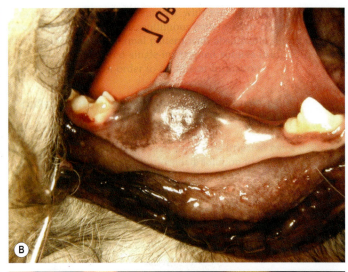

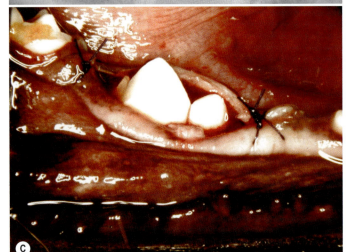

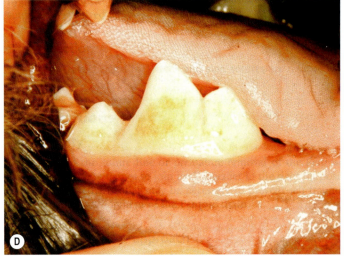

Fig. 54.1 (**A**) Radiograph of a right mandibular first molar tooth in a 7-month-old dog impacted under a thin shelf of bone. Clinically, a thick layer of keratinized tissue overlying the tooth was present. (**B**) Right mandibular first molar tooth impacted under a cover of gingiva. (**C**) Two-thirds of the crown of the mandibular right first molar tooth are exposed following gingivectomy. Note that more than 2 mm of attached gingiva is left around the impacted crown. (**D**) The tooth has erupted spontaneously. One month after being exposed, it is in its anatomic position and requires no further treatment. Note that the full crown is now exposed.

if it carries greater risks than potential benefits, if the medical status of the patient is compromised, and if extraction can result in extensive damage to adjacent structures.[2] Often, secondary lesions are present at time of diagnosis and the operator needs to be prepared to deal with complications such as cyst or tumor formation that will necessitate an en-bloc excision rather than simple extraction. The algorithm in Figure 54.3 summarizes the correct decision-making process.

SURGICAL TECHNIQUES

Surgical exposure

A surgical approach is necessary to expose the crown of the tooth before orthodontically moving it. Various procedures have been described, depending on the depth of the impaction. In cases of shallow impaction when only keratinized tissue is covering the tooth (see Fig. 54.1B), an operculectomy is indicated. Exposure of one-half to two-thirds of the crown is sufficient. A minimum of 2 mm of

attached gingiva is left at the base of the treated tooth to prevent gingival recession (see Fig. 54.1C).[3,9] If there is little attached gingiva present, an apically positioned flap procedure is preferred to preserve the maximum amount of keratinized tissue. Because the gingiva present is often thicker than normal, a partial-thickness flap is recommended to correct this problem. Once the crown of the tooth is exposed, the flap is sutured in a more apical position.

In cases where the tooth is deeper, an open eruption technique or a closed eruption technique is used. The open eruption technique consists of an apically-positioned flap combined with an ostectomy. Half to two-thirds of the crown is exposed before reattaching the flap. Exposing the crown down to the cemento-enamel junction leads to periodontal attachment loss following orthodontic treatment.[10] An attachment device, such as a small button or a hook, is then bonded to the crown to commence the orthodontic part of the treatment.[4] The closed technique is reserved for deep impactions or where an apically-positioned flap is impractical. It consists of making an alveolar margin incision over the location of the tooth (see Fig. 54.2C). Vertical incisions are extended mesially and distally to allow exposure of the area without tearing the flap. Bone is removed to expose enough of the

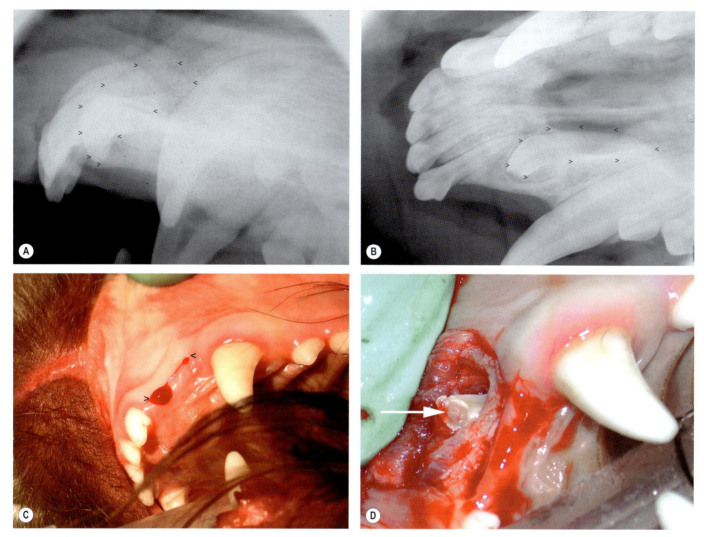

Fig. 54.2 (**A**) First view of a vertical tube shift technique to localize the impacted incisor tooth. The tube is nearly horizontal in alignment. (**B**) Second view, the tube is moved ventrally and the tooth that is furthest from the tube moves in the same direction. (**C**) A mid-marginal incision is made over the area of the impacted tooth. (**D**) An osteoplasty is performed to expose half to two-thirds of the crown. The arrow shows where the attachment will be bonded to the crown to facilitate extrusion of the tooth.

crown to bond an attachment connected to a traction wire (see Fig. 54.2D). The flap is sutured back in place and the wire exits through the incision. This ensures that the tooth will erupt through attached gingiva. If the tooth erupts through oral mucosa, it will be periodontally compromised.[4]

Orthodontic management

Before starting the surgical exposure, the operator should make sure that there is sufficient space for the tooth to be extruded into. If the space does not exist, it must be created prior to exposing the impacted tooth. When the impaction is shallow, an immature tooth may complete its eruption without aid (see Fig. 54.1D).[3,4] Orthodontic treatment may only be necessary to tip it into its correct position. When the impaction is deeper, the orthodontic treatment consists of two phases: extrusion and final placement. Traction is applied to the affected tooth using an elastic chain and adjacent teeth as anchor. Sometimes, a rigid arm is created to direct the force on the tooth in the appropriate direction. The arm also increases the range of movement and the consistency of the force applied.[4] Extrusion by means

of a small magnet bonded to the crown of the impacted tooth and a larger anchor magnet incorporated into an acrylic appliance has been used in humans.[4,11] Extrusion requires light forces, similar to those used in tipping movements.[4] Once erupted, the tooth is moved or tipped by orthodontic means; once the tooth is in place, a retainer is indicated to prevent relapse.[4]

Extraction of unerupted teeth

A surgical extraction technique is used for the extraction of unerupted teeth. This must be carefully planned, given the fact that the tooth may be covered by a considerable amount of bone, its anatomical location may be abnormal, and its shape may be distorted. A wide pedicle or triangle flap is indicated to obtain adequate exposure. The amount of bone removal should be sufficient to allow atraumatic delivery of the tooth, taking care not to weaken the jaw bone unduly. This may be challenging, especially when extracting an unerupted mandibular canine or first molar tooth. If cystic changes surrounding the unerupted tooth are apparent, the soft tissue lining must be completely removed and submitted for histopathological examination.

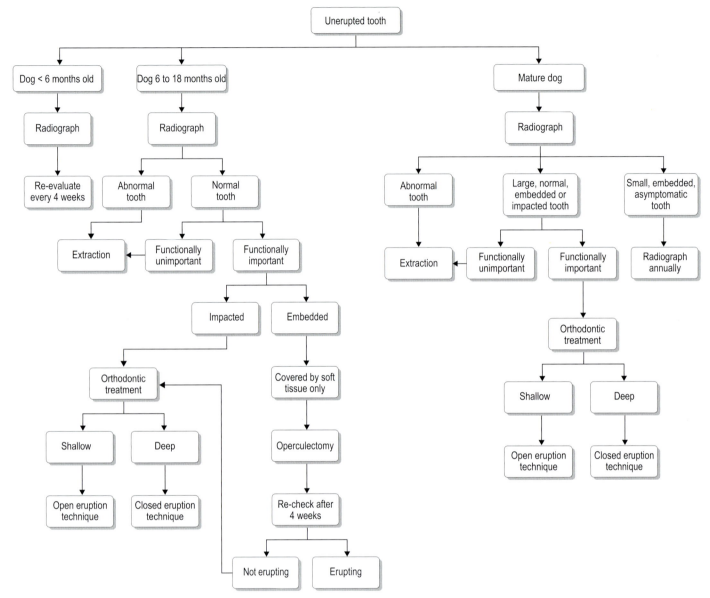

Fig. 54.3 Algorithm depicting the decision-making process when faced with an unerupted tooth.

Bone grafting may be indicated to promote healing of the alveolectomy site.

POSTOPERATIVE CARE

Pain management is very important but routine (see Ch. 4). The client is instructed to observe for postoperative signs of swelling, bleeding, discoloration and inappetence. It is essential for the client to keep the surgical area clean at all times. This is achieved by daily, gentle cleaning of the area using toothpaste or mouthwash and a toothbrush or a cotton swab. Debris, plaque and calculus deposition will interfere with healing and may result in severe inflammation that can lead to dehiscence and failure of the procedure. The patient is examined at 5 to 7 days postoperatively to ascertain that the flap is healing correctly.

COMPLICATIONS

Three types of complications are encountered: intraoperative, postoperative and complications associated with the orthodontic treatment. Intraoperative complications include hemorrhage, damage to the unerupted crown, fracture of tooth and fracture of adjacent bone. Postoperative complications include dehiscence of suture line, flap necrosis and infection of surgical site. Some complications are specific to the orthodontic treatment. Lack of movement may be due to ankylosis of the unerupted tooth, which should have been diagnosed prior to treatment by gently luxating the tooth following exposure. Trying to move an ankylosed tooth is impossible and would cause the anchor teeth to tip.[3,4] Most common are the periodontal problems associated with the extruded tooth. Unless an adequate band of keratinized tissue is left attached around the base of the crown, the incidence of attachment loss, gingival recession and inflammation is high.

Extrusion and further orthodontic movement have been found to result in impairment of the pulpal blood flow and subsequent necrosis in over 20% of human patients.[12] Endodontic treatment is required to correct this complication. Damage to the orthodontic appliance is also a common complication. Alterations to the design of the appliance may be necessary to prevent repeat breakage. Vertical relapse may occur and an appropriate method and length of retention should be included in the treatment plan.

REFERENCES

1. Shafer WG, Hine MK, Levy BM. Developmental disturbances of oral and paraoral structures. In: Shafer WG, Hine MK, Levy BM, editors. A textbook of oral pathology. 4th ed. Philadelphia, PA: W.B. Saunders; 1983. p. 2–85.

2. Peterson LJ, Ellis III E, Hupp JR, et al, editors. Contemporary oral and maxillofacial surgery. 2nd ed. St Louis, MO: Mosby; 1993.

3. Jarjoura K, Crespo P, Fine JB. Maxillary canine impactions: orthodontic and surgical management. Compend Contin Educ Dent 2002; 23:23–40.

4. Proffit WR, Fields HW, Ackerman JL, et al. Contemporary orthodontics. 2nd ed. St. Louis, MO: Mosby; 1993.

5. Wiggs RB, Lobprise HB. Veterinary dentistry principles and practice. Philadelphia, PA: Lippincott-Raven; 1997. p. 235.

6. Boucher CO, Zwemer TJ. Boucher's clinical dental terminology – a glossary of accepted terms in all disciplines of dentistry. 4th ed. St. Louis, MO: Mosby; 1993.

7. Jacobs SG. Localization of the unerupted maxillary canine: how to and when to. Am J Orthod Dentofacial Orthop 1999; 115:314–22.

8. Jacobs SG. Radiographic localization of unerupted teeth: further findings about the vertical tube shift method and other localization techniques. Am J Orthod Dentofacial Orthop 2000;118:439–47.

9. Pini Prato G, Bacetti T, Magnani C, et al. Mucogingival interceptive surgery of bucally-erupted premolars in patients scheduled for orthodontic treatment. J Periodontol 2000;71:172–81.

10. Quirynen M, Op Heij DG, Adriansens A, et al. Periodontal health of orthodontically extruded impacted teeth. A split-mouth long-term evaluation. J Periodontol 2000; 71:1708–14.

11. Sandler JP. An attractive solution to unerupted teeth. Am J Orthod Dentofacial Orthop 1991;100:489–93.

12. Woloshyn H, Artun J, Kennedy DB, et al. Pulpal and periodontal reactions to orthodontic alignment of palatally impacted canines. Angle Orthod 1994; 64:257–64.

Chapter 55

Temporomandibular joint dysplasia

Gary C. Lantz

DEFINITIONS

Dysplasia is an abnormal development of tissue.[1] Temporomandibular joint (TMJ) dysplasia is an infrequently reported condition that results in subluxation and subsequent lateral and/or rostral shifting of the mandibles which usually allows abnormal contact of a coronoid process with the adjacent zygomatic arch. Dysplasia of the TMJ may involve abnormalities of the bone and/or soft tissues.[2] The resulting clinical findings are intermittent episodes of inability to voluntarily close the mouth, or joint sensitivity without locking episodes.

BACKGROUND

Temporomandibular joint dysplasia and the surgical correction of open-mouth jaw locking by partial zygomatic arch resection was originally reported in an Irish setter by Stewart, Baker and Lee in 1975.[3] Robbins and Grandage reported the condition and similar surgical correction in two basset hounds and proposed a mechanism of jaw locking.[4] These and subsequent reports suggest a breed predisposition toward basset hounds and Irish setters, although the condition has been reported in several dog breeds and in cats.[2,5–9] Radiographic evidence of TMJ dysplasia in six related cocker spaniels suggested a genetic component.[10] Bennett and Prymak presented three cases treated by mandibular condylectomy.[5] Lobprise and Wiggs discussed surgical treatment in a cat using partial zygomatic arch excision and height reduction of the adjacent coronoid process.[9] Open-mouth jaw locking has been reported possibly resulting from malocclusion-induced TMJ soft tissue laxity.[11,12]

FUNCTIONAL ANATOMY OF THE TEMPOROMANDIBULAR JOINT[4,13,14]

The TMJ is a synovial joint. The head of the mandible (*caput mandibulae*) on the condylar process (*processus condylaris*) articulates with the mandibular fossa (*fossa mandibularis*) of the squamous part of the temporal bone. An articular disk separates the fossa and articular surface of the head of the mandible. The disk attaches laterally to the head and medially to the temporal bone by ligamentous extensions. Capsular attachments to the disk are found circumferentially. The lateral aspect of the joint capsule is strengthened by the lateral temporomandibular ligament. This ligament originates from the caudoventral aspect of the zygomatic arch and inserts on the lateral aspect of the condylar process and retroarticular process. Each mandible rotates about a common transverse axis that passes through the center of each condylar process. The long axis of each condylar process is, generally, nearly parallel to the transverse axis, although specific breed studies of this relationship are lacking. This relationship results in a small angle between the axis of rotation and long axis. The medial aspect of the mandibular head is seated firmly in the fossa during full-range opening. The lateral aspect of the mandibular head moves in a rostral and ventral arc during mouth opening. At maximal jaw opening, the joint capsule and lateral ligament are tense. The masseter, temporalis and pterygoid muscles hold the condylar process tight in the fossa. There is a small amount of lateral movement that occurs during mastication which is limited by the TMJ ligaments and normal occlusal relationship of the caudal maxillary and mandibular teeth.

PATHOPHYSIOLOGY

Temporomandibular joint abnormalities may be unilateral or bilateral, and include a shallow mandibular fossa, flattened mandibular head, abnormal obliquity of the mandibular head and fossa, and joint capsule and ligamentous laxity.[2–7] A large angle between the axis of rotation and long axis of the mandibular head suggests an abnormal obliquity of the TMJ which results in excessive movement of the lateral aspect of the condylar process.[4] Stretching of the lateral ligament and capsule occurs. The joint incongruity and soft tissue laxity results in subluxation of the involved joint and contralateral shifting on the mandibles.[4] The contralateral coronoid process contacts the ventral aspect of the adjacent zygomatic arch or moves lateral to the arch. The resulting mechanical interference with the coronoid process motion prevents mouth

DOI: 10.1016/B978-0-7020-4618-6.00055-5

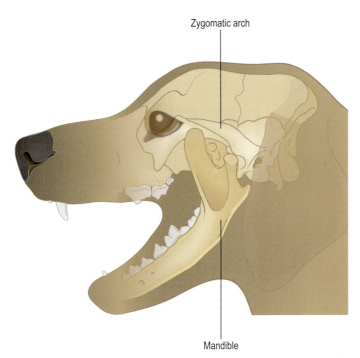

Zygomatic arch

Mandible

Fig. 55.1 The coronoid process is displaced lateral to the zygomatic arch as a result of a dysplastic contralateral temporomandibular joint. The lower jaw is locked in an open position.

closure (Fig. 55.1). Variable severity of TMJ dysplasia apparently occurs, which may account for the variable age of onset, frequency and duration of open-mouth locking episodes, and inconsistent radiographic findings.[2] The lax TMJ(s) may allow rostral displacement of the coronoid process(es) such that the rostral dorsal aspect of the process contacts the junction area of the zygomatic and maxillary bones when the mouth is opened. The abnormal bone contact may result in locking episodes or only clinical signs related to oral sensitivity. It is possible that these clinical signs may be due to an abnormally tall coronoid process(es) with or without concurrent TMJ dysplasia.

CLINICAL PRESENTATION

Signalment and history

Age of onset ranges from approximately 6 months to 5 years. The initial observation of clinical signs often starts in young adults.[2–9,12] Observed locking episodes may occur multiple times daily or occasionally over several weeks or months. Most dogs will vocalize, shake the head, paw at the muzzle and rub the muzzle on the ground until the locking is spontaneously reduced. Cats may seek seclusion. Most locking episodes are of short duration and corrected by spontaneous reduction. This reduction occurs by opening the mouth wider, thereby allowing the coronoid process to disengage the zygomatic arch. Failure of spontaneous reduction results in the client seeking medical care for the animal. There is usually no history of trauma. However, healed depressed fractures of the zygomatic arch may interfere with the movement of the coronoid process and produce locking episodes that mimic those caused by TMJ dysplasia.[2] Slow deliberate mastication and a change from hard to soft food may be reported, and may be caused by TMJ sensitivity secondary to degenerative joint disease and/or from contact of the rostrodorsal aspect of the coronoid process with the zygomatic and maxillary bone junction area.

Physical examination

Examination of a patient that has spontaneously reduced the locked jaw may reveal no abnormalities. Resistance to head palpation and manipulation of the lower jaw may be noted. Neurological evaluation of the cranial nerves yields no abnormalities. Chronic oral sensitivity may result in visible temporal muscle disuse atrophy.[5] Examination during an open-mouth lock episode finds an open mouth and a patient very resistant to manipulation of the lower jaw. A palpable and usually visible bulge on the side of the face is present when the coronoid process is displaced ventrally or laterally to the zygomatic arch. The lower jaw is shifted toward the side where the lock has occurred and is tilted such that the mandibular body on the lock side is displaced slightly ventral compared to the opposite mandibular body.

Manipulation of the mandibles

Open-mouth locking can usually be reproduced by manipulation of the lower jaw.[2] After induction of general anesthesia and endotracheal intubation, the patient is placed in left lateral recumbency. The mouth is widely opened to see whether the lower jaw tends to shift toward one side. Laterally directed digital pressure is placed on the medial aspect of the right coronoid process and the jaw rotated counterclockwise to lower the right coronoid process ventral to the right zygomatic arch as the mouth is widely opened. The manipulation is repeated on the left side with the patient in right lateral recumbency and clockwise rotation of the mandible. Clinical experience suggests that successful displacement of the coronoid process to engage the ventral or lateral aspect of the adjacent zygomatic arch and create the lock on one side indicates laxity of the contralateral and/or ipsilateral side TMJ (Fig. 55.2). Locking cannot be recreated if joints are normal. Locking may not be recreated in every patient with a history of open-mouth locking episodes. It is important to manipulate the right and left sides even if a unilateral lock was observed in the awake patient, as bilateral TMJ dysplasia may be present that could result in alternating right and left locking episodes. Crepitus secondary to degenerative TMJ disease may be noted during manipulation. Manual reduction of open-mouth locking is accomplished by opening the mouth further, pressing the laterally displaced coronoid process in a medial direction then closing the mouth. It is possible that diagnostic manipulation of the mandible may not cause locking. However, the TMJ laxity is often apparent on manipulation and the coronoid process(es) may be displaced laterally to contact the ventral aspect of the zygomatic arch then slip medially when manipulation is stopped. Neither of these findings is present in normal animals.

The patient is then placed in dorsal recumbency to assess for contact between the rostrodorsal aspect of the coronoid process and zygomatic and maxilla bone junction. Opening the mouth with counterclockwise rotation of the mandible will cause the left coronoid process to contact the zygomatic and maxillary bone junction. Opening with clockwise rotation will test the right side. During this manipulation, intraoral digital palpation of the caudal maxilla immediately caudal to the second molar tooth may reveal crepitus, contact between the bone structures, or the vibration of contact and disengagement, all of which suggest TMJ dysplasia and possibly an abnormally tall coronoid process. The normal patient should exhibit no bone contact.

DIAGNOSTIC IMAGING

Radiographic findings

The radiographic anatomy and patient positioning for TMJ radiographs have been described.[15–19] Skull radiographs include

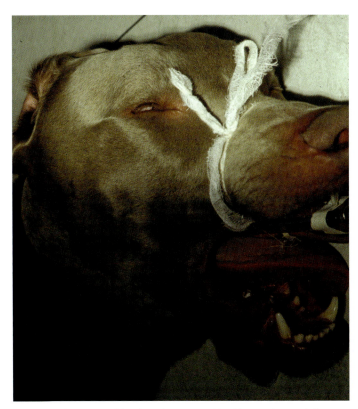

Fig. 55.2 Three-year-old male Weimaraner with a history of once-daily open-mouth jaw locking of 1-month duration. Each episode was spontaneously reduced. This photograph shows the patient with the mouth locked open after manual manipulation. Only a right side lock could be created. A right facial bulge is noted from the displaced right coronoid process. Right partial zygomatic arch resection prevented further locking episodes.

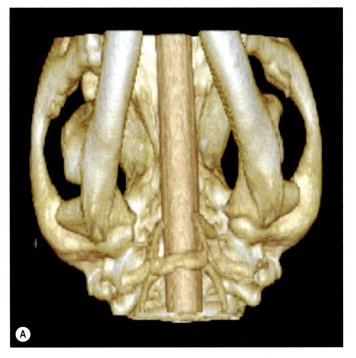

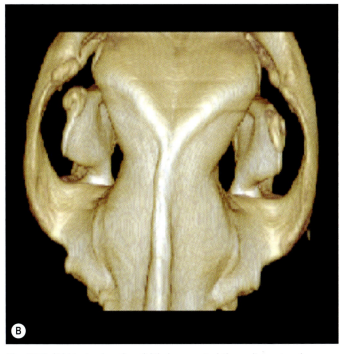

Fig. 55.3 (**A**) Ventrodorsal and (**B**) dorsoventral three-dimensional computed tomography reconstruction of a dog showing osteophyte production on the rostral aspect of each zygomatic arch and coronoid process.

ventrodorsal, lateral and open-mouth projections. Right and left lateral oblique projections are made to isolate each TMJ. Radiographic findings of TMJ dysplasia may include claw-shaped or widened joint spaces, flattened mandibular heads, short flattened mandibular fossae resulting in decreased coverage of the heads, increased obliquity of the condylar process long axis, and enlarged, hypoplastic or absent retro-articular processes.[2–7] Radiographic signs of degenerative joint disease may also be present.[5] Periosteal proliferation may be visible along the ventral margin of the involved zygomatic arch (Fig. 55.3).[2] Evidence of a zygomatic arch fracture may be present in patients with previous history of trauma. Radiographic findings may also be normal.[2,8] Radio-graphs made during a locking episode may reveal zygomatic arch and coronoid process contact (Fig. 55.4) and a widened joint space of the joint opposite to the locking side, or may not reveal any contact between the zygomatic arch and coronoid processes.[5] The latter finding suggests a possible TMJ internal derangement or possibly coronoid process contact with the caudal maxilla causing the locking.

Computed tomography and magnetic resonance imaging

Computed tomography for the diagnosis of TMJ dysplasia has been reported as a complement to radiographs[3,7,11,12] and may be of benefit when radiographic findings are normal in a patient with a history of locking episodes or oral sensitivity.[3,7] Advanced imaging may allow detection of subtle anatomic abnormalities and a comparison between both joints of one patient (see Figs 55.3 and 55.4). Computed tomographical anatomy for the canine TMJ has been described.[19,20]

In humans, magnetic resonance imaging is used to study TMJ function.[21]

SURGICAL ANATOMY[13,22]

The function of the zygomatic arch is protection of the eye, origin for the masseter and part of the temporal muscles, and to provide an

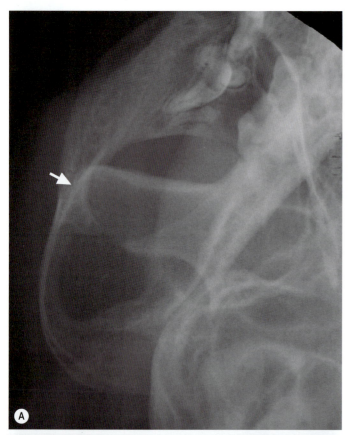

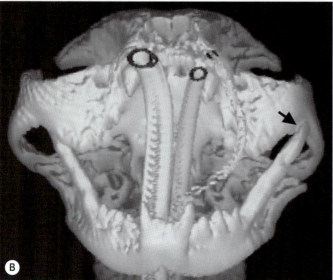

Fig. 55.4 (**A**) Ventrodorsal radiograph of a cat showing abnormal contact between the coronoid process and zygomatic arch with the mouth locked open. (**B**) Three-dimensional reconstruction of the cat showing left coronoid process and zygomatic arch contact. *(From: Reiter AM. Symphysiotomy, symphysiectomy, and intermandibular arthrodesis in a cat with open-mouth jaw locking – case report and literature review. J Vet Dent 2004;21:147–158)*

mandibular nerve and small branches of the transverse facial artery and vein cross the incision site. The superficial and middle layers of the masseter muscle originate along the ventral border of the zygomatic arch. The origin on the deep layer of the masseter muscle is intermingled with the lateral aspect of the temporal muscle. The temporal muscle inserts on the medial and lateral aspect of the coronoid process to surround the process. Its lateral ventral extent is the ventral aspect of the masseteric fossa. The muscle contacts the pterygoid muscles on the medial aspect of the coronoid process. The body of the masseter muscle lies in the masseteric fossa of the mandibular ramus. The rostral border of the coronoid process, the coronoid crest, is thick cortical bone.

THERAPEUTIC DECISION-MAKING

Differential diagnoses

Differential diagnoses include conditions that result in acute or chronic inability to completely close the mouth. These include traumatic unilateral or bilateral temporomandibular subluxation or luxation, mandibular fracture, oral foreign body, periodontal disease resulting in extrusion of a tooth with subsequent malocclusion, and trigeminal neuropraxia.

Surgical technique and unilateral or bilateral surgery

The goal of surgical treatment is to prevent further locking episodes. Partial zygomatic arch excision has been most commonly reported.[2–4,6–8] Mandibular condylectomy has also been described.[5] Unilateral partial arch excision is considered when (1) the clinical observation of an open-mouth locking episode with a facial bulge is duplicated by jaw manipulation that can only reproduce the same unilateral lock and facial bulge, and (2) history and diagnostic findings support a tentative diagnosis of open-mouth jaw locking and jaw manipulation that can only produce a unilateral lock (with or without a facial bulge). Bilateral surgery should be considered when (1) the history and diagnostic findings support a tentative diagnosis of open-mouth jaw locking, and jaw manipulation results in bilateral locking, and (2) the history and diagnostic findings support a tentative diagnosis and locking cannot be reproduced by jaw manipulation. Radiographic findings may or may not help with these decisions. Mandibular condylectomy is considered when locking is recreated but there is no evidence of zygomatic and coronoid process contact or of coronoid process and zygomatic arch/maxilla junction contact. Condylectomy is also performed when oral sensitivity and radiographic evidence of degenerative joint disease are present. Partial coronoidectomy is indicated for coronoid process height reduction when the history documents episodes of open-mouth jaw locking or behavior suggesting oral sensitivity and diagnostic mandible manipulation confirms contact between the process and junction of the zygomatic and maxillary bones. Clinical experience suggests that partial coronoidectomy may be more commonly indicated in brachycephalic dogs. Surgical decision-making is summarized in Figure 55.6.

SURGICAL TECHNIQUES

Partial zygomatic arch excision[3,4]

With the dog or cat in lateral recumbency, a skin and subcutaneous tissue incision is made along the rostroventral border of the zygomatic arch for approximately two-thirds of the arch length. Thin fiber

articulation for the mandible. The zygomatic arch is approached by an incision made along its ventral border (Fig. 55.5). The palpebral and dorsal buccal branches of the facial nerve lie near the dorsal and ventral borders of the zygomatic arch, respectively. The zygomatic and deep sphincter colli muscles, small sensory branches from the

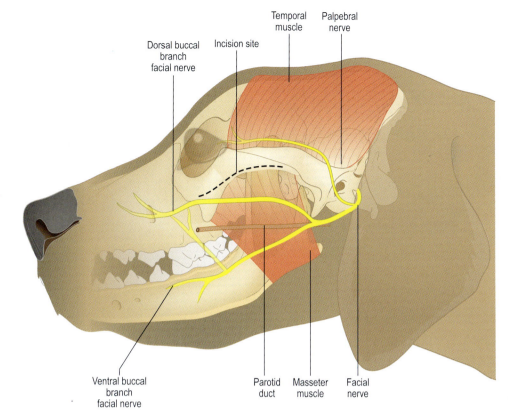

Fig. 55.5 Surgical anatomy for partial zygomatic arch resection. The incision (*dotted line*) is made along the ventral border of the arch.

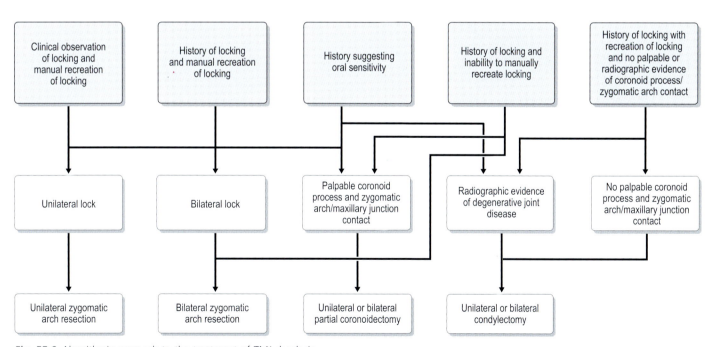

Fig. 55.6 Algorithmic approach to the treatment of TMJ dysplasia.

bundles of the zygomatic and deep sphincter colli muscles are incised. The mouth is opened and closed by a nonsterile assistant to allow the surgeon to observe the movement of the coronoid process evidenced by lateral displacement of the masseter muscle. The masseter fascia is incised at the muscle origin along the ventral arch border. The muscle is subperiosteally elevated and ventrally retracted.

Mouth opening and closing is performed as needed to help determine the extent of partial arch excision. Usually, ostectomy of the rostral one-half to two-thirds of the arch length and one-half to two-thirds of the arch height is sufficient. Ostectomy is performed using a rongeur, osteotome and mallet, or surgical handpiece with bur (Fig. 55.7). The ostectomy site is enlarged as needed, based on coronoid

535

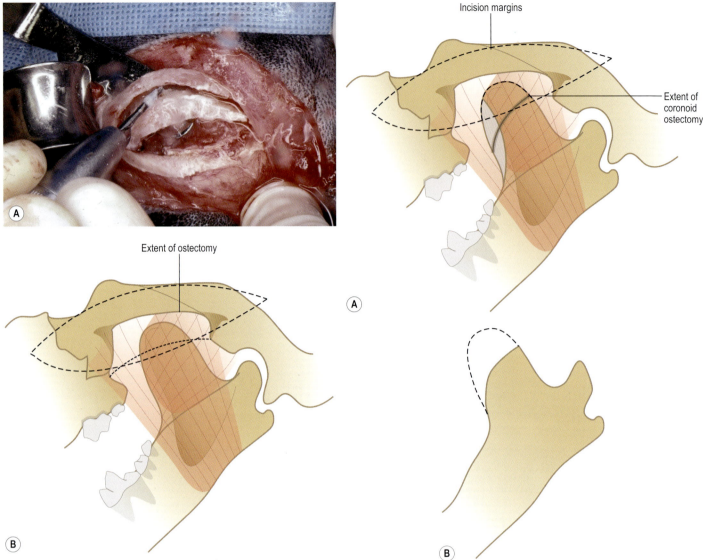

Fig. 55.7 (**A**) Partial zygomatic arch excision. (**B**) The rostral ventral aspect of the zygomatic arch is excised. The resection size is determined during surgery by lower jaw manipulation by a nonsterile assistant and should provide an unimpaired range of motion for the coronoid process.

Fig. 55.8 (**A**) The rostral extent of the partial zygomatic arch excision is the suture between the zygomatic bone and maxilla. Zygomatic arch excision is needed to provide adequate exposure for coronoid process height reduction. The temporal muscle is subperiosteally elevated from the process. (**B**) The extent of coronoid process height reduction is determined in surgery during manipulation of the mandible by a nonsterile assistant. The process is cut and the rostral border tapered in a caudodorsal direction.

process movement. The dorsal aspect of the ostectomy site is beveled in a dorsomedial direction. The lateral aspect of the coronoid process is covered by the blended deep layer of the masseter and temporal muscles. Local thickening and fibrosis of this muscle may be seen. The muscle has been chronically traumatized by compression between the process and arch. This fibrous tissue is left intact. The masseter fascia is apposed to the periosteal/fascia tissue covering the remaining zygomatic arch using horizontal mattress sutures. The subcutaneous tissue and skin are routinely closed.

Reduction of the coronoid process height

This procedure is performed in conjunction with partial zygomatic arch ostectomy to provide access to the coronoid process. It is considered if preoperative or intraoperative manipulation of the mandible reveals the coronoid process contacting or locking at the junction of the rostral arch and maxillary bone. Removal of this thicker maxillary

bone may injure pterygoid fossa neurovascular structures and caudal maxillary teeth. To avoid injury to these structures, the rostral extent of zygomatic arch resection should stop at the visible suture between the zygomatic and maxillary bones. Partial coronoid process excision will also avoid removal of the complete height of the zygomatic arch segment when a tall coronoid process is present.[9] Zygomatic arch function is maintained.

After partial zygomatic arch ostectomy, the fibers of the deep leaf of the masseter muscle are separated, temporal muscle fascia is incised parallel to the coronoid crest and temporal muscle fibers are longitudinally split immediately lateral to the coronoid crest. The muscles on the lateral aspect are subperiosteally elevated to expose the dorsal half of the coronoid process (Fig. 55.8A). The fibrous muscle insertion along the coronoid crest is incised and the temporal muscle is subperiosteally elevated from the medial aspect of the coronoid process. The appropriate height reduction of the process is determined by palpation during mandible manipulation by a nonsterile assistant. The bone is cut and separated from any remaining temporal muscle fiber attachments. The rostral aspect of the remaining coronoid process is tapered in a dorsocaudal direction (Fig. 55.8B). The temporal fascia is closed and the surgical site is closed as previously described.

Mandibular condylectomy

This procedure is discussed in Chapter 33.

POSTOPERATIVE CARE AND ASSESSMENT

Soft food is recommended and oral activity is limited to eating and drinking for the first 2 postoperative weeks. Thereafter, normal oral activity may resume.

COMPLICATIONS

A small seroma may develop at the surgery site secondary to jaw movement. These usually do not require treatment. If the entire height of the zygomatic arch is excised, some facial asymmetry may result, with the operated side appearing flatter compared to the normal side. Recurrence of locking episodes after a unilateral surgery indicates possible inadequate removal of zygomatic arch, inadequate reduction of coronoid process height, possible undetected bilateral disease and the need for surgery on the opposite side, or an initial misdiagnosis of the involved side. Results and complications of mandibular condylectomy are discussed in Chapter 33.

PROGNOSIS

The prognosis is generally good after unilateral surgery. Clients should be warned about possible undetected bilateral disease and the need for additional surgery should locking episodes recur. The prognosis is generally good with bilateral surgery. Long-term results do not indicate further clinical complications associated with the dysplastic temporomandibular joints.[2]

REFERENCES

1. Venes D, Thomas CL, editors. Taber's cyclopedic medical dictionary. 21st ed. Philadelphia, PA: FA Davis; 2001. p. 652.
2. Lantz GC, Cantwell HD. Intermittent open-mouth lower jaw locking in five dogs. J Am Vet Med Assoc 1986;188:1403–5.
3. Stewart WC, Baker GJ, Lee R. Temporomandibular subluxation in the dog: a case report. J Small Anim Pract 1975;16:345–9.
4. Robins G, Grandage J. Temporomandibular joint dysplasia and open-mouth jaw locking in the dog. J Am Vet Med Assoc 1977;171:1072–6.
5. Bennett D, Prymak C. Excision arthroplasty as a treatment for temporomandibular dysplasia. J Small Anim Pract 1986;27:361–70.
6. Johnson KA. Temporomandibular joint dysplasia in an Irish Setter. J Small Anim Pract 1979;20:209–18.
7. Thomas RE. Temporo-mandibular joint dysplasia and open-mouth jaw locking in Bassett Hound: a case report. J Small Anim Pract 1979;20:697–701.
8. Lantz GC. Intermittent open-mouth locking of the temporomandibular joint in a cat. J Am Vet Med Assoc 1987;190:1574.

9. Lobprise HB, Wiggs RB. Modified surgical treatment of intermittent open-mouth mandibular locking in a cat. J Vet Dent 1992;9:8–12.
10. Hoppe F, Svalastoga E. Temporomandibular dysplasia in American Cocker Spaniels. J Small Anim Pract 1980;21:675–8.
11. Reiter AM. Symphysiotomy, symphysiectomy, and intermandibular arthrodesis in a cat with open-mouth jaw locking – case report and literature review. J Vet Dent 2004;21:147–58.
12. Beam RC, Kunz DA, Cook CR, et al. Use of three-dimensional computed tomography for diagnosis and treatment planning for open-mouth jaw locking in a cat. J Am Vet Med Assoc 2007;230:59–63.
13. Evans HE. Miller's anatomy of the dog. 3rd ed. Philadelphia: WB Saunders; 1993.
14. Scapino RP. The third joint of the canine jaw. J Morphol 1965;116:23–50.
15. Kealy JD, McAllister H. The skull and vertebral column. In: Kealy JD, McAllister H, editors. Diagnostic radiology and ultrasonography of the dog and cat. 3rd ed. Philadelphia: WB Saunders; 2000. p. 339–411.
16. Schebitz H, Wilkens H. In: Schebitz H, Wilkens H, editors. An atlas of

radiographic anatomy of the dog and cat. 4th ed. Philadelphia, PA: WB Saunders; 1986. p. 12–33.
17. Dickie AM, Sullivan M. The effect of obliquity on the radiographic appearance of the temporomandibular joint in dogs. Vet Radiol Ultrasound 2001;42:205–17.
18. Ticer JW, Spencer CP. Injury of the feline temporomandibular joint: radiographic signs. J Am Vet Rad Soc 1978;19:146–56.
19. Schwarz t, Weller R, Dickie A, et al. Imaging of the canine and feline temporomandibular joint: a review. Vet Radiol Ultrasound 2002;43:85–97.
20. Assheuer J, Sager M. Abdomen. In: Assheuer J, Sager M, editors. MRI and CT atlas of the dog. Berlin: Blackwell Science; 1997. p. 1–80.
21. Shellock FG. Kinematic MRI of the temporomandibular joint. In: Shellock FG, Powers CM, editors. Kinematic MRI of the joints. functional anatomy, kinesiology and clinical applications. Boca Raton, FL: CRC Press; 2001. p. 277–95.
22. Piermattei DL. The head, approach to the temporomandibular joint. In: Piermattei DL editor. An atlas of surgical approaches to the bones and joints of the dog and cat. 3rd ed. Philadelphia, PA: WB Saunders; 1993. p. 38–9.

Chapter | 56 |

Correction of overlong soft palate

Kyle G. Mathews

SURGICAL ANATOMY

The soft palate extends caudally from the hard palate to just beyond the tip of the epiglottis in mesaticephalic breeds. It separates the oropharynx ventrally from the nasopharynx dorsally. The elongated soft palate of many brachycephalic dogs may be so long as to reach the vocal folds and thereby partially obstruct airflow (Fig. 56.1). The soft palate is covered with a stratified squamous epithelium ventrally and along its caudal margin, while it is covered by a pseudostratified ciliated columnar epithelium over most of its dorsal surface.[1] Numerous palatine glands open to the ventral surface of the soft palate. The number of glands decreases caudally. The bulk of the soft palate consists of the paired palatine muscles, which are separated at the midline. Dorsal to the palatine muscles and ventral to the nasopharyngeal epithelium there is a palatine aponeurosis which blends with the terminal fibers of several muscles including the palatopharyngeal, tensor and levator veli palatini muscles. Arteries feeding the soft palate include the paired minor palatine arteries, and to a lesser extent the ascending pharyngeal branches which arise from the major palatine arteries. Efferent blood flow occurs via the laterally located paired venous plexi.

SPECIAL INSTRUMENTS AND MATERIALS

All instruments should have handles that are at least 180 mm in length. Kelly hemostats, Metzenbaum scissors or angled (Potts) scissors, DeBakey forceps, long-handled needle holders, head lamp or other supplemental light source, 3–0 to 4–0 Monocryl (Ethicon, Inc. Somerville, NJ) or Vicryl (Ethicon, Inc. Somerville, NJ) suture are used. If a CO_2 laser is to be used, matted nonreflective instruments and protective eyewear are required (see Ch. 8).

THERAPEUTIC DECISION-MAKING

Most brachycephalic dogs suffer from some degree of airway obstruction. The English bulldog is the most commonly affected breed.[2] Stenotic nares, and everted laryngeal ventricles are commonly present

in association with an overlong soft palate.[2-5,9-11] This triad of congenital abnormalities is referred to as brachycephalic syndrome. Many brachycephalic dogs, English bulldogs in particular, also have redundant pharyngeal mucosa and a hypoplastic trachea, which exacerbate the problem.[3,6-8,12] With time, the increased negative pressure that must be generated by the affected animal during inspiration may not only cause laryngeal ventricle eversion, but may ultimately result in laryngeal collapse. Laryngeal collapse is the end-stage result of brachycephalic syndrome.[13,14] Weakening of the laryngeal cartilages results in their collapse toward the midline, narrowing of the rima glottidis and further airway obstruction. A vicious cycle of obstruction, increased work of breathing, increased inspiratory strain on the laryngeal cartilages, and further collapse ensues. Treatment at this stage may require a permanent tracheostomy with all of the inherent problems associated with a tracheostomy in a loose-skinned dog.[15,16]

Affected animals are typically presented with a history of inspiratory stridor, snoring, and exercise intolerance. Severely affected dogs may

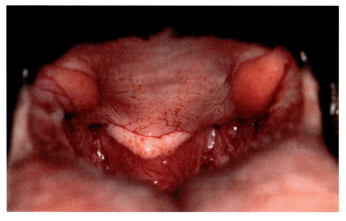

Fig. 56.1 Preoperative photograph of a pug with elongated soft palate. Oropharyngeal tissues are erythematous and the palatine tonsils are everted from their fossae. Ventral retraction of the epiglottis with a laryngoscope allowed visualization of the caudal tip of the soft palate, which extended to the level of the vocal folds. The laryngeal ventricles were also everted.

© 2012 Elsevier Ltd
DOI: 10.1016/B0123456789123(09)12345-1

have a history of collapse or syncope, and present in respiratory distress, especially during hot and humid weather. They may be cyanotic, acidotic, hyperthermic, have exaggerated thoracic wall movements consistent with airway obstruction, and may develop secondary pulmonary edema.[17,18] Cyanosis is only evident when the PaO_2 is at or less than 60 mmHg.[3,19] Myocardial ischemia may result in arrhythmias. Additionally, some dogs will have vomited as a result of acidosis and stimulation of a gag reflex by the elongated palate.[5] This may compound matters if the vomitus is aspirated. Oxygen therapy, intravenous fluids, diuretics, sedation and cooling are often needed to stabilize the patient that presents in distress.[3-5,19] Monitoring with an ECG, serial blood gas analysis (if available) and pulse-oximetry (SpO_2) should be considered. In severe cases, endotracheal intubation or a temporary tracheostomy may be needed.

Once the patient is stable enough, thoracic radiographs are performed and evaluated for evidence of pulmonary edema and hypovolemia. Tracheal diameter is measured, and other conditions which may result in similar clinical signs, such as laryngeal neoplasia, are investigated.

Chronic hypoxia secondary to brachycephalic syndrome may also result in pulmonary vasoconstriction with resultant pulmonary hypertension, *cor pulmonale* and eventual right heart failure.[3] With these things in mind, owners of brachycephalic dogs should be counseled about warning signs (stridor, etc.) that indicate there is some degree of airway obstruction. The soft palate should be examined at the time of routine neuter or spay to aid in this counseling process. Correction of overlong soft palate (staphylectomy), nasal wedge resection and resection of everted laryngeal ventricles, if present, should be done before the animal experiences a respiratory crisis.

In stable patients, a thorough pharyngeal examination is performed under general anesthesia with the plan to surgically correct an overlong soft palate, if present, during the same anesthetic episode. The patient should be preoxygenated prior to induction. Cefazolin (22 mg/kg, IV) and prednisolone (1 mg/kg, IV) are typically administered at induction. Using a laryngoscope, the pharynx, tonsils, soft palate and larynx are carefully examined. In affected dogs, the soft palate and larynx are often erythematous and edematous. As previously mentioned, the soft palate extends just beyond the tip of the epiglottis in the normal dog.

Indications for surgery

Any brachycephalic dog with inspiratory stridor or exercise intolerance should have its soft palate examined, and if elongated it should be shortened (staphylectomy). Stenotic nares and everted laryngeal ventricles are corrected, if present, and a tonsillectomy performed if the palatine tonsils are significantly enlarged and contributing to airway obstruction (see Ch. 59).[2-5,9,10] Simultaneous neutering should also be considered.

SURGICAL TECHNIQUE

With the dog's maxilla suspended with gauze between two IV poles, a known number of pharyngeal sponges are placed, and the cuff of the endotracheal tube is inflated to prevent aspiration of blood. Adequate lighting is required – a headlamp is preferable. An assistant grasps the dog's tongue with one hand and retracts the epiglottis and endotracheal tube ventrally (if present) with a laryngoscope. Some surgeons prefer to perform this procedure after placing a temporary tracheostomy tube to improve exposure of the soft palate and laryngeal ventricles. The author has found this to be unnecessary in most cases as long as adequate assistance is available. If right-handed, first

place a surgical knot in the left lateral edge of the dog's soft palate just caudal to the ipsilateral palatine tonsil. A hemostat is placed on the tag end of the suture, which is left long to aid in the manipulation of the palate (some surgeons prefer to place a stay suture at the palatal margins bilaterally). The assistant places tension on this end of the suture while the surgeon grasps the tip of the soft palate, pulling it ventrally and to the dog's right. This maneuver tenses the soft palate, making it easier to cut. The palate is shortened using sharp dissection with Metzenbaum scissors (Fig. 56.2). A transverse cut is made across one-third of the soft palate near the tip of the epiglottis. By pulling the tip of the soft palate rostrally, the nasopharyngeal mucosa, which may have retracted dorsally, is easy to locate (Fig. 56.3). The oral and nasopharyngeal mucosa of this segment are then sutured together with a simple continuous pattern (e.g., using 4–0 Monocryl (Ethicon, Inc. Somerville, NJ) or Vicryl (Ethicon, Inc. Somerville, NJ)) (Fig. 56.4). This process is repeated in sections to limit hemorrhage. Grasping the mucosa with forceps should be avoided, if possible, to limit swelling. The palatine muscles are not included in the suture. To

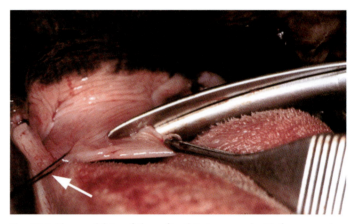

Fig. 56.2 The caudal tip of the soft palate is grasped with forceps and retracted ventrally and rostrally. Lateral tension is applied to the caudolateral margins of the soft palate with uni- or bilateral stay sutures (*arrow*). Metzenbaum scissors are used to cut transversely across approximately one-third of the soft palate. The naso- and oropharyngeal mucosa are sutured together before continuing with the transection.

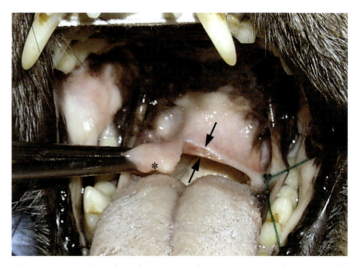

Fig. 56.3 By applying lateral tension to the stay suture, and rostroventral tension to the tip of the soft palate (***), the naso- and oropharyngeal mucosa (*arrows*) can be identified.

lost if performing the cut-and-sew method described above. Electrocautery is not needed and, if used, would predispose to tissue swelling and postoperative airway obstruction. Crushing the soft palate with a hemostat will also likely increase postoperative swelling. It is unclear if this predisposes to clinical difficulties. Others prefer to mark the location of the epiglottis on the soft palate with a sterile marker prior to resection.[5]

Laser staphylectomy is another viable alternative (see Ch. 8).[20,21] Hemorrhage is minimal since the laser seals small blood vessels as it cuts. In one study, surgery time was shorter with CO_2 laser staphylectomy than with a conventional sharp dissection technique. There were few other differences between the two groups in postoperative clinical or histological response.[21] The use of a laser in the oral cavity requires special precautions to avoid airway fires, and inadvertent injury to other tissues and personnel. A similar study compared the CO_2 laser to a bipolar sealing device (Ligasure, Valleylab, Tyco Healthcare, Boulder, CO) for performing a staphylectomy on normal dogs. Few differences between the two techniques were noted other than a decreased operative time when using the bipolar device.[22]

When using the conventional technique, primary repair is important to limit inflammation. Postoperative dysphagia following suture failure and subsequent granulation tissue formation at the edge of the palate is possible. Overshortening the palate prevents the dog from occluding its nasopharynx; the net result of this will be the nasal return of food during swallowing and a severe rhinitis.[10]

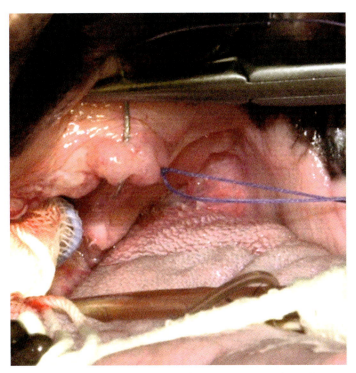

Fig. 56.4 The naso- and oropharyngeal mucosa are sutured together with a simple continuous pattern. The palatine muscles are not included in the sutures.

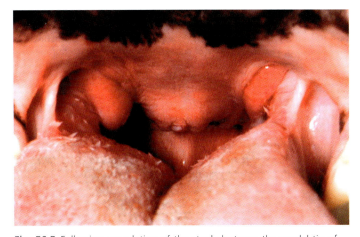

Fig. 56.5 Following completion of the staphylectomy, the caudal tip of the soft palate should lay just caudal to the tip of the epiglottis. The tip of the epiglottis has been pushed dorsal to the soft palate in this photograph for illustration purposes.

complete the suture pattern, a second knot is started at the left lateral edge of the soft palate (a mirror image of the right side), a final small attachment of the end of the soft palate is transected, and the knot is finished. All suture ends are then trimmed (Fig. 56.5). Sponges are recounted and the pharynx is suctioned prior to recovery from anesthesia.

Some surgeons prefer to place a hemostat across the soft palate to crush the tissues and to mark the line of resection so as to prevent overcorrection.[3] Another potential benefit of this technique is decreased hemorrhage, although there is surprisingly little blood

POSTOPERATIVE CARE AND ASSESSMENT

Despite contamination at the time of surgery, prolonged antibiotic therapy is not indicated. As previously noted, a single dose of corticosteroids is generally given at induction, prior to manipulation of the tissues, to diminish postoperative swelling. Because postoperative laryngeal/pharyngeal edema can result in airway obstruction, continuous monitoring for the first 12–24 hours is highly recommended. If edema is significant at the time of surgery, a temporary tracheostomy tube is placed prior to recovery. Frequent suctioning of the tube will be needed to prevent obstruction.[15,16] The tube is removed when the patient can breathe around it during trial occlusion. Oxygen should be readily available for all dogs undergoing correction for an overlong soft palate. Some prefer to place a nasal oxygen line prior to recovery if there is edema present. Induction drugs and a tracheostomy tube should also be kept nearby so that rapid induction followed by intubation can be performed if needed. Retching and vomiting may occur postoperatively.[3,10] If vomiting occurs, the patient should be evaluated for the possible development of aspiration pneumonia. Soft food is fed for the first 3–7 days.

PROGNOSIS

The prognosis for a full recovery is generally good if brachycephalic syndrome has not resulted in laryngeal collapse or right-sided heart failure. However, owners of affected dogs must be warned about the possibility of postoperative obstruction. English bulldogs may have a worse prognosis than other brachycephalic breeds.[4] They are more likely to have redundant pharyngeal mucosa and a hypoplastic trachea than other breeds. One report indicated good to excellent results in 67% of nonbulldog breeds, and similar results in 45% of English bulldogs.[4] The fact that only 56 of 118 owners returned questionnaires in this study likely affected the results. Still, most feel that English

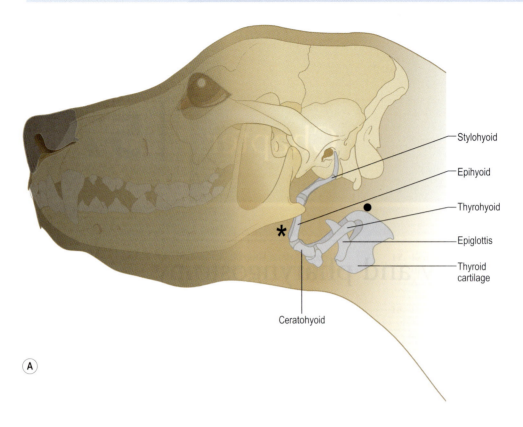

Stylohyoid

Epihyoid

Thyrohyoid

Epiglottis

Thyroid cartilage

Ceratohyoid

(A)

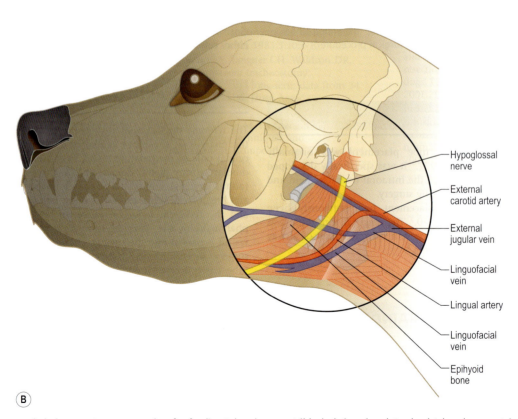

Hypoglossal nerve

External carotid artery

External jugular vein

Linguofacial vein

Lingual artery

Linguofacial vein

Epihyoid bone

(B)

Fig. 57.1 (**A**) Recommended pharyngotomy approaches for feeding tube placement (*black dot*) and endotracheal tube placement (*asterisk*). Placement of the feeding tube in a more caudal position prevents epiglottic entrapment. The endotracheal tube placed through this pharyngotomy site is removed immediately after surgery. (**B**) Neurovasular anatomy adjacent to the pharyngotomy sites.

Feeding tube

Generally recommended tube diameters are as follows: 10 to 12 F for cats and small dogs; 16 to 18 F for animals with a body weight of 10 to 15 kg, and 18 to 20 F for larger dogs. The relatively small-sized tube in relation to patient size reduces the risk of injury to anatomic structures during tube insertion and maintenance. Commercial liquid diets or commercial canned foods made into a liquid consistency in a food blender pass through these tubes. Appropriate tube materials include rubber (Sovereign, Kendall Co., Mansfield, MA) and silicone (Cook Veterinary Products, Eight Mile Plains, Queensland, AUS) feeding catheters, and Foley catheters (Foley Catheter, American Hospital Supply Corp., Valencia, CA) (without distension of the bulb). The ends of tubes with side ports are cut off to minimize tube obstruction. Mushroom tips are also cut off.

SURGICAL TECHNIQUE[4,7,8]

Tubes are placed in the right or left pharyngeal wall according to the surgeon's preference, or as determined by the surgical procedure planned; for example, for caudal mandibular fracture repair the contralateral pharyngeal wall is preferred. The skin surface is prepared for surgery. The external jugular vein is occluded at the thoracic inlet to cause distention of the maxillary and linguofacial veins to confirm their location so as to avoid inadvertent trauma. A gloved hand is placed into the oral cavity and the hyoid apparatus palpated. The joint between the thyrohyoid bone and thyroid cartilage is found. If an endotracheal tube is to be placed without postoperative conversion to feeding tube placement, then the epihyoid bone is palpated and the tube is placed immediately rostral to this bone. The index finger is flexed and moved laterally to create a visible bulge of the skin at this level.

A small incision is made in the skin and subcutaneous tissue over the index finger parallel to the adjacent veins. Curved Kelly or Carmalt forceps (Miltex Surgical Instruments. Tuttlingen, Germany) is placed in the incision and blunt dissection is used to gently separate tissues until the instrument tips are palpated to rest on the pharyngeal wall at the finger tip. The blunt dissection is performed by opening the instrument tips after each repeated insertion into the tissues. The instrument tips are opened parallel to the adjacent veins. Care is taken to avoid all neurovascular structures.

The forceps' tips and index finger are moved medially and the interposed segment of pharyngeal wall is deviated into the pharyngeal lumen. As the pharyngeal wall is viewed via the oral cavity, a small mucosal incision is made in this area and the forceps' tips are advanced into the pharyngeal lumen. The mucosal opening is made the appropriate diameter for the tube by stretching the tissue by repeated opening of the forceps jaws. A second pair of forceps is placed in the oral cavity and the tips placed in the open jaws of the first pair. As the first pair of forceps is withdrawn, the second 'follows' it into the oral incision and is advanced until its tips are visible at the skin incision. The caudal end of the tube is grasped with the second forceps and the tube drawn through the pharyngeal wall, leaving the rostral portion of the tube exterior to the skin. Depending on patient size, the second forceps may be a curved Kelly, Carmalt or a long (203-mm) curved forceps such as Johns Hopkins gallbladder forceps (Johnson and Johnson Hospital Services, New Brunswick, NJ) (Fig. 57.2) in order to reach into the pharyngeal lumen.

Alternatively, the finger used for identifying the landmarks for the skin incision can be replaced by the curved Johns Hopkins gallbladder forceps. The forceps is subsequently pushed in a closed fashion from within the oral cavity through the pharyngeal wall and overlying tissues. As the forceps becomes visible in the skin wound, the

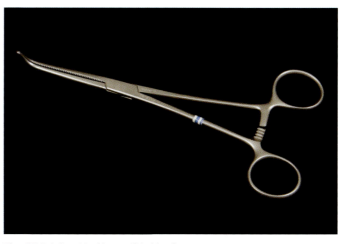

Fig. 57.2 Johns Hopkins gallbladder forceps. *(Johnson and Johnson Hospital Services, New Brunswick, NJ.)*

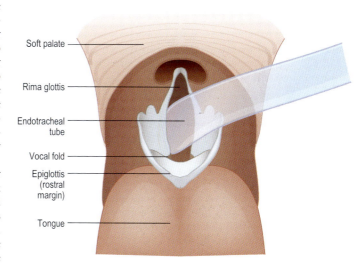

Soft palate

Rima glottis

Endotracheal tube

Vocal fold

Epiglottis (rostral margin)

Tongue

Fig. 57.3 Intraoral view showing placement of an endotracheal tube.

instrument tips are opened to separate the subcutaneous tissues and widen the pharyngotomy. The pharyngotomy should be wide enough to draw the tube atraumatically through the opened tissues. The distal end of the tube is grasped with the forceps and pulled through the pharyngeal wall into the pharyngeal lumen.

An endotracheal tube is gently guided into the tracheal lumen (Fig. 57.3). The wire-reinforced tubes are fairly stiff and care is taken to not injure mucosa and cartilages of the epiglottis and larynx during tube manipulation. The tube is palpated via the cervical trachea to ensure adequate placement. It is secured into place by a gauze tie around the neck or by means of a tape butterfly attached to the tube and sutured to the skin. The anesthesia hoses can also be taped to the surgery table.

A feeding tube is gently passed into the esophagus and advanced to the mid-thoracic esophagus at the level of rib 6 or 7. The tube must be premeasured and cut to length before placement. Secondary esophageal peristaltic waves will propel nutrient material into the stomach from this point. Placement of the tube at this level will not promote gastric reflux or interfere with esophageal clearance of refluxed gastric acid as may happen if the tube was advanced into the gastric lumen.[9] Laryngeal obstruction and epiglottic entrapment are

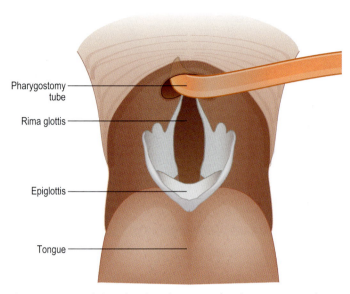

Pharyngostomy tube
Rima glottis
Epiglottis
Tongue

Fig. 57.4 Intraoral view showing placement of a pharyngostomy tube.

minimized by passing the tube at the correct level on the pharyngeal wall (Fig. 57.4, and see Fig. 57.1). To secure the tube, a tape butterfly is attached to the tube and sutured to the skin or a Chinese finger trap suture is placed. The tube is capped.

POSTOPERATIVE CARE AND ASSESSMENT

Pharyngotomy

The pharyngotomy endotracheal tube is removed immediately after surgery and replaced by a conventional oral endotracheal tube until final extubation is indicated. The pharyngotomy opening is generally left unsutured. Intravenous fluids are continued for 24 hours to allow a fibrin 'seal' to develop in the tissue tract. Eating and drinking are allowed in 24 hours. If possible, a light bandage is placed to cover the skin incision. If bandaging is not possible, as is often the case, the skin surface is kept clean and dry as needed. A small amount of serosanguineous drainage occurs for 2 to 4 days then ceases. If needed, one skin suture may be placed to prevent wide skin gapping during head

and neck movement and still allow drainage through an open wound. The wound heals by second intention in 10 to 14 days.

Pharyngostomy

The skin surface around the pharyngostomy tube is cleaned and dried as necessary. Some wound drainage occurs. A bandage is not placed. Eventually, a 'cuff' of granulation tissue may be seen between the tube and skin surface. After tube removal, the pharyngocutaneous fistula is not sutured and heals by second intention in 10 to 14 days.

COMPLICATIONS

Hemorrhage is the major intraoperative complication. This results from inaccurate placement of the incision and dissection. Observing the distended veins and deviating the index finger to tent the skin laterally before making the incision will displace the neurovascular structures from the incision site. The incision and subsequent blunt dissection must be performed parallel to the veins.

Injury to the mucosal surfaces during excessively traumatic endotracheal tube placement may result in postoperative cough secondary to laryngitis. Fracture of cartilages may result in abnormal epiglottic movement and laryngeal airway obstruction. However, this is normally a very safe technique with no complications.

Pharyngostomy tubes have potential to cause several complications.[4,10] Epiglottic entrapment or reduced movement due to the tube increases the risk of aspiration pneumonia. Larger-diameter tubes may obstruct the aditus laryngis. These complications can be minimized by accurate tube placement.[4] The tube is located in an area of normal movement and the exterior part of the tube may contact the side of the head during movement. The presence of the tube may create stress and discomfort for the patient. The tube may become dislodged from the esophagus, resulting in excess tube in the oropharyngeal area or hanging from the mouth. Patients may not voluntarily eat with the tube placed. It may be difficult to assess ability to adequately eat and drink during the course of recovery. Local infection and swelling may occur. Larger stiff tubes may cause pressure necrosis.

The advent of improved techniques and instrumentation for placement of esophagostomy and gastrostomy tubes has essentially replaced the use of the pharyngostomy tube (see Ch. 5).[11-13]

REFERENCES

1. Stedman TL. Stedman's medical dictionary. 27th ed. Philadelphia, PA: Lippincott Williams & Wilkins; 2000. p. 1703, 1842.
2. Hartsfield SM, Genfreau CL, Smith CW, et al. Endotracheal intubation by pharyngotomy. J Am Anim Hosp Assoc 1977;13:71–4.
3. Bohning RH, DeHoff WD, McElhinney A, et al. Pharyngostomy for maintenance of the anorectic animal. J Am Vet Med Assoc 1970;156:611–15.
4. Crowe DT, Downs MO. Pharyngostomy complications in dogs and cats and recommended technical modifications: experimental and clinical investigations. J Am Anim Hosp Assoc 1986;22: 493–503.

5. Verstraete FJM. Self-assessment color review of veterinary dentistry. Ames, IA: Iowa State University Press; 1999. p. 180.
6. Evans HE. Miller's anatomy of the dog. 3rd ed. Philadelphia, PA: WB Saunders; 1993.
7. Lantz GC. Pharyngostomy tube placement. In: Bojrab MJ, editor. Current techniques in small animal surgery. 3rd ed. Philadelphia, PA: Lea and Febiger; 1990. p. 189–91.
8. Smith MM. Pharyngostomy endotracheal tube. J Vet Dent 2004;21:191–4.
9. Lantz GC, Cantwell HD, VanVleet JF, et al. Pharyngostomy tube initiated gastric reflux and esophagitis. J Am Anim Hosp Assoc 1982;18:883–90.

10. Bartges JW. Enteral nutritional support. In: Lipowitz AJ, Caywood DD, Newton CD, et al, editors. Complications in small animal surgery. Baltimore, MD: Williams and Wilkins; 1996. p. 44–72.
11. Rawlings CA. Percutaneous placement of a medcervical esophagostomy tube: new technique and representative cases. J Am Anim Hosp Assoc 1993;29:526–30.
12. Crowe DT, Devey JJ. Esophagostomy tubes for feeding and decompression: clinical experience in 29 small animal patients. J Am Anim Hosp Assoc 1997;33:393–403.
13. Bright RM, Okrasinski Eb, Pardo AD, et al. Percutaneous tube gastrostomy for enteral alimentation in small animals. Compend Contin Educ Pract Vet 1991;13:15–23.

Chapter 58

Oral approaches to the nasal cavity and nasopharynx

Kyle G. Mathews

SURGICAL ANATOMY

The bony portion of the hard palate is made up of the paired palatine processes of the incisive bones rostrally, the palatine processes of the maxillae centrally, and the horizontal laminae of the palatine bones caudally.[1] There is a midline eminence at the caudal border of the hard palate referred to as the caudal nasal spine. The bones of the hard palate are covered with a thick, durable and vascular mucoperiosteum ventrally, and a pseudostratified ciliated columnar epithelium on the nasal surface. Blood supply to the hard palate is supplied primarily from the paired major palatine arteries, and to a lesser extent from the minor palatine arteries caudally, and the sphenopalatine arteries dorsally. Each major palatine artery runs through a major palatine foramen, between the maxillae and palatine bones, and then rostrally beneath the mucoperiosteum within a groove, called the palatine sulcus, in the ventral surface of the hard palate. Numerous anastomoses exist between these paired arteries. Venous drainage is via a diffuse venous plexus to the maxillary vein. Sensory innervation is supplied to the oral surface of the hard palate by the major palatine branch of the maxillary division of the trigeminal nerve, which runs along with the major palatine artery in the palatine canal. For details of soft palate anatomy, see Chapter 56.

SPECIAL INSTRUMENTS AND MATERIALS

An oral surgery drill unit (see Ch. 6), or an orthopedic nitrogen or battery-powered unit (e.g., Surgairtome (Hall Surgical, Linvatec Corporation. Largo, FL)), headlamp or other supplemental light source, electrocautery unit, Lempert rongeurs, curettes, small Gelpi retractors, cold saline, suction, 2–0 to 3–0 Monocryl (Ethicon, Inc. Somerville, NJ) or Vicryl (Ethicon, Inc. Somerville, NJ) suture are required. For temporary carotid artery occlusion, umbilical tape, 22 G orthopedic wire, 10–12 F red rubber catheter are used.

THERAPEUTIC DECISION MAKING

Nasal or nasopharyngeal disease should be suspected in any animal with nasal discharge, sneezing, stertorous respiration, nasal planum ulceration, epistaxis, or changes in phonation. Appropriate diagnostic tests may include nasal and oral (including hard and soft palate) palpation, nasal and thoracic radiography, computed tomography, and rhinoscopy in addition to a complete blood count, serum chemistry panel, fungal titers, bacterial and fungal cultures and cytology/histopathology.

Indications for surgery

The ventral approach to the nasal cavity can be used as an alternative to dorsal rhinotomy for the removal of foreign bodies that are not retrievable via rhinoscopy and that are located fairly ventrally, to debulk fungal granulomas as an adjunct to topical or systemic antifungal therapy, and potentially as an adjunct to radiation therapy for nasal tumors.[2,3] Subcutaneous emphysema, which can occur following a dorsal rhinotomy, is not a problem with the ventral approach. Clients may consider the ventral approach to be cosmetically more acceptable since the incision is hidden from view. Also, if carotid artery ligation is to be performed, repositioning the animal is not necessary. The decision to approach a nasal lesion ventrally should be based on preoperative radiography, computed tomography or rhinoscopy. Fungal granulomas in the frontal sinuses are more common than those in the ventral nasal cavity, and should be approached via a dorsal sinusotomy. Lesions in the ventral ethmoid turbinates, or rostral to the ethmoid turbinates, can be approached through the hard palate.

Access to the nasopharynx can be gained by incision of the soft palate alone. Fifty-four percent (20/37) of dogs with nasopharyngeal disorders in one study were diagnosed with neoplasia.[4] The other dogs in this study had either noninfectious inflammatory tissue or benign cysts obstructing the nasopharynx. Nasopharyngeal granulomas associated with cryptococcal infection have also been reported in both cats and dogs.[5,6] If the granuloma is large, removal with a flexible bronchoscope is usually not possible. Removal of large nasopharyngeal foreign bodies and surgical excision of nasopharyngeal stenosis may also require splitting of the soft palate. Nasopharyngeal stenosis is most common in cats and is thought to be acquired secondary to chronic upper respiratory tract infections.[7] The author has seen it occur in a dog secondary to vomiting, which presumably resulted in irritation of the nasopharynx. Resection of the stenosis and temporary stenting with a large-diameter nasal Foley catheter resulted in resolution of the problem. Congenital choanal atresia has also been reported in the dog.[8] Successful correction of nasopharyngeal stenosis has been reported following excision with or without a mucosal flap, excision with placement of a nasopharyngeal stent, following balloon dilation, and following placement of a balloon-expandable stent.[7,9-12]

SURGICAL TECHNIQUE

Control of hemorrhage

Because hemorrhage during ventral approaches to the nasal cavity is expected, coagulation profiles, cross-matching and the potential need for a transfusion should be considered prior to surgery.

Hemorrhage during a ventral approach to the nasal cavity (ventral rhinotomy) may be diminished by temporary bilateral carotid artery ligation. Because of well-developed collateral circulation originating from the vertebral arteries in dogs, this procedure can be performed with no notable adverse effects. There are at least five described sites of anastomoses between the internal and external carotid arteries in a normal dog, allowing them to survive with no residual effect following long-term ligation of one or both carotid arteries and other major vessels supplying the head.[13-17] Bilateral carotid ligation may result in death in cats; therefore ligation is limited to one side.[3,18] Carotid artery ligation has been shown to decrease lingual arterial pressures in dogs.[19] Similar diminution in blood pressure should occur in the major and minor palatine arteries since they arise from the maxillary artery which, as with the lingual artery, arises from the common carotid artery. Although the ventral approach through the hard and soft palates will likely be associated with less hemorrhage following carotid artery ligation, it is unclear if the same is true when performing nasal turbinate resection.[1,20]

The common carotid arteries are approached by making a ventral midline incision in the mid-cervical region, or two smaller parasagittal incisions ventral to the jugular groove. The carotid sheath is identified and opened longitudinally with Metzenbaum scissors. Care must be taken to avoid stretching or otherwise damaging the vagosympathetic trunk and internal jugular vein, which also lie within the carotid sheath. Once the carotid artery has been isolated, a Rumel tourniquet is fashioned by passing a strand of moistened 6-mm umbilical tape around the artery (Fig. 58.1A). The two ends of the umbilical tape are drawn through a 60–100-mm section of red-rubber catheter (Fig. 58.1B). This is accomplished by first passing some thin orthopedic wire through the catheter segment. The tourniquet is tightened by pushing the catheter against the artery while maintaining tension on the umbilical tape. A hemostat is placed across the catheter to maintain occlusion of blood flow, and the incision is closed around the tourniquet (Fig. 58.1C). When the oral procedure has been completed, the hemostat, catheter and umbilical tape are easily removed.

After penetrating the hard palate, further hemorrhage can be expected from the nasal mucosa, which is richly endowed with blood vessels. Lavage of the nasal cavity with cold saline will improve visualization. Several bottles of saline should be refrigerated the day prior to surgery. Instillation of epinephrine (1 : 100,000) may also improve

visualization, but the application of cold saline is usually sufficient. Suction should be used; however, the surgeon must keep track of blood loss through the suction unit. Direct pressure can be obtained by temporarily packing the surgery site with cold saline-soaked sponges before proceeding. Bone wax can be applied to the bleeding edges of the palatine bone in larger animals where bone thickness will allow its use. Bipolar electrocautery can be used to cauterize individual vessels.

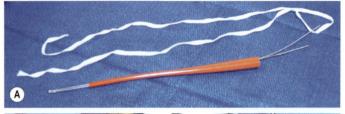

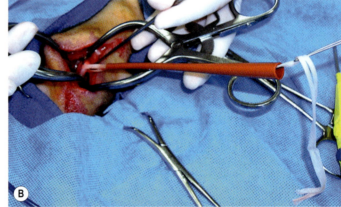

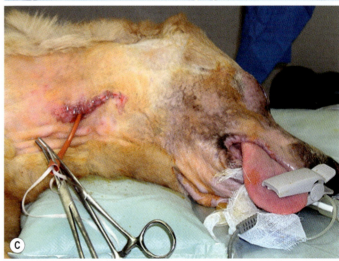

Fig. 58.1 Temporary carotid artery occlusion in the dog: (**A**) Supplies needed for the Rumel tourniquet (*see text*). (**B**) After carefully dissecting the carotid artery out of its sheath, the umbilical tape is passed around the artery. The ends of the umbilical tape are passed through the doubled-over orthopedic wire and pulled through the red-rubber catheter. (**C**) The carotid artery is occluded by pushing the catheter against the artery while applying tension to the umbilical tape. Occlusion is maintained by placing hemostats across the catheter and umbilical tape. The incision is closed around the Rumel tourniquet, which is easily removed following the rhinotomy.

Ventral approach to the rostral nasal passages

Following anesthetic induction, a single dose of antibiotic is given (e.g., cefazolin 22 mg/kg, IV). An infraorbital nerve block is performed as outlined in Chapter 4. The patient is placed in dorsal recumbency with the surgical table positioned to form a trough. The thoracic limbs are tied caudally. A rolled towel is placed under the patient's neck for support. If carotid artery ligation is planned, the ventral and lateral cervical area is clipped and aseptically prepared. The palate is maintained in a horizontal position by placing a long strip of tape from the table over the maxillary canine teeth. The mouth is held open by tying or taping the mandible up to an IV pole on either side of the surgical table. The endotracheal tube should be elevated along with the mandible away from the hard palate. Gauze sponges are counted and placed in the pharynx, and the endotracheal tube is inflated to prevent aspiration of blood and saline flush during the procedure. The palate is then aseptically prepared for surgery.

Following carotid artery ligation, if performed, a midline incision is made through the mucoperiosteum directly over the area of interest, identified with radiography or computed tomography. The mucoperiosteum is elevated from the hard palate with a periosteal elevator. The paired major palatine arteries penetrate the hard palate approximately half way between the midline and the caudal aspects of the fourth premolar teeth. Lateral mucoperiosteal elevation to the level of the palatine arteries usually achieves adequate exposure. Exposure is maintained by placing small Gelpi retractors into the incision, or by use of several stay sutures placed through the cut edges of the mucoperiosteum (Fig. 58.2A).

A longitudinally oriented trough is then created in the hard palate with a round bur on an oral surgery unit or nitrogen or battery-powered orthopedic drill (Fig. 58.2B). The trough is centered on the midline for bilateral lesions, or can be started to the side of midline for unilateral lesions. Once through the hard palate into the ventral nasal cavity, the trough may be extended in any direction to improve access to the tissues of interest. If irrigation is not provided through the handpiece, cold saline should be continuously dripped on the bur during bone removal to prevent overheating. Continuous suction is used to remove bone debris and improve visibility. Hemorrhage is controlled as outlined above. The vertically oriented vomer and/or nasal septum may be trimmed if necessary with Lempert rongeurs (Fig. 58.2C). Diseased tissues, fungal granulomas and foreign bodies within the nasal cavity are removed with curettes and/or rongeurs.

Once the objectives of the surgery have been achieved, hemorrhage is under control, and the nasal cavity has been thoroughly flushed with saline, the tissues are closed. A single row of simple interrupted absorbable sutures (e.g., Monocryl (Ethicon, Inc. Somerville, NJ) or Vicryl (Ethicon, Inc. Somerville, NJ)) are placed in the mucoperiosteum overlying the hard palate (Fig. 58.2D). Extra throws are placed on these knots to keep them from untying due to tongue motion. The pharyngeal gauze sponges are recounted and the pharynx is suctioned prior to recovery from anesthesia.

Ventral approach to the caudal nasal passages and nasopharynx

Positioning of the patient is identical to that described for ventral approach to the rostral nasal passages.

A midline incision is made through the mucosa of the soft palate. The caudal edge of the soft palate should be preserved to simplify closure. The incision is continued through the full thickness of the soft palate between the paired palatine muscles, and through the nasopharyngeal mucosa. Exposure to this area is improved by placing

stay sutures along the incision margins to retract the tissues laterally. Small Gelpi retractors are also quite helpful. If the nasopharyngeal area of interest is near the caudal edge of the hard palate, the two approaches may be combined. The incision may be extended cranially through the palatine mucoperiosteum. A portion of the caudal hard palate is then removed along the midline.

Once the nasopharyngeal obstruction (stricture, mass, fungal granuloma, foreign body) has been removed, closure of the soft palate is accomplished in two or three layers. Absorbable continuous sutures are placed in the nasopharyngeal mucosa, followed by similar apposition of the palatine muscles. Simple interrupted or continuous absorbable sutures (e.g., Monocryl or Vicryl) are placed in the oropharyngeal mucosa. As before, extra throws are generally placed on these knots to keep them from untying due to tongue motion.

POSTOPERATIVE CARE AND ASSESSMENT

Most animals will begin eating the day following surgery and can be discharged from the hospital within 1–2 days. A soft diet is fed for 2 weeks. A gastrostomy or esophagostomy tube may need to be placed in some animals. Cats with caudal nasal disease, in particular, may not eat and will require caloric supplementation for several days postoperatively (see Ch. 5). A fentanyl patch should be considered, placed the day prior to surgery if possible, and removed 3–5 days postoperatively (see Ch. 4). Additional analgesia should be provided with an injectable narcotic (e.g., hydromorphone, as needed) while in the hospital. Nonsteroidal antiinflammatory drugs should also be considered (e.g., dogs: carprofen 2 mg/kg, PO, BID for 1 week, then q24 h as needed; cats: ketoprofen 1 mg/kg, PO, q24h for 5 days). The surgical site should be inspected weekly for 2–3 weeks so that areas of dehiscence may be detected early and resutured.

PROGNOSIS

Ventral rhinotomy was performed on 11 cats and 47 dogs in one study.[3] Two cats died in the postoperative period. Both had significant hemorrhage intraoperatively, requiring temporary carotid artery ligation. Decreased blood flow to the brain during surgery likely contributed to their deaths. Persistent mucopurulent or serous nasal discharge occurred in the majority of animals. The cause of postoperative nasal discharge is not understood, although it also occurs following dorsal rhinotomy with turbinectomy. Dehiscence was rarely a problem, with one patient developing an oronasal fistula.

Long-term prognosis depends on the underlying disease process. Most cases of canine and feline fungal rhinitis can be cured with topical and/or systemic antifungal therapy with surgical removal of granulomas, when present.[5,21] Nasopharyngeal cysts and stenoses respond favorably to surgical intervention. Nasal and nasopharyngeal neoplasia carries a guarded to poor prognosis. Performing rhinotomy and aggressive surgical debulking prior to orthovoltage radiation for the treatment of nasal carcinomas has improved survival times compared to orthovoltage therapy alone in several studies.[22,23] Affected animals may also temporarily benefit from surgical debulking of tumors that impede airflow through the nasal cavity or nasopharynx. Megavoltage therapy of canine nasal carcinoma is now more commonly performed, and survival times are similar to those reported for combined surgery and orthovoltage therapy.[24–26] Surgical debulking prior to megavoltage therapy is not recommended as it may result in uneven dose distribution within the tumor.[25] The potential benefits of surgical debulking of selected tumors following megavoltage therapy is unclear at present.[26,27]

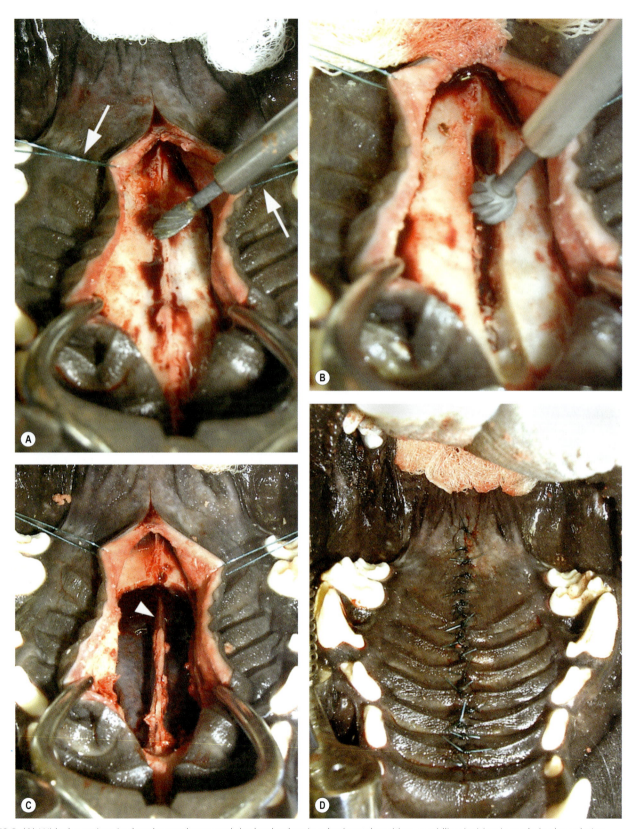

Fig. 58.2 (**A**) With the patient in dorsal recumbency and the hard palate in a horizontal position, a midline incision is made in the palatine mucoperiosteum. The edges of the mucoperiosteum are retracted with Gelpi retractors and stay sutures (*arrows*) to expose the hard palate, which is then penetrated with a rotating bur. Extension of the midline incision caudally through the soft palate may be performed, if necessary. (**B**) The hard palate is removed with a rotating bur over the area of interest. Continuous lavage and suction are required to prevent overheating and improve visibility. (**C**) The nasal cavity is exposed. The vomer (*arrowhead*) and affected turbinates are removed with rongeurs and curettes, if necessary. (**D**) The mucoperiosteum is closed with numerous simple interrupted absorbable sutures. Extra throws are placed on the sutures to prevent premature untying.

REFERENCES

1. Evans HE. The pharynx. In: Evans HE, editor. Miller's Anatomy of the dog. 3rd ed. Philadelphia, PA: WB Saunders Co; 1993. p. 421–3.

2. Holmberg DL, Fries D, Cockshutt J, et al. Ventral rhinotomy in the dog and cat. Vet Surg 1989;18:446–9.

3. Holmberg DL. Sequelae of ventral rhinotomy in dogs and cats with inflammatory and neoplastic nasal pathology: a retrospective study. Can Vet J 1996;37:483–5.

4. Hunt GB, Perkins MC, Foster SF, et al. Nasopharyngeal disorders of dogs and cats: a review and retrospective study. Compend Cont Ed Pract Vet 2002;24:184–99.

5. Malik R, Martin P, Wigney DI, et al. Nasopharyngeal cryptococcosis. Aust Vet J 1997;75:483–8.

6. Malik R, Dill-Macky E, Martin P, et al. Cryptococcosis in dogs: a retrospective study of 20 consecutive cases. J Med Vet Mycol 1995;33:291–7.

7. Mitten RW. Nasopharyngeal stenosis in four cats. J Small Anim Pract 1998;29:341–5.

8. Coolman BR, Manfra Marretta S, McKiernan BC, et al. Choanal atresia and secondary nasopharyngeal stenosis in a dog. J Am Anim Hosp Assoc 1998;34:497–501.

9. Griffon DJ, Tasker S. Use of a mucosal advancement flap for the treatment of nasopharyngeal stenosis in a cat. J Small Anim Pract 2000;41:71–3.

10. Glaus TM, Tomsa K, Reusch CE. Balloon dilation for the treatment of chronic recurrent nasopharyngeal stenosis in a cat. J Small Anim Pract 2002;43:88–90.

11. Novo RE, Kramek B. Surgical repair of nasopharyngeal stenosis in a cat using a stent. J Am Anim Hosp Assoc 1999;35:251–6.

12. Berent AC, Weisse C, Todd K, et al. Use of a balloon-expandable metallic stent for treatment of nasopharyngeal stenosis in dogs and cats: six cases (2005–2007). J Am Vet Med Assoc 2008;233:1432–40.

13. Whisnant JP, Millikan CH, Wakim KG, et al. Collateral circulation to the brain of the dog following bilateral ligation of the carotid and vertebral arteries. Am J Physiol 1956;186:275–7.

14. Clandenin MA, Conrad MC. Collateral vessel development after chronic bilateral common carotid artery occlusion in the dog. Am J Vet Res 1979;40:1244–8.

15. Clendinin MA, Conrad MC: Collateral vessel development, following unilateral chronic carotid occlusion in the dog. Am J Vet Res 1979;40:84–8.

16. Jewell PA: The anastomoses between internal and external carotid circulations in the dog. J Anat 1952;86:83–94.

17. Moss G: The adequacy of the cerebral collateral circulation: tolerance of awake experimental animals to acute bilateral common carotid artery occlusion. J Surg Res 1974;16:337–8.

18. King AS. Arterial supply to the central nervous system. In: Physiological and clinical anatomy of the domestic mammals, vol. 1. Oxford, UK: Oxford University Press; 1987. p. 1–8.

19. Holmberg DL, Pettifer GR. Effect of carotid artery occlusion on lingual arterial blood pressure in dogs. Can Vet J 1997;38:629–31.

20. Done SH, Goody PC, Evans SA, et al.: Color atlas of veterinary anatomy Volume 3: The dog and cat. London: Mosby-Wolfe; 1996.

21. Mathews KG, Davidson AP, Koblik PD, et al. Comparison of topical administration of clotrimazole through surgically placed versus nonsurgically placed catheters for treatment of nasal aspergillosis in dogs: 60 cases (1990–1996). J Am Vet Med Assoc 1998;213:501–6.

22. Thrall DE, Harvey CE. Radiotherapy of malignant nasal tumors in 21 dogs. J Am Vet Med Assoc 1983;183:663–6.

23. Adams WM, Withrow SJ, Walshaw R, et al. Radiotherapy of malignant nasal tumours in 67 dogs. J Am Vet Med Assoc 1987;191:311–15.

24. Theon AP, Madewell BR, Harb MF, et al. Megavoltage irradiation of neoplasms of the nasal and paranasal cavities in 77 dogs. J Am Vet Med Assoc 1993;202:1469–75.

25. McEntee MC, Page RL, Heidner GL, et al. A retrospective study of 27 dogs with intranasal neoplasms treated with cobalt radiation. Vet Radiol 1991;32:135–9.

26. LaDue TA, Dodge R, Page RL, et al. Factors influencing survival after radiotherapy of nasal tumors in 130 dogs. Vet Radiol Ultrasound 1999;40:312–17.

27. Henry CJ, Brewer WG, Tyler JW, et al. Survival in dogs with nasal adenocarcinoma: 64 cases (1981–1995). J Vet Int Med 1998;12:436–9.

Chapter | 59 |

Tonsillectomy

Kyle G. Mathews

SURGICAL ANATOMY

The palatine tonsils are located in the dorsolateral walls of the oropharynx just caudal to the caudolateral borders of the soft palate (palatoglossal folds) and are recessed within the tonsillar fossa in normal dogs.[1] They have no afferent lymphatics, but numerous efferents which empty into the medial retropharyngeal lymph nodes. The lingual artery gives rise to the tonsillar artery which branches 2–3 times as it enters the base of each tonsil. Numerous small veins leave each tonsil and empty into the palatine venous plexus.

SPECIAL INSTRUMENTS AND MATERIALS

All instruments should have handles that are at least 180 mm in length: Kelly hemostats, right angled forceps, or hemostatic tonsil forceps (e.g., Schnidt or Sawtell forceps (Sklar, West Chester, PA)); Metzenbaum scissors or tonsil scissors (e.g., Dean or Boettcher tonsil scissors (Sklar, West Chester, PA)); DeBakey forceps or tonsil forceps (e.g., White or Colver-Coakley forceps (Sklar, West Chester, PA)); long-handled needle holders. A head lamp or other supplemental light source is very useful. Recommended suture material is 3–0 to 4–0 Monocryl (Ethicon, Inc. Somerville, NJ) or Vicryl (Ethicon, Inc. Somerville, NJ). An electrocautery unit (bipolar preferred) is often needed, while a tonsillar snare is optional.

THERAPEUTIC DECISION-MAKING

Indications for surgery

Tonsillectomy is indicated in cases of chronic recurrent tonsillitis unresponsive to antibiotic therapy, as an adjunct to radiation therapy for dogs with tonsillar squamous cell carcinoma, and for removal of benign tonsillar polyps and cysts.[2,3] It may also be required in dogs with brachycephalic syndrome if the tonsils have enlarged to the point

where they contribute to airway obstruction.[4] Some surgeons prefer to remove the tonsils in all dogs presented for soft palate and everted laryngeal ventricle resection (Fig. 59.1).[5] The author has not found tonsillectomy to be necessary in the large majority of dogs with this condition. Correction of the airway obstruction due to brachycephalic syndrome presumably results in diminution of negative pressure generated during inhalation, and return of the tonsils to their fossae.

Malignant lymphoma may also affect the tonsils, but animals with tonsillar lymphoma tend to have uniform bilateral enlargement (Fig. 59.2A) rather than the irregular, firm, unilateral enlargement seen with tonsillar carcinoma (Fig. 59.2B).[6] In addition, animals with lymphoma generally have multiple other sites of involvement, including distant lymph nodes such as the mediastinal and sternal nodes, seen on thoracic radiography. Dogs with tonsillar carcinoma, which

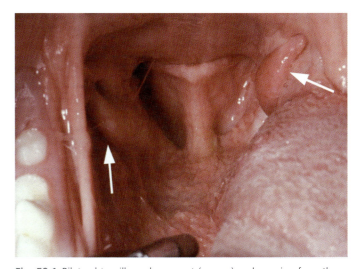

Fig. 59.1 Bilateral tonsillar enlargement (*arrows*) and eversion from the tonsillar fossae is frequently seen in dogs with brachycephalic syndrome. Resection is only necessary if the enlarged tonsils are contributing to airway obstruction.

© 2012 Elsevier Ltd
DOI: 10.1016/B0123456789123(09)12345-1

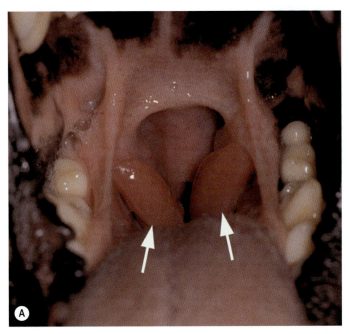
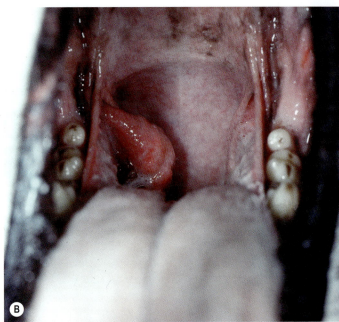

Fig. 59.2 Tonsillar neoplasia: (**A**) Bilateral tonsillar enlargement (*arrows*) in a dog with malignant lymphoma. (**B**) Unilateral tonsillar squamous cell carcinoma in a dog.

is rare in cats, often have only local pharyngeal and mandibular lymphadenopathy, although they may have lung metastases at diagnosis. Both occur in older animals. The mean age for tonsillar carcinomas is between 8 and 11 years.[6–10] A diagnosis of malignant lymphoma is based on nodal or tonsillar fine needle aspirates and biopsies. Chemotherapy is instituted. Tonsillectomy is not indicated.

Squamous cell carcinoma (SCC) is the most commonly reported tonsillar tumor in dogs.[6–13] Several studies have reported a higher incidence of tonsillar SCC in urban areas, presumably due to increased exposure to environmental carcinogens.[6,7,10,13] This tumor may also occur more frequently in male dogs than in females.[6–9] Tonsillar squamous cell carcinomas are rapidly growing, infiltrative and rarely resectable. Because the tonsils have multiple efferent lymphatics, and because most tumors go unnoticed until they are large enough to cause clinical symptoms (dysphagia, ptyalism, cough, gagging, anorexia, dyspnea, cervical swelling, voice change) most affected animals have regional lymph node metastasis at the time of diagnosis. Distant metastases to the lungs, liver and other sites are also commonly reported.[6–8]

Surgery for dogs with tonsillar SCC is limited to debulking prior to radiotherapy. Radical neck dissection to remove all gross tumor and affected nodes is generally not performed in dogs due to the risk to local structures. Biopsy of the ipsi- and contralateral mandibular lymph nodes, and the contralateral tonsil, for staging purposes should be considered. One study reported that 8 of 24 dogs had involvement of the contralateral lymph nodes.[6] Contralateral tonsillar involvement has also been reported[7] without gross enlargement of the tonsil. Affected nodes are generally included in the radiation field.

Chronic tonsillitis (bacterial or viral) is a disease of young animals, usually <1 year of age. It is usually a component of viral pharyngitis.[14,15] The tonsils can be 2–3 times their normal size, firm and hyperemic. The animal may be systemically ill with a fever, leukocytosis or leukopenia, and be malnourished and dehydrated. If pharyngitis is present, the animal may hold its neck in an extended position, exhibit pain on palpation and have difficulty swallowing. Once stabilized with fluid therapy, antibiotics and nutritional support, tonsillectomy may be considered if prior medical management has not resulted in more than temporary resolution of the problem.

SURGICAL TECHNIQUE

Although shortening of the soft palate with a CO_2 laser has been reported in dogs, laser tonsillectomy has not. Laser tonsillectomy results in less intraoperative hemorrhage and is commonly and successfully performed in humans.[16,17] The use of lasers for this procedure in dogs would be a logical next step and is described in Chapter 8.

A variety of conventional tonsillectomy techniques have been reported in dogs. In each case, the animal is placed in sternal recumbency with its head elevated. A tape or gauze sling is created between two IV poles. The sling is placed just caudal to the maxillary canine teeth so that the dorsal aspect of the animal's nose is horizontal. A mouth gag is placed as well as a known number of pharyngeal sponges. The cuff of the endotracheal tube is inflated to prevent aspiration of blood. Adequate lighting is required – a head lamp is preferable. While an assistant pulls the tongue out and downward, the surgeon grasps the tonsil with forceps or hemostats and elevates it from its fossa. At this point the tonsil can be pulled through a tonsil snare and the base cauterized.[18] Alternative techniques include transection of the base of the tonsil with Metzenbaum scissors, followed by ligation or bipolar cauterization of tonsillar artery branches and/or digital pressure.[4,19,20] Others prefer to cross-clamp the base of the tonsil with hemostats prior to transection.[5] Continuous sutures are then placed around the hemostats (Parker-Kerr suture pattern) (Fig. 59.3). Upon removal of the hemostat, the suture line is tightened and tied. If individual vessel ligation or cauterization is performed, some surgeons prefer to oversew the fossa with continuous sutures,[4,20,21] while others leave the site open.[18] Transection of the tonsillar base with monopolar cautery has also been suggested, although concerns regarding tissue swelling should limit its use.[22]

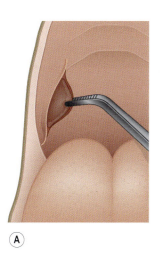 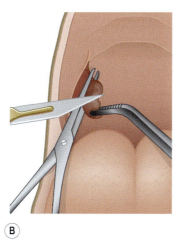 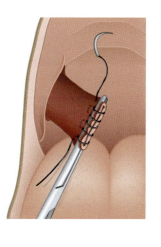 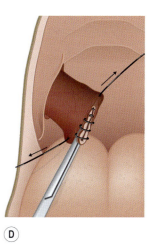

(A) (B) (C) (D)

Fig. 59.3 Tonsillectomy technique: (**A**) The base of the affected tonsil is clamped with hemostats or right-angled forceps after applying traction to the tonsil. (**B**) The tonsil is resected. (**C**) The base of the tonsil and clamp are oversewn with a Parker-Kerr suture pattern. (**D**) Following clamp removal, the suture line is tightened and tied.

The use of epinephrine injections (1:5000) into the base of the tonsil followed by digital pressure with epinephrine-soaked sponges has also been reported to control hemorrhage.[23] There is some theoretical concern with injecting epinephrine into a highly vascular region,[15] although complications with this technique have not been reported. In the end, technique is based on personal preference and available materials.

POSTOPERATIVE CARE AND ASSESSMENT

Despite contamination at the time of surgery, prolonged antibiotic therapy is rarely indicated unless the animal is systemically affected by bacterial tonsillitis/pharyngitis. If tonsillectomy is to be performed for noninfectious reasons, a single dose of corticosteroids is generally given at induction, prior to manipulation of the tissues, to diminish postoperative swelling. Prior to recovery from anesthesia the pharynx is thoroughly suctioned, and the pharyngeal sponges counted. Patients should be monitored closely for the first 24 hours for evidence of respiratory distress secondary to swelling. An emergency tracheostomy

kit and supplemental oxygen should be readily available, if needed. Soft food is fed for the first 3–7 days.

PROGNOSIS

The prognosis for uneventful recovery following tonsillectomy is good for dogs in which it is performed as an adjunct to soft palate resection, and for the treatment of chronic tonsillitis. Postoperative complications such as excessive hemorrhage and infection are uncommon.

Tonsillar squamous cell carcinoma carries a poor prognosis even following tonsillectomy and radiation therapy. Many dogs respond to radiation therapy, but because most tonsillar carcinomas have infiltrated local tissues and metastasized by the time of diagnosis, survival is often short.[9,11] Median survival in eight dogs treated with 35–42.5 Gy of megavoltage radiation following tonsillectomy was 110 days.[11] In two other studies, median survival from the time of diagnosis was 211 and 270 days following tonsillectomy, radiotherapy and chemotherapy.[9,24] There is evidence to suggest that some dogs with tonsillar squamous cell carcinoma may benefit from the administration of piroxicam, although a large prospective study is needed.[25]

REFERENCES

1. Evans HE. The pharynx. In: Evans HE, editor. Miller's Anatomy of the dog. 3rd ed. Philadelphia, PA: WB Saunders Co; 1993. p. 421–3.

2. Lucke VM, Pearson GR, Gregory SP, et al. Tonsillar polyps in the dog. J Small Anim Pract 1988;29:373–9.

3. Degner DA, Bauer MS, Ehrhart EJ. Palatine tonsil cyst in a dog. J Am Vet Med Assoc 1995;204:1041–2.

4. Harvey CE, Venker van Haagen A. Surgical management of pharyngeal and laryngeal airway obstruction in the dog. Vet Clin North Am Small Anim Pract 1975;5: 515–35.

5. Dorn AS. Soft tissue surgery of the head and neck. Tijdschr Diergeneesk 1987; 112:67S–72S.

6. Brodey RS. A clinical and pathologic study of 130 neoplasms of the mouth and pharynx in the dog. Am J Vet Res 1960;21:787–812.

7. Brodey RS. The biological behavior of canine oral and pharyngeal neoplasia. J Small Anim Pract 1970;11:45–53.

8. Todoroff RJ, Brodey RS. Oral and pharyngeal neoplasia in the dog: a retrospective survey in 361 cases. J Am Vet Med Assoc 1979;175:567–71.

9. Brooks MB, Matus RE, Leifer CE, et al. Chemotherapy versus chemotherapy plus radiotherapy in the treatment of tonsillar squamous cell carcinoma in the dog. J Vet Int Med 1988;2:206–11.

10. White RAS, Jeffries AR, Freedman LS. Clinical staging for oropharyngeal

malignancies in the dog. J Small Anim Pract 1985;26:581–94.

11. MacMillan R, Withrow SJ, Gillette EL. Surgery and regional irradiation for treatment of canine tonsillar squamous cell carcinoma: retrospective review of eight cases. J Am Anim Hosp Assoc 1982;18:311–14.

12. Dorn CR, Priester WA. Epidemiologic analysis of oral and pharyngeal cancers in dogs, cats, horses, and cattle. J Am Vet Med Assoc 1976;169:1202–6.

13. Bostock DE, Curtis R. Comparison of canine oropharyngeal malignancy in various geographical locations. Vet Rec 1984;114:341–2.

14. Venker-van Haagen AJ. Diseases of the throat. In: Ettinger SE, Feldman EC,

editors. Textbook of veterinary internal medicine. 5th ed. Philadelphia, PA: WB Saunders Co; 2000. p. 1028–9.

15. Dulisch ML. The tonsils. In: Slatter DH, editor. Textbook of small animal surgery. 2nd ed. Philadelphia, PA: WB Saunders Co; 1993. p. 973–7.

16. Linder A, Markström A, Hultcrantz E. Using the carbon dioxide laser for tonsillectomy in children. Int J Pediatr Otorhinolaryngol 1999;50:31–6.

17. Kothari P, Patel S, Brown P, et al. A prospective double-blind randomized controlled trial comparing the suitability of KTP laser tonsillectomy for day case surgery. Clin Otolaryngol Allied Sci 2002; 27:369–73.

18. Rickards DA. Tonsillectomy and soft palate resection. Canine Pract 1974;1:29–33.

19. Hofmeyr CFB. Surgery of the pharynx. Vet Clin North Am Small Anim Pract 1972;2:3–16.

20. Hedlund CS. Tonsillectomy. In: Welch Fossum T, editor. Small Animal Surgery. 2nd ed. St. Louis, MO: CV Mosby Co; 2002. p. 281–2.

21. Dean PW. Surgery of the tonsils. Probl Vet Med 1991;3:298–303.

22. Leonard EP. Tonsillectomy. In: Leonard EP, editor. Fundamentals of small animal surgery. Philadelphia, PA: WB Saunders Co; 1968. p. 176–7.

23. Kaplan B. A technic for tonsillectomy in the dog. Vet Med Small Anim Clin 1969; 64:805–10.

24. Murphy S, Hayes A, Adams V, et al. Role of carboplatin in multi-modality treatment of canine tonsillar squamous cell carcinoma – a case series of five dogs. J Small Anim Pract 2006;47:216–20.

25. Schmidt BR, Glickman NW, DeNicola DB, et al. Evaluation of piroxicam for the treatment of oral squamous cell carcinoma in dogs. J Am Vet Med Assoc 2001;218: 1783–6.

Index

Index

Index

Power density (irradiance), 81–82, 81t
    defined, 79
Power equipment, 60–61
Prehension, 477
Premaxilla, defined, 451
Premaxillectomy, defined, 423, 451
Premolar teeth
    anatomy, 116, 116f, 131–132
    extraction, 119–120, 132–135, 133f–137f,
        147
Premolar-molar extractions, 143–144, 147,
        148f–149f
Prevotella strains, 17
Prilocaine, 28, 28t
Primary palate, defined, 343
Prolene sutures, 73
Proliferation phase, wound healing, 2
Proliferative lesions, infectious origin, 413–414
Promagic, 50
Promod, 50
Promote, 50
Pronova sutures, 73
Pseudopocket, defined, 161
Pulmonary aspiration, 52, 53
Pulp necrosis, 97, 210–211, 211f, 218
Pulpal healing complications, 209f, 210–211,
        211f
Pulse mode, 79, 79f
Pulse oximetry, 27–28
Pyogenic granuloma, 412

R

Radical excision, 426
Radiosurgery, 61, 169–170, 170f
Random-pattern flap-closure, 250–254,
        253f–255f
Ranula, 477
    defined, 501
    intraoral marsupialization, 509
Reactive exostosis, 412
Reactive lesions, 409
Reattachment, defined, 161
Reconstruction, 487–494
    planning, 487
    postoperative care, 493
    techniques, 447, 487–493
Rectangular excision, 433, 437f–438f
Rectus abdominis myoperitoneal flap, 491
Regeneration
    defined, 1, 161
    procedures, 178
Remifentanil, 25–26
Remodeling phase, wound healing, 2
Renal function, anesthesia, 28
Repair, defined, 1
Replacement resorption, 212–213
Replantation, 203, 212f
    complications, 210–213
    pretreatment, 207
Research *see* Experimental research
Resorption *see* Root resorption; Tooth resorption
Respiratory function, anesthesia, 27–28
Retractors, 57–58, 58f, 103
Retrograde filling, 229–230
    failure, 231
Reverse (internal) bevel incision, defined, 175

Rim excision, 473
    defined, 423–424, 467
Risdon wiring technique, 277, 278f
Rochester–Carmalt forceps, 45–46
Root amputation
    defined, 217, 221
    /hemisection, 217–218
Root canal obliteration, 211–212
Root canal therapy, 217–219
    anatomical problems, 218
    complications, 219
    failed, 218–219
    indications, 218–219
    pain following, 218
    standard, 217, 221
    surgical anatomy, 221–224, 222f
    surgical, defined, 221
Root resorption, 212
    advanced apical, 218
    inflammatory, 212, 212f
    replacement, 212–213
    surface, 212
Roots, tooth, 101, 102f
    displacement, 154, 154f
    fractures, 153–154, 154f
    fragment removal, 110–111
    retention, intentional, 111, 111f
    tip picks, 104–105, 105f
    wiring damage, 291
    see also Extractions, multirooted teeth;
        Extractions, single-rooted teeth
Ropivacaine, 28, 28t
Rotary instruments, 60–61, 61f
Rotation flap, 244–245, 245f, 254f–255f
    defined, 243

S

S. typhimurium, 18
Salivary gland, 398–399
    biopsies, 497, 497f
    complications, 499
    definitions, 495
    diagnostic imaging, 496, 497f
    diseases, 497–499
    principles, 495–500
    surgical anatomy, 495–496
Sanitization, 62
    defined, 55
Scaling and root planing (SRP), 17–18
Scalpel handles/blades, 55, 56f
Schnidt forceps, 45–46
Scissors, 55–56, 57f
Second intention, defined, 343
Secondary palate, defined, 343
Securos system, 311, 313
Segmental mandibulectomy, 423–424
Seldin #304 elevator, 104f
Seldin retractor, 57, 58f
Semilunar flap, 226f–227f, 227
Senn retractor, 58, 58f
Shar-Pei, 516–518, 516f
Sialoadenectomy, 508–509
    zygomatic, 509, 510f
Sialoceles, 501–510
    definitions, 501
    diagnosis, 504, 504f

Sialoceles *(Continued)*
    epidemiology, 502b
    general anatomy, 504–505
    pathogenesis, 501–503, 502f–503f
    postoperative care, 509
    surgical objectives, 504
    surgical techniques, 505–509
    topographical anatomy, 505
Sialography, defined, 495
Sialoliths, 495, 497
Siberian huskies, 415–416
Silk sutures, 71t, 73
Single-pedicle advancement flap, 246,
        246f–247f, 249, 252f–253f
    defined, 243
Sinuses, extraoral approach, 263, 263f
SK ESF System, 311
'Skewer pin' wire, 289f
Skin
    grafts, 491, 492f
    preparation, 66
    substitutes, 4
    sutures, 75
Skin resection, 518
    complications, 518
    postoperative care, 518
Skull trauma, 265
Sliding flap, 178–180, 181f
Soft palate, cleft, defined, 351
Soft palate correction, 84, 85f, 539–542
    equipment, 539
    indications, 540
    planning, 539–540
    postoperative care, 541
    prognosis, 541–542
    surgical anatomy, 539, 539f
    surgical technique, 540–541, 540f–541f
Soft tissue injuries, 154–155, 243–257
    biopsies, 377, 377f
    complications, 256–257
    definitions, 243
    dehiscence, 291
    flaps, design, 106, 106f
    implant coverage, 305–306
    preoperative concerns, 243
    postoperative care, 255
    surgical techniques, 243–255, 243f
    see also Wound healing
'Soudure autogène', 10
Speculum, mouth, 65, 66f
Splinting, 207–210, 208f–209f, 212f
    see also Intraoral acrylic/composite splints
Split palatal U-flap, 367–368, 368f
    defined, 363
Split/partial-thickness flap, defined, 175
Split-thickness flap, defined, 343
Squamous cell carcinoma (SCC), 388–392,
        388f
    tonsillar, 554
Stainless steel, 296
    sutures, 71t, 73
Staphylococci, 15
Staphylococcus aureus, 72
Staphylococcus epidermidis, 72
Staphylococcus intermedius, 18
Staples, surgical, 75
Steinmann pins, 268